Practical
Gynecologic
Oncology

Practical Gynecologic Oncology

Second Edition

Jonathan S. Berek, M.D., M.M.Sc.

Professor and Vice-Chair
Director, Gynecologic Oncology Service
Chief of Gynecology
Department of Obstetrics and Gynecology
UCLA School of Medicine
Jonsson Comprehensive Cancer Center
Los Angeles, California

Neville F. Hacker, M.D.

Director of Gynaecologic Oncology
Royal Hospital for Women
Associate Professor
Obstetrics and Gynaecology
University of New South Wales
Sydney, Australia

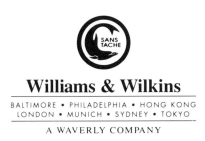

Williams & Wilkins

BALTIMORE • PHILADELPHIA • HONG KONG
LONDON • MUNICH • SYDNEY • TOKYO

A WAVERLY COMPANY

Editor: Charles Mitchell
Project Manager: Victoria Vaughn

Copyright © 1994
Williams & Wilkins
428 East Preston Street
Baltimore, Maryland 21202, USA

Accurate indications, adverse reactions, and dosage schedules for drugs are provided in this book, but it is possible that they may change. The reader is urged to review the package information data of the manufacturers of the medications mentioned.

Printed in the United States of America

First Edition 1989

Library of Congress Cataloging in Publication Data

Practical gynecologic oncology /   edited by Jonathan S. Berek, Neville
  F. Hacker.—2nd ed.
        p.   cm.
    Includes bibliographical references and index.
    ISBN 0-683-07899-2
    1. Generative organs, Female—Cancer.   I. Berek, Jonathan S.
  II. Hacker, Neville F.
    [DNLM: 1. Genital Neoplasms, Female.   WP 145 P895 1994]
  RC280.G5P73   1994
  616.99′465—dc20
  DNLM/DLC
  for Library of Congress   94-6101
                                                                                   CIP

                                                        90 91 92 93 94
                                          1   2   3   4   5   6   7   8   9   10

*To our wives, Deborah and Estelle,
whose patience and support made this
endeavor possible.*

Foreword to the First Edition

Close to the beginning of this century, William Osler observed that "The practice of medicine is an art, based on science." That brief characterization of our profession rings true even as we approach the next century in the midst of brilliant, accelerating scientific discovery.

Some aspects of the art—including compassion and the basic skills of history taking and physical examination—are, or should be, common to all physicians and remain largely unchanged by a century of research. In other ways the "art," which can also be translated as "craft" from the original Greek word "techne," has been greatly enlarged and diversified by science and technology. Thus the special skills required by a gynecologic oncologist derive not only from experience and practice, but also from the proliferation of knowledge in many branches of science. Indeed, it is mainly the developments of science in obstetrics and gynecology—and in some other disciplines—that have evolved the clinical subspecialty of gynecologic oncology.

The art and the science are connected not only by ancestry, however. Their relationship continues to be an interdependent one. One of the ever-expanding glories of medicine is that what is learned in the laboratory can enhance learning at the bedside and what is learned from experience with patients helps to shape and direct scientific inquiry.

Doctors who remain lifelong students are exhilarated by these interconnections and make the best teachers of clinical medicine. It is in this scholary tradition that Jonathan S. Berek and Neville F. Hacker, with contributions from distinguished colleagues in their own discipline and in fields that bear upon it, have brought together the salient information required to develop the acumen and skills that enable clinicians to understand and to care for women suffering from tumors.

Practical Gynecologic Oncology reflects the indivisibility of art and science in medicine. The two editors—one in Los Angeles and one in Sydney—worked and studied together for 7 years in the same hospital and laboratories and remain mutually helpful intellectual allies on opposite shores of the Pacific Ocean.

Sherman M. Mellinkoff, M.D.
Dean Emeritus
Professor of Medicine
UCLA School of Medicine
Los Angeles, California

Preface to the Second Edition

The first edition of *Practical Gynecologic Oncology* was so well received that we have been encouraged to produce this second edition. We have maintained the objectives of the first edition but have made some alterations in the format and broadened the scope of the book somewhat by adding a chapter on palliative care and pain management.

During the 5 years since the publication of the first edition, the subspecialty of gynecologic oncology has continued to expand internationally to the betterment of care for women suffering from gynecologic malignancies. New national societies have been founded, and the international exchange of ideas has accelerated. A significant catalyst for this exchange has been the International Gynecologic Cancer Society, founded in 1987, which meets every other year.

With an ever-increasing number of clinicians and basic scientists devoting their professional careers to gynecologic oncology, research into all aspects of the discipline has continued to flourish. We have attempted to critically review the recent literature and provide a practical guide to current evaluation and treatment strategies for gynecologic malignancies. We acknowledge that some positions taken in the book may be controversial, but it has not been our intention to exhaustively debate the various options but rather to support our preferred option with adequate reference to the literature.

The modern practice of gynecologic oncology requires a multidisciplinary team approach, and the book would not have been possible without the valued input from our coauthors, all of whom are internationally acknowledged experts in the field. We are most grateful to Gwynne Gloege for her outstanding illustrations. Special thanks are due to Karen Kannmacher, who superbly coordinated and performed most of the word processing and, with considerable finesse, prepared the final manuscript. We would also like to thank Kathleen Agbayani and Daphne Blackman, both of whom assisted in the preparation of the manuscript. We gratefully acknowledge the excellent work of Joy Moore, Vicki Vaughn, and Charles Mitchell who guided the book through the publication process.

We trust that this second edition will contribute to improved care for women suffering from a gynecologic malignancy.

Jonathan S. Berek

Neville F. Hacker

Preface to the First Edition

Gynecologic Oncology was officially recognized as a subspecialty of Obstetrics and Gynecology in the United States in 1973, and subsequently almost 360 gynecologic oncologists have been certified by the American College of Obstetricians and Gynecologists. The specialty is established in some centers in Europe and has recently been given official recognition by the relevant colleges in Britain and Australia. Hence, an increasing number of physicians are devoting their professional careers to the management of patients with gynecologic malignancies.

Since the development of the subspecialty, there has been a proliferation of societies and journals devoted to gynecologic cancer, and the field has been the subject of more intense clinical and basic research than ever before. New treatment strategies are constantly being devised, and many traditional concepts have been challenged. For example, radical vulvectomy is no longer considered necessary for all patients with early vulvar cancer, and unilateral salpingo-oophorectomy is now considered appropriate for selected patients with ovarian tumors. Individualization of treatment is regarded as desirable, and an increasing emphasis is being placed on the quality of the patient's life. It is not surprising that such issues as pelvic reconstruction and sexual rehabilitation are increasingly becoming legitimate concerns of the practicing gynecologic oncologist.

This book was written to provide a practical guide to current evaluation and treatment strategies for patients with preinvasive and invasive malignancies of the female genital tract. It is a culmination of our collaborative teaching, clinical, and research activities during the 7 years we worked together in the Division of Gynecologic Oncology at the UCLA School of Medicine. We undoubtedly have interjected some personal biases but have tried to justify our points of view with adequate reference to the literature.

We have made no attempt to cover basic research issues but have included chapters on the principles of cancer therapy, because an understanding of these principles is mandatory for proper patient care. The bibliography is not intended to be exhaustive but rather to be sufficiently comprehensive to allow each subject to be adequately reviewed. Similarly, the brief descriptions of some surgical procedures are not intended to replace a large surgical atlas. They are intended merely to help facilitate a better understanding of the basic steps involved in the particular operation.

The text has been written primarily for fellows undertaking postgraduate training in gynecologic oncology, but it also should be of interest to gynecology residents, consultant gynecologists, and physicians in allied fields whose practice involves a significant component of gynecologic oncology. The book is divided into three sections. The first section discusses general principles of oncology, particularly as they relate to gynecologic malignancies. This section includes chapters on chemotherapy, radiation, immunology, pathology, and biostatistics. The second section deals with the primary disease sites, and the third section presents topics of special interest to the gynecologic oncologist. Such topics include relevant aspects of medicine, surgery, nutrition, and psychology.

We would like to acknowledge the contribution of our colleagues who have written chapters for this book. All are respected authorities in their particular fields. We are most grateful to Gwynne Gloege for her outstanding illustrations and to Norman Chang for preparing the photography. Drs. Yao S. Fu and Fredrick Montz provided valuable suggestions regarding the preparation of the manuscript. Special thanks are due to Monique Etcheverry, who superbly coordinated and performed most of the initial word processing, and to Kathleen Agbayani who, with considerable finesse, prepared the final manuscript. Additional manuscript preparation was performed by Chris Poirier.

Finally, we are most grateful for the encouragement and support we have received over the years from our mentors: Dr. Sherman Mellinkoff, Dean Emeritus of the UCLA School of Medicine; Dr. J. George Moore, former Chairman of the Department of Obstetrics and Gynecology at UCLA; and Professor Eric Mackay, Chairman of the Department of Obstetrics and Gynecology at the University of Queensland.

We trust that this book will make a contribution toward the improved care for women with gynecologic malignancies.

Jonathan S. Berek

Neville F. Hacker

Contributors

Barbara L. Andersen, Ph.D.

Professor
Department of Psychology, and
Obstetrics and Gynecology
Ohio State University
Columbus, Ohio

Robert C. Bast, Jr., M.D.

R. Wayne Rundles Professor of Medicine
Director, Duke Comprehensive Cancer Center
Duke University Medical Center
Durham, North Carolina

Ross S. Berkowitz, M.D.

Professor of Obstetrics, Gynecology and Reproductive Biology
Director, Division of Gynecologic Oncology
Harvard Medical School
Brigham and Women's Hospital
Dana Farber Cancer Institute
Co-Director, New England Trophoblastic Disease Center
Boston, Massachusetts

Cinda M. Boyer, Ph.D.

Assistant Research Professor
Department of Medicine
Duke University Medical Center
Durham, North Carolina

Daniel W. Cramer, M.D., Sc.D.

Associate Professor
Department of Obstetrics and Gynecology
Harvard Medical School
Brigham and Women's Hospital
Boston, Massachusetts

Yao S. Fu, M.D.

Professor and Chief of Surgical Pathology
Department of Pathology
UCLA School of Medicine
Los Angeles, California

Armando E. Giuliano, M.D.

Clinical Professor
Department of Surgery
UCLA School of Medicine
Director, Joyce Eisenberg Keefer Breast Center
John Wayne Cancer Institute
Saint John's Hospital
Los Angeles, California

John A. Glaspy, M.D.

Assistant Professor
Department of Medicine
Division of Hematology and Oncology
UCLA School of Medicine
Los Angeles, California

Donald P. Goldstein, M.D.

Assistant Clinical Professor
Department of Obstetrics and Gynecology
Harvard Medical School
Director, New England Trophoblastic Disease Center
Boston, Massachusetts

Kenneth D. Hatch, M.D.

Professor and Director
Division of Gynecologic Oncology
Department of Obstetrics and Gynecology
University of Arizona Health Sciences Center
Tucson, Arizona

David Heber, M.D., Ph.D.

Professor of Medicine
Department of Medicine
Chief, Division of Clinical Nutrition
UCLA School of Medicine
Los Angeles, California

Robert C. Knapp, M.D.

William H. Baker Professor of Gynecology
Department of Obstetrics and Gynecology
Harvard Medical School
Brigham and Women's Hospital
Dana Farber Cancer Institute
Boston, Massachusetts

J. Norelle Lickliss, M.D.

Associate Professor of Medicine
University of Sydney, and
University of New South Wales
Director of Palliative Care
Royal Prince Alfred, Prince of Wales, and
Royal Hospital for Women
Sydney, Australia

Frederick Naftolin, M.D., D. Phil.

Professor and Chairman
Department of Obstetrics and Gynecology
Yale University School of Medicine
New Haven, Connecticut

Richard Reid, M.D.

Assistant Professor
Department of Obstetrics and Gynecology
Wayne State University
Director of Gynecologic Laser Services
Sinai Hospital of Detroit
Detroit, Michigan

Peter E. Schwartz, M.D.

Professor and Director
Division of Gynecologic Oncology
Department of Obstetrics and Gynecology
Yale University School of Medicine
New Haven, Connecticut

Samuel Skootsky, M.D.

Associate Clinical Professor of Medicine
Department of Medicine
Director, Consultation Service
UCLA School of Medicine
Los Angeles, California

Gillian M. Thomas, M.D.

Associate Professor
Department of Radiation Oncology, and Obstetrics and Gynecology
University of Toronto
Toronto Bayview Regional Cancer Center
Toronto, Ontario, Canada

J. Donald Woodruff, M.D.
The Richard W. TeLinde Professor Emeritus of Gynecologic Pathology
Department of Gynecology and Obstetrics
The Johns Hopkins University School of Medicine
Baltimore, Maryland

Robert C. Young, M.D.
President
Fox Chase Cancer Center
Philadelphia, Pennsylvania

Contents

GENERAL PRINCIPLES OF ONCOLOGY

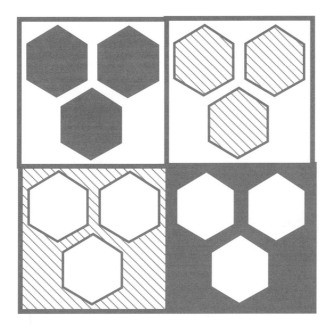

1

Chemotherapy

Robert C. Young

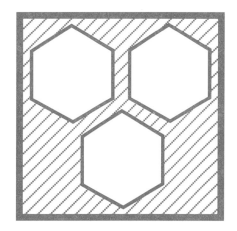

General Principles

Selection of Chemotherapy

Drugs capable of the relatively selective destruction of malignant cells are now used routinely in patients with cancer. A wide variety of such agents are available, and the selection of drugs is often difficult. Furthermore, because the vast majority of antineoplastic agents have a narrower therapeutic index than drugs of other types, careful thought should be given to the factors outlined in Table 1.1 before the institution of antineoplastic chemotherapy.

It is important to understand clearly the natural history of each patient's malignancy. The use of chemotherapeutic agents should be restricted to patients whose malignancies have been proven by biopsy. In some instances, second opinions regarding definitive histologic diagnoses should be obtained before the institution of chemotherapy. When doubt exists concerning the diagnosis, it is preferable to delay initial therapy and not use response to chemotherapy as a diagnostic trial.

The decision to use chemotherapy is also dependent on a thorough knowledge of the extent of the patient's disease as well as the rate of progression of that disease. Limited evidence of metastatic spread or documented slow disease progression may warrant withholding chemotherapy for a period. Because all chemotherapeutic agents produce toxicity, it is important that there be an evaluable tumor so that one can assess response. It is inappropriate, in general, to administer antineoplastic agents unless one can objectively determine benefit to the patient. Thus, except in rare instances, the ability to determine tumor response to chemotherapy is an important factor in treatment decisions.

The patient's particular circumstances may play a major role in decisions regarding chemotherapy. The extent of previous therapy and the patient's age, general health, and other complicating illnesses form an important part of the physician's decision and may substantially affect tolerance to antineoplastic drug treatment. In addition, the patient's emotional, social, and even financial status must be respected and evaluated before a final decision is made.

3

Table 1.1   Issues To Be Considered Before Using Antineoplastic Drugs

---

1. *Natural History of the Particular Malignancy*
   a. Diagnosis of a malignancy made by biopsy
   b. Rate of disease progression
   c. Extent of disease spread

---

2. *Patient's Circumstances and Tolerance*
   a. Age, general health, underlying diseases
   b. Extent of previous treatment
   c. Adequate facilities to evaluate, monitor, and treat potential drug toxicities
   d. The patient's emotional, social, and financial situation

---

3. *Likelihood of Achieving a Beneficial Response*
   a. Cancers in which chemotherapy is curative in some patients, e.g., ovarian germ cell tumors
   b. Cancers in which chemotherapy has demonstrated improvement in survival, e.g., epithelial ovarian cancer
   c. Cancers that respond to treatment but in which improved survival has not been clearly demonstrated, e.g., cervical cancer
   d. Cancers with marginal or no response to chemotherapy, e.g., melanoma

---

Chemotherapy should not be used unless facilities are available for careful monitoring and treatment of the resulting toxicities. If such facilities are not available and chemotherapy clearly is required, the patient should be referred to a physician or another facility that has that capability.

The decision to use chemotherapy depends heavily on the probability of achieving a useful response. Not all cancers respond to chemotherapy in similar quantitative and qualitative ways. Nevertheless, tumors can be grouped into four categories by their likelihood of chemotherapeutic response:

1. In the first group of tumors (e.g., ovarian germ cell tumors, choriocarcinoma), antineoplastic therapy is curative for most patients. Obviously, a decision not to treat patients with diseases known to be curable with chemotherapy is, with rare exceptions, inappropriate. Even substantial toxicity is acceptable if the probability of cure is high.

2. In the second group (e.g., epithelial ovarian cancer), chemotherapy improves patient survival but does not restore a normal life expectancy. Patients with these tumors usually benefit from chemotherapy, and it should be offered unless there are exceptional circumstances.

3. In the third group (e.g., cervical carcinoma, uterine sarcoma), responses to chemotherapy occur, but improved survival has not yet been achieved for a significant number of patients.

4. In the fourth group (e.g., melanoma), few, if any, responses to chemotherapy are seen. In such cases the use of chemotherapy should be restricted, and every effort should be made to include these patients in well-designed prospective clinical trials testing new treatment approaches.

Differential Sensitivity   For any particular antineoplastic agent to be effective, it must have greater toxicity for the malignant cells than for the patient's normal cells. In that sense, all useful chemotherapeutic agents have greater activity against tumors than against normal tissues. The window between antitumor effect and normal

4

tissue toxicity may be small, because most chemotherapeutic agents work by disrupting DNA or RNA synthesis, affecting crucial cellular enzymes, or by altering protein synthesis.

Normal cells also use these vital cellular processes in ways similar to that of malignant cells, particularly fetal or regenerating tissue or normal cell populations in which constant cell proliferation is required (e.g., bone marrow, gastrointestinal epithelium, and hair follicles). As a result, the differential effect of antineoplastic drugs on tumors as compared with normal tissues is quantitative rather than qualitative, and some degree of injury to normal tissue is produced by every chemotherapeutic agent. The normal tissue toxicity produced by most chemotherapeutic agents correlates with the intrinsic cellular proliferation of the target tissue. This explains why toxicities, such as blood count suppression, mucosal injury, and alopecia, are commonly seen with most chemotherapeutic regimens.

Therapeutic Index

For any particular chemotherapeutic agent, the net effect on the patient is often referred to as the drug's therapeutic index (i.e., a ratio of the doses at which therapeutic effect and toxicity occur). Cancer chemotherapy requires a balance of therapeutic effect and toxicity to optimize the therapeutic index. Because the window of toxicity is often narrow for currently available chemotherapeutic agents, successful chemotherapy depends on pharmacologic and biologic factors.

Biologic Factors Influencing Treatment

Cell Kinetic Concepts

Both normal and tumorous tissues have a certain growth capacity and are influenced and regulated by various internal and external forces. The differential growth and regulatory influences occurring in both normal and tumorous tissues form the basis of effective cancer treatment. The exploitation of these differences forms the basis for the effective use of both radiation therapy and chemotherapy in cancer management (1).

Patterns of Normal Growth

All normal tissues have the capacity for cellular division and growth. However, normal tissues grow in substantially different patterns. There are three general types of normal tissue growth, classified as *static, renewing,* and *expanding.*

1. The *static* population is comprised of relatively well-differentiated cells which, after initial proliferative activity in the embryonic and neonatal period, rarely undergo cell division. Typical examples are striated muscle and neurons.

2. The *expanding* population of cells is characterized by the capacity to proliferate under special stimuli (e.g., tissue injury). Under those circumstances, the normally quiescent tissue (e.g., liver or kidney) undergoes a surge of proliferation with regrowth.

3. The *renewing* population of cells is constantly in a proliferative state. There is constant cell division, a high degree of cell turnover, and constant cell loss. This occurs in bone marrow, epidermis, and gastrointestinal mucosa.

Understanding these patterns of normal tissue growth partially explains some of the most common types of toxicity seen with cancer treatments. Normal tissues with a static pattern of growth are rarely seriously injured by drug therapy, whereas renewing cell populations, such as bone marrow, gastrointestinal mucosa, and spermatozoa, are commonly injured.

Cancer Cell Growth

Tumor cell growth represents a disruption in the normal cellular brake mechanisms that exist; consequently, continued proliferation and eventual death of the host result. Although cell proliferation occurs continuously in human tumors, there is evidence that it does not take place more rapidly in cancers than in their normal-tissue counterparts. It is not the speed of cell proliferation but the failure of the regulated balance between cell loss and cell proliferation that differentiates tumorous tissues from normal tissues.

Gompertzian Growth

The characteristics of cancer growth have been assessed by multiple studies in animals and more limited studies in humans. When tumors are extremely small, growth follows an exponential pattern but later seems to slow. Such a growth pattern is known as *Gompertzian growth*. Strictly speaking, this means exponential growth with exponential growth retardation over the entire duration of tumor growth. More simply, **Gompertzian growth means that as a tumor mass increases, the time required to double the tumor's volume also increases.**

Doubling Time

The doubling time of a human tumor is the time it takes for the mass to double its size. There is considerable variation in doubling times of human tumors. For example, embryonal tumors, lymphomas, and some malignant mesenchymal tumors have relatively fast doubling times (20–40 days), whereas adenocarcinomas and squamous cell carcinomas have relatively slow doubling times (50–150 days). Metastases generally have faster doubling times than primary lesions.

If it is assumed that exponential growth occurs early in a tumor's history and that a tumor starts from a single malignant cell, then

1. A 1 mm mass will have undergone approximately 20 tumor doublings.

2. A 5 mm mass (a size that might be first visualized on x-ray film) will have undergone 27 doublings.

3. A 1 cm mass will have undergone 30 doublings. Were such a lesion discovered clinically, the physician would assume that the tumor had been detected early. The reality is that it would have already undergone 30 doublings, or been present approximately 60% of its life span.

Unfortunately, our current clinical techniques recognize tumors late in their growth, and metastasis may well have occurred long before there is obvious evidence of the primary lesion. The second implication from this kinetic information is that in late stages of tumor growth, a very few doublings in tumor mass have a dramatic impact on the size of the tumor. Once a tumor becomes palpable (1 cm in diameter), only three more doublings would produce an enormous tumor mass (8 cm in diameter).

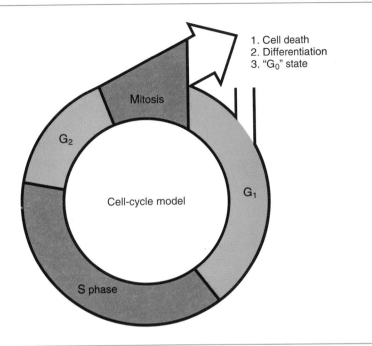

1. Cell death
2. Differentiation
3. "G_0" state

Figure 1.1   The cell cycle. After cell division, a cell can either (1) die, (2) differentiate, or (3) enter resting (G_0) phase. The latter two can reenter the cycle at G_1.

Cell Cycle

Information on growth patterns and doubling times relates to the growth of the tumor mass as a whole. The kinetic behavior of individual tumor cells has been well described and a classic cell cycle model has been produced (Fig. 1.1).

1. *M phase—mitotic phase*—of the cell cycle is the phase of cell division.

2. *G_1 phase—postmitotic phase*—is a period of variable duration when cellular activities and protein and RNA synthesis continue. These G_1 cells can differentiate or continue in the proliferative cycle.

3. *S phase—DNA synthetic phase*—is the period in which new DNA replication occurs.

4. *G_2 phase—postsynthetic phase*—is the period in which the cell has a diploid number of chromosomes and twice the DNA content of the normal cell. The cell remains in this phase for a relatively short time and then enters the mitotic phase again.

5. *G_0 phase—the resting phase*—is the time during which cells do not divide. Cells may move in and out of the G_0 phase.

The generation time is the duration of the cycle from M phase to M phase. Variation occurs in all phases of the cell cycle, but the variation is greatest during the G_1 period. The events controlling this variation are not well understood.

These cell cycle events have important implications for the cancer therapist (2). Differential sensitivities to chemotherapy and radiotherapy are associated with different proliferative states. Dividing cancer cells that are actively traversing the cell cycle are very sensitive to chemotherapeutic agents. Cells in a resting state

(G^0) are relatively insensitive to chemotherapeutic agents, although they occupy space and contribute to the bulk of the tumor.

Cell Kinetics

In cell kinetic studies performed on human tumors, the duration of the S phase (DNA synthesis phase) is relatively similar for most human tumors, ranging from a low of 10 hours to a high of approximately 31 hours. The length of the cell cycle in human tumors varies from slightly more than ½ day to perhaps 5 days. With cell cycle times in the range of 24 hours and doubling times in the range of 10–1000 days, it is clear that only a small proportion of tumor cells are in active cell division at any one time.

Two major factors that affect the rate at which tumors grow are the *growth fraction* and *cell death*. **The growth fraction is the number of cells in the tumor mass that are actively undergoing cell division.** There is a marked variation in the growth fraction of tumors in human beings, ranging from 25% to almost 95%. In the past it was thought that human tumors contained billions of cells, all growing slowly. In actuality, only a small fraction of cells within a tumor mass are rapidly proliferating; the remainder are out of the cell cycle and quiescent.

Tumor growth may be altered by the following:

1. *Cytotoxic chemotherapy*, which alters both the generation time and the growth fraction of tumors.

2. *Hormones*, which appear to alter the growth fraction without changing the generation time.

3. *X-ray therapy*, which alters both the generation time and the growth fraction.

4. *Alterations in oxygen tension and vascular supply*, which alter the growth fraction without altering generation time.

5. *Immunologic therapies*, which seem to alter both generation time and growth fraction.

Cell Cycle-Specific Versus Nonspecific Drugs

Antineoplastic agents have complex mechanisms of action and alter cells in a wide variety of ways. Different drugs have different sites of action in the cell

Table 1.2   Cell Cycle-Specificity of Chemotherapeutic Agents

Classification	Examples
Cell cycle-specific, proliferation-dependent	Hydroxyurea, Ara-C*
Cell cycle-specific, less proliferation-dependent	5-FU*, methotrexate
Cell cycle-nonspecific, proliferation-dependent	Cytoxan, actinomycin D, cisplatin
Cell cycle-nonspecific, less proliferation-dependent	Nitrogen mustard

*Ara-C = cytosine arabinoside; 5-FU = 5-fluorouracil.

Table 1.3   Site of Action in the Cell Cycle

Portion of Cell Cycle	Drugs
G_1	Actinomycin D
Early S	Hydroxyurea, Ara-C*, 5-FU*, methotrexate
Late S	Adriamycin, daunomycin
G_2	Bleomycin, radiation, etoposide, teniposide
M	Vincristine, vinblastine

*Ara-C = cytosine arabinoside; 5-FU = 5-fluorouracil.

cycle, and their effectiveness is also a function of the proliferative capacity of the tissue involved. With the use of some of these kinetic concepts, it is possible to classify chemotherapeutic agents on the basis of their cell cycle specificity and their site of maximal drug action within the cell cycle (Table 1.2).

Cell Cycle-Nonspecific   Cell cycle–nonspecific agents kill in all phases of the cell cycle and are not too dependent on proliferative capacity.

Cell Cycle-Specific   At the other end of the spectrum, cell cycle–specific agents, such as hydroxyurea, depend for their action on the proliferative capacity and on the phase of the cell cycle. The agents kill in only one portion of the cell cycle, and cells not in that phase will not be injured. They tend to be most effective against tumors with relatively long S phases and those tumors in which there is a relatively high growth fraction and a rapid proliferation rate. Between these two broad classifications, there is a spectrum of drugs with variable degrees of cell cycle and proliferation dependence.

In addition to cell cycle and proliferation sensitivity, chemotherapeutic agents may exert a greater effect in a particular phase of the cell cycle. Thus, chemotherapeutic agents can be grouped according to their site of action in the cell cycle and the extent of their dependence on proliferative activity (Table 1.3).

Log Kill Hypothesis

From knowledge of basic cellular kinetics, there have emerged certain concepts of chemotherapy that have proved useful in the design of chemotherapeutic regimens. In experimental tumor systems in animals, the survival of an animal is inversely proportional to the number of cells implanted or to the size of the tumor at the time treatment is initiated (3). Treatment immediately after tumor implantation or when the tumor is subclinical in size results in more cures than when the tumor is clinically obvious and large.

Chemotherapeutic agents appear to work by first-order kinetics; i.e., they kill a constant fraction of cells rather than a constant number. This concept has important conceptual implications in cancer treatment. For instance, a single exposure of tumor cells to an antineoplastic drug might be capable of producing 2–5 logs of cell kill. With typical body tumor burdens of 10^{12} cells (1 kg), a single dose of chemotherapy is unlikely to be curative. This explains the need for intermittent courses of chemotherapy to achieve the magnitude of cell kill necessary to produce tumor regression and cure. It also provides a rationale for multiple drug or combination chemotherapy.

9

The cure rate would be significantly improved if small tumors were present, but cell masses of 10^1–10^4 cells are too small for clinical detection. This is the basis for using *adjuvant chemotherapy* in early stages of disease when subclinical numbers of cancer cells are suspected.

Drug Resistance and Tumor Cell Heterogeneity

The clinical utility of a particular chemotherapeutic agent or drug combination may be compromised severely when *drug resistance* develops. Chemotherapeutic agents often are active when initially used in cancer treatment, but tumors commonly become resistant during chemotherapy. Hence patients often have an initial remission followed by a recurrence that is no longer responsive to the drugs that were initially effective.

A variety of cellular mechanisms are involved in drug resistance. Resistant tumor cells may display increased deactivation or decreased activation of drugs; they may be associated with increased drug efflux; or they may resist normal drug uptake. In some instances, altered specificity to an inhibiting enzyme or increased production of the target enzyme occurs to explain drug resistance on a pharmacologic basis.

Goldie-Coldman Hypothesis

It has been suggested that spontaneous mutation to phenotypic drug resistance occurs in rapidly growing malignant tumors, *the somatic mutation theory* (4). **This theory suggests that most mammalian cells start with intrinsic sensitivity to antineoplastic drugs but develop spontaneous resistance at variable rates.** This concept—the Goldie-Coldman hypothesis—has been applied to the growth of malignant tumors and has important clinical implications.

Goldie and Coldman have developed a mathematical model that relates curability to the time of appearance of singly or doubly resistant cells. Assuming a natural mutation rate, the model predicts a variation in size of the resistant fraction in tumors of the same size and type, depending on the mutation rate and the point at which the first mutation develops. Given such assumptions, the proportion of resistant cells in any untreated tumor is likely to be small, and the initial response to treatment would not be influenced by the number of resistant cells. In clinical practice, this means that a complete remission could be obtained even if a resistant cell line were present. The failure to cure such a patient, however, would be directly dependent on the presence of resistant cell lines.

This model of spontaneous drug resistance implies that:

1. Tumors are curable with chemotherapy if no permanently resistant cell lines are present and if chemotherapy is begun before such cells develop.

2. If only one antineoplastic agent is used, the probability of cure diminishes rapidly with the development of a single resistant line.

3. Minimizing the emergence of drug-resistant clones requires multiple effective drugs or therapies and requires that they be applied as early as possible in the course of the patient's malignant disease.

4. The rate of spontaneous mutation to resistance occurs at about the natural frequency of 1 in 10,000 to 1 in 1,000,000 cell divisions.

This model predicts that alternating cycles of treatment should be superior to the sequential use of particular agents because sequential use of antineoplastic drugs would allow for the development and regrowth of a doubly resistant line. The intrinsic frequency of spontaneous mutation to drug resistance is also likely to be influenced by etiologic factors responsible for tumor development. Lung or bladder cancers, for instance, result from exposure to multiple carcinogenic chemicals and may have a higher spontaneous mutation rate than is seen in other tumors. Under these circumstances, numerous drug-resistant clones may be present even before the tumors are clinically evident. This would explain the inability of antineoplastic therapy to cure a number of the common malignancies.

Pleiotropic Drug Resistance

The Goldie-Coldman model has focused attention on mechanisms of drug resistance. If the failure of drug treatment depends on the spontaneous appearance of resistant cells, an understanding of drug resistance is crucial to therapeutic success. A wide variety of mechanisms for drug resistance have been described, although these mechanisms generally confer resistance to a particular drug or drug family. The phenomenon of pleiotropic drug resistance occurs when certain drug-resistance mechanisms confer cross-resistance to structurally dissimilar drugs with different mechanisms of action (5).

Some pleiotropic resistant cells contain a cell-surface P-glycoprotein with a molecular weight of 170 kilodaltons (kd). Generally, the appearance of pleiotropic drug resistance is associated with impaired ability of the cell to accumulate and retain antineoplastic drugs. It has been further demonstrated that this P-glycoprotein is directly related to the expression of resistance, and cells that revert to sensitive ones lose this membrane glycoprotein.

DNA can be transferred from resistant cells into sensitive cells, producing a transfer of pleiotropic resistance to unexposed cells. The gene responsible for this multidrug resistance has been isolated, and the production of monoclonal antibodies offers a possible approach to reversing this pleiotropic resistance.

Dose Intensity

For many years, it has been taught that full doses of chemotherapy were necessary to obtain optimal clinical results. Substantial laboratory and clinical evidence now exists to support this concept. Studies in human solid tumors *in vitro* frequently demonstrate steep dose-response curves, suggesting the importance of full drug dosage. In clinical trials, higher doses of certain chemotherapeutic agents often produce responses after conventional doses have failed. In testicular and ovarian cancer, for example, twofold or threefold increases in cisplatin dosage will produce clinical responses in patients who have relapsed after conventional doses.

A systematic analysis of dose intensity has been performed for breast and ovarian cancer (6), and it is now possible to compare different chemotherapeutic regimens by converting the drug dosage within each individual program to milligrams per meter squared per week.

$$\text{Dose Intensity} = \text{Drug (mg)}/\text{Surface Area (M}^2)/\text{Time (week)}$$

When results of chemotherapy trials are analyzed and compared, it is important that dose intensity be optimized and that drug intensity be reported.

11

Most of the data on the clinical impact of dose intensity come from retrospective analyses, but several prospective trials of dose intensity in ovarian cancer have produced mixed results. A large GOG trial of dose-intensive versus standard-dose cisplatin and Cytoxan in patients with advanced ovarian cancer failed to demonstrate improved duration of remission or survival, although the dose-intense regimen was double the relative dose intensity of the standard regimen (7). In contrast, a randomized trial from the Scottish Ovarian Cancer Study Group that included 190 patients was closed prematurely because of a highly significant survival difference between six cycles of 50 mg/M^2 and 100 mg/M^2 of cisplatin, each combined with Cytoxan 750 mg/M^2 every 3 weeks (8). More studies will be necessary to define precisely the role of dose intensity in optimal management of ovarian cancer.

Other approaches are now being explored to increase the intensity of drug regimens so as to increase remission rates and durations. These have included intensifying chemotherapy with the use of bone marrow or stem cell transplantation or hematopoietic growth factors to enhance marrow recovery.

Bone marrow transplantation is being used on an experimental basis in advanced, poor-prognosis, and refractory ovarian cancer. Although higher response rates are often achieved, the toxicity of these regimens often has been severe (mortality 10%–35%), and as yet no survival benefit has been documented. Peripheral stem cell transplantations are also being studied and offer the advantage of not requiring marrow harvest under general anesthesia.

Attempts are also being made to reduce dose-limiting myelotoxicity by using *granulocyte-macrophage colony-stimulating factor (GM-CSF)*, or *G-CSF*. Although these therapies will accelerate the recovery of granulocytes after treatment and will often reduce the duration of hospitalization after bone marrow transplantation, they are expensive and have yet to be shown to alter the therapeutic outcome. In addition, there is no study that documents any benefit from the routine prophylactic use of these hematopoietic growth factors during conventional chemotherapy. Furthermore, none of the growth factors currently available have any significant impact on platelet recovery, which is often the dose-limiting toxicity of platinum-based chemotherapy.

Pharmacologic Factors Influencing Treatment

Pharmacologically, it is useful to describe effective chemotherapy as concentration over time of the active agent or its metabolite at the primary site of antitumor action. Although it is not possible to determine exact pericellular pharmacokinetics, substantial information on important pharmacokinetic factors is available (9).

Drug Effect = Drug Concentration × Duration of Exposure = C × T

Because direct measurements often are not possible, considerable focus is given to the plasma concentration × time (C × T) analyses. A number of important factors influence this pharmacokinetic result, including route of administration, drug absorption, drug transport, distribution, biotransformation, inactivation, excretion, and interactions with other drugs.

Route of Administration and Absorption

Traditionally, drugs have been given *orally, intravenously, intramuscularly,* or *intraarterially.* More recently, considerable attention has been given to the *intrapleural* or *intraperitoneal* administration of chemotherapeutic agents, particularly in ovarian cancer (10). The intraperitoneal approach is based on the concept that the pleural or peritoneal clearance of the agent is slower than its plasma clearance and, as a result, an increased concentration of the drug in the pleural or peritoneal cavity is maintained while plasma concentrations are low.

Studies of a wide variety of chemotherapeutic agents have demonstrated a differential concentration of 30–500-fold, depending on the molecular weight, charge, and lipid solubility of the particular drug. Clinical trials in ovarian cancer have been performed with *cisplatin, paclitaxel (Taxol)* and drug combinations. Clinical trials using intraperitoneal cisplatin have resulted in 30% negative third-look laparotomies in patients with minimal residual disease. Although these approaches remain experimental, they illustrate the importance of route of administration in the ultimate outcome of therapy (11).

Drug Distribution

Antineoplastic agents generally produce their antitumor effect by interacting with intracellular target molecules. As a result, the ability of a particular drug or active metabolite to arrive at the cancer cell in sufficient concentration for lethal effect is of major importance. After absorption, drugs may be bound to serum albumin or other blood components; their ability to penetrate various body compartments, vascular spaces, and extracellular sites is highly influenced by plasma protein binding, relative ionization at physiologic pH, molecular size, and lipid solubility.

Sanctuary Sites   Unique circumstances may produce sanctuary sites, which are areas where the tumor is inaccessible to anticancer drugs and the drug concentration over time is insufficient for cell kill. Examples of such sanctuary sites include the cerebrospinal fluid and areas of large tumor masses with central tumor necrosis and low oxygen tension.

Cell Penetration   Although some drugs enter the target cell by simple diffusion, in some instances cellular penetration is an active process. As an example, many of the alkylating agents depend on a carrier transport system for cellular penetration. For large macromolecules, it may be necessary for pinocytosis to accomplish cellular entry.

Drug Metabolism

Many antineoplastic agents are active as intact molecules, but some require metabolism to an active form. Many of the antimetabolites require phosphorylation for cell entry. The alkylating agent, cyclophosphamide, requires absorption and liver metabolism in order to be activated. Attention to these unique metabolic requirements is needed for appropriate drug selection. For example, if direct installation of an alkylating agent is required, an agent that is active as an intact drug should be selected (e.g., *thiotepa* or *nitrogen mustard*), rather than *Cytoxan (cyclophosphamide)*, because the latter drug requires hepatic biotransformation and would not be active locally. Not only is initial activation important, but the rate of metabolic degradation of the active drug or metabolite is important in determining antitumor activity. As an example, a major mechanism of drug resistance in ovarian cancer is increased metabolism of alkylating agents due to increased intracellular enzymes (e.g., glutathione-S-transferase).

13

Excretion

Most chemotherapeutic agents are excreted through the kidney or the liver. Because overall kidney or liver function is critical to normal drug excretion, it is necessary to modify the dosage of certain agents when either of these organs is functionally impaired. Certain drugs (e.g., *vincristine, Adriamycin*), are excreted primarily through the liver, and others (e.g., *methotrexate*) are excreted almost entirely by the kidney. Most experimental protocols and cooperative group trials contain formulas for dose modification for specific organ impairments that influence drug excretion.

Drug Interactions

Commonly, multiple drugs are administered to patients during a hospital stay. These include chemotherapeutic agents as well as non-cancer-related drugs. Consequently, there are multiple opportunities for clinically important drug interactions to occur during cancer treatment. These interactions may increase or decrease the antitumor activity of a particular agent, or they may increase or modify its toxicity (12). Types of drug interaction of potential importance include those listed in Table 1.4.

Important drug interactions with antineoplastic drugs include:

1. The alkylating agents are highly reactive compounds and may produce direct chemical or physical inactivation when multiple drugs are mixed.

2. Intestinal absorption of certain chemotherapeutic agents is altered by antibiotics that suppress bowel flora (e.g., reduced absorption of oral *methotrexate*), resulting in its decreased circulating level.

3. Drugs such as *cisplatin* or *methotrexate* bind to albumin or plasma proteins and may be displaced from that binding by drugs that bind to similar sites, such as aspirin or sulfa, thereby increasing the circulating level of bioavailable *cisplatin* or *methotrexate*.

4. Alterations in drug activation may occur, as when *methotrexate* increases *5-fluorouracil* activation; conversely, drug interaction may antagonize

---

Table 1.4   Drug Interactions in Cancer Chemotherapy

	Effect		Interaction		
		Caused by:		*Resulting in:*	*Bioavailable Drug*
↓	**Renal function/excretion**	Nephrotoxic antibiotics	Methotrexate cisplatin	↓ excretion	↑
↓	**Hepatic metabolism/biliary excretion**	Vincristine	Adriamycin	↓ excretion	↑
↑	**Displacement from albumin or plasma proteins**	Sulfonamides; salicylates	Methotrexate; cisplatin	↓ binding	↑
↑	**Intestinal absorption**	Neomycin	Methotrexate	↓ absorption	↓
↑	**Direct chemical interaction**	Mannitol	Cisplatin	↑ excretion	↓
↑	**Direct effect on metabolism**	Phenobarbitol Methotrexate 5-Fluorouracil	Cytoxan 5-Fluorouracil Methotrexate	↑ metabolism ↑ activation ↓ metabolism	↑ ↑ ↓

antitumor effect, as when *5-fluorouracil* impairs the antifolate action of *methotrexate*.

5. The nephrotoxic antibiotics frequently alter *methotrexate* excretion and may increase the renal toxicity of *cisplatin*.

Principles of Combination Chemotherapy

Antineoplastic agents are now commonly used in combinations (13). Combination chemotherapy has become the standard approach to management of ovarian germ cell tumors as well as many other adult solid tumors, including Hodgkin's disease, non-Hodgkin's lymphomas, breast cancer, and testicular cancer. The enthusiasm for combinations results from several significant limitations inherent in single-agent chemotherapy. In addition, there is a solid theoretic basis for combination chemotherapy from a knowledge of cellular kinetics, drug metabolism, drug resistance, and tumor heterogeneity.

Limitations of Single-Drug Therapy

The major limitations of single-agent chemotherapy are:

1. Toxicity limits the dose and duration of drug administration and thus restricts the tumor cell kill achievable.

2. Adoptive mechanisms allow cell survival and eventual regrowth of resistant tumor cells in spite of lethal effects produced in the bulk of the tumor.

3. Spontaneous development of drug resistance.

4. Multidrug or pleiotropic drug resistance.

Several different mechanisms of resistance are seen with antineoplastic agents, and some of these are listed in Table 1.5. Most problems inherent in single-drug therapy cannot be corrected by simply altering the dose or schedule of that single

Table 1.5   Mechanisms of Resistance to Anticancer Drugs

Mechanism	Example Drug
Insufficient activation of drug	Intraperitoneal Cytoxan, 6-mercapto-purine, 5-fluorouracil
Insufficient drug intake or defective drug transport	Methotrexate, daunomycin
Increased activation	Cytosine arabinoside
Increased utilization of an alternative biochemical pathway (salvage)	Cytosine arabinoside, 5-fluorouracil
Increased concentration of the target enzyme	Methotrexate
Decreased requirement for a specific metabolic product	L-asparaginase
Rapid DNA repair of a drug-related lesion	Alkylating agents, cisplatin, carbo-platin
Gene amplification	Methotrexate

15

drug. As a result, increasing use has been made of multidrug combination chemotherapy.

Combination Chemotherapy Mechanisms

Different chemotherapeutic agents may act in different phases of the tumor cell cycle. Use of multiple drugs with different cellular kinetic characteristics reduces the tumor mass more completely than any individual chemotherapeutic agent while minimizing the impact of single-drug resistance. For instance, if a cell cycle-nonspecific agent is administered, producing a 2 log cell kill in a tumor mass with 10^9 cells and no further therapy is given, a minor tumor response will occur, followed by tumor regrowth and no impact on survival. If a cell cycle-specific agent produces a similar degree of cell kill, only the cells coming into cell cycle will be affected by such an agent. Simply by using combinations or sequences of cell cycle-specific and nonspecific agents, log kill can be enhanced in tumors. With identification of appropriate combinations and proper sequencing, sufficient log kill may be achieved to produce a cure.

Drug Resistance

Combination chemotherapy can help to circumvent spontaneous mutations to drug resistance. After initial cell kill, the residual tumor may contain drug-resistant cells. **The probability of the emergence of drug-resistant cells in any given population is reduced if two or more agents with different mechanisms of action can be used in a tightly sequenced treatment scheme.**

Biochemical Actions

Different mechanisms of drug action and biochemical effects also provide a rationale for drug combinations. Although there appear to be very few exploitable biochemical differences between tumor and normal cells, there is evidence of some differential sensitivity. Combinations can be designed with the use of agents that produce differential biochemical injury and work by attacking multiple sites in the biosynthetic pathways.

Several biochemical concepts have been important in designing drug combinations. These include sequential blockade, concurrent blockade, and complementary inhibition.

Sequential Blockade Sequential blockade uses the simultaneous inhibition of sequential enzymes in a single biochemical pathway. An example of sequential blockade is the inhibition of *de novo* purine synthesis by the combination of *azaserine* and *6–mercaptopurine*.

Concurrent Blockade Concurrent blockade involves the simultaneous inhibition of parallel enzymatic pathways leading to the same end product. An example is the interaction of azaserine, a glutamine antagonist that inhibits *de novo* purine biosynthesis, and *6-thioguanine,* which inhibits reutilization of preformed purines.

Complementary Inhibition Complementary inhibition employs drugs that produce biochemical lesions at different sites in the synthesis of DNA, RNA, or protein. Certain drugs, such as antimetabolites, inhibit the synthesis of vital intracellular molecules. Alkylating agents or antitumor antibiotics, on the other hand, directly attack a preformed molecule.

Combinations based on complementary inhibition interfere with both the synthesis and the function of DNA, RNA, or protein at multiple sites. Many regimens have been designed according to the concept of complementary inhibition. Examples include *methotrexate* and *Cytoxan (MeCy)* in ovarian cancer and *CMF (Cytoxan, methotrexate, and 5-fluorouracil)* in adjuvant treatment of breast cancer.

Drug Interaction

Drug interactions may be additive, synergistic, or antagonistic. Combinations that result in improved therapy because of increased antitumor activity or decreased toxicity are said to be *synergistic*. *Additive* therapies produce enhanced antitumor activity equivalent to the sum of both agents acting singly. Finally, antitumor agents may actually *antagonize* the effect of each other, producing a lesser therapeutic effect than when used singly. For example, *5-fluorouracil* prevents the antifolate action of *methotrexate* when used before *methotrexate* administration.

Schedule Dependency

In some instances, the same drugs used in different sequences may produce a widely varied effect, suggesting the importance of schedule dependency. An example is the reduced cardiac toxicity demonstrated for weekly low-dose *Adriamycin* compared with high-dose bolus *Adriamycin*. Although schedule dependency has been an important, well-documented phenomenon in experimental tumors, its importance is less well defined for human cancer chemotherapy.

The general principles that allowed the development of successful combinations are shown in Table 1.6. Although these cannot be used in every regimen and some overlap in toxicities is common, these concepts are a central feature of most of the regimens now being used successfully in cancer treatment.

Remission

Once a treatment regimen has been selected, it is necessary to have some standardized way to evaluate the response to drug treatment. The terms "complete remission" and "partial remission" are used frequently and provide a convenient way to describe responses and compare various published regimens.

Complete Remission **Complete remission is the complete disappearance of all objective evidence of tumor as well as the resolution of all signs and symptoms referable to the tumor.** Complete regressions of cancer are generally those associated with significant prolongation of survival.

Table 1.6   Important Factors in the Design of Drug Combinations

1. The drugs used must be active as single agents against the particular tumor.

2. The drugs should have different mechanisms of action to minimize emergence of drug resistance.

3. The drugs should have a biochemical basis of at least additive and preferably synergistic effects.

4. The drugs chosen should have a different spectrum of toxicity so they can be used for maximum cell kill at full doses.

5. The drugs chosen should be administered intermittently so that cell kill is enhanced and prolonged immunosuppression is minimized.

Partial Remission **Partial remission is a ≥ 50% reduction in the size of all measurable lesions along with some degree of subjective improvement and the absence of any new lesions during therapy.** Partial remissions generally translate into improved well-being for the patient but only occasionally are associated with longer overall survival.

Finally, various terms indicate lesser responses, such as "objective response" or "minor response," but such responses rarely result in any significant improvement in survival.

Dose Adjustment

Patients vary in their tolerance to chemotherapy, and thus some mechanism for tailoring the treatment to a particular patient is necessary. One convenient method involves the use of a "sliding scale." A typical scheme for adjusting chemotherapy based on myelosuppression is presented in Table 1.7. Doses of myelosuppressive agents are reduced if the patient proves very sensitive to the regimen but can be returned to full levels if tolerance improves in subsequent courses.

Many experimental protocols provide for an escalation of drug dose if no significant toxicity is experienced with initial courses of therapy. A sliding scale offers the best opportunity to give the maximum amount of therapy possible. The sliding scale presented is based only on bone marrow toxicity. If the drugs used in any particular combination have other serious toxicities, such as renal or hepatic toxicity, then sliding scales based on the other toxicities are used to minimize toxicity but maximize therapeutic effect.

As an example, carboplatin is generally given at 300 mg/M^2 intravenously every 4 weeks to patients with good bone marrow reserve. Because the drug is cleared renally and occasional severe marrow toxicity occurs, dose-adjustment scales based on renal function have been developed. Dose adjustments are based on glomerular filtration rate (GFR) or creatinine clearance and the target serum

Table 1.7 Drug Dose Adjustments for Combination Chemotherapy (Sliding Scale Based on Bone Marrow Toxicity)

If White Blood Count Before Starting the Next Course Is:	Then Dosage Is:
>4000/mm³	100% of all drugs
3999–3000/mm³	100% of nonmyelotoxic agents and 50% of each myelotoxic agent
2999–2000/mm³	100% of nonmyelotoxic agents and 25% of each myelotoxic agent
1999–1000/mm³	50% of nonmyelotoxic agents and 25% of myelotoxic agents
999–0/mm³	No drug until blood counts recover

If the Platelet Count Before Starting Next Course Is:	Then Dosage Is:
>100,000/mm³	100% of all drugs
50,000–100,000/mm³	100% of nonmyelotoxic drugs and 50% of myelotoxic drugs
<50,000/mm³	No drug until blood counts recover

concentration multiplied by the "area under curve" (AUC) for the drugs' antitumor activity (14). The formula is

$$\text{Dose (mg)} = \text{Target AUC} \times (\text{GFR} + 25)$$

The desired target AUC is 4–6 mg/mL for previously treated patients and 6–8 mg/mL for those previously untreated. The use of these dose-adjustment schemes tailored to the particular toxicity will allow for safer administration of chemotherapeutic agents.

Treatment Evaluation

A great number of combination regimens are currently in use in gynecologic malignancies. Many are established as treatments of choice for particular tumors, and others are experimental. In evaluating any particular combination, several important points should be considered:

1. Has the regimen been used for a number of years, and has it been demonstrated to be effective by more than one investigator for a particular stage or stages of disease?

2. Has the regimen been published with adequate discussion of the toxicities inherent in the treatment?

3. Does the regimen contain unusual forms of treatment that require unique facilities?

4. Is the combination made up of drugs that are available commercially?

Drug Toxicity

Antineoplastic drugs are among the most toxic agents used in modern medicine. Many of the toxic side effects, particularly those to organ systems with a rapidly proliferating cell population, are dose related and predictable. Usually the mechanism of toxicity is similar to the mechanism that produces the desired cytocidal effect on tumors. Even organs with limited cell proliferation can be damaged by chemotherapeutic agents in either a dose-related or an idiosyncratic fashion. In almost all instances, chemotherapeutic agents are used in doses that produce some degree of toxicity to normal tissues.

Severe systemic debility, advanced age, poor nutritional status, or direct organ involvement by primary or metastatic tumor can result in unexpectedly severe side effects of chemotherapy. Idiosyncratic drug reactions also can have severe and unexpected consequences. As a result, careful monitoring of patients receiving cancer chemotherapy is a major responsibility of physicians who elect to use this approach to cancer management (15, 16).

Hematologic Toxicity

The proliferating cells of the erythroid, myeloid, and megakaryocytic series of the bone marrow are highly susceptible to damage by many of the commonly employed antineoplastic agents. Granulocytopenia and thrombocytopenia are predictable side effects of most of the commonly employed antitumor agents and are seen with all effective regimens of combination chemotherapy. The severity and duration of these side effects are quite variable and depend on the drugs, the dose, the schedule, and the patient's previous radiation or chemotherapy.

19

In general, acute granulocytopenia occurs 6–12 days after administration of most myelosuppressive chemotherapeutic agents and recovery occurs in 21–24 days; platelet suppression occurs 4–5 days later, with recovery after white cell count recovery. Several agents are unique in producing delayed bone marrow suppression, among them *mitomycin C* and the *nitrosoureas*. Marrow suppression from these drugs commonly occurs at 28–42 days, with recovery 40–60 days after treatment.

Granulocytopenia **Patients with an absolute granulocyte count < 500/mm³ for 5 days or longer are at high risk of rapidly fatal sepsis.** The wide use of prophylactic, empiric, broad-spectrum antibiotics in febrile cancer patients with granulocytopenia has significantly decreased the incidence of life-threatening infections. Granulocytopenic patients should have their temperature checked every 4 hours and must be examined frequently for evidence of infection. Recent availability of hematopoietic growth factors such as G-CSF and GM-CSF have enabled physicians to reduce the duration of granulocytopenia in certain patients. However, thrombocytopenia is not reversed.

Thrombocytopenia **Patients with sustained thrombocytopenia who have platelet counts < 20,000/mm³ are at risk of spontaneous hemorrhage, particularly gastrointestinal or acute intracranial hemorrhage.** Routine platelet transfusions for platelet counts < 20,000/mm³ have significantly reduced the risk of spontaneous hemorrhage. It is common to transfuse 6–10 units of random donor platelets to the patient with a platelet count < 20,000/mm³. Repeat transfusions at intervals of 2–3 days for the duration of the severe thrombocytopenia are indicated. Although patients with platelet counts > 50,000/mm³ do not commonly experience severe bleeding, transfusion at this level is indicated

1. If the patient manifests active bleeding

2. If the patient has active peptic ulcer disease

3. Before and during surgical procedures

A posttransfusion platelet count performed 1 hour after platelet administration should show an appropriate incremental increase. If no posttransfusion platelet increase occurs, it is likely that there has been previous sensitization to random donor platelets and the patient will require single-donor HLA (human lymphocyte antigen) matched platelets for future transfusions.

Gastrointestinal Toxicity The gastrointestinal tract is a frequent site of serious toxicity of antineoplastic drug treatment. Mucositis caused by a direct effect on the rapidly dividing epithelial mucosal cells is common; concomitant granulocytopenia allows the injured mucosa to become infected and serves as a portal of entry for bacteria and fungi into the bloodstream. Impaired cellular immunity due to underlying disease or corticosteroid therapy also can contribute to extensive infection of the gastrointestinal tract. Other side effects related to the gastrointestinal tract include impaired intestinal motility resulting from the autonomic neuropathic effect of vinca alkaloids (*vincristine* and *vinblastine*) and nausea and vomiting, induced by many anticancer drugs.

Upper Gastrointestinal   The onset of mucositis is frequently 3–5 days earlier than the myelosuppression. Lesions of the mouth and pharynx are difficult to distinguish from candidiasis and herpes simplex. Esophagitis due to direct drug toxicity can be confused with radiation esophagitis or infections with bacteria, fungi, or herpes simplex because they all produce dysphagia and retrosternal burning pain. Oral candidiasis (thrush) responds to oral *chlortrimazole*, 10 mg five times daily. Esophageal or severe oral candidiasis usually responds to a 7-day course of intravenous *amphotericin B*, 0.5 mg/kg/day. Mucocutaneous herpes simplex clears more rapidly with intravenous *acyclovir*, 750 mg/m^2/day. Symptomatic management of painful upper gastrointestinal inflammation includes warm saline mouth rinses and topical anesthetics, such as viscous *lidocaine*. Intravenous fluids or hyperalimentation may be required.

Lower Gastrointestinal   Mucositis in the lower gastrointestinal tract is invariably associated with diarrhea. Serious complications include bowel perforation, hemorrhage, and necrotizing enterocolitis.

Necrotizing enterocolitis includes a spectrum of severe diarrheal illnesses that can be fatal in a granulocytopenic patient. Broad-spectrum antibiotic therapy may predispose the patient to necrotizing enterocolitis. Symptoms of necrotizing enterocolitis include watery or bloody diarrhea, abdominal pain, sore throat, nausea, vomiting, and fever. Physical examination usually reveals abdominal tenderness and distention. Most necrotizing enterocolitis is seen in patients who are treated with clindamycin and is caused by the anaerobic bacteria *Clostridium difficile*. The treatment of choice for a *C. difficile* infection is oral vancomycin, 125 mg four times daily for 10–14 days.

Immunosuppression

Most anticancer drugs are capable of producing suppression of cellular and, to a lesser extent, humoral immunity. The magnitude and duration of the immunosuppression vary with the dose and schedule of drug administration and have been inadequately characterized for most chemotherapeutic agents. However, most of the acute immunosuppressive side effects do not persist after completion of drug treatment. Laboratory studies suggest a marked decrease in host defenses during treatment associated with a rebound to complete or nearly complete restoration 2–3 days after treatment is completed. This short-term immunosuppressive effect has led to increased use of intermittent chemotherapy regimens to allow immunologic recovery during courses of treatment.

Dermatologic Reactions

Several important drug toxicities involve skin reactions. These include alopecia, local necrosis from drug extravasation, and allergic or hypersensitivity reactions. Skin necrosis and sloughing may result from extravasation of certain particularly irritating chemotherapeutic agents, such as *Adriamycin, actinomycin D, mitomycin C, vinblastine, vincristine,* and *nitrogen mustard*. The extent of necrosis is dependent on the quantity of drug extravasated and can vary from local erythema to chronic ulcerative necrosis. Management often includes immediate removal of the intravenous line, local infiltration of corticosteroids, ice pack therapy four times a day for 3 days, and elevation of the affected limb. Long-term monitoring of the affected area is required, and surgical debridement and full-thickness skin grafting are often necessary for severe lesions.

Alopecia is the most common side effect of many anticancer drugs. Although not intrinsically injurious, it has major emotional consequences for patients. Agents commonly associated with severe hair loss include the anthracycline antibiotics, the vinca alkaloids, *Taxol,* and *Cytoxan,* but most commonly used drug combinations produce variable degrees of alopecia. Alopecia is virtually always reversible if the patient is able to discontinue chemotherapy. Generally, hair regrowth begins 10 days to several weeks after treatment is completed. Attempts to minimize alopecia by using cold caps have been variably effective.

Generalized allergic skin reactions can occur with chemotherapeutic agents, as they do with other drugs, and can sometimes be severe. Other skin reactions occasionally seen with chemotherapeutic agents include increased skin pigmentation *(bleomycin)*, photosensitivity reactions, transverse banding or nail loss, folliculitis *(actinomycin D, methotrexate)*, and radiation recall reactions *(Adriamycin)*.

Hepatic Toxicity

Modest elevations in transaminase, alkaline phosphatase, and bilirubin levels are frequently seen with many anticancer agents, but they resolve soon after treatment is completed. Nevertheless, more severe reactions do occur. Long-term administration of methotrexate induces hepatic fibrosis that can progress to frank cirrhosis. The cirrhosis and drug-induced hepatitis should be managed by withdrawal of the toxic agent, with the same supportive measures that are used for hepatitis or cirrhosis of any cause.

Preexisting liver disease or exposure to other hepatotoxins may increase the risk. Antimetabolites, such as *6–mercaptopurine* and *6–thioguanine,* can produce reversible cholestatic jaundice. Transient liver enzyme abnormalities are seen with *cytosine arabinoside,* the *nitrosoureas,* and L-*asparaginase. Mithramycin,* an agent used to control hypercalcemia, frequently causes marked elevations in liver enzyme levels associated with clotting disorders and renal insufficiency. Interim lactic dehydrogenase (LDH) and prothrombin time should be followed if multiple courses of *mithramycin* are to be used.

Pulmonary Complications

Patients with cancer have a wide variety of problems that can manifest as pulmonary complications. Respiratory compromise due to lung metastases, pulmonary emboli, radiation pneumonitis, tumor-induced neuromuscular dysfunction, and pneumonia all may be significant complications. In addition, direct pulmonary toxicity from commonly used anticancer drugs sometimes is seen.

Interstitial Pneumonitis Interstitial pneumonitis with pulmonary fibrosis is the usual pattern of lung damage associated with cytotoxic drugs. Agents likely to cause such an effect are *bleomycin, alkylating agents,* and the *nitrosoureas.* The physical and chest x-ray findings are not easily distinguishable from those of interstitial pneumonitis resulting from infectious agents, viruses, or lymphangitic spread of cancer.

Management of drug-induced interstitial pneumonitis includes discontinuation of the suspected agent and supportive care. Steroids may have some benefit in the hypersensitivity to *mitomycin C* and *procarbazine.* There is little evidence of benefit in cases of pneumonitis and fibrosis secondary to alkylating agents, the nitrosoureas, and the antitumor antibiotics.

Cardiac Toxicity

Cardiac toxicity is seen with several important cancer chemotherapeutic agents. Although the myocardium consists of largely nondividing cells, drugs of the anthracycline antibiotic class, specifically *Adriamycin* and *daunomycin,* can cause severe cardiomyopathy.

The risk of cardiac toxicity increases with the total cumulative dose of *Adriamycin*. For this reason, a cumulative dose of 500 mg/m^2 of ideal body surface area is now widely used as the maximum tolerable dose of *Adriamycin*. With careful and frequent monitoring of left ventricular function by means of ejection fraction studies, therapy can be continued to higher doses if no satisfactory alternative exists. More infrequently, anthracyclines and *Taxol* can cause acute arrhythmias that generally disappear within a few days of drug treatment. They appear not to be related to total drug dose. Anthracycline cardiac toxicity is potentiated by radiation.

The medical management of cardiomyopathy induced by anthracyclines is supportive but generally unsatisfactory. Early detection of cardiac compromise with radionuclide cardiac scintigraphy before the clinical manifestations of congestive heart failure appear is important. Discontinuation of the drug at the first indication of decreasing left ventricular function will minimize the risk of cardiovascular decompensation.

Rarely, *Cytoxan* has been reported to produce cardiotoxicity, particularly in the massive doses used in conjunction with bone marrow transplantation. With conventional doses of *Cytoxan,* this complication is unlikely. *Busulfan* and *mitomycin C* have been reported to cause endocardial fibrosis and myocardial fibrosis, respectively. In some patients, *5-fluorouracil* has been reported to be a rare cause of angina pectoris.

Genitourinary Toxicity

In addition to chemotherapeutic agents, various other cancer-related complications may produce chronic azotemia or acute renal failure, including fluid depletion, infection, tumor infiltration of the kidney, ureteral obstruction by tumor, radiation damage, and tumor lysis syndrome.

Drugs that cause kidney damage include:

1. *Cisplatin*, which produces renal tubular toxicity associated with azotemia and magnesium wasting.

2. *Methotrexate*, which can precipitate in the renal tubules, causing oliguric renal failure. *Methotrexate* toxicity can be prevented by maintenance of a high urine volume and alkalinization of the urine.

3. *Nitrosoureas*, which cause a chronic interstitial nephritis with chronic renal failure.

4. *Mitomycin C*, which causes a systemic microangiopathic hemolysis and acute renal failure.

Metabolites of *Cytoxan* are irritants to the bladder mucosa and cause a *chronic hemorrhagic cystitis,* particularly during high-dose or prolonged treatment. Vigorous hydration and diuresis can reduce the risk of this complication.

23

Treatment of drug-related genitourinary toxicity requires discontinuation of the possibly nephrotoxic drugs and volume expansion to increase glomerular filtration. Specific metabolic abnormalities, such as hyperuricemia and hypomagnesemia, should be corrected. If oliguria develops or if medical management is unsuccessful in restoring acceptable kidney function, short-term peritoneal dialysis or hemodialysis may be required. Daily administration of 3 liters of fluid containing 100–150 mEq of sodium bicarbonate per liter will maintain the urinary pH above 7. Because *methotrexate* is poorly dialyzed, prolonged toxic levels can result if *leucovorin* rescue therapy is not continued until the methotrexate concentration is less than 5×10^{-8} M.

Recently, *n*-acetylcysteine or *mesna* (sodium mercaptoethanesulfonate) has been used in conjunction with very high doses of *Cytoxan* (cyclophosphamide) or *Ifex* (iphosphamide) to prevent bladder toxicity by inactivating the toxic metabolite *(acrolein)*. Persistent hemorrhagic cystitis that does not respond to conservative management may be treated with ε-*aminocaproic acid*.

Neurotoxicity

Many antineoplastic drugs are associated with some central or peripheral neurotoxicity. Generally, these neurologic side effects are mild, but occasionally they can be severe.

Vinca Alkaloids The vinca alkaloids (*vincristine, vinblastine,* and *vindesine*) are commonly associated with peripheral motor, sensory, and autonomic neuropathies, which are the major side effects of vincristine. Toxicity first appears as loss of deep tendon reflexes with distal paresthesias. Cranial nerves can be affected, and the autonomic neuropathy can appear as adynamic ileus, urinary bladder atony with retention, or hypotension. All of these neurologic toxicities from the vinca alkaloids are slowly reversible after cessation of the offending drug.

Cisplatin *Cisplatin* produces ototoxicity, peripheral neuropathy, and, rarely, retrobulbar neuritis and blindness. High doses of *cisplatin*, often used in ovarian cancer therapy, are particularly likely to produce a progressive and somewhat delayed peripheral neuropathy. This defect is characterized by sensory impairment and loss of proprioception, whereas motor strength generally is preserved. Progression of this neuropathy 1–2 months after cessation of high-dose cisplatin has been reported.

Other Drugs *5-Fluorouracil (5-FU)* rarely can be associated with an acute cerebellar toxicity, apparently related to its metabolism to fluorocitrate, a neurotoxic metabolite of the parent compound. *Hexamethylmelamine* has been reported to produce peripheral neuropathy and encephalopathy. Some improvement in the peripheral neuropathy has been reported with administration of B vitamin supplements, but therapeutic effectiveness may be reduced. High-dose *cytosine arabinoside (Ara-C)* has been associated with somnolence, ataxia, and confusion.

Vascular and Hypersensitivity Reactions

Occasionally, severe hypersensitivity reactions in the form of anaphylaxis develop with chemotherapeutic agents. In rare cases this has been associated with *Cytoxan, Adriamycin, cisplatin,* intravenous *melphalan,* and high-dose *methotrexate.* *Bleomycin* administration may be associated with marked fever reactions, anaphylaxis,

Raynaud's phenomenon, and a chronic scleroderma-like reaction. The same re-actions have been reported with *procarbazine, etoposide (VP-16), and teniposide (VM-26).* Hypersensitivity reactions have been seen with *Taxol* and are believed to be due to hypersensitivity to the *cremophor* vehicle. They can be ameliorated with intravenous infusions of dexamethasone 20 mg, diphenhydramine 50 mg, and cimetidine 300 mg 30 minutes before *Taxol* is administered.

Second Malignancies

Many antineoplastic agents in current use are mutagenic and teratogenic. The potential of these agents to induce second malignancies appears to vary with the class of agent (17). Alkylating agents (especially *melphalan*), *procarbazine,* and the *nitrosoureas* seem to be the major offenders. The cumulative 7-year risk of acute nonlymphocytic leukemia (ANL) developing in patients treated primarily with oral *melphalan* for ovarian cancer is as high as 9.6% in patients receiving therapy for more than 1 year (17). Antimetabolites, in contrast, seem to be less risky. Evidence from long-term studies of Hodgkin's disease suggests a major risk with combined chemotherapy and radiation therapy. In such patients, there is a risk of acute leukemia as well as an increase in solid tumors, seen particularly in the radiation ports. An increase in the frequency of acute leukemia has been reported in patients treated for Hodgkin's disease, multiple myeloma, and ovarian cancer.

The second malignancy commonly occurs 4–7 years after successful therapy. Encouragingly, recent evidence suggests that after 11 years the risk of acute leukemia in patients treated for Hodgkin's disease decreases to that of the normal population. Also encouraging are the long-term follow-up studies in women cured of choriocarcinoma, primarily with antimetabolite therapy. In such patient populations there is no evidence of an increased risk of second malignancy. Radiation alone appears to produce a relatively low risk of late leukemia. Chemotherapeutic regimens alone, particularly those without alkylating agents or *procarbazine,* are also associated with relatively little risk. Combination chemotherapy and limited-field radiation therapy increase the risk only slightly.

Particularly high risks are associated with:

1. Extensive radiation therapy plus combination chemotherapy

2. Prolonged alkylating agent therapy (> 1 year)

3. Prolonged maintenance therapy

4. Age at initial treatment > 40 years

Gonadal Dysfunction

Many cancer chemotherapeutic agents have profound and lasting effects on tes-ticular and ovarian function. Chemotherapeutic agents, particularly alkylating agents, can cause azoospermia and amenorrhea. Secondary sexual characteristics related to hormonal function are generally less disturbed. Prolonged intensive combination chemotherapy commonly produces azoospermia in males, and re-covery is uncommon.

The onset of amenorrhea and ovarian failure is accompanied by an elevation of the serum follicle-stimulating hormone (FSH) and luteinizing hormone (LH) and

25

a decrease in the serum estradiol level. Occasionally, this hormonal pattern can be seen before the onset of amenorrhea. If the characteristic pattern is seen, patients should be advised to consider conception, because these findings predict premature ovarian failure and early menopause.

When short-term intensive chemotherapy is used, particularly with antimetabolites, vinca alkaloids, or antitumor antibiotics, injury to the reproductive system is less common. For example, males treated for testicular cancer, children with acute leukemia, and women cured of gestational trophoblastic disease or ovarian germ cell malignancies generally have recovered reproductive capacity after therapy.

Chemotherapy in Pregnancy   Risk of congenital abnormalities from these drugs is highest during the first trimester of pregnancy, especially when antimetabolites (e.g., *cytosine arabinoside* or *methotrexate*) and alkylating agents are used. Chemotherapy administered during the second or third trimesters is generally not associated with an increase in fetal abnormalities, although the number of patients studied is relatively small.

Metabolic Abnormalities

Inappropriate Antidiuretic Hormone Secretion   Inappropriate antidiuretic hormone (ADH) secretion is characterized by hyponatremia, high urine osmolality, and high urinary sodium values and is associated with several malignancies, most commonly small cell carcinoma of the lung. It can also be seen as a complication of vinca alkaloid chemotherapy. Symptoms are primarily neurologic and include altered mental status, confusion, lethargy, seizures, and coma. The severity of symptoms is related to the rapidity of development of hyponatremia. The diagnosis rests on

1. The documentation of hyponatremia

2. The presence of a urine that is hypertonic to plasma

3. The exclusion of hypothyroidism or adrenal insufficiency

Hyperuricemia   Hyperuricemia may be a complication of effective cancer chemotherapy in certain tumors, particularly hematologic malignancies where rapid tumor lysis is seen in response to initial treatment. Rapid tumor lysis produces release of predominant intracellular ions and uric acid and can result in life-threatening hyperkalemia, hyperphosphatemia, hypocalcemia, and hyperuricemia. Renal failure associated with hyperuricemia can be severe. Prevention of the *tumor lysis syndrome* requires maintenance of a high urinary output, maintenance of high urinary pH (above 7.0), and prophylactic use of the xanthine oxidase inhibitor, *allopurinol,* as discussed in Chapter 16.

Antineoplastic Drugs

Alkylating Agents

This class of antineoplastic agent acts primarily by chemically interacting with DNA (18). These drugs form extremely unstable alkyl groups that react with nucleophilic (electron-rich) sites on many important organic compounds, such as nucleic acids, proteins, and amino acids. These interactions produce the primary cytotoxic effects.

Mechanism

Alkylating agents commonly bind to the N-7 position of guanine and to other key DNA sites. In doing so, they interfere with accurate base pairing, cross-link DNA, and produce single- and double-stranded breaks. This results in the inhibition of DNA, RNA, and protein synthesis.

Because alkylating agents share some effects similar to irradiation, they are often called *radiomimetic*. Most of the effective alkylating agents are bifunctional or polyfunctional and have two or more potentially unstable alkyl groups per molecule. These bifunctional alkylating agents allow cross-linkage of DNA that results in cellular disruption.

Because all alkylating agents have similar mechanisms of action, there tends to be cross-resistance to other agents of the same class.

Drugs

Although several hundred alkylating agents exist, those most commonly in use include *nitrogen mustard (Mustargen), cyclophosphamide (Cytoxan), melphalan (Alkeran), thiotepa, chlorambucil (Leukeran), busulfan (Myleran)*, and *Ifex*.

In addition to the more common alkylating agents, several antineoplastic agents of different types are generally classified as alkylating-like agents, although their precise mechanism of action is less well understood and is probably not exclusively alkylation (19). These include the *nitrosoureas, BCNU (carmustine), methyl-CCNU (semustine), CCNU (lomustine), DTIC (decarbazine)*, and the platinum analogs, *cisplatin* and *carboplatin*.

The characteristics of the commonly used alkylating agents are listed in Table 1.8. The alkylating-like agents are listed in Table 1.9.

Antitumor Antibiotics

The antitumor antibiotics are antineoplastic drugs that, in general, have been isolated as natural products from fungi found in the soil (20). These natural products generally have extremely complex and different chemical structures, although they generally function by forming complexes with DNA.

Mechanism

The interaction between these drugs and DNA often involves intercalation in which the compound is inserted between DNA base pairs. A second mechanism thought to be important in their antitumor action is the formation of free radicals capable of damaging DNA, RNA, and vital proteins. Other effects include metal ion chelation and alteration of tumor cell membranes. This class of antineoplastic agents is generally thought to be *cell cycle-nonspecific*.

Drugs

Major drugs in this family include the anthracycline antibiotics *doxorubicin (Adriamycin)* and *daunorubicin (Daunomycin)* as well as *actinomycin D (Dactinomycin), bleomycin (Blenoxane), mitomycin C (Mutamycin)*, and *mithramycin*.

Anthracyclines The anthracyclines are antibiotics isolated from the fungi, *Streptomyces*. These pigmented compounds have an anthraquinone nucleus attached to an amino sugar and have multiple mechanisms of action. Because of

27

Table 1.8   Alkylating Agents Used for Gynecologic Cancer

Drug	Route of Administration	Common Treatment Schedules	Common Toxicities	Diseases Treated
Nitrogen mustard (**Mustargen, HN₂**)	I.V. Intracavitary	I.V.: 0.4 mg/kg as a single dose or 0.1 mg/kg every day × 4 Intracavitary: 0.2–0.4 mg/kg	Nausea and vomiting, myelosuppression	Ovary, malignant pleural or pericardial effusions
Cyclophosphamide (**Cytoxan**)	Oral, I.V.	1.5–3.0 mg/kg/day p.o. 10–50 mg/kg I.V. every 1–4 weeks	Myelosuppression, cystitis ± bladder fibrosis, alopecia, hepatits, amenorrhea, azoospermia	Breast, ovary, soft tissue sarcomas
Chlorambucil (**Leukeran**)	Oral	0.03–0.1 mg/kg/day	Myelosuppression, gastrointestinal distress, dermatitis, hepatotoxicity	Ovary
Melphalan (**Alkeran, L-PAM**)	Oral	0.2 mg/kg/day × 5 days every 4–6 weeks	Myelosuppression, nausea and vomiting (rare), mucosal ulceration (rare), second malignancies	Ovary, breast
Triethylene thiophosphoramide (**TSPA, Thiotepa**)	I.V. Intracavitary	I.V.: 0.8 mg/kg every 4–6 weeks Intracavitary: 45–60 mg	Myelosuppression, nausea and vomiting, headaches, fever (rare)	Ovary, breast; intracavitary for malignant effusions
Iphosphamide (**Ifex**)	I.V.	1.0 or 1.2 g/m²/day × 5 days With mesna: 200 mg/m² immediately before and 4 and 8 hr after iphosphamide	Myelosuppression, bladder toxicity, CNS dysfunction, renal toxicity	Cervix, ovary

Table 1.9   Alkylating-Like Agents Used for Gynecologic Cancer

Drug	Route of Administration	Common Treatment Schedules	Common Toxicities	Diseases Treated
Cis-dichlorodiaminoplatinum (**cisplatin**)	I.V.	10–20 mg/m²/day × 5 every 3 weeks or 50–75 mg/m² every 1–3 weeks	Nephrotoxicity, tinnitis and hearing loss, nausea and vomiting, myelosuppression, peripheral neuropathy	Ovarian and germ cell carcinomas, cervical cancer
Carboplatin	I.V.	300–400 mg/m² × 6 every 3–4 weeks	Less neuropathy, ototoxicity, and nephrotoxicity than cisplatin; more hematopoeitic toxicity, especially thrombocytopenia, than cisplatin	Ovarian and germ cell carcinomas
Decarbazine (**DTIC**)	I.V.	2–4.5 mg/kg/day × 10 days every 4 weeks	Myelosuppression, nausea and vomiting, flulike syndrome, hepatotoxicity	Uterine sarcomas, soft tissue sarcomas

the planar structure of the anthraquinone moiety, these agents act as intercalators in the DNA double helix. In addition, they are known to chelate divalent cations and are avid calcium binders. These agents cause single-stranded DNA breaks, inhibit DNA repair, and actively generate free radicals that are capable of producing DNA damage. Recent evidence suggests that anthracyclines are capable of reacting directly with cell membranes, disrupting membrane structure, and altering membrane function.

Bleomycin   *Bleomycin* was also isolated from the *Streptomyces* fungus. Its structure contains a DNA-binding fragment and an ion-binding unit. It appears to produce its antitumor action primarily by producing single- and double-stranded breaks in DNA, mainly at sites of guanine bases. The drug is primarily excreted in the urine, and increased toxicity may be seen in patients with impaired renal function.

Mitomycin C   *Mitomycin C* is another antibiotic that was isolated from the *Streptomyces* fungus. It is activated *in vivo* into an alkylating agent that can bind DNA, producing cross-links and inhibition of DNA synthesis. In addition, it has a quinone moiety that can generate free radical reactions similar to those seen with the anthracycline antibiotics. It is administered intravenously and is degraded primarily by metabolism. Renal clearance is not a major mechanism of excretion.

Mithramycin   *Mithramycin* is an antitumor antibiotic isolated from another *Streptomyces* species. It has intrinsic antitumor properties and is also effective in the management of hypercalcemia. Its primary mechanism of action seems to be the inhibition of RNA synthesis, although it binds to DNA and produces inhibition of DNA and protein synthesis.

Some of the important characteristics of the antitumor antibiotics are listed in Table 1.10.

Antimetabolites

The antimetabolite family of antineoplastic agents interacts with vital intracellular enzymes, leading to their inactivation or to the production of fraudulent products incapable of normal intracellular function (21, 22). In general, their structures resemble analogs of normal purines and pyrimidines, or they resemble normal substances that are vital for cell function. Some antimetabolites are active as intact drugs, and others require biotransformation to active agents.

Mechanism

Although many of these agents act at different sites in biosynthetic pathways, they appear to exert their antitumor activity by disruption of functions crucial to the viability of the cell. These effects are generally more disruptive to actively proliferating cells; thus the antimetabolites are generally classed as *cell cycle-specific* agents.

Drugs

Although hundreds of antimetabolites have been investigated in cancer treatment, only a few are commonly used. They include:

1. The folate antagonist, *methotrexate,* which inhibits the enzyme dihydrofolate reductase

29

Table 1.10   Antitumor Antibiotics Used for Gynecologic Cancer

Drug	Route of Administration	Common Treatment Schedules	Common Toxicities	Diseases Treated
Actinomycin D (dactinomycin, Cosmegen)	I.V.	0.3–0.5 mg/m² I.V. × 5 days every 3–4 weeks	Nausea and vomiting, skin necrosis, mucosal ulceration, myelosuppression	Germ cell ovarian tumors, choriocarcinoma, soft tissue sarcoma
Bleomycin (Blenoxane)	I.V., S.C., I.M., I.P.	10–20 units/m² 1–2 times/week to total dose of 400 units; for effusions: 60–120 units	Fever, dermatologic reactions, pulmonary toxicity, anaphylactic reactions	Cervix, germ cell ovarian tumors, malignant effusions
Mitomycin-C (Mutamycin)	I.V.	10–20 mg/m² every 6–8 weeks	Myelosuppression, local vesicant, nausea and vomiting, mucosal ulcerations, nephrotoxicity	Breast, cervix, ovary
Doxorubicin (Adriamycin)	I.V.	60–90 mg/m² every 3 weeks or 20–35 mg/m² every day × 3 every 3 weeks	Myelosuppression, alopecia, cardiotoxicity, local vesicant, nausea and vomiting, mucosal ulcerations	Ovary, breast, endometrium
Mithramycin (Mithracin)	I.V.	20–50 mg/kg/day every 4–6 weeks; Hypercalcemia: 25 mg/kg every 3–4 days	Nausea and vomiting, hemorrhagic diathesis, hepatotoxicity, renal toxicity, fever, myelosuppression, facial flushing	Hypercalcemia of malignancy

2. The purine antagonists, *6-mercaptopurine (6-MP, Purinethol)* and *6-thioguanine*

3. The pyrimidine antagonists, *5-fluorouracil (5-FU, fluorouracil)* and *cytosine arabinoside (Ara-C, Cytosar-U)*

4. The ribonucleotide reductase inhibitor, *hydroxyurea (Hydrea)*

In most instances the antimetabolites are used not as single drugs but in combinations because of their cell cycle specificity and their capacity for complementary inhibition. Antimetabolites commonly used in the treatment of gynecologic malignancies are summarized in Table 1.11.

Plant Alkaloids

The most common plant alkaloids in use are the vinca alkaloids, natural products derived from the common periwinkle plant *(Vinca rosea)*, although the epipodophyllotoxins and, recently, *Taxol* are used frequently in gynecologic malignancies (Table 1.12) (23). Like most natural products, these compounds are large and complex molecules, but *vincristine* and *vinblastine* differ only by a single methyl group on one side chain.

Mechanism

Vincristine and vinblastine act primarily by binding to vital intracellular microtubular proteins, particularly tubulin. Tubulin binding produces inhibition of microtubule assembly and destruction of the mitotic spindle, and cells are arrested

Table 1.11   Antimetabolites Used for Gynecologic Cancer

Drug	Route of Administration	Common Treatment Schedules	Common Toxicities	Diseases Treated
5-Fluorouracil (Fluorouracil, 5-FU)	I.V.	10–15 mg/kg/week	Myelosuppression, nausea and vomiting, anorexia, alopecia	Breast, ovary
Methotrexate (MTX, amethopterin)	P.O., I.V., Intrathecal	Oral: 15–40 mg/day × 5 days; I.V.: 240 mg/m² with leucovorin rescue; Intrathecal: 12–15 mg/m²/week	Mucosal ulceration, myelosuppression, hepatotoxicity, allergic pneumonitis; with intrathecal: meningeal irritation	Choriocarcinoma, breast, ovary
Hydroxyurea (Hydrea)	P.O., I.V.	1–2 gm/m²/daily for 2–6 weeks	Myelosuppression, nausea and vomiting, anorexia	Cervix

Table 1.12   Plant Alkaloids

Drug	Route of Administration	Common Treatment Schedules	Common Toxicities	Diseases Treated
Vincristine (Oncovin)	I.V.	0.01–0.03 mg/kg/week	Neurotoxicity, alopecia, myelosuppression, cranial nerve palsies, gastrointestinal	Ovarian germ cell, sarcomas, cervical cancer
Vinblastine (Velban)	I.V.	5–6 mg/m² every 1–2 weeks	Myelosuppression, alopecia, nausea and vomiting, neurotoxicity	Ovarian germ cell, choriocarcinoma
Epipodophyllotoxin (Etoposide, VP-16)	I.V.	300–600 mg/m² divided over 3–4 days every 3–4 weeks	Myelosuppression, alopecia, hypotension	Ovarian germ cell, choriocarcinoma
Paclitaxel (Taxol)	I.V.	135–250 mg/m² as a 3–24 hour infusion every 3 weeks	Myelosuppression, alopecia, allergic reactions, cardiac arrhythmias	Ovarian cancer, breast cancer

in mitosis. Generally, this class of antineoplastic agent is believed to be *cell cycle-specific*. At high concentrations, these drugs also have effects on nucleic acid and protein synthesis.

Taxol has a unique mechanism of action; it binds preferentially to microtubules and results in their polymerization and stabilization. *Taxol*-treated cells contain large numbers of microtubules, free and in bundles, that result in disruption of microtubule function and, ultimately, in cell death. Renal clearance is minimal (5%).

Drugs

Vinblastine is used primarily in the treatment of breast cancer and ovarian germ cell tumors. Its primary toxicity is myelosuppression. In contrast, *vincristine* causes little myelosuppression. Its primary dose-limiting toxicity is peripheral neuropathy. Vincristine is used primarily in cervical carcinoma and genital tract sarcomas.

Table 1.13   Miscellaneous Agent

Drug	Route of Administration	Common Treatment Schedules	Common Toxicities	Diseases Treated
Hexamethylmelamine, Altretamine **(Hexalen)**	Oral	120 mg/m^2/day × 14 days every 4 weeks	Nausea and vomiting, myelosuppression, neurotoxicity, skin rashes	Ovary, breast

Recently, a new family of plant alkaloids has been documented to have significant antitumor properties. Members of this family, known as the *epipodophyllotoxins*, are extracts from the mandrake plant. Although the primary plant extracts had tubulin-binding properties similar to those of the vinca alkaloids, the active derivatives, *etoposide (VP-16)* and *teniposide (VM-26)*, do not seem to function either by inhibiting mitotic spindle formation or by tubulin binding. They appear to function by causing single-stranded DNA breaks. Unlike many of the other compounds that act primarily by DNA interactions, these agents appear to be *cell cycle-specific* and *schedule-dependent*. The drugs are poorly water soluble and thus are administered intravenously. The dose-limiting toxicity is myelosuppression. Other toxicities include an infusion rate–limited hypotension, nausea, vomiting, anorexia, and alopecia.

Taxol is an extract from the bark of the Pacific yew tree. Its chemical formula is complex, and it has not yet been synthesized. Toxic effects of Taxol include bone marrow suppression, alopecia, myalgias, arthralgias, and hypersensitivity reactions. The most common dose-limiting toxic effect is granulocytopenia. Taxol was available initially as a salvage agent through NCI-designated Comprehensive Cancer Centers at 135 mg/M^2 every 3 weeks for advanced ovarian cancer. It has been recently approved for use in women with ovarian cancer (see Chapter 9). It is also active in breast and lung cancer.

Other Agents

In addition to the antineoplastic agents summarized above, there is another group of commonly used drugs that do not fall into any particular class. They have unique or poorly understood mechanisms. The only agent commonly used in gynecologic malignancies is hexamethylmelamine (Hexalen) (Table 1.13).

New Drug Trials

A number of chemotherapeutic agents have been studied experimentally but are not commercially available. Many of these agents have already demonstrated activity against human tumors, but sufficient evidence to allow human experimentation has not yet been acquired. In addition, many investigational agents are currently being studied in phase I and phase II trials.

Phase I Trials   These studies define the spectrum of toxicity of a new chemotherapeutic agent and are complete when the dose-limiting toxicity of any particular dose and schedule has been defined.

Phase II Trials   These studies generally use the dose established from phase I trials and apply this dose and schedule to selected tumor types of importance.

Phase III Trials   These studies compare one effective treatment with another in a randomized fashion.

References

1. **Silver RT, Young RC, Holland J:** Some new aspects of modern cancer chemotherapy. *Am J Med* 63:772, 1977.

2. **Young RC:** Principles of chemotherapy in gynecologic cancer. In Hoskins WJ, Perez CA, Young RC (eds): *Principles and Practices of Gynecologic Oncology.* Philadelphia, JB Lippincott, 1992, pp 333–349.

3. **Skipper HE, Schabel FM Jr, Mullett LB, et al:** Implications of biochemical, cytokinetic, pharmacologic, and toxicologic relationships in the design of optimal therapeutic schedules. *Cancer Chemother Rep* 54:431, 1950.

4. **Goldie JH, Coldman AJ:** A mathematical model for relating the drug sensitivity of tumors to their spontaneous mutation rate. *Cancer Treat Rep* 63:1727, 1979.

5. **Ling V:** Drug resistance and membrane mutants of mammalian cells. *Can J Genet Cytol* 17:503, 1975.

6. **Hryniuk W, Busch H:** The importance of dose intensity in chemotherapy of metastatic breast cancer. *J Clin Oncol* 2:1281, 1984.

7. **McGuire WP, Hoskins WJ, Brady MS, et al:** A phase III trial of dose intense versus standard dose cisplatin and cytoxan in advanced ovarian cancer. *Proc Int Soc Gynecol Oncol* 2:35, 1991.

8. **Kaye SB, Lewis CR, Paul J, et al:** Randomised study of two doses of cisplatin with cyclophosphamide in epithelial ovarian cancer. *Lancet* 340:329, 1992.

9. **Chabner BA (ed):** Clinical strategies for cancer treatment: the role of drugs. In Chabner BA, Collins JM (eds): *Cancer Chemotherapy: Principles and Practice.* Philadelphia, JB Lippincott, 1990, pp 1–16.

10. **Myers C:** The use of intraperitoneal chemotherapy in the treatment of ovarian cancer. *Semin Oncol* 11:275, 1984.

11. **Markman M:** Intraperitoneal chemotherapy. In Rubin SC, Sutton GP (eds): *Ovarian Cancer.* New York, McGraw-Hill, 1993, p 325.

12. **Haskell CM:** Principles and practice of cancer chemotherapy. In Haskell CM (ed): *Cancer Treatment*, ed 3. Philadelphia, WB Saunders, 1990, pp 21–44.

13. **Frei E III:** Combination cancer therapy. Presidential Address. *Cancer Res* 32:2593, 1972.

14. **Calvert AH, Newell DR, Gumbrell LA, et al:** Carboplatin dosage: prospective evaluation of a simple formula based on renal function. *J Clin Oncol* 7:1748, 1989.

15. **Calabresi P, Parks RE Jr:** Chemotherapy of neoplastic diseases. In Goodman LS, Gilman A (eds): *Goodman and Gilman's The Pharmacological Basis of Therapeutics*, ed 6. New York, Macmillan, 1980, p 1249.

16. **Kaufman D, Rosen N, Young RC:** Clinical consequences and management of antineoplastic agents. In Parrillo JE, Masur H (eds): *The Critically Ill Immunosuppressed Patient: Diagnosis and Management.* Rockville, Maryland, Aspen Press, 1986.

17. **Schilsky RL, Erlichman C:** Late complications of chemotherapy: infertility and carcinogenesis. In Chabner BA (ed): *Pharmacologic Principles of Cancer Treatment.* Philadelphia, WB Saunders, 1982, pp 109–131.

18. **Greene MH, Boice JD, Greer BE, et al:** Acute nonlymphocytic leukemia after therapy with alkylating agents for ovarian cancer. *N Engl J Med* 307:1416, 1982.

19. **Colvin M, Chabner BA:** Alkylating agents. In Chabner BA, Collins JM (eds): *Cancer Chemotherapy: Principles and Practice.* Philadelphia, JB Lippincott, 1990, pp 276–314.

20. **Chabner BA, Myer CE:** Clinical pharmacology of cancer chemotherapy. In DeVita VT, Hellman S, Rosenberg SA (eds): *Cancer: Principles and Practice of Oncology*, ed 3. Philadelphia, JB Lippincott, 1989, pp 349–396.

21. **Chabner BA (ed):** Cytadine analogues. In *Cancer Chemotherapy: Principles and Practice*. Philadelphia, JB Lippincott, 1990, pp 154–180.

22. **McCormick JJ, Johns DG:** Purine and purine nucleoside antimetabolites. In Chabner BA, Collins JM (eds): *Cancer Chemotherapy: Principles and Practice*. Philadelphia, JB Lippincott, 1990, pp 234–253.

23. **Bender RA, Hamel E, Hande KR:** Plant alkaloids. In Chabner BA, Collins JM (eds): *Cancer Chemotherapy: Principles and Practice*. Philadelphia, JB Lippincott, 1990, pp 253–276.

2 Radiation Therapy

Gillian M. Thomas

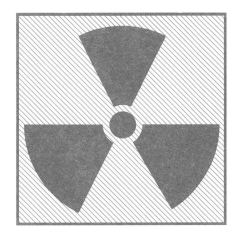

Radiation therapy plays a major role in the management of patients with gynecologic malignancies. Its specific curative role has been established for cervical cancer (1, 2); when surgery is not possible, radiation therapy also may be curative for localized endometrial cancer (3). For selected patients with ovarian cancer, postoperative adjuvant radiation therapy may be curative (4, 5). It improves pelvic control when used as adjuvant therapy after surgery for high-risk endometrial cancer (6) and has an expanding role in the management of carcinomas of the vagina and vulva (7, 8).

Recently, our understanding of the principles of radiation biology has improved. Although the clinical practice of radiation therapy has evolved empirically, new concepts of radiobiology, particularly the significance of radiation *dose fractionation schedules* (9) and the use of *combined modality therapy* (10), have allowed a better understanding of the usefulness of radiation therapy as a modality for the treatment of gynecologic cancer. The basic principles of radiation therapy, including physics and radiobiology, and the specific use of radiation therapy in gynecologic malignancies are presented.

Radiobiology

Ionizing Radiation

Cellular Effects

Cell death in the context of radiation biology is defined as the loss of clonogenic capacity (i.e., the ability of the cell to undergo continued reproduction). Ionizing radiation in sufficient dosage will produce cell death, which is the basis for its use in treating malignancies. The critical target for radiation injury for most cell types is DNA. Thus the damage caused by ionizing radiation is expressed when cells attempt to undergo mitosis. Ionizing radiation produces free radical formation, which disrupts the reproductive integrity of DNA and produces mitotic death. After DNA damage, the cell may undergo a limited number of mitoses, but cellular death ultimately ensues because the cell can no longer reproduce indefinitely. Although the cell may appear normal morphologically, it may have lost its reproductive capacity. Disruption of plasma membranes is the other form of cell damage that may result from ionizing radiation, and it is not linked to cell division.

The effect of ionizing radiation of any type is not selective for neoplastic cells, and this interaction with matter occurs in both the normal and neoplastic tissues in the path of the radiation beam. Interaction with the normal tissues and cells is responsible for both the acute and chronic complications associated with radiation therapy.

Rad and Gray

The rad has been the unit commonly used to measure the amount of energy absorbed per unit mass of tissue. The new standard nomenclature for measuring absorbed dose is the Gray (1 joule/kg); 1 Gray = 100 rad. Current practice uses the term *centigray* **(cGy), because 1 cGy = 1 rad.**

Cell Survival Curves

Typical survival curves for various single doses of radiation have been generated for established tumor and normal tissue cell lines grown both *in vitro* and *in vivo* in animal models (11) (Fig. 2.1). These curves show the number of cells surviving a particular dose of radiation therapy and are plotted on a semilogarithmic scale: the radiation dose is plotted on the linear scale and the surviving fraction of cells on a logarithmic scale. For sparsely ionizing radiation, such as beams of x-rays, gamma rays, electrons, and protons, the survival curve has two components:

1. The *shoulder* region

2. The straight-line or *exponential* region

For most mammalian cells, the width of the shoulder region (Dq) may be considered as a measure of the amount of wasted irradiation attributable to sublethal damage from radiation. The straight-line portion of the curve implies that *for any constant incremental increase in dosage, a constant proportion of the cells is killed*. Therefore, if 500 cGy kills 50% of the remaining viable cells, an additional 500 cGy will kill 50% of the cells surviving the previous dose.

The slope of the straight-line portion of the curve is a measure of the amount of radiation required to reduce the surviving number of clonogenic cells by a given percentage. This implies that the larger the number of clonogenic cells present, the higher the dose of radiation required to reduce the probability of clonogenic cells remaining.

Fractionation

Conventional radiation therapy usually is given in a fractionated course using daily doses of 180–200 cGy per fraction. The resultant survival curve after fractionated radiation therapy has a smaller gradient than that seen after a single dose. (Fig. 2.2).

Comparison of these curves reveals that a single dose of radiation (e.g., 600 cGy) will result in fewer surviving cells than the same total dose given in several smaller fractions (e.g., three fractions of 200 cGy each). This "sparing" effect

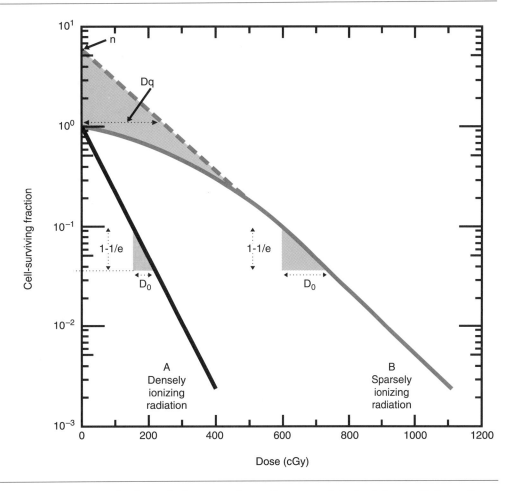

Figure 2.1   Typical survival curves for cells exposed to ionizing radiation. *Curve A* is for high LET radiation. The shoulder is absent or small. *Curve B* has two parts: an initial shoulder whose "width" is specified by the extrapolation number *n* or by the "quasithreshold dose" *Dq*, and the straight-line portion whose slope is $1/D_0$, e = natural logarithm. (Reproduced, with permission, from Hall EJ: *Radiobiology for the Radiologist,* ed 4. Philadelphia, Harper & Row, 1994.)

results from repetition of the shoulder region of the curve with each fraction of radiation. The shoulder region has been interpreted to represent the presence of *repair of sublethal damage* in an irradiated cell population (12).

Two biologic models have been used to explain the implication that radiation does not totally destroy the clonogenic capacity of all cells (11):

1. The multitarget single-hit model

2. The single-target multihit model

In the first model, the cell has a number of sensitive target structures, each requiring activation by single ionizing events. In the second model, there is a single target that requires multiple ionizing hits before the cell loses its clonogenic capacity. Biologically, this shoulder region is important because repair of normal tissue damage between fractions can occur with fractionated radiation. Where the fraction size is considerably smaller than the conventional 180 or 200 cGy frac-

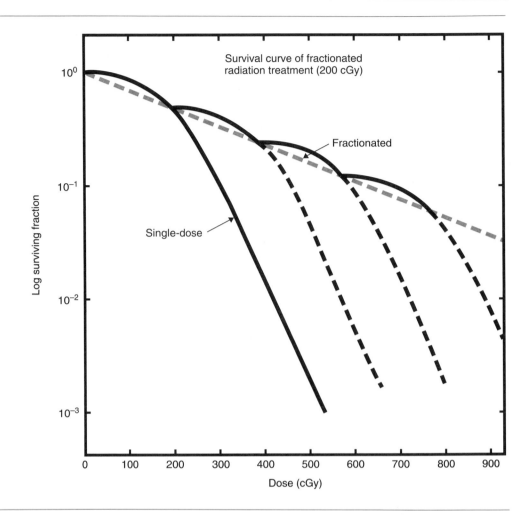

Figure 2.2   Idealized survival curve for fractionated radiation therapy. The time interval between fractions is sufficient to allow repair of sublethal damage, and the shoulder is repeated with each fraction. The resultant slope of the survival curve with *fractionated* radiation is more shallow than that of the *single dose*. Reduction of the surviving fraction to 10^{-1} requires 350 cGy in a single fraction or 600 cGy in three fractions.

tions, the resultant surviving fraction remains on the early part of the shoulder, and the resultant slope of several small fractions will be less than that of the same total dose given in larger fractions.

Radiosensitivity

Many factors can modify the biologic effect of ionizing radiation on the cellular radiosensitivity. Therefore the amount of cell kill produced by a given dose of radiation may vary, depending on the following factors:

1. The "four R's of radiobiology," which are (*a*) repair, (*b*) reoxygenation, (*c*) repopulation, and (*d*) redistribution

2. The quality of radiation

3. The temperature of the tissues

4. The presence of various drugs

The same biologic effect on tumor can be achieved by different doses of radiation with the use of different fractionation schedules. A typical "isoeffect" curve (11) is shown in Figure 2.3.

For example, 90% of squamous cell cancers of the skin measuring 2 cm or less in diameter will be controlled with 2800 cGy in one fraction or 4100 cGy in ten fractions. The magnitude of the dose required to produce a given level of biologic damage depends on the manner in which the radiation is fractionated. The explanation for this isoeffect phenomenon is related to *the four R's of radiobiology.*

Repair

With increased shoulder width, the slope of the isoeffect curve will increase, i.e., the wider the shoulder, the more repair of sublethal damage will occur (12). Thus a higher total dose of radiation will be required to produce the same effect

Figure 2.3   Isoeffect curves relating the total radiation dose to the overall treatment time for normal tissue end points (erythema, desquamation, necrosis) and 90% cure of skin cancer. (Redrawn from Strandquvist M: *Acta Radiol* [Suppl] 55:1, 1944.)

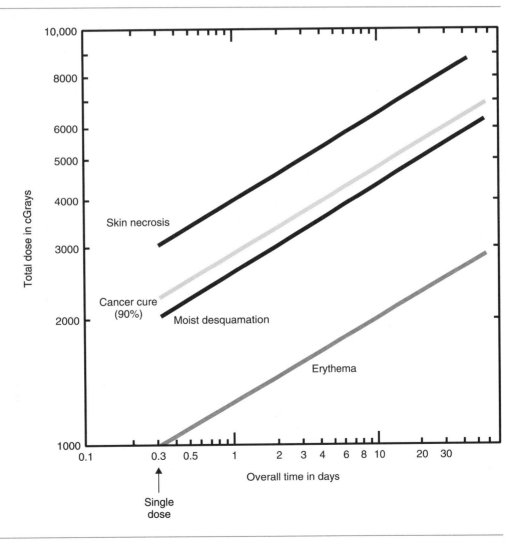

if more fractions are given. A higher total dose also will be required when the shoulder is wider.

Repopulation

The magnitude of the effect of repopulation on the dose required to produce a given level of cell kill depends on the doubling time of the cells involved. The phenomenon of cellular repopulation causes an increase in the slope of the isoeffect curve. For cells with a long doubling time relative to the time required to give a fractionated course of radiation, little repopulation will occur during a course of radiation treatment. If doubling times are relatively short, however, a higher dose will be required to achieve the same level of cell kill. The phenomenon of repopulation may be an important practical consideration in the application of fractionated radiation therapy in gynecologic malignancies. Because it is believed that radiation therapy may produce accelerated tumor doubling times, the introduction of a rest period may protract the time over which a radiation course is given, and this may allow some tumor repopulation, which could be detrimental to the outcome (13).

Redistribution

Studies in synchronized cell populations have shown significant differences in the radiosensitivity of the same cell type throughout the cellular division cycle (14). In most cells, the late G^2 and mitotic phases are the most sensitive and the late S and early G^1 phases the most resistant. Delivering radiation in a fractionated schedule increases the chance that a given cell will be in a sensitive phase of the division cycle at some time during radiation therapy. This is especially true if the cell population has a moderately rapid turnover time. Cellular redistribution may lead to a decrease in the slope of the isoeffect curve. This applies both to normal tissues with a rapid turnover time (such as the gut mucosa) and to tumors.

Reoxygenation

The phenomenon of reoxygenation results in a decrease in the slope of the isoeffect curve as a result of the oxygen effect (15). Radiosensitivity correlates with the presence of oxygen, because oxygen appears to inhibit repair of radiation injury to DNA. Survival curves for cultured mammalian cells exposed to x-rays under oxygenated and hypoxic conditions reveal similar shapes, but the magnitude of the dose required to produce a given degree of cell damage is modified by the presence of oxygen (Fig. 2.4).

Oxygen Enhancement Ratio (OER) **The dose of radiation required under hypoxic conditions is approximately three times greater than the dose required under fully oxygenated conditions. The ratio of these doses is referred to as the oxygen enhancement ratio (OER).** Most of the changes in radiosensitivity occur as the oxygen concentration increases from 0 to 30 mm Hg, well below the PO_2 of venous blood. Nevertheless, clinically significant hypoxia does exist in human solid tumors, and the hypoxic cells are relatively radioresistant when compared with fully oxygenated ones. During a fractionated course of radiation therapy, relatively hypoxic cells may become more oxygenated and therefore more sensitive to the effects of ionizing radiation; thus fractionation may allow reoxygenation and therefore increased tumor destruction (15).

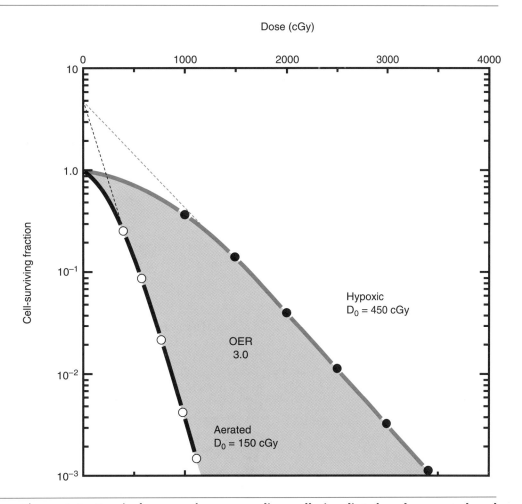

Figure 2.4   Survival curves for mammalian cells irradiated under aerated and hypoxic conditions. Oxygen is dose modifying. The dose required to produce a given level of damage is three times greater under *hypoxic* than under aerated conditions. The ratio of doses is the oxygen enhancement ratio (*OER*). Sometimes the shoulder also is reduced under hypoxic conditions. (Reproduced, with permission, from Hall EJ: *Radiobiology for the Radiologist,* ed 2. Philadelphia, Harper & Row, 1978.)

Treatment Strategies   Because of the importance of the oxygen effect, many treatment strategies have been used to try to overcome the relative radioresistance of hypoxic cells in solid human tumors (16–19). These include:

1. Modifications of fractionation schedules

2. Carbogen breathing during radiation therapy

3. Selective vasoconstriction of normal tissues by tourniquet application

4. Various pharmacologic agents (e.g., misonidasole) that can act as hypoxic cell radiation sensitizers

5. Use of hyperbaric oxygen

6. Use of high linear energy transfer (LET) radiation

Tumor hypoxia continues to be one probable cause of the failure of radiation to control some tumors (e.g., advanced cervical cancers with a significant population of hypoxic tumor cells) (20).

Quality of Radiation

Whereas photons and high-energy electrons produce sparsely ionizing radiation, larger atomic particles (e.g., neutrons) produce more densely ionizing radiation.

Linear Energy Transfer The term *linear energy transfer* (LET) is used to describe the rate of deposition of energy along the path of the beam (19). For densely ionizing radiation, the LET will be higher than for sparsely ionizing radiation. Thus equal doses of different types of ionizing radiation do not produce equal biologic effects.

Relative Biologic Effectiveness To compare the biologic effects of different radiation beams, the term *relative biologic effectiveness* (RBE) is used. The RBE is defined as the ratio of the dose of some test radiation compared with the dose

Figure 2.5 Survival curves for cells of human origin exposed to irradiation of *increasing LET.* As the LET increases, the size of the shoulder decreases and the terminal slope increases. The dose of radiation required to produce the same level of cell kill decreases with increasing LET. (Reproduced with permission from Hall EJ: *Radiobiology for the Radiologist*, ed 2. Philadelphia, Harper & Row, 1978.)

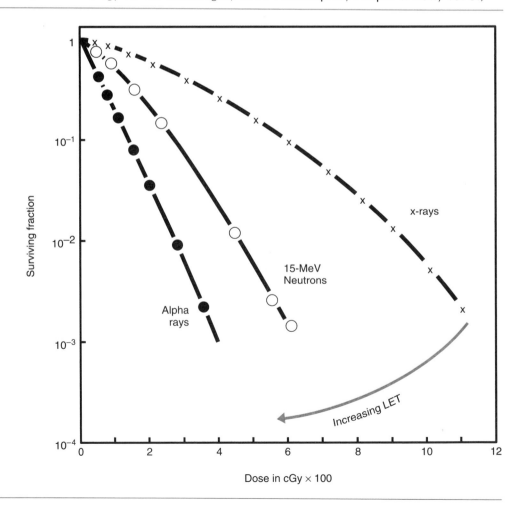

of 250 kiloelectron volt (kV) x-rays required to produce an equal biologic effect (Fig. 2.5). High LET radiation is associated with an increasing RBE and a decreasing OER (21).

High LET radiation is potentially useful in therapy because

1. It reduces or abolishes the shoulder on the cell survival curve, thus reducing tumor repair.

2. It increases the terminal slope of the curve, thus increasing cell kill.

3. It diminishes the significance of the oxygen effect.

In practice, few facilities exist for the production of high LET beams, and their use has had no major impact on the results of treatment for gynecologic malignancies.

Hyperthermia

Hyperthermia is another factor that modifies the effect of ionizing radiation (22). Heat itself may be cytotoxic because it is preferentially toxic to cells at low pH (which may correspond to areas of hypoxia) and to cells in the relatively resistant S phase of the division cycle. Hyperthermia in the range of 42–43°C sensitizes cells to radiation both by reducing the shoulder and by increasing the slope of the survival curve. Preferential heating may occur in tumors compared with the surrounding normal tissues. Thus hyperthermia may offer a therapeutic advantage in combination with radiation therapy. The technology necessary to produce the deep-seated heating for this biologic effect is not presently available.

Radiation Effects and Drugs

Some drugs can modify the response to radiation. This may result from the independent cytotoxicity of the two modalities or from the direct interaction between the drug and the radiation (22). Four terms are used to describe the types of possible interactions:

Independent Action   Drugs and radiation may act independently when their mechanisms of action are different, so that the total effect of the combination is equal to that of each agent separately.

Additivity   The agents may act at the same site in the cell; therefore, sublethal damage inflicted by each agent interacts to cause greater cell kill than with either agent alone.

Synergism (Superadditivity)   The interaction between the two agents results in greater cell kill than that seen with additivity. An example is the interaction of actinomycin-D and radiation.

Antagonism (Subadditivity)   The cell kill that results from the use of the two agents is less than that expected by independent action.

Clinically, it is difficult to determine which mode of interaction occurs when two agents are used. When an increased reaction is observed, the term *synergism* often is used, but the mechanism of interaction may be simply independent action or additivity.

43

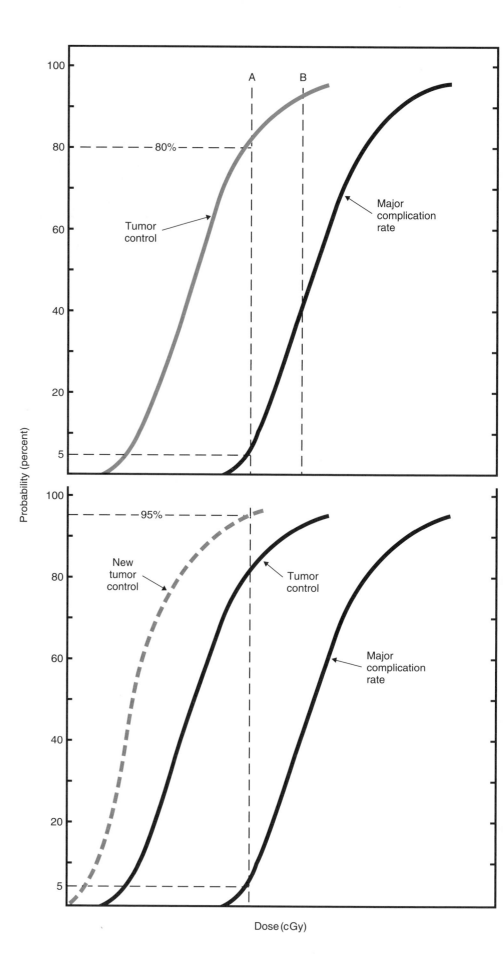

The addition of a cytotoxic drug to radiation may be useful if the dose-limiting tissue toxicity of the drug is different from that of radiation therapy; i.e., it may provide an improvement in the therapeutic index. The addition of the two agents can separate the dose-response curves for cure and toxicity. The drug may be independently cytotoxic or act additively to increase tumor cell kill without increasing the toxicity to normal tissues that would require reduction in the radiation dose. Clinical trials are being conducted with a combination of radiation and cytotoxic drugs, e.g., 5-fluorouracil (5-FU) and cisplatin, in advanced carcinomas of the cervix and vulva (10).

Therapeutic Ratio

All cells in the path of radiation, including those of the normal tissues, suffer radiation injury. If the dose of radiation given is plotted against the likelihood of cure for a given tumor, a sigmoid curve is generated (Fig. 2.6).

At low radiation doses, there is insufficient cell kill to produce tumor cure, but as the dose is increased, the likelihood of cure rises rapidly and plateaus. The shape and steepness of the dose-response curve vary for different tumors (23, 24). A similar sigmoid relationship is seen when the likelihood of complications is plotted against the dose of radiation. A simultaneous plot of the dose-control curve for the tumor and the dose-complication curve for the normal tissues allows an examination of the therapuetic ratio. This term indicates that, for a given dose of radiation, there is an expected rate of tumor control and an expected complication rate. In the optimistic situation, the complication curve is placed to the right of the cure curve, and the difference between these curves is a measure of the therapeutic gain of a given dose of radiation. Radiation research efforts are concerned with attempts to improve the therapeutic ratio by separating these curves.

The extent of radiation damage to normal tissues depends on the rate of division of the irradiated cells (25). Tissues that are turning over rapidly (i.e., whose functional activity requires constant cell renewal) manifest radiation injury acutely soon after exposure. Examples of *acutely reacting* tissues include most epithelia (e.g., the skin, the gastrointestinal mucosa, bone marrow, and reproductive tissues). In contrast, tissues whose cells are characterized by low cellular turnover rates and whose functional activity does not require rapid cell renewal do not manifest any early radiation injury. Examples of *late-reacting* tissues are the connective tissues, muscle, and neural tissues.

Acute Reactions

With pelvic irradiation, acute reactions, such as diarrhea, are usually associated with denudation of the intestinal mucosa, which in turn causes an increased regenerative response (26). The regenerative response usually can keep pace with weekly doses of 900–1000 cGy in five fractions. This empirically derived weekly dose continues to be in common use because it produces acceptable acute com-

Figure 2.6   Theoretical sigmoid dose-response curves for tumor control and severe complications. The farther apart the two curves are, the higher the therapeutic ratio. *Top:* Dose *A* produces cure in 80% with 5% complications. Dose *B* falls on the steep part of the complication curve and produces a much higher rise in the complication rate than in the cure rate. *Bottom:* This shows a shift to the left in the dose-cure curve (e.g., by the addition of sensitizing drugs). Dose *A* produces 95% cure with 5% complications.

45

plications. If an increased dose is given over shorter periods, the regenerative capacity of the epithelium may be overwhelmed (27), and the acute reaction so severe that it may be necessary to introduce a *split-treatment course* to enable the epithelial regeneration to catch up before therapy is resumed. The severity of the acute reactions also depends on the *volume* of the normal tissues irradiated and the specific *nature* of the tissues.

Late Reactions

The pathogenesis of late-developing reactions (i.e., those that occur months to years after radiation therapy is completed) differs from that of the acute reactions (25, 28). One hypothesis to explain the late effects of radiation is that there is damage to the vascular connective tissue stroma that causes an epithelial proliferation with decreased blood supply and subsequent fibrosis. Another hypothesis is that some stem cells have a limited proliferative capacity, and extensive destruction of these cells may result in eventual tissue loss (26). Because these late-reacting tissues are not proliferating rapidly, the duration of a course of radiation treatment does not alter the late tolerance to radiation therapy. However, there is ample evidence to suggest that the sensitivity of these late-reacting tissues is markedly dependent on the size of the dose per fraction of radiation used.

The larger the dose per fraction used, the greater the risk of late complications. Thus if a few fractions of large size are used rather than a greater number of smaller fractions, there is an increased risk of overdosage for the late-reacting tissues if the doses are adjusted to equalize the acute reactions. The effect of fraction size on the development of acute and late reactions has been summarized by Peters (9, 29) (Fig. 2.7).

If the overall treatment time is held constant and the dose per fraction is increased, there will be a relatively greater effect on the isoeffect doses for the late-reacting tissues than for the acutely reacting tissues. If the overall time of treatment is varied while the number of fractions is held constant, the effect is different. If treatment time is extended, the acute reactions may be preferentially spared because of the regenerative capacity of the acutely reacting tissues. Therefore, a total dose of radiation that produces an equal effect on the acutely reacting tissues may lead to excessive late effects. Thus radiation schemes that produce similar acute reactions but use larger than normal doses per fraction or protracted treatment times may produce excessive late normal tissue reactions.

Figure 2.7 *Top:* **The effect of changing the number (and size) of dose fractions when overall treatment time is constant.** The curves are isoeffect curves for a given level of reaction compared with a point designated *conventional fractionation* (1.8 to 2.0 Gy, five fractions weekly). The size of the dose per fraction has a greater effect on the late reactions than on acute reactions. If the total dose is adjusted to produce the same level of acute reaction, *hypofractionation* (larger dose per fraction) results in increased late effects. *Hyperfractionation* may spare late effects. *Bottom:* **The effect of changing the overall treatment time using the same number of fractions.** The influence on late effects is small. If the total time is protracted, the total dose that can be delivered will be higher to produce the same level of acute reactions, but this may produce increased late effects. (Reproduced with permission from Peters LJ: Biology of radiation therapy. In Thawley S, Panje W (eds): *Comprehensive Management of Head and Neck Tumours.* Philadelphia, WB Saunders, 1985.)

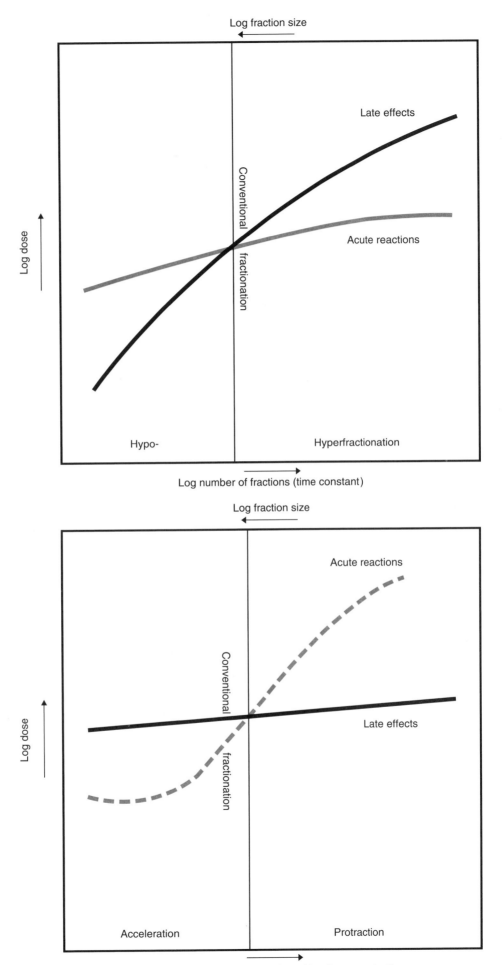

Two possible nonconventional fractionation schedules—hyperfractionation and accelerated fractionation—offer theoretic improvements in the therapeutic ratio for tumor control versus late normal injury (16, 30).

Hyperfractionation

The term *hyperfractionation* refers to an altered fractionation scheme where (31):

1. The size of the dose per fraction is reduced.

2. The number of dosage fractions is increased.

3. The total dose is increased.

4. The overall time is relatively unchanged.

With hyperfractionation, treatment usually is given two or more times daily with at least 4–6 hours between fractions to allow repair. The rationale behind anticipating an improvement in the therapeutic ratio with hyperfractionation is that an increase in the total dose may be given without exceeding the tolerance of the late-reacting normal tissues. The increased dose can be given because a smaller dose per fraction is used, which allows preferential sparing of the late-reacting normal tissues. With an increase in the number of fractions, redistribution of cells into the sensitive phases of the cell cycle may occur and therefore produce increased cell kill. With lower doses per fraction, there may be a lower OER. Because hyperfractionation does not use an increase in the overall time of treatment, there should be no increased repopulation compared with a conventional fractionation scheme.

Accelerated Fractionation

In an accelerated fractionation scheme, the overall time of treatment is shortened, whereas the number of dose fractions is unchanged (16). Treatment is given two or more times daily, using fraction sizes that are unchanged or only slightly reduced and a total dose that is unchanged or slightly reduced. The result of accelerated fractionation is the delivery of the same dose of radiation in a shorter overall time. The theoretic benefits of an accelerated fractionation scheme are that a decrease in the overall time reduces the chance of tumor cell repopulation during treatment, and this may increase the likelihood of tumor control for a given total dose. Shortening treatment time should not influence the likelihood of late normal tissue damage if the size of the dose per fraction is not increased. However, the shortened time means that the reaction of the acutely reacting normal tissues may be worsened; as a result, the total dose may have to be reduced or introduction of a split-treatment regimen may be necessary. Both of these changes could be detrimental to tumor control.

Combination of Surgery and Radiation

There are theoretic reasons why the combination of surgery and radiation therapy may provide better tumor control. The two modalities may be complementary in some situations, because the mechanisms of failure for the two techniques are different. Surgery may remove gross tumor masses, but the extent of surgical dissection may be limited. Even when all gross tumor is resected, tumor regrowth may occur because of residual microscopic tumor in the periphery of the lesion. Radiation therapy, on the other hand, is more likely to control effectively microscopic disease at the periphery of tumors, where the cell numbers are small

Table 2.1   Preoperative and Postoperative Radiation

Advantages	Disadvantages
Preoperative 1. Surgically undisturbed tumor bed: intact vascularity (good oxygenation) 2. May facilitate surgical dissection, allowing a lesser procedure 3. May decrease the risk of implantation or dissemination of viable tumor cells by surgery, e.g., tumor marginally resectable or cut-through	1. Precludes accurate pretreatment staging 2. May be given unnecessarily to patients with limited disease with high likelihood of cure with surgery alone 3. Delays wound healing
Postoperative 1. Extent of locoregional disease accurately defined 2. Radiation therapy may be used more selectively or omitted in some patients	1. Surgery may change tumor proliferation kinetics 2. Surgery may disturb vascularity and increase risk of hypoxia

and the vascularity is good (2). When radiation fails, it is often because of the inability to control bulky central tumor masses in which the number of clonogenic cells and the probability of hypoxia are high. The choice of sequence of radiation and surgery depends on the specific tumor and the clinical situation. The potential advantages and disadvantages of preoperative and postoperative irradiation are presented in Table 2.1.

When surgery and radiation are combined, the initial plan of treatment must exploit the complementary features of the two modalities. Some examples of the usefulness of planned combined surgery and radiation in gynecologic malignancies are:

1. *Vulvar Cancer*—The addition of postoperative pelvic and groin irradiation provides a survival advantage to patients with multiple positive inguinal nodes over that achieved with pelvic node dissection (7).

2. *Endometrial Cancer*—Postoperative pelvic irradiation reduces the incidence of pelvic recurrence in patients with high-risk stage I disease, presumably by sterilizing microscopic residual tumor cells in the pelvis and pelvic lymph nodes (6, 32).

3. *Cervical Cancer*—In patients with "bulky" or "barrel-shaped" stage Ib disease, hysterectomy may be required to remove residual central disease that has not been sterilized by the radiation therapy (2).

Radiation Techniques

Radiation therapy is delivered in three ways:

1. *Teletherapy,* (i.e., external beam)

2. *Brachytherapy,* in which the radiation device is placed either within or close to the target volume (i.e., interstitial and intracavitary irradiation)

3. *Intracavitary radioisotopes*

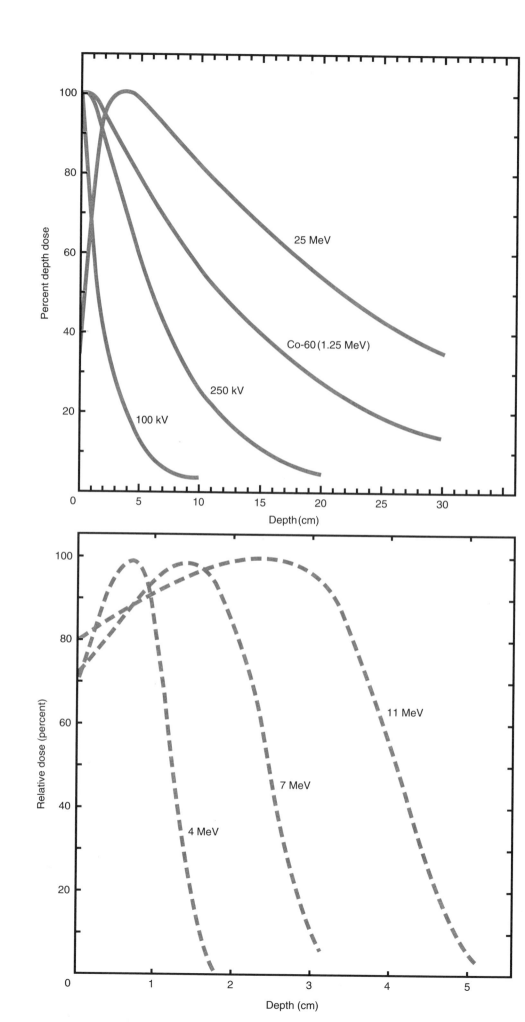

Teletherapy

Many factors influence the deposition of external radiation into deep tissues (33). The beam energy is defined by its voltage; the higher the beam energy, the more deeply it penetrates into tissues. In modern radiation therapy, external beam treatment is largely given with megavoltage or supervoltage equipment.

Photons

A photon is a quantum of high-energy electromagnetic radiation that travels at the speed of light, and its interaction with tissues causes ionization. Photons may be x-rays or gamma rays: x-rays are produced by bombardment of an anode by a high-speed electron beam; gamma rays result from the decay of radioactive isotopes. The average energy of the photons produced by the decay of radioactive cobalt is 1.2 million electron volts (MeV). Higher-energy x-ray beams in the 2–35 MeV range are produced mainly from linear accelerators. High-energy electron beams also can be generated from linear accelerators. Comparative isodose distributions for typical beams of varying energies are presented in Figure 2.8.

Ideally designed, external radiation therapy will maximize the dose of radiation delivered to the target while minimizing the dose delivered outside the target. It will also produce a relatively homogeneous dose within the volume of interest. This is important because wide variation of dose within the volume (> 5–10%) can result in either low-dose areas that could lead to tumor recurrence or high-dose areas that increase the risk of complications. For irradiation of tumor volumes in this homogeneous fashion, multiple external fields are usually required. The use of multiple beams may tend to decrease the dose to the normal tissues in transit toward the tumor. The isodose distributions for two opposing parallel portals and a four-field technique used for the treatment of cervical cancer are presented in Figure 2.9.

The radiation beam may be modified to conform better to a specific tumor while protecting normal tissues by shielding or blocking part of the beam. Sometimes, particularly with angulated beams, it is desirable to have a beam that is more intense on one side than on the other, and this can be achieved with the positioning of wedges of metal within the beam (33). These wedges absorb the beam differentially, depending on their thickness, and will produce angled isodose curves. Specific anatomic volumes may be treated with protection of the surrounding vital structures by means of individually fashioned blocks that are made to conform to the patient's tumor.

Figure 2.8 *Top:* **Depth-dose curves for x-ray and γ-ray beams of increasing energy.** As the energy increases, the depth of maximum dose (100%) increases; thus, for 100 keV and 250 keV, it is at the skin surface. With ⁶⁰Co and 25 MeV, it moves below the surface, minimizing the skin reactions; as the energy increases, the beam penetrates more deeply. At a depth of 10 cm from the surface, the depth dose is approximately 25% for 250 kV, 60% for ⁶⁰Co, and 80% for 25 MeV. Thus, deep pelvic tumors are treated more appropriately with higher-energy beams. *Bottom:* **Depth-dose curves for various electron energies.** The depth of maximum dose increases with increasing energy. At depths just beyond the maximum, the dose falls off rapidly and therefore may spare deeper underlying tissues. An approximate way to choose optimal electron energy is to determine the depth of the tumor from the surface and use an electron energy of three times the depth (e.g., with a tumor at 2 cm, choose electron energy of 6 to 7 MeV).

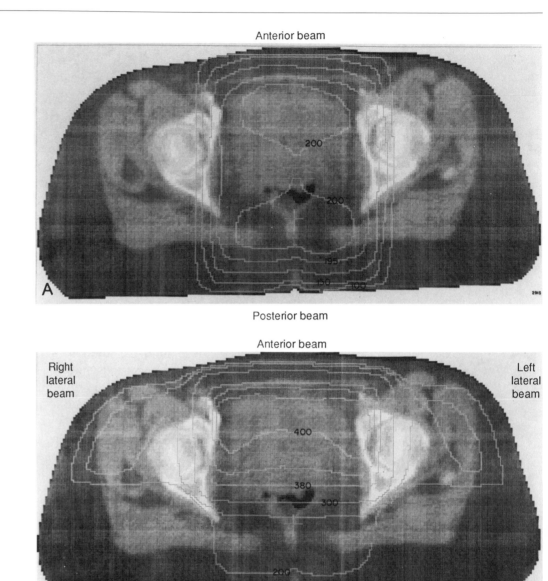

Figure 2.9   Isodose distribution for external radiation using 25 MeV. *A,* parallel pair (anterior-posterior) fields; *B,* box field arrangement superimposed on a CT scan showing a large cervical cancer. The parallel pair essentially treats the bladder and rectum to full tumor dose. The positioning and size of the lateral beams in the box technique determine where the high-dose volume is located. In this arrangement, the dose to the rectum (*dark shadow*) is significantly reduced. The isodose distribution may be tailored to almost any desired by varying the beam angles, numbers, energies, and arrangements.

Electrons

In addition to x-ray and photon beams for external radiation therapy, electron beams are available. These usually are generated from betatrons or high-energy accelerators, and the depth dose characteristics differ substantially from those of photon or x-ray beams. Electron beams may have much less skin sparing. The maximum dose is reached at a depth that depends on the energy of the beam, and then there is a rapid falloff.

Electron beams are most useful in the treatment of superficially placed tumors where it is desirable to spare the deeper tissues, (e.g., irradiation of the inguinal nodes in vulvar cancer). The choice of beam energy is tailored to the estimated depth of the nodes. Considerably more sparing of the underlying femoral heads may be achieved while an adequate dose is delivered to a superficially placed tumor.

Brachytherapy

Intracavitary

The intrauterine and intravaginal *intracavitary* devices used in the treatment of cervical and endometrial cancer are examples of brachytherapy used for gynecologic malignancies. These devices vary in their appearance and configuration, but their general construction is similar despite the great number and variety of applicators used. They usually consist of a hollow stem, such as the classic intrauterine tandem, which often carries the name of the designer of the applicator (e.g., Fletcher-Delclos and Fletcher-Suit) (2) (Fig. 2.10).

These intrauterine tandems may be placed within the uterine cavity, and the hollow center may be afterloaded with radioactive sources such as radium or cesium. Similarly, various afterloading applicators (e.g., vaginal ovoids or colpostats) have been designed for placement in the vaginal vault. Other applicators that

Figure 2.10   Intrauterine stem and vaginal colpostats used for intracavitary irradiation in cervical cancer.

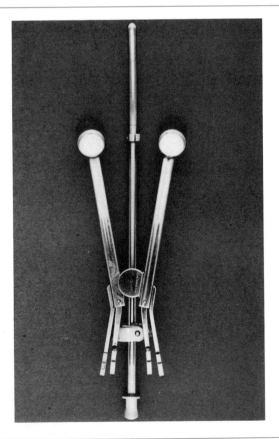

hold line sources of radioactivity may be used to treat varying lengths of the vagina.

To minimize the exposure of personnel to radiation, most applicators used currently are *afterloaded* with radioactive sources once their positioning has been proven satisfactory by x-ray. The more recent use of *remote afterloading devices* (e.g., the Selectron) can further protect personnel from radiation. With these remote afterloading devices, radioactive sources are stored in a lead-lined safe in the patient's room and connected to the intrauterine or intravaginal devices by hollow tubes. The sources then may be remotely afterloaded after the personnel caring for the patient have left the room. Although these devices do offer further protection of personnel, they may prolong the intracavitary radiation treatment time because of the intermittent automatic removal of sources.

Inverse Square Law

The inverse square law states that the dose of radiation at a given point is inversely proportional to the square of the distance from the source of ra-

Figure 2.11 **Treatment plan for cervical carcinoma showing a radiograph of the intracavitary irradiation** in situ **with its isodose distribution in cGy per hour.** The stem is loaded with ^{137}Cs sources of radium equivalent strengths of 15 mg, 10 mg, and 10 mg from proximal to distal. Each of the colpostats contains 15 mg radium equivalent sources. The dose to point A is 50 cGy per hour. The duration of the application is determined by the dose required. The usual external beam edges are superimposed on the x-ray and include the pelvic nodes as visualized on lymphography.

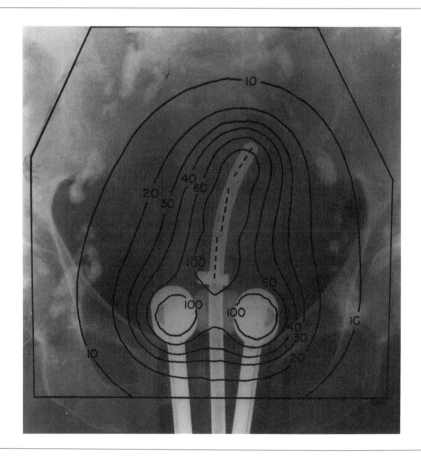

diation (33). Therefore, with brachytherapy, the dose at a distance from the source is determined largely by the inverse square law.

A typical isodose distribution around a line source and colpostats loaded with radioactive *cesium-137* used for the treatment of cervical cancer is shown in Figure 2.11. The dose decreases rapidly as the distance from the applicator increases. Because of this rapid change of dose over short distances, accurate positioning of intracavitary sources is very important. The advantage of intracavitary therapy is that a very high dose of radiation can be achieved in a very small volume. Thus, in the treatment of cervical cancer, high doses of radiation can be delivered centrally within the tumor and also within the adjacent paracervical tissues. However, the rapid falloff of dose means that many of the sensitive normal tissues within the pelvis, particularly the rectum and bladder, may be spared an excessive radiation dose.

Dose Rate of Intracavitary Irradiation

Conventionally, intracavitary brachytherapy has been delivered with the use of *low-dose-rate (LDR) irradiation* with rates ranging from about 0.4 to 1.2 Gy per hour. Low-dose-rate therapy necessitates relatively lengthy intracavitary insertions, often totaling 2 or 3 days, with considerable inconvenience and discomfort for the patient. LDR schedules differentially spare late-responding tissues compared with early-responding normal tissues and tumor cells.

High-dose-rate (HDR) brachytherapy for cervical cancer was first used about 25 years ago. It offers practical advantages for the patient, because treatment is typically done on an outpatient basis, and it is also less expensive. HDR equipment has become more available in the past 5 years, but many centers have been reluctant to change to HDR therapy because of the lack of randomized controlled clinical trials designed to compare high- and low-dose-rate regimens. It is important that dose fractionation schemes used for HDR equipment give efficacy and morbidity approximately equivalent to those of LDR equipment. Because of the nature of the dose-response curves for late effects, it would be expected that dosages using HDR equipment that provide equivalent early effects (including tumor control) might result in an increased incidence of late complications. However, for the special case of brachytherapy of the cervix, the tissues responsible for late effects (primarily the rectum and bladder) are at some distance from the tumor site and thus receive a dose that is significantly lower than the prescribed tumor dose. Therefore, if the HDR intracavitary dose is calculated to yield equivalent early effects (tumor control), the rectum and bladder receive relatively less than the prescribed tumor dose and the late effects may be comparable or less at HDR than LDR. In a retrospective analysis of more than 17,000 cervical cancer patients treated with high-dose-rate remote afterloading equipment in 56 institutions, 5-year survival rates were comparable and late effects appeared to be no worse than those observed in LDR regimens, provided the corresponding doses were matched to produce equal early effects (34). *Fractionation* of HDR treatment significantly influenced morbidity. Moderate and severe toxicity was significantly lower if the dose per fraction at Point A was ≤ 7 Gy. The most commonly used fractionation regimen is now five fractions of 7 Gy each to Point A.

On average, most centers have reduced the total dose by a factor of 0.54 ± 0.06 to convert from LDR to HDR regimens. It is not known what constitutes the optimal dose per fraction, although increasing the number of fractions and concomitantly decreasing the dose per fraction significantly reduces the rate of moderate and severe complications. The effect on survival is equivocal. Without randomized trials to compare the efficacy of HDR and LDR regimens, it is difficult to know how best to integrate HDR intracavitary radiation into clinical trials that examine other primary questions regarding therapy for carcinoma of the cervix.

Before the development of supervoltage radiation equipment, most patients with cervical cancer were treated with brachytherapy. As supervoltage equipment became available, "deep" tumors could be treated more readily with external beams while sparing the skin from excessive acute reactions. In some centers in the late 1950s, intracavitary radiation was abandoned in favor of external beam therapy, but it became obvious that brachytherapy was vital for the central control of tumors.

Interstitial Implants

Interstitial sources are another form of brachytherapy. The term *interstitial* implies the placement of radioactive sources within tissues. Various sources of radiation, such as *iridium-192*, *iodine-125*, and *tantalum-182*, may be available as radioactive wires or seeds. Hollow guide needles are placed in a specified geometric pattern that will deliver a known, relatively uniform dose of radiation to a target volume. The position of these guides is checked radiologically and, when sat-

Figure 2.12 Interstitial implant for an advanced cervical cancer. (Reproduced with permission from Dr. Mark Schray, Division of Radiation Oncology, Mayo Clinic.)

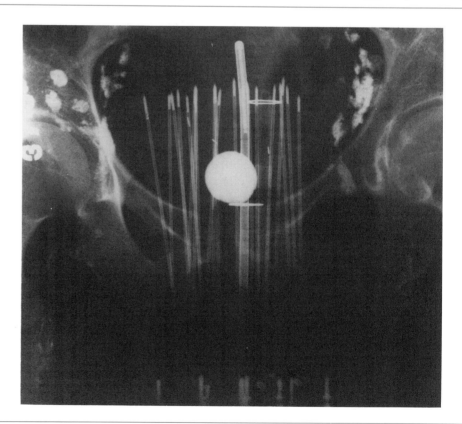

isfactory, they can be threaded with the radioactive sources that are left in the tissues; the hollow guides then are removed.

The interstitial therapy used in gynecologic malignancies usually involves a temporary implant. The implant will be left in the tissues for a period determined by the strength of the sources and the radiation dose required. Interstitial therapy has the advantage of delivering a relatively high dose of radiation to a relatively small volume (the tumor) and therefore offers a theoretic advantage over external beam therapy. The disadvantage is the greater potential damage to normal tissues in or near the tumor, especially if there is difficulty in accurately placing the needles. This may cause an increased incidence of severe late complications. Interstitial implants to the parametrial areas have been used with some success in the treatment of advanced or recurrent carcinoma of the cervix (34) (Fig. 2.12).

The use of interstitial implants is increasing, particularly for patients with advanced pelvic malignancy. With greater clinical experience and refinements of templates for transperineal applications, there has been an apparent decrease in serious morbidity (35). The radiation oncology community remains polarized as to the appropriateness of interstitial therapy, and as yet no randomized trials have been conducted to compare the therapeutic ratio of conventional intracavitary irradiation with interstitial parametrial treatment.

Perineal templates theoretically allow greater control of placement of the sources relative to the tumor volume and normal structures. Computerized optimization of source placement and strengths during the planning phase should improve the therapeutic ratio (Fig. 2.12).

Recurrences after conventional radical therapy cannot be retreated to a satisfactory dose with external beam radiation because of the limited tolerance of the surrounding normal tissues. Limited parametrial implants have been used and have produced tumor control in some patients and occasional cures of recurrent disease (2), but vesicovaginal and rectovaginal fistula rates may be excessive. Interstitial implants also may be used to treat selected vaginal or vulvar malignancies, either primarily or secondarily. The choice of interstitial radiation in combination with external beam radiation may be made to achieve a high tumor dose while sparing the surrounding normal tissues from unnecessary irradiation.

Intracavitary Radioisotopes

Radioisotopes have been used to treat epithelial ovarian cancer because of the pattern of dissemination throughout the peritoneal cavity (36). On theoretic grounds, if the tumor remains confined to this body cavity, the even distribution of a radioisotope in the peritoneum could irradiate all structures within the cavity. The pattern of energy deposition and the depth of penetration from the surface that the isotope contacts depend on many factors, including the physical characteristics of the particular isotope used, the energies of the decay products, and the distribution of the isotope within the peritoneal cavity.

Radioactive *chromic phosphate* (^{32}P) has largely replaced *colloidal gold* (^{198}Au) for intracavitary irradiation. Its longer half-life (14.3 days) and its pure β decay with a mean energy of 0.698 MeV allow deeper penetration into tissues (8 mm compared with 3.8 mm for ^{198}Au), a slightly longer exposure, and fewer radiation

Isotope		Half-Life	γ-Ray Energy (MeV)	β-Ray Average Energy at 1 cm	γ-Factor* R/mc/hr
Phosphorus	³²P	14.3 days		0.698	
Technesium	⁹⁹Tc	6.0 hours	0.14	0.014	0.56
Iodine	¹³¹I	8.07 days	Many 0.08–0.72	0.188	2.24
Cesium	¹³⁷Cs	30 years	0.662	0.242	3.2
Iridium	¹⁹²Ir	74 days	Several 0.32–0.61		5.0
Gold	¹⁹⁸Au	2.7 days	Several 0.41–1.1	0.328	2.43
Radium	²²⁶Ra	1620 years	Several 0.19–0.6		8.25

Table 2.2 Isotopes

*γ(gamma) factor: Dose rate from a γ-emitting isotope expressed as the exposure rate in roentgens per hour at 1 cm from a point source of 1 mc.

protection problems. After instillation, most of the isotope is adsorbed onto the peritoneal surface, but some is phagocytosed by macrophages and taken up by lymphatics (37).

Although theoretically sound, studies reveal that, in practice, the isotope seldom is delivered uniformly to the peritoneal and omental surfaces (37). Postsurgical adhesions may limit the free flow of colloid, and this nonuniform distribution may result in significant underdosage of some tumor sites and significant overdosage of some normal tissues. This may result in unacceptable complications. **The curative potential of radiocolloid in the treatment of ovarian cancer has not been established.**

The most commonly employed radioisotopes in gynecologic oncology and their half-lives are presented in Table 2.2.

Clinical Uses

Cervical Cancer

Radiation therapy techniques for the curative treatment of cervical cancer usually combine both external pelvic irradiation and brachytherapy (2). Because of the wide variation in radiation techniques, it is sometimes difficult to understand the basic principles on which the radiation treatment is formulated.

Radiation therapy, like surgery, is local therapy and therefore influences cancer only within the applied radiation volume. Thus, radiation will not be curative for those with disease outside the volume treated, although it may provide worthwhile control of disease that would otherwise cause pelvic symptoms. Curative doses of radiation therapy may be applied to treat the pelvic tissues and also to treat involved para-aortic nodes.

The principle of radiation therapy for cervical cancer is the delivery of curative doses of radiation to the primary tumor and its local extensions, as well as to the regional lymph nodes (i.e., the obturator nodes and the internal, external, and common iliac nodes). The tolerance of the normal tissues within the pelvis limits the dose that can be applied to the described volume. The dose-limiting normal tissues in the pelvis are the rectum posteriorly, the bladder anteriorly, and any loops of small bowel within the pelvic radiation fields. Because the bulk of tumor usually lies centrally within the pelvis, higher central tumor doses can be achieved by the judicious application of brachytherapy.

Treatment Dosage

The doses of radiation prescribed usually are tailored to the volume of cancer present in the primary tumor and regional nodes (2). Microscopic or occult tumor deposits from epithelial cancers require 4000–5000 cGy for local control, whereas clinically obvious tumor will require in excess of 6000 cGy (23, 24).

Reference Points

Two reference points in the pelvis are used to describe the dose prescription:

1. *Point A*—This point is 2 cm lateral and 2 cm superior to the external cervical os.

2. *Point B*—This point is 3 cm lateral to point A and corresponds to the pelvic sidewall.

Although the cGy doses from intracavitary and external radiation therapy may not be biologically equivalent, it is common practice to sum these doses to express the dose prescription for points A and B.

1. The summated dose to point A believed to be adequate for central control is usually between 7500 and 8500 cGy.

2. The prescribed dose to point B is 4500–6500 cGy, depending on the bulk of parametrial and sidewall disease.

Milligram-Hours

Some centers continue to express the dose of radiation from the intracavitary application in milligram-hours. The term "milligram-hours" does not express the radiation prescription well: it refers to the number of milligrams of radium or radium equivalent present and the duration over which the insertion is left *in situ*. For purposes of communication between various centers, the term "milligram-hours" to express radiation dose is transferable only if the geometry and volume of the intracavitary system used are identical. The dose that any given system of radiation delivers to various points in the pelvis should be expressed in terms of the Gray (cGy) and can be derived from the appropriate isodose distributions related to the specific intracavitary or interstitial techniques used.

Treatment Volume

The term *treatment volume* describes the volume receiving the prescribed tumor dose ± 5%. It is not coincident with the marked borders of the field on check films. The treatment volume is usually smaller than those borders, and the degree of constriction of the high-dose volume is related to the number of beams used, the energy of the beams, and various other technical factors. The treatment volume is designed to encompass the primary tumor in the pelvis and its possible adjacent extensions, in addition to the appropriate first- and second-echelon draining lymph nodes. The pelvis is usually treated to within acceptable tolerance of the normal tissues.

The borders of the treatment field used to achieve the appropriate treatment volumes are as follows:

1. *Inferior border*—this usually lies at the inferior aspect of the obturator foramina and thus encompasses the obturator nodes. If vaginal extension has occurred, the border is moved inferiorly to 2 cm below visible and palpable tumor. Usually no attempt is made to encompass the entire vaginal tube unless disease extends into the lower third of the vagina.

2. *Superior border*—this is usually between L4 and L5 or in the midvertebral level of L5. The only reason to treat up to this level is to provide some dose to the common iliac nodes, although it is unclear whether there is additional therapeutic benefit in most cases in taking the fields up to this level as opposed to the L5/S1 junction.

3. *Lateral borders*—these are 1 cm lateral to the pelvic lymph nodes as visualized on a lymphogram or at least 1 cm lateral to the margins of the bony pelvis. Appropriate shielding along the common iliac nodes decreases the volume of normal tissue irradiated.

The incidence of late complications depends on the specific tolerance of the normal tissues irradiated, the dose that they receive, and the volume of radiation (39). Every effort should be made to minimize the high-dose treatment volume while adequately encompassing the tumor and its regional lymph nodes. The volume is significantly less using a *box technique* rather than an anterior and posterior parallel opposed pair of beams (Fig. 2.9). If there is no tumor extension along the uterosacral ligaments, a box technique may spare some of the rectum and sigmoid colon posteriorly. Even when there is posterior tumor extension and the rectum cannot be spared, a box technique may allow significant sparing of anteriorly placed small bowel if an anterior/superior corner shield is used to exclude structures in front of the external iliac lymph nodes.

In general, particularly for bulky lesions, external radiation therapy is given first to decrease the size of the primary tumor. One or two applications of intracavitary irradiation are performed after external radiation therapy to achieve the desired radiation dose levels. The amount of radiation delivered by each technique is determined by the tumor extent (2). Where disease is mainly central (e.g., in the cervix only or in the medial parametria), a higher proportion of the total dose will be prescribed for the intracavitary radiation; less external radiation will be used, because the lateral disease will be microscopic. Where bulky lateral parametrial or sidewall disease is present, a greater proportion of the dose will be delivered with the external beam.

A small group of patients with stage Ib disease without apparent nodal involvement and with tumors < 2 cm in diameter are curable without external radiation therapy but with two applications of intracavitary radiation (39). Such patients should have an extremely low risk of parametrial or nodal involvement. In addition to small tumor volume, the patient should have a low-grade tumor with no evidence of capillary or lymphatic space involvement.

Radiation therapy is highly successful in controlling pelvic disease in stage Ib lesions, with < 5% of patients having pelvic recurrence of disease only (1).

However, as the FIGO stage advances, the control of pelvic disease becomes inadequate. Clinical research efforts to improve the outcome for patients with cervical cancer are now directed to modifications of existing radiation schemes and to their combination either with preradiation chemotherapy (41) or concurrent chemotherapy (10) with agents such as *5-FU* or *cisplatin.*

For patients with carcinoma of the cervix who have vaginal hemorrhage, external radiation therapy usually will produce hemostasis. The practice of using trans-vaginal kilovoltage irradiation to achieve hemostasis (2) has been abandoned by many, because it is not likely to be more beneficial than the immediate commencement of a planned course of external radiation therapy using standard fraction sizes.

Adjuvant Pelvic Radiotherapy After Radical Hysterectomy

An extensive review of patients with Stage Ib and IIa cervical cancer managed by radical hysterectomy and pelvic lymphadenectomy revealed that nodal involvement is the strongest predictor of outcome, with survival rates approximately twice as good in node-negative patients (90% vs 46%) (42). For this reason, postoperative adjuvant pelvic radiotherapy has been used in patients with three or more positive pelvic lymph nodes. While this approach improves pelvic control, it does not increase survival because of the propensity for systemic dissemination (43). It is now recognized that, even in node-negative patients, certain tumor factors such as large tumor size, deep stromal invasion (> 10 mm or > 50%), or lymph vascular space involvement can predict pelvic recurrence after radical hysterectomy and pelvic lymphadenectomy (44). The Gynecologic Oncology Group is currently conducting a phase III trial in which patients with high-risk, lymph node−negative tumors are randomized between observation and postoperative adjuvant pelvic radiation.

Recurrent Cervical Cancer

Radiation in combination with infusional 5-fluorouracil has been used to treat patients with carcinoma of the cervix that has recurred after radical hysterectomy and pelvic lymphadenectomy. Where disease is confined to the pelvis or pelvic and para-aortic nodes, long-term survival has been reported in 45% of the patients (45).

Complications

Late complications of radical irradiation for cervical cancer occur in 5–15% of patients and are related to the size of the daily dose per fraction, the total dose administered, and the volume irradiated (46). The positioning of the intracavitary system also may influence complications. Late effects may be seen in the bladder with hematuria, fibrosis and contraction, or fistulas. Similar effects may occur in the rectosigmoid or terminal ileum with bleeding, stricture, obstruction, or perforation. Although late effects may increase with time, 75% of the late complications develop within 30 months of radiation therapy (47).

Interstitial Implants

Interstitial therapy with iridium-192 is being used increasingly in the management of cervical cancer, despite the lack of controlled clinical trials. It has been used to provide a small volume boost in patients with bulky cervical stump carcinomas after external therapy. Both central and pelvic sidewall implants have been used in the management of recurrent pelvic cancer after previous radiation therapy (48,

49). This treatment is being used more frequently in a number of centers for patients with bulky primary cervical cancer, Stages Ib to III (48). The Syed-Neblett template has been used as a guide for afterloading interstitial sources to deliver a relatively uniform dose to the implanted volume. The risk of complications is considerably higher than with conventional external and intracavitary therapy, particularly in the hands of inexperienced operators. However, recent reports claim high local control rates with acceptable morbidity (35).

Palliation

Because cervical cancer is generally a radioresponsive lesion, radiation therapy has an important role in the palliation of metastatic disease. Short courses of palliative radiation, such as 2000 cGy in five fractions or 3000 cGy in ten fractions, usually will alleviate symptoms related to bony metastases or para-aortic nodal disease. It also may relieve symptoms related to pressure from enlarging mediastinal or supraclavicular nodal disease. In rare circumstances, disease recurrent in the pelvis after initial radiation therapy may be palliated with further external beam radiation. Such circumstances may include the patient who has a late recurrence years after primary radiation therapy or the patient in whom inadequate initial doses of radiation were used.

Endometrial Cancer

The role of radiation therapy in the treatment of endometrial carcinoma is discussed in Chapter 8, but its roles may be summarized as follows:

1. As an adjunct to surgery to prevent pelvic recurrence after bilateral salpingo-oophorectomy and hysterectomy.

2. With curative intent in some patients whose preexisting medical problems preclude surgery.

3. With curative intent in patients with isolated vaginal or vaginal and pelvic recurrence. Therapy is directed to the whole pelvis and the entire vagina with the use of both external and intracavitary or interstitial radiation.

4. For palliative treatment of nonresectable intrapelvic or metastatic disease.

In the past, disease confined to the uterus often was treated with the routine application of preoperative irradiation with tumor doses of 40–60 Gy. An intracavitary line source was placed in the uterus, or the uterus was packed with mutiple radioactive capsules (Heyman's capsules) in an attempt to distribute the dose more uniformly throughout the myometrium (50). If routine preoperative intracavitary irradiation was not used, routine postoperative vault irradiation was given. **The use of preoperative or postoperative irradiation decreases the overall incidence of recurrence at the vaginal vault, but no significant survival benefit has been demonstrated** (6, 50–52).

Approximately 75–80% of patients with Stage I disease fall into a low-risk category in which the chance of recurrence is in the order of 5% after surgery alone (Fig. 2.13). In this group, it is unlikely that adjuvant radiation therapy will provide measurable improvement in pelvic control or survival rates. **At present,**

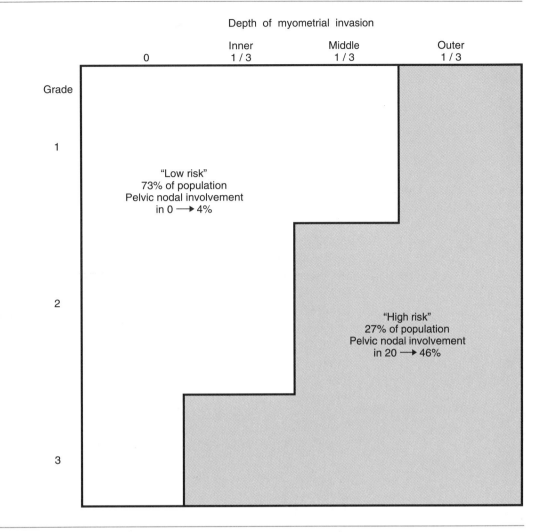

Depth of myometrial invasion

Figure 2.13   The risk of pelvic lymph node metastasis with grade and depth of myometrial penetration in clinical Stage I endometrial cancer. Adjuvant pelvic irradiation is recommended for the *high-risk* group but not for the *low-risk* group. (Reproduced with permission from DiSaia PJ, Creasman WT: Management of endometrial adenocarcinoma, Stage I with surgical staging followed by tailored adjuvant radiation therapy. *Clin Obstet Gynecol* 13:751, 1986.)

the role of adjuvant pelvic radiation therapy appears to be in the reduction of pelvic recurrences in high-risk patients (6, 32). Previously, this treatment included both whole pelvic irradiation to 45–50 Gy and vault colpostats to boost the dose to the vaginal cuff. The additional benefit of the vault boost has been questioned, but its usefulness has not been tested formally. Many have abandoned its routine use.

Ovarian Cancer

A curative role for whole abdominal and pelvic irradiation has been established for some subsets of patients with epithelial ovarian cancer by several independent investigators (53–57). Because most studies of radiotherapy in ovarian cancer include patients with no macroscopic residual disease after primary surgery, reports do not indicate how many patients were cured by the radiotherapy; some may have been cured by surgery alone. An assessment of the curative potential of radiotherapy can be made by assessing the outcome in patients with known macroscopic residual tumor. The long-term or relapse-free survival rates from five such published series are summarized in Table 2.3. The proportion of survivors is very similar in the four studies and appears to be determined by the presenting stage and volume of residual disease. Approximately 40–50% of patients with small residual lesions are cured; most of these are derived from Stage II and most from patients in whom the tumor residuum was confined to the pelvis, where a higher radiation dose can be delivered. With larger residual lesions, the probability of cure with radiotherapy is in the neighborhood of only 5–15%.

Whole Abdominopelvic Radiation

Clinical experience and staging studies have demonstrated that transperitoneal spread is the most common route of dissemination of ovarian cancer (58, 59). Furthermore, at the time of first relapse, tumor is confined to the abdominal cavity in about 85% of patients. Thus techniques of radiation encompassing the whole peritoneal cavity are more likely to be curative than those that treat the pelvis alone or the lower abdomen. The dose of radiation that can be given to the upper abdomen is considerably lower than that considered "radical" for solid tumors. It would be expected, therefore, that whole abdominal irradiation would produce a modest improvement in tumor control in the upper abdomen and that this benefit would be seen only in patients with microscopic volumes of tumor. Although a curative benefit has been established for radiation therapy, the literature at this time does not resolve for us the relative effectiveness of abdominopelvic radiotherapy and combination platinum-based chemotherapy in patients with small or no macroscopic residual disease.

Choice of Radiation Technique

In general, two techniques have been used to treat the whole abdomen. The *moving-strip technique* employs a 10 cm high field that is moved by 2.5 cm increments (strips), so that each strip receives 8 or 10 fractions (60, 61). Although the concept originally arose in an era when radiotherapy equipment could not

Table 2.3   Evidence of Long-Term Control of Stages II and III Ovarian Cancer with Macroscopic Residual Disease Using Abdominopelvic Radiotherapy

Center	End Point	Size of Residual Disease	
		< 2 cm	**> 2 cm**
Princess Margaret Hospital (53)	(n)	(91)	(91)
	% 10-year RFR	38	6
Stanford (54)	(n)	(42)	(54)
	% 15-year FFR	50	14
Salt Lake City (55)	(n)	(12)	(10)
	% 10-year RFS	62	0
Walter Reed Hospital (56)	(n)	(24)	(20)
	% 10-year SR	42	10
Yale (57)	(n)	(27)	—
	~6-year SF	.41	

RFR = relapse-free rate; FFR = failure-free rate; SR = survival rate; RFS = relapse-free survival rate; SF = surviving fraction; n = number.
Reproduced and modified, with permission, from Dembo AJ: Epithelial ovarian cancer: The role of radiotherapy. *Int J Rad Oncol Biol Phys* 22:835, 1992.

Table 2.4   Technical Principles of Curative Radiotherapy

1. The entire peritoneal cavity must be encompassed, and radiologic verification is required.
2. The moving-strip and open-field techniques are equally effective, but the latter is less morbid.
3. No liver shielding is used; this limits the upper abdominal dose to 2500–2800 cGy in 100–120 cGy daily fractions.
4. Partial kidney shielding is used to keep the renal dose at 1800–2000 cGy.
5. The true pelvis is given a boost dose in 180–220 cGy fractions to a total dose of 4500 cGy.
6. Parallel opposing portals should be used, with beam energy sufficient to ensure a dosage variation no greater than 5%.

Reproduced and modified, with permission, from Dembo AJ: Epithelial ovarian cancer: The role of radiotherapy. *Int J Rad Oncol Biol Phys* 22:835, 1992.

adequately irradiate large volumes in one portal, the major justification for use of the moving-strip technique has been that it can deliver a biologically higher dose than the open-field technique. In the *open-field technique,* the whole volume is treated each day, usually in a single portal. This requires a reduction in the size of the daily dose. Arguments against the use of the moving strip technique are as follows:

1. The treatment course takes approximately twice as long as does the open-field technique

2. Tumor metastases theoretically may reseed during treatment

3. Abdominal contents may move from day to day so that the actual dose delivered to a given area is uncertain.

Randomized studies that compare the two techniques have been undertaken (62, 63). In both studies, the difference in 5-year survival was less than 1% between the treatment arms. A detailed subgroup analysis of the Princess Margaret Hospital study showed that the two techniques were comparable in all patient subgroups, regardless of stage, histology, grade, or residual disease. Acute toxicity was similar for both techniques, although thrombocytopenia was more common with the moving-strip technique. Late complications were more frequent with the strip technique, 6% of patients requiring bowel surgery compared with only 1% of those who received open-field radiation. These toxicity observations are in keeping with the linear quadratic model of acute- and late-reacting tissues (30, 62). For reasons of shorter treatment duration, simplicity, reduced toxicity, and equal efficacy, the open-field technique has become the standard in most centers. Modifications to the open-field technique include the addition of a "T boost" to the para-aortics and medial domes of diaphragms (54) and the treatment of the upper and lower abdomen through separate portals (65, 66). The technical principles of abdominopelvic radiotherapy are summarized in Table 2.4, and the treatment volume is shown in Figure 2.14.

Toxicity   Side effects of open-field whole abdominal radiation are (51):

1. 60% of patients experience abdominal cramps and diarrhea, which are usually mild and controlled with antidiarrhea medications

2. 75% experience anorexia, nausea, or vomiting

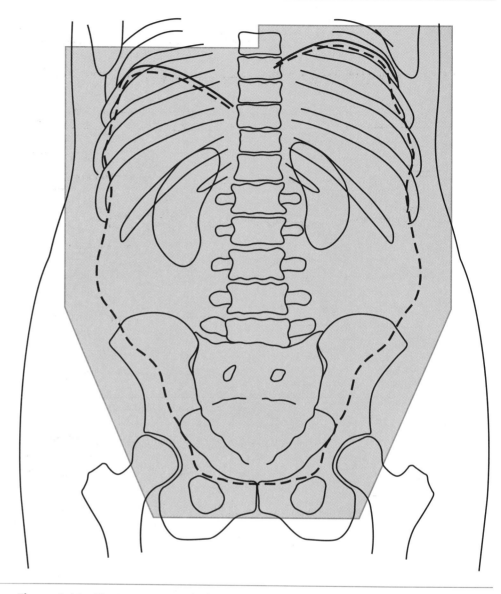

Figure 2.14   Treatment portals for carcinoma of the ovary. The entire peritoneal cavity is encompassed by the field.

3. 100% develop general fatigue

4. 10% develop significant thrombocytopenia (platelet count < 100,000) or neutropenia (neutrophil count < 1500). After chemotherapy, about one-third will have significant myelotoxicity.

5. 15% develop radiologic evidence of basal pneumonitis, and it is symptomatic in 1%. The condition is self-limiting and resolves spontaneously.

6. 40% have transient biochemical evidence of liver damage with increased serum alkaline phosphatase levels, but symptomatic hepatitis is not observed.

7. 10% have mild abdominal bloating.

The incidence of bowel complications after postoperative abdominopelvic irradiation is shown in Table 2.5. In the Princess Margaret Hospital experience, fewer than 2% required operative correction of bowel obstruction. The frequency of bowel complications will increase if higher total doses or larger fraction sizes are used. The extent and number of previous abdominal operations, especially if a para-aortic lymphadenectomy has been performed, may add to the risk of bowel damage (67).

Indications Postoperative whole abdominopelvic irradiation should be limited to those patients who are most likely to benefit. In addition to the general medical condition of the patients, their suitability for abdominopelvic radiotherapy is determined by the extent of disease at presentation, the amount and site of residual disease, and the grade of the tumor (68, 69). Abdominopelvic radiotherapy encompasses only the peritoneal cavity and retroperitoneum, so its use as primary treatment is restricted to Stages I, II, and III. It should be used only in patients with no macroscopic disease in the upper abdomen and small (< 2 cm) or no macroscopic residual disease in the pelvis (57, 67, 69–72).

Radiotherapy After Chemotherapy in Advanced Disease

Fuks and coworkers stated the rationale for sequential cisplatin-based chemotherapy, secondary exploration, and cytoreductive surgery, followed by radiotherapy in advanced ovarian cancer (73). Twenty-four reports of sequential multimodality therapy have appeared in the literature, most of which are single-arm studies with no satisfactory controls. Four randomized studies have been performed (74–77). Generally, the results of the studies have been disappointing, and the balance of evidence is against a significant curative benefit for radiotherapy as salvage or consolidation treatment. Although there appears to be an advantage for patients with no macroscopic residual disease or residual disease < 5 mm, the observed outcomes are compatible with the natural history of the disease and do not establish a treatment effect. About one-fourth to one-half of the patients are not able to receive a therapeutic dose of irradiation after chemotherapy because of myelotoxicity (78, 79).

A recent retrospective analysis of the Toronto data suggested an improved overall survival and relapse-free survival for high-risk patients treated with sequential chemotherapy and whole abdominal radiation compared with historical controls

---

Table 2.5   Bowel Complications of Abdominopelvic Irradiation as Primary Treatment for Ovarian Cancer

Number of patients	1098*
Surgery for radiation complications	61 (5.6%)
Deaths related to radiation-induced bowel injury	4 (0.4%)
Lowest bowel complication rate:	1.4%
• Radiation dose 2250 cGy in 22 fractions. Open-field technique with additional pelvic boost of 2250 cGy in 10 more fractions	
Highest bowel complication rate:	14.3%
• Radiation dose 3000 in 8 fractions of moving-strip with an additional pelvic boost of 1500 cGy in 10 more fractions by open-field technique	

*Combined data (references 53–57, 60–68).

treated with radiation alone (80). Randomized studies would be necessary to establish superiority of this approach over chemotherapy alone.

Vulvar Cancer

The role of radiation therapy in the treatment of vulvar cancer has remained largely unexplored until recently (8, 54). Historically, radiation therapy was delivered with non-skin-sparing orthovoltage equipment in relatively high doses per fraction, and this produced extensive acute morbidity with desquamation of the skin of the vulva and groins. Vulvar irradiation thus fell into disrepute.

The curative value of radiation therapy in the control of squamous cell cancers of other sites, including the head and neck and anal canal, is well established. Because the radiosensitivity of squamous cell carcinomas of the vulva should be inherently the same as that of other squamous cell cancers, the use of radiation in this disease is being redefined with newer techniques (81–86). Current concepts in the integration of more limited surgery and adjunctive or primary radiation therapy in vulvar cancer are discussed in Chapter 11.

The aims of integrated multimodality therapy, including surgery, radiation, and possibly concurrent chemoradiation therapy, are:

1. To reduce the risks of postoperative locoregional failure in patients with advanced primary or nodal disease

2. To obviate the need for exenteration in patients with disease involving the anus or proximal urethra (85).

Where radiation is used in vulvar cancer, the following guidelines with respect to radiation technique and dosage should be followed:

1. The total dose of radiation should be tailored to the volume of tumor with doses in the order of 45–50 Gy for microscopic disease and 60–64 Gy for macroscopic disease.

2. When the vulva is irradiated, the fraction size should be limited to 160–175 cGy to minimize late radiation sequelae.

3. When disease is macroscopic, vulvar or nodal, concurrent "sensitizing" chemotherapy (e.g., with infusional *5-FU* or *cisplatin*) may be a useful adjunct and is being explored in current and future studies of the Gynecologic Oncology Group.

4. When concurrent infusional chemotherapy is used, two radiation fractions per day may be advantageous to maximize drug-radiation interaction and shorten the overall treatment time.

5. Treatment interruptions (split) should be kept to a minimum to avoid possible tumor proliferation during rests in radiation therapy.

6. A perineal port should be used when technically feasible. It is recommended that the vulvar lesion be encompassed with an adequate margin. No attempt should be made to include the entire vulva in the radiation field if disease is unifocal and can be included in smaller fields. The beam energies to be used for treatment of the primary tumor by direct

fields should be cobalt or 4–6 MeV photons. Appropriate energy electrons may be used, tailored to the thickness of the lesion, but the dose from electrons to the primary lesion should probably be limited to 30–50% of the dose in view of the subcutaneous fibrosis that is commonly seen when all electron therapy is given. Advanced or very bulky disease may require whole vulvar irradiation using anterior-posterior parallel opposed fields.

7. Inguinopelvic nodal irradiation should be delivered with the use of energies greater than 6 MeV photons. Appropriate use of bolus or mixed beams should be employed to ensure that the inguinal nodal regions lying 0–4 cm below the skin receive full tumor dosage.

Acute moist desquamation of the skin of the inguinal creases and vulva is expected. The severity and duration of this acute reaction may be minimized by the choice of daily fraction sizes of 150–175 cGy. Late complications may include lymphedema, atrophy, and fibrosis of the skin and subcutaneous tissues in the treatment field. The risk of hip fracture in elderly women may be increased. Fractures have been reported in 4 of 13 women over the age of 50 years treated with cobalt irradiation in doses of 2600–4500 cGy (53).

References

1. **Perez CA, Breaux S, Madoc-Jones H, et al:** Radiation therapy alone in the treatment of carcinoma of the uterine cervix. *Cancer* 51:1393, 1983.

2. **Fletcher GH:** *Textbook of Radiotherapy.* Philadelphia, Lea & Febiger, 1980, pp 720–789.

3. **Landgren RD, Fletcher GH, Delclos L, et al:** Irradiation of endometrial cancer in patients with medical contraindications to surgery or with unresectable lesions. *Am J Roentgenol Radium Ther Nucl Med* 126:148, 1976.

4. **Dembo AJ, Bush RS, Beale FA, et al:** Ovarian carcinoma: Improved survival following abdominopelvic irradiation in patients with a completed pelvic operation. *Am J Obstet Gynecol* 134:793, 1979.

5. **Dembo AJ:** Radiotherapeutic management of ovarian cancer. *Semin Oncol* 11:238, 1984.

6. **Aalders J, Abeler V, Kolstad P, Onsrud M:** Postoperative external irradiation and prognostic parameters in Stage I endometrial carcinoma. *Obstet Gynecol* 55:419, 1980.

7. **Homesley HD, Bundy BN, Sedlis A, Adcock L:** Radiation therapy versus pelvic node resection for carcinoma of the vulva with positive groin nodes. *Obstet Gynecol* 68:733, 1986.

8. **Boronow RC:** Combined therapy as an alternative to exenteration for locally advanced vulvo-vaginal cancer. *Cancer* 49:1085, 1982.

9. **Peters LJ, Ang KK:** Unconventional fractionation schemes in radiotherapy. In *Important Advances in Oncology 1986.* Philadelphia, JB Lippincott, 1986, pp 269–285.

10. **Thomas GM, Dembo AJ, Beale F, et al:** Concurrent radiation, mitomycin-C and 5-fluorouracil in poor prognosis carcinoma of the cervix: preliminary results of a Phase I-II study. *Int J Radiat Oncol Biol Phys* 10:1785, 1984.

11. **Hall EJ:** *Radiobiology for the Radiologist,* ed 2. Philadelphia, Harper & Row, 1978.

12. **Elkind MM, Sutton H:** Radiation response of mammalian cells grown in culture: 1. Repair of x-ray damage in surviving Chinese hamster cells. *Radiat Res* 13:556, 1960.

13. **Parsons JT, Bova FJ, Million RR:** A re-evaluation of the University of Florida split-course technique for squamous carcinoma of the head and neck. *Int J Radiat Oncol Biol Phys* 6:1645, 1980.

14. **Terasima R, Tolmach LJ:** X-ray sensitivity and DNA synthesis in synchronous population of HeLa cells. *Sciences* 140:490, 1963.

15. **Kallman RF:** The phenomenon of reoxygenation and its implications for fractionated radiotherapy. *Radiology* 105:135, 1972.

16. **Thames HD Jr, Peters LJ, Withers HR, Fletcher GH:** Accelerated fractionation vs. hyperfractionation: rationales for several treatments per day. *Int J Radiat Oncol Biol Phys* 11:87, 1985.

17. **Adams GE, Ahmed L, Felden, et al:** The development of some mitronidazoles as hypoxic cell sensitizers. *Cancer Clin Trials* 3:37, 1980.

18. **Watson R, Dische S, Cade I, et al:** Hyperbaric oxygen and radiotherapy: a Medical Research Council trial in carcinoma of the cervix. *Br J Radiol* 51:879, 1978.

19. **Barendsen GW: :** Response of cultured cells, tumors and normal tissues to radiations of different linear energy transfer. *Curr Topics Radiat Res* 4:293, 1968.

20. **Bush RS, Jenkin RP, Allt WE, et al:** Definitive evidence for hypoxic cells influencing cure in cancer therapy. *Br J Cancer* 37:302, 1978.

21. **Steel GG, Peckham MJ:** Exploitable mechanisms in combined radiotherapy and chemotherapy: the concept of additivity. *Int J Radiat Oncol Biol Phys* 9:1145, 1979.

22. **Manning MR, Cetas TC, Miller RC, et al:** Clinical hyperthermia: results of a Phase I trial employing hyperthermia alone or in combination with external beam or interstitial radiotherapy. *Cancer* 49:205, 1982.

23. **Fletcher GH:** Clinical dose-response curves of human malignant epithelial tumours. *Br J Radiol* 46:1, 1973.

24. **Shukovsky LJ:** Dose, time volume relationships in squamous cell carcinoma of the supraglottic larynx. *Am J Roentgenol Radium Ther Nucl Med* 108:27, 1970.

25. **Rubin P, Casarett GW:** *Clinical Radiation Pathology.* Philadelphia, WB Saunders, 1968.

26. **Withers HR, Mason KA:** The kinetics of recovery in irradiated colonic mucosa in the mouse. *Cancer* 34:896, 1974.

27. **Reinche U, Hannon EC, Rosenblatt M, Hellman S:** Proliferative capacity of murine hematopoietic stem cells in vitro. *Science* 215:1619, 1982.

28. **Withers HR, Peters LJ, Kogelnik HD:** The pathobiology of late effects of irradiation. In Meyn RE, Withers HR (eds): *Radiation Biology in Cancer Research.* New York, Raven Press, 1980, pp 439–448.

29. **Peters LJ:** Biology of radiation therapy. In Thawley S, Panje W (eds): *Comprehensive Management of Head and Neck Tumours.* Philadelphia, WB Saunders, 1985, pp 132–152.

30. **Thames HD, Withers HR, Peters LJ, Fletcher GH:** Changes in early and late radiation response with altered dose fractionation: implications for dose-survival relationships. *Int J Rad Oncol Biol Phys* 8:219, 1982.

31. **Withers HR, Peters LJ, Thames HD, Fletcher GH:** Hyperfractionation. *Int J Radiat Oncol Biol Phys* 8:1807, 1982.

32. **Onsrud M, Kolstad P, Normann T:** Postoperative external pelvic irradiation in carcinoma of the corpus Stage I: a controlled clinical trial. *Gynecol Oncol* 4:222, 1976.

33. **Johns HE, Cunningham JR:** The physics of radiology. Springfield, Illinois, Charles C Thomas, 1977.

34. **Orton GG, Seyedsadr M, Somnay A:** Comparison of high and low dose rate remote afterloading for cervix cancer and the importance of fractionation. *Int J Rad Oncol Biol Phys* 21:1425, 1992.

35. **Martinez A, Edmundson GK, Cox RS, et al:** Combination of external beam irradiation and multiple-site perineal applicator (MUPIT) for treatment of locally advanced or recurrent prostatic, anorectal and gynecologic malignancies. *Int J Rad Oncol Biol Phys* 11:391, 1985.

36. **Rosenshein NB:** Radioisotopes in the treatment of ovarian cancer. *Clin Obstet Gynaecol* 10:279, 1983.

37. **Reed GW, Watson ER, Chesters MS:** A note on the distribution of radioactive colloidal gold following intraperitoneal injection. *Br J Radiol* 34:323, 1961.

38. **Tewfik HH, Gruber H, Tewfik FA, et al:** Intraperitoneal distribution of ^{32}P chromic phosphate suspension in the dog. *Int J Rad Oncol Biol Phys* 5:1907, 1979.

39. **Allt WEC:** Supervoltage radiation treatment in advanced cancer of the uterine cervix. *Can Med Assoc J* 100:792, 1963.

40. **Bush RS:** Carcinoma of the cervix: Management. In Peckham MJ, Carter RL (eds): *The Management of Malignant Disease*, series 2. London, E Arnold Publishers, 1979, pp 183–216.

41. **Friedlander ML, Atkinson K, Coppleson JVM, et al:** The integration of chemotherapy into the management of locally advanced cervical cancer: a pilot study. *Gynecol Oncol* 19:1, 1984.

42. **van Bommel P, van Lindert A, Kock H, et al:** A review of prognostic factors in early-stage carcinoma of the cervix (FIGO Ib and IIa) and implications for treatment strategy. *Eur J Obstet Gynecol Reprod Biol* 26:69, 1987.

43. **Kinney WK, Alvarez RD, Reid GC, et al:** Value of adjuvant whole-pelvic irradiation after Wertheim hysterectomy for early-stage squamous carcinoma of the cervix with pelvic nodal metastasis: a matched-control study. *Gynecol Oncol* 34:258, 1989.

44. **Delgado G, Bundy BN, Fowler WC, et al:** A prospective surgical pathological study of stage I squamous carcinoma of the cervix: a Gynecologic Oncology Group study. *Gynecol Oncol* 35:314, 1989.

45. **Thomas GM, Dembo AJ, Myhr T, et al:** Long-term results of concurrent radiation and chemotherapy for carcinoma of the cervix recurrent after surgery. *Int J Gynecol Cancer* 3:193, 1993.

46. **Hamberger AD, Abdurrahman U, Jershenson DM, Fletcher GH:** Analysis of the severe complications of irradiation of carcinoma of the cervix. Whole pelvis irradiation and intracavitary radium. *Int J Rad Oncol Biol Phys* 9:367, 1982.

47. **Covens A, Thomas GM, DePetrillo A, Jamieson C:** The prognostic importance of site and type of radiation-induced bowel injury in patients requiring surgical management. *Gynecol Oncol* 43:270, 1991.

48. **Prempree T:** Parametrial implant in Stage IIIb cancer of the cervix. *Cancer* 52:748, 1983.

49. **Randall ME:** Results of interstitial reradiation for recurrent gynecologic malignancies. *Proc Int Gynecol Cancer Soc* 3:266, 1991.

50. **Heyman J, Reuterwell O, Benner S:** The Radiumhemmet experience with radiotherapy in cancer of the corpus of the uterus. *Acta Radiol* 22:14, 1941.

51. **Piver SM, Yazigi R, Blumenson L, Tsukada Y:** A prospective trial comparing hysterectomy, hysterectomy plus vaginal radium, and uterine radium plus hysterectomy in Stage I endometrial carcinoma. *Obstet Gynecol* 54:85, 1979.

52. **Boronow RC, Morrow CP, Creasman WT, et al:** Surgical staging in endometrial cancer: clinical-pathological findings of a prospective study. *Obstet Gynecol* 63:825, 1984.

53. **Dembo AJ:** Abdominopelvic radiotherapy in ovarian cancer: a 10 year experience. *Cancer* 55:2285, 1980.

54. **Martinez A, Schray MF, Howes AE, Bagshaw MA:** Postoperative radiation therapy for epithelial ovarian cancer: the curative role based on a 24-year experience. *J Clin Oncol* 3:901, 1985.

55. **Fuller DB, Sause WT, Plenk H, Menlove RL:** Analysis of post-operative radiation therapy in Stage I through III epithelial ovarian carcinoma. *J Clin Oncol* 5:897, 1987.

56. **Weiser EB, Burke TW, Heller PB, et al:** Determinants of survival of patients with epithelial ovarian carcinoma following whole abdominal irradiation (WAR). *Gynecol Oncol* 30:201, 1988.

57. **Goldberg N, Peschel RE:** Postoperative abdominopelvic radiation therapy for ovarian cancer. *Int J Rad Oncol Phys* 14(3):425, 1988.

58. **Piver MS, Barlow JJ, Lele SB: :** Incidence of subclinical metastasis in stage I and II ovarian carcinoma. *Obstet Gynecol* 52:100, 1978.

59. **Rosenoff SH, Young RC, Anderson T, et al:** Peritoneoscopy: a valuable staging tool in ovarian carcinoma. *Ann Intern Med* 83:37, 1975.

60. **Delclos L, Smith JP:** Ovarian cancer, with special regard to types of radiotherapy. *Natl Cancer Inst Monogr* 42:129, 1975.

61. **Dembo AJ, Van Dyk J, Japp B, et al:** Whole abdominal irradiation by a moving strip technique for patients with ovarian cancer. *Int J Rad Oncol Biol Phys* 5:1933, 1982.

62. **Dembo AJ, Bush RS, Beale FA, et al:** A randomized clinical trial of moving strip versus open field whole abdominal irradiation in patients with invasive epithelial cancer of ovary. *Int J Rad Oncol Biol Phys* 9 (Suppl):97, 1983.

63. **Fazekas JT, Maier JG:** Irradiation of ovarian carcinomas: a prospective comparison of the open-field and moving-strip techniques. *Am J Roentgenol* 120:118, 1974.

64. **Dembo AJ, Balogh JM:** Advances in radiotherapy in the gynecologic malignancies. *Semin Surg Oncol* 6:323, 1990.

65. **Einhorn N, von Hamos K, Hindmarsh T, et al:** Radiation therapy of ovarian carcinoma: presentation of a six-field technique. *Radiother Oncol* 7(2):125, 1986.

66. **Order SE, Rosenshein NB, Klein JL, et al:** New methods applied to the analysis and treatment of ovarian cancer. *Int J Rad Oncol Biol Phys* 5:861, 1979.

67. **van Bunnigen B, Bouma J, Kooijman C, et al:** Total abdominal irradiation in stage I and II carcinoma of the ovary. *Radiother Oncol* 11:305, 1988.

68. **Dembo AJ, Bush RS, Brown TC:** Clinicopathological correlates in ovarian cancer. *Bull Cancer* (Paris) 69:292, 1982.

69. **Carey MS, Dembo AJ, Simm JE, et al:** Testing the validity of a prognostic classification in patients with surgically optimal ovarian carcinoma: a 15-year review. *Int J Gynecol Cancer* 3:24, 1993.

70. **Dembo AJ, Bush RS:** Choice of postoperative therapy based on prognostic factors. *Int J Rad Oncol Biol Phys* 8:893, 1982.

71. **Sell A, Bertelsen K, Anderson JE, et al:** Randomized study of whole abdomen irradiation versus pelvic irradiation plus cyclophosphamide in treatment of early ovarian cancer. *Gynecol Oncol* 37:367, 1990.

72. **Lindner H, Willich H, Atzinger A:** Primary adjuvant whole abdominal irradiation in ovarian carcinoma. *Int J Rad Oncol Biol Phys* 19:1203, 1990.

73. **Fuks Z, Rizel S, Anteby SO, Biran S:** The multimodal approach to the treatment of stage III ovarian carcinoma. *Int J Rad Oncol Biol Phys* 89:903, 1982.

74. **Bruzzone M, Repetto L, Chiara S, et al:** Chemotherapy versus radiotherapy in the management of ovarian cancer patients with pathological complete response or minimal residual disease at second look. *Gynecol Oncol* 38:392, 1990.

75. **Lambert HE, Rustin GJS, Gregory WM, Nelstrop AE:** A randomised trial comparing single agent carboplatin with carboplatin followed by radiotherapy for advanced ovarian cancer. *A North Thames Ovary Group Study.* Annual Meeting British Oncol Association, 1991.

76. **Mangioni C, Epis A, Vassena L, et al:** Radiotherapy (RT) versus chemotherapy (CH) as second line treatment of minimal residual disease (MRD) in advanced epithelial ovarian cancer (EOC). *Proc Int Gynecol Cancer Soc* 1:49, 1987.

77. **Lawton F, Luesley D, Blackledge G, et al:** A randomized trial comparing whole abdominal radiotherapy with chemotherapy following cisplatinum cytoreduction in epithelial ovarian cancer. West Midlands Ovarian Cancer Group Trial II. *Clin Oncol* 2:409, 1990.

78. **Dembo AJ:** The sequential multiple modality treatment of ovarian cancer. *Radiother Oncol* 3:187, 1985.

79. **Hacker NF, Berek JS, Burnison MG, et al:** Whole abdominal radiation as salvage therapy for epithelial ovarian cancer. *Obstet Gynecol* 65:60, 1985.

80. **Ledermann JA, Dembo AJ, Sturgeon JFG, et al:** Outcome of patients with unfavorable optimally cytoreduced ovarian cancer treated with chemotherapy and whole abdominal radiation. *Gynecol Oncol* 41:30, 1991.

81. **Neijt JP, ten Bokkel Huinink WW, van den Burg MEL, et al:** Randomized trial comparing two combination chemotherapy regimens (CHAP-5 vs CP) in advanced ovarian carcinoma. *J Clin Oncol* 6:893, 1988.

82. **Way S:** Carcinoma of the vulva. *Am J Obstet Gynecol* 79:692, 1960.

83. **Pirtoli L, Rottoli ML:** Results of radiation therapy for vulvar cancer. *Acta Radiol Oncol* 21:45, 1982.

84. **Prempree T, Amornmarn R:** Radiation treatment of recurrent carcinoma of the vulva. *Cancer* 54:1943, 1984.

85. **Thomas GM, Dembo AJ, Bryson SCO, et al:** Changing concepts in the management of vulvar cancer. *Gynecol Oncol* 42:9, 1991.

86. **Guarishi A, Keane TJ, Elhakim T:** Metastatic inguinal nodes from an unknown primary neoplasm. *Cancer* 59:572, 1987.

3

Biology and Immunology

Cinda M. Boyer
Robert C. Knapp
Robert C. Bast, Jr.

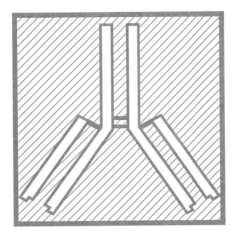

Biology of Gynecologic Cancers

Malignant Phenotype

All cancers share certain characteristics that set them apart from the normal cells from which they arise. The malignant phenotype is associated with morphologic changes, anchorage-independent growth, and loss of contact inhibition *in vitro* as well as growth in nude mice *in vivo*. Malignant cells are capable of invading adjacent normal tissue and metastasizing to distant organ sites. Although the malignant phenotype persists through many generations, tumor cells are genetically unstable. In most cancers, four or five genetic alterations are required to transform benign precursors into cells with a fully malignant phenotype.

Clonality

Most epithelial cancers arise from single cells and consequently are "clonal" diseases. Among the gynecologic cancers, the issue of clonality has been most thoroughly studied in ovarian cancer. More than 90% of ovarian malignancies arise from the surface epithelium of the ovary. Whether epithelial ovarian cancer develops from a single cell has been debated. Epithelial ovarian cancer often affects both ovaries. Relatively small amounts of tumor may be found on the ovaries; yet numerous and large bulky tumor deposits may be found elsewhere in the peritoneum. Occasionally, peritoneal carcinomatosis, indistinguishable histologically from ovarian cancer, occurs after oophorectomy. These factors, as well as the common embryologic origin of the ovarian surface epithelium and the peritoneal mesothelium, led to the "field change" hypothesis of ovarian carcinogenesis (1). This hypothesis suggested that ovarian cancer was a polyclonal disease arising at multiple sites that shared a susceptibility to events leading to malignant transformation. However, recent molecular analyses of epithelial ovarian cancers using mutation of the p53 gene (2,3), allelic deletion (2), and X-chromosome inactivation (2,3) have found that the primary tumor deposits in the ovary, as well as deposits found elsewhere in the peritoneum, share the same

75

genetic markers, suggesting monoclonality. Twenty-four of 26 sporadic cases of ovarian cancers studied by these techniques were found to be monoclonal (2,3).

Pathogenesis and Genetics of Gynecologic Cancers

The pathogenesis of different gynecologic cancers is poorly understood. Protracted proliferation of epithelial cells may be one factor that contributes to the development of cancers at several different sites. Multiple genetic errors are more likely to occur or to be expressed during cell proliferation. In the case of cervical cancer, expression of viral proteins can inactivate critical host molecules that ordinarily suppress proliferation. In the pathogenesis of endometrial cancer, unopposed estrogenic stimulation favors proliferation of the endometrial epithelium. In epithelial ovarian cancer, persistent ovulation correlates with disease incidence. Early menarche and late menopause increase the risk of ovarian cancer, whereas pregnancy, lactation, and oral contraceptive medication decrease the incidence. Although hormonal factors may be important, proliferation of epithelial cells to repair ovulatory damage may permit development or expression of genetic alterations.

Malignant transformation of normal cells is likely to involve genes that regulate cell growth. Proliferation of normal ovarian, endometrial, and cervical epithelium is ordinarily under tight control that is lost during malignant transformation. Alterations in growth factors, oncogenes, and tumor suppressor genes may all contribute to the pathogenesis of gynecologic cancers (Fig. 3.1).

Oncogenes are normal growth regulatory genes that have undergone activation via mutation, amplification, or translocation (4). More than 60 oncogenes have been described. Many of the oncogenes thus far identified encode proteins homologous to growth factors or transmembrane growth factor receptors with tyrosine kinase activity (Table 3.1) (Fig. 3.2). Some intracellular oncogenes are part of growth regulatory signal transduction pathways involving either ty-

Figure 3.1. Oncogenes and tumor supressor genes may contribute to the growth and development of gynecologic cancers.

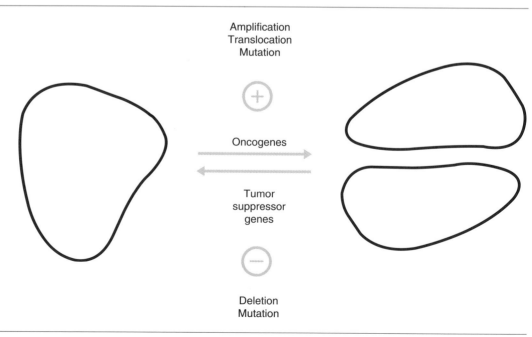

Amplification
Translocation
Mutation

+

Oncogenes

Tumor suppressor genes

−

Deletion
Mutation

Table 3.1 Properties and Functions of Selected Oncogenes

Oncogene	Functional Activity	Molecular Weight (Kd)	Cellular Location
sis	Growth factor (B chain of PDGF)	28–35	Extracellular
int-2	Growth factor (FGF family)	28–32	Extracellular
erbB	Receptor tyrosine kinase (truncated EGF receptor)	72	Transmembrane
erbB-2	Receptor tyrosine kinase	185	Transmembrane
fms	Receptor tyrosine kinase (intact M-CSF receptor)	165	Transmembrane
src	Nonreceptor tyrosine kinase	60	Intracellular membrane associated
abl	Nonreceptor tyrosine kinase	145	Cytoplasmic
raf-1	Serine/threonine kinase	75	Cytoplasmic
ras	Guanine nucleotide binding protein	21	Intracellular membrane associated
myc	DNA binding protein	62–64	Nuclear
jun	DNA binding protein (AP-1 transcription factor component)	47	Nuclear
fos	DNA binding protein (AP-1 transcription factor component)	62	Nuclear

rosine or serine/threonine phosphorylation. Other families of oncogenes have guanine nucleotide or DNA binding activity.

Tumor-suppressor genes are normal genes whose products limit proliferation or maintain differentiation. Relatively few tumor suppressor genes have been characterized. Both retinoblastoma (Rb) and p53 genes encode nuclear DNA binding proteins, but not all tumor suppressor genes act directly on DNA. The DCC (deleted in colon carcinoma) tumor-suppressor gene, for example, encodes a protein with homology to cell surface adhesion molecules. Protein tyrosine phosphatases that can remove the phosphotyrosine added by tyrosine kinases are also candidates for tumor suppressor genes.

By regulating the cell cycle, proto-oncogenes and tumor suppressor genes play important roles in controlling cell growth and differentiation. The primary points in the cell cycle where some of these gene loci exert their control are presented in Figure 3.3. **Carcinogenesis is almost certainly a multistep process resulting from activation of several oncogenes and loss of multiple tumor suppressor genes within a single cell** (5). The order in which these changes occurs may not be important, although some changes are associated statistically with more advanced or aggressive malignancy. Different patterns of genetic change have been observed in tumors that arise from different sites.

Genes that predispose to the development of cancer might be carried in the germ line. **Fewer than 5% of ovarian cancers arise in women with a strong family history of the disease (6), but recent studies have mapped to chromosome 17q an abnormal gene in families with a history of breast-ovarian cancer syndrome.** A majority of sporadic ovarian cancers have aneuploid DNA content and have lost one or both alleles at certain chromosomal sites. No single karyotypic abnormality has been consistently associated with ovarian cancer, but alterations of chromosomes 1, 3, 6, and 11 have been frequently observed (6). Allelic loss

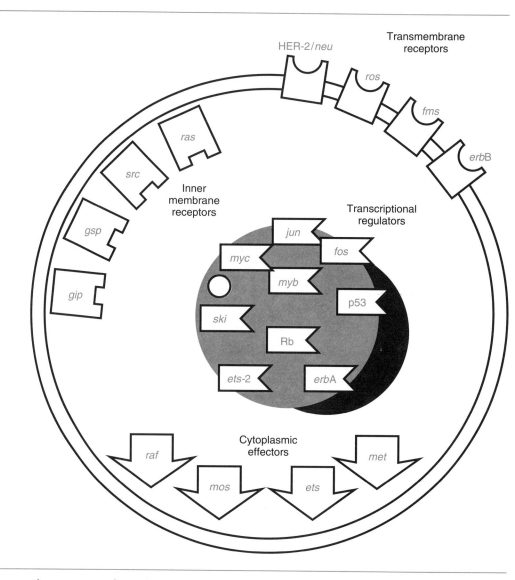

Figure 3.2. The cellular locations of selected proto-oncogenes and tumor suppressor gene protein products are shown. (Reproduced, with permission, from Baker V: Oncogenes and tumor suppressor genes in gynecologic cancer. *Contemp Obstet Gynecol* Sept.:75, 1992.)

detected by polymorphic genetic markers has been described for loci on chromosomes 3p, 4p, 6p, 6q, 7p, 8q, 11p, 12p, 12q, 16p, 16q, 17p, 17q, and 19p (7,8). Loci where genes are inactivated or heterozygosity is lost may be sites of tumor suppressor genes.

Aneuploidy and allelic loss are less frequently detected in endometrial cancers. In one study, only 16% of tumors were aneuploid or tetraploid, although the patients with these tumors had a poorer prognosis than did patients with diploid tumors (9). Another study reported loss of heterozygosity in 30% of endometrial cancers, with the most frequent loss of alleles being on chromosome 17p (10). In cervical cancer the most frequent site of allelic loss discovered to date has been on chromosome 3p (11).

Growth Factors in Gynecologic Cancers

A number of peptide growth factors that may be involved in the growth regulation of gynecologic cancers have been identified (Table 3.2). **Peptide growth factors**

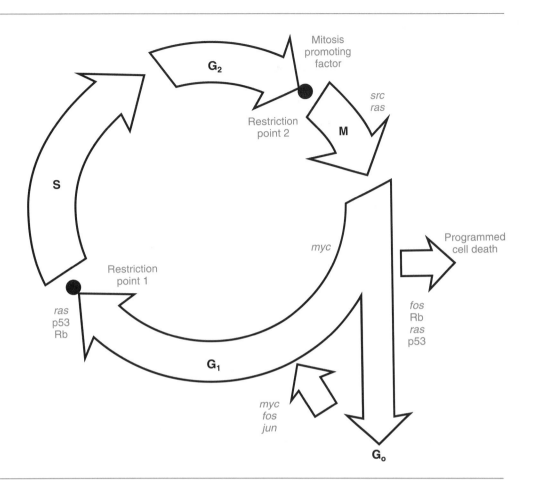

Figure 3.3.   The regulation of the cell cycle by proto-oncogenes and tumor suppressor genes. (Reproduced, with permission, from Baker V: Oncogenes and tumor suppressor genes in gynecologic cancer. *Contemp Obstet Gynecol* Sept.: 75, 1992.)

Table 3.2   Selected Peptide Growth Factors and Their Receptors

Growth Factor	Molecular Weight (Kd)	Receptor	Receptor Kinase Activity	Molecular Weight (Kd)
EGF	6	EGF receptor	Tyrosine	170
TGF-α	6	EGF receptor	Tyrosine	170
TGF-β	26	TGF-β receptor	Serine	53
PDGF	28–35	PDGF receptor	Tyrosine	160–180
FGF (acidic)	15.5	FGF receptor	Tyrosine	125
FGF (basic)	18–29	FGF receptor	Tyrosine	125
IGF	7.5	IGF receptor (α, β)	Tyrosine	130, 95
M-CSF	70	*fms*	Tyrosine	165
c-*erb*B-2 ligands	30	c-*erb*B-2	Tyrosine	185
	5	c-*erb*B-2	Tyrosine	185

are polypeptides that regulate cell proliferation by binding to specific cell surface receptor proteins that have intracellular domains with tyrosine or serine/threonine kinase activity. Peptide growth factors can initiate autocrine or paracrine growth regulation of normal or malignant cells (Fig. 3.4). In *autocrine growth regulation,* the growth factor is produced by the cell that it regulates. In *paracrine growth stimulation,* the growth factor is produced by a neighboring cell. Different autocrine and paracrine factors can either stimulate or inhibit growth of cells. In benign and some malignant epithelial cells, *transforming growth factor-alpha (TGF-α)* and the *epidermal growth factor (EGF)* stimulate proliferation, whereas *transforming growth factor-beta (TGF-β)* inhibits proliferation.

Both EGF and TGF-α must bind to the *epidermal growth factor receptor (EGFR)* to stimulate epithelial cell growth. Malignant ovarian epithelial cells are less responsive to EGF than normal ovarian epithelial cells *in vitro* (12), but cancer cells that maintain functional EGFR can still be stimulated by EGF or TGF-α. As some ovarian cancer cells can produce TGF-α, autocrine growth stimulation could drive proliferation of those cancers that express both EGFR and TGF-α. Consistent with this possibility, antibodies that neutralize TGF-α have been shown to inhibit growth of ovarian cancer cell lines (13).

Normal and malignant endometrium express EGFR and the receptor for *insulin-derived growth factor (IGFR)* (14,15). In endometrial cancers, hormones can modulate the response to peptide growth factors. Progesterone treatment of endometrial gland cultures increases expression of both EGFR and IGFR (16). Squamous cell carcinoma of the cervix, carcinoma *in situ,* and dysplastic epithelium have higher levels of EGFR expression than does normal cervical epithelium (17).

TGF-β inhibits the growth of epithelial cells. Many epithelial cancers have lost responsiveness to the inhibitory effects of TGF-β. An autocrine growth inhibitory pathway initiated by TGF-β can be lost in ovarian cancer. Normal ovarian epithelial cultures are regularly inhibited by TGF-β and produce active TGF-β (18), whereas ovarian cancer cells are often refractory to inhibition with exogenous TGF-β, fail to express TGF-β, or produce inactive TGF-β. A fraction of endometrial cancer cell lines are also refractory to inhibition with TGF-β (19). *Fibroblast growth factor (FGF)* and *platelet-derived growth factor (PDGF)* have stimulated cancers that arise at other sites, but a role in gynecologic malignancies has yet to be documented.

Oncogenes in Gynecologic Cancers

Expression of different oncogenes and tumor suppressor genes has been observed in gynecologic cancers. Oncogenes can be analyzed for amplification, deletion, or rearrangement of DNA by *Southern blot analysis*. DNA from cancer tissue is digested with restriction endonucleases, electrophoresed and transferred to a nitrocellulose or nylon membrane by capillary diffusion. Radiolabeled nucleic acid sequences that are complementary to the oncogene sequences are incubated with the membrane, permitting specific binding. After washing, the membrane is autoradiographed to reveal oncogene sequences present in the cancer that have bound the specific DNA probe.

The level of expression of oncogenic RNA is analyzed by *northern blotting*. This technique is analogous to Southern blotting except that RNA rather than

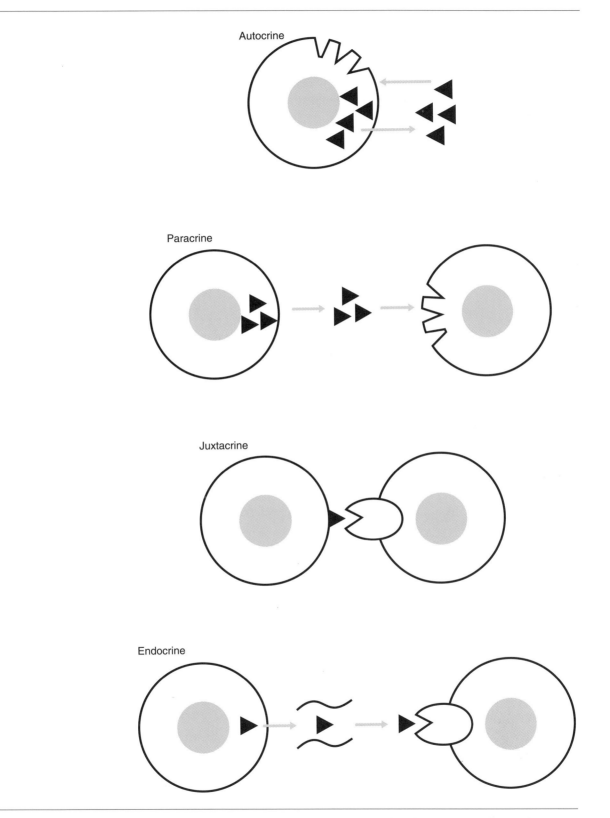

Figure 3.4.   Autocrine, paracrine, juxtacrine, and endocrine growth regulation. In autocrine growth regulation the growth factor is produced by the same cell it regulates, whereas in paracrine growth regulation the growth factor is produced by a neighboring cell. Juxtacrine growth regulation requires direct cell-to-cell contact as compared with classic endocrine growth regulation.

DNA is electrophoresed, transferred to a solid support, and hybridized to the radiolabeled nucleic acid sequences specific for the oncogene. Endonuclease digestion is not required. If antibodies that bind to the proteins encoded by oncogenes or tumor suppressor genes are available, expression of these products by cancer cells can be evaluated by immunohistochemical staining of frozen or paraffin-embedded tissue sections.

Oncogenes that encode membrane spanning *tyrosine kinase growth factor receptors* have been detected in several different gynecologic cancers. In the case of EGFR, c-*erb*B-2, and *fms,* tumors are thought to express both the receptors and their ligands, permitting autocrine growth stimulation. The EGFR has been found in normal ovarian surface epithelium and continued expression of EGFR has been associated with a poor prognosis in ovarian cancer (20). Approximately one-third of ovarian cancers overexpress the c-*erb*B-2 gene product that resembles the EGFR but has different ligands and a different amino acid sequence (Fig. 3.5) (21, 22).

Overexpression of c-*erb*B-2 (p185) is also associated with a poor prognosis in ovarian cancer (21, 22). The recently described p30 and p75 ligands stimulate anchorage independent growth of cells expressing p185 at low concentration and are inhibitory at high concentration (23, 24). More studies are needed to define the distribution and activities of ligands that bind to p185, but the poor prognosis associated with overexpression of p185 in ovarian and breast cancers may be related to an aberrant growth regulatory pathway. Overexpression of c-*erb*B-2 by endometrial cancers has been observed less frequently (9%) but, when present, has generally been associated with advanced-stage disease (25).

Figure 3.5. Oncogene encoding a tyrosine kinase growth factor receptor. In expression of c-*erb* B-2 and *fms,* the oncogene expression activates both the receptors and their ligands. (Reproduced, with permission, from Berchuck A, Bast RC: Overexpression of HER-2/*neu* in gyn cancer. *Contemp Obstet Gynecol,* March: 25, 1992.)

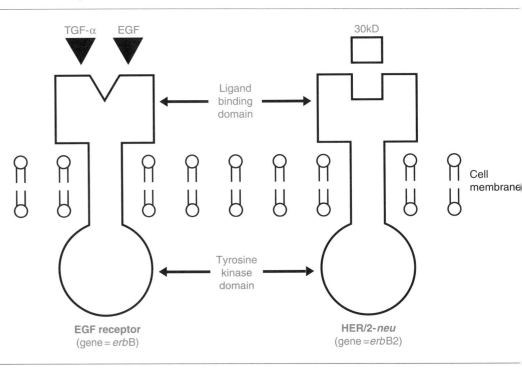

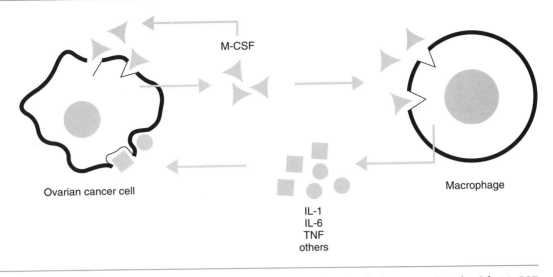

Figure 3.6. Autocrine and paracrine growth stimulation associated with M-CSF binding to the *fms* receptor. Note interaction of cytokines M-CSF, TNF-α, IL-1, and IL-6.

Expression of *fms* has been associated with clinically aggressive endometrial and ovarian cancers (26, 27). A majority of ovarian and endometrial cancers also express *macrophage colony stimulating factor (M-CSF)*. Autocrine growth stimulation may occur when endogenously produced M-CSF binds to the *fms* receptor. In addition to its possible role as an autocrine growth factor, M-CSF released by tumor cells can recruit macrophages to produce paracrine growth factors including *interleukin 1 (IL-1), tumor necrosis factor-α (TNF-α)* and *interleukin 6 (IL-6)* (Fig. 3.6) (28, 29). Besides stimulating proliferation of ovarian cancer cells, IL-1 also induces production of TNF-α messenger RNA and protein (30). Because TNF-α itself stimulates growth of ovarian cancer cells, TNF-α may function as both an autocrine and a paracrine growth factor in ovarian cancer (30).

Among the oncogenes that encode cytoplasmic transducing proteins, mutations in the *ras* oncogene have been found in 40–50% of endometrial cancers (31). In cervical cancer, expression of *ras* protein has been associated with a higher incidence of lymph node metastasis (32). By contrast, in ovarian cancer, only 2–12% of tumors have had *ras* amplification or mutation (33). Among the nuclear binding proteins, overexpression of c-*myc* has been observed in about 30% of cervical cancers and in early-stage patients has been related to a higher risk of relapse (34). Although c-*myc* can be amplified in 23% of ovarian cancers, no consistent prognostic significance has been found.

Tumor Suppressor Genes in Gynecologic Cancer

There have been fewer studies of tumor suppressor genes such as Rb and p53 in gynecologic cancers. Homozygous deletion of the endogenous Rb tumor suppressor gene has not been observed in gynecologic cancers (35). Sequences of human papilloma virus (HPV) types 16 and 18 are found in more than 80% of cervical carcinomas (36). HPV 16 and 18 contain two genes, E6 and E7, with transforming properties. The E6 and E7 gene products bind to the p53 and Rb tumor suppressor gene products, respectively, providing a means to inactivate p53 and Rb (37, 38). In those cervical cancers that lack expression of HPV proteins, mutant p53 has been detected. Consequently, interruption of growth regulation by p53 may occur in nearly all cervical cancers, either through infection with an oncogenic virus or through mutation of the host's endogenous p53 gene.

In ovarian and endometrial cancers, mutation of p53 may be a relatively late event that precedes metastasis. About half of stage II–IV ovarian cancers overexpress mutant p53 protein (39), whereas 14% of Stage I tumors have mutant p53 (40). In cases studied to date, the primary tumor and peritoneal metastases generally have had identical p53 mutations, consistent with a genetic alteration, before tumor spread (2). In endometrial cancers, p53 mutation has been observed more frequently in Stages III and IV (41%) than in Stage I disease (9%) (41).

Tumor-Associated Antigens

Tumor-Specific Antigens

Tumor immunology is based on the premise that tumors express unique antigens that are not found on normal cells and can be recognized as "foreign" by the host. Antigens that mediate tumor rejection have been defined only for animal tumors that can be transplanted between members of inbred strains. Some *tumor-specific transplantation resistance antigens* are proteins encoded by the oncogenic viruses that have transformed cells. Others arise during malignant transformation, through the inappropriate expression of endogenous host genes or the mutation of genes normally expressed by the host.

Immunity

Immunization of animals can be achieved by repeated injection of irradiated tumor cells or by excision of progressively growing tumor transplants. *Preimmunization* with tumor cells can protect inbred mice from subsequent injection of tumor cells that would grow progressively in nonimmune mice. *Tumor rejection* depends on immunologic recognition of antigens expressed by the cells used for immunization. *Immunity* is limited in strength, however, and resistance usually can be overcome by increasing the number of viable tumor cells used to challenge the immune animal.

Injection of *T lymphocytes*, but not immune serum, from immune donors, protects unimmunized animals from subsequent tumor challenge, indicating that T lymphocytes are critical for tumor-specific transplantation resistance (42). T lymphocytes recognize many foreign antigens at the cell surface in association with the host's own *major histocompatibility complex antigens (MHC)* (43). MHC antigens on tumor cells are important for T cell recognition of virus-induced murine tumors (44) and are likely to be important in the recognition of tumors induced by other agents. If putative human tumor-specific antigens were individually specific to each neoplasm and were recognized in the context of "self-MHC" antigens, the *autologous* (i.e., the patient's own) tumor cells may be the best target for initiation or amplification of an immune response.

Different animal tumors can express a variety of tumor-specific antigens. Each tumor induced by a single chemical carcinogen has an individually specific antigen that mediates rejection only of the tumor used for immunization. All tumors induced by a single oncogenic virus can share antigens that mediate rejection of any tumor induced by the same virus. *Oncofetal antigens* sometimes are found on chemically induced tumors, and unique antigens also can be expressed by virally induced tumors.

Tumors vary widely in their *immunogenicity*, ranging from strongly immunogenic to nonimmunogenic. *Tumor-specific transplantation resistance* originally was demonstrated with strongly immunogenic murine tumors induced by chemicals or viruses. Among spontaneously arising rat tumors, however, tumor-specific antigens have been expressed in only 16% (45). It is not known whether human tumors resemble the strongly *immunogenic* murine tumors induced by viruses or chemicals or whether they resemble the more weakly immunogenic "spontaneous" tumors induced by unknown agents.

Specific Immunotherapy

Strategies for *specific immunotherapy* of human cancer may apply only to those few patients whose tumors express the relevant antigens. *Tumor-associated antigens* may be recognized in the context of the patient's own MHC antigens. Components present on autologous tumor cells may be required to prepare relevant vaccines. Specific immunotherapy is most likely to eliminate small numbers of tumor cells in an adjuvant setting.

Clinically, transplantation of viable tumor cells is not an acceptable approach to demonstrate whether tumor-specific antigens are associated with human tumors. Efforts to detect tumor-specific antigens on human tumors have included *in vivo* skin testing with tumor extracts as well as *in vitro* assays using lymphoid cells and sera. Some cancer patients have had delayed cutaneous reactions toward extracts of their own tumors. However, autologous normal tissue extracts are not always available for testing. As tumor extracts contain a complex mixture of antigens, it is not clear whether the responses they elicit are tumor specific. Immunization with a vaccine containing autologous colorectal cancer cells and *bacillus Calmette-Guerin (BCG)* has enhanced skin test reactivity to autologous tumor extracts but not to extracts of autologous normal bowel mucosa (46). Genes for human tumor-associated antigens have now been cloned into vaccinia virus vectors to permit immunization with a single defined human protein at the site of an immune response to the virus. Immunogenicity of tumor cells has also been enhanced by transfer of genes for different cytokines, including interleukin-2 (IL-2), interleukin-6 (IL-6), and gamma interferon. Whether such strategies will permit detection of latent antigens remains to be resolved.

Lymphocytes   Lymphocytes from about 70% of patients with a variety of cancers proliferate when mixed with *autologous* tumor cells *in vitro* (47). In about 35% of cases, cancer patients' lymphocytes can kill fresh autologous tumor cells (48). *Allogeneic* (i.e., other donor) tumor cells have been lysed in as few as 7% of cases (48).The question of whether lymphocytes react only with tumor cells has remained unresolved because autologous normal tissues usually are not available for testing. Proliferative responses to normal cells obtained from other autologous tissues sometimes have been observed (49).

Antibodies   Sera of cancer patients have been tested for antibodies that recognize tumor-specific antigens. Antibodies have been classified into three groups on the basis of whether they bind to autologous tumor cells alone, to autologous and allogeneic tumor cells of the same histologic type, or to a variety of normal as well as malignant cells (50). Antibodies to proteins from the human T cell leukemia virus, the Epstein-Barr virus, the herpes simplex virus, and the papillomavirus have been detected in serum from patients with malignancies that may be linked etiologically to these agents (51).

Oncofetal Antigens

Although tumor-specific transplantation antigens have not been demonstrated definitively in human tumors, a large number of antigens have been found in human neoplasms that also are detected in normal and fetal tissues. Expression of these antigens on other cell types does not necessarily preclude use of an antigen in diagnosis, monitoring, or treatment of cancer. Some tumor-associated antigens have been defined with the use of *polyclonal heteroantisera*, but the amount of antiserum usually has been limited, and reactivity of different antisera has not always been reproducible.

Monoclonal Antibodies

In the last decade, *monoclonal antibodies* have provided an unlimited supply of antibody with reproducible reactivity. These reagents have contributed greatly to the definition and biochemical characterization of tumor-associated antigens. Monoclonal antibodies of rodent origin do, however, have certain limitations. Murine monoclonal antibodies, for example, define only those tumor-associated antigens that can be recognized by the mouse as immunologically foreign. *Epitopes* (i.e., the specific molecular composition of the antigen) recognized by murine antibodies may or may not elicit an immune response in human beings (52). Monoclonal antibodies of human origin have been more difficult to generate.

In addition to facilitating the isolation and biochemical characterization of tumor-associated antigens, monoclonal antibodies have permitted studies of their cellular localization and functional significance. Antigens expressed at the cell surface are thought to be particularly important as targets for antibody binding *in situ*. Whether a cell surface antigen is shed or is engulfed by the cell can affect its usefulness as a target for immunodiagnosis or immunotherapy. Patterns of monoclonal antibodies are beginning to distinguish subsets of neoplasms, only some of which correspond to conventional histopathologic categories.

Major Histocompatibility Complex (MHC) Antigens of Gynecologic Cancers

MHC antigens in human beings are distributed widely on body cells. *Class I MHC antigens (HLA-A, B, and C)* are found on almost all body cells, whereas *class II MHC antigens (HLA-DR, DP, and DQ)* have a more restricted distribution, being limited largely to lymphoreticular and endothelial cells. Both class I and class II MHC antigens are important for recognition of foreign antigens by T lymphocytes (53). Endogenous peptides produced by tumor cells are recognized in association with class I MHC antigens on the tumor cell surface, whereas exogenous peptides shed by tumor cells can be recognized only after they associate with class II antigens of macrophages or other antigen-presenting cells. Among the T lymphocytes, CD4 cells recognize antigenic peptides in the context of class II MHC antigens and CD8 cells recognize antigenic peptides in the context of class I determinants. As both T cell subsets may be required for effective immunity, expression of both class I and class II determinants within tumors may be important. **Thus the expression of MHC molecules on tumors may influence immune recognition of tumor-associated antigens by the host. Normal epithelial cells express class I MHC determinants but usually do not express class II MHC antigens.**

Class I MHC

Class I MHC antigens are expressed by ovarian surface epithelium, stroma, and follicles, as well as by the epithelium and glands of the endometrium and the endocervix. In epithelial tumor tissues, expression of class I MHC antigens can be lost. Class I MHC antigens have been detected in only 80% of ovarian, 50% of endometrial, and 40% of cervical cancers (54, 55).

Class II MHC   Among gynecologic tissues, class II MHC antigens are found in endocervical and endometrial glands from some patients but not in the normal ovary. Anomalous expression of class II MHC has been observed in some epithelial cancers. Class II MHC antigens are expressed ectopically in 16–40% of epithelial ovarian cancers, 25% of endometrial carcinomas, and 20% of cervical cancers (54, 55). The increase of class II MHC antigen expression is most notable in epithelial ovarian carcinomas relative to normal ovarian epithelium (54). Changes in MHC expression by tumors may limit or enhance immune recognition by the host. Class II determinants also have been found in papillomavirus-infected cells and in cervical intraepithelial neoplasia (56). Inflammation, immunologic reactions, and hormonal stimuli induce expression of HLA-DR in epithelial tissue (55). *In vitro* treatment with gamma interferon can increase MHC antigen expression on a number of cell types, including epithelial cells.

In *gestational trophoblastic neoplasia (GTN)*, paternal MHC antigens could be highly specific markers, provided that the trophoblastic tissue expressed the antigens and that the maternal MHC antigens were phenotypically distinct. In a normal placenta, there are no detectable class I or II MHC antigens on the villous trophoblast from 7 weeks' gestation until term. Class I antigens are observed, however, on villous stromal cells just under the MHC-negative trophoblastic layer (57). Cytotrophoblastic cells derived from chorionic villi that infiltrate the decidua early in pregnancy are also MHC positive (57). Similarly, MHC antigens are detected on stromal cells but not on trophoblasts in chorionic villi from molar pregnancies (58). Even though MHC-positive stromal cells in the chorionic villi of both normal and molar pregnancies are shielded by the MHC-negative villous trophoblast, sensitization to paternal HLA antigens occurs, possibly by exposure to MHC-positive cytotrophoblastic cell columns, as evidenced by antibody formation to paternal antigens in primiparous women. Some choriocarcinomas express class I MHC antigens, although the strength of antigen expression varies among different tumor specimens and cell lines. The intensity of lymphocytic infiltration at the tumor-host interface has correlated with a good prognosis for patients with invasive moles (59).

Paternal polymorphic HLA antigen fragments have been identified in immune complexes from serum after chemotherapy-induced regression of trophoblastic tumors (60). The immune response to paternal MHC antigens often has been cited as one plausible explanation for the high rate of cures achieved by single-agent chemotherapy in GTN, even when widespread metastases have occurred (59). Several studies have evaluated MHC compatibility of patients with GTN and their partners, because it has been suggested that MHC compatibility might contribute to the development and/or progression of the disease. Greater MHC compatibility might prevent recognition and elimination of cells which bear paternal antigens, although recent data do not support this possibility (59).

Viral Antigens of Gynecologic Cancers   Human papillomavirus (HPV) DNA is integrated into the cellular DNA in cervical carcinomas but can remain extrachromosomal in condylomas. Papillomaviruses share a group-specific antigen and also have type-specific antigens. Immunologic techniques have proved useful in identifying viral products, and patients have recognized several viral proteins as foreign antigens. Antibodies against the E7 viral protein are observed more frequently in patients with cervical cancer than in control subjects. HSV-2 may be a cofactor in cervical carcinoma, perhaps potentiating the progression of HPV-induced lesions. An immune response to HSV-2–associated antigens has also been documented in a majority of patients with cervical cancer (61-63). The role of HPV and HSV-2 in cervical neoplasia is discussed in Chapter 6.

Oncofetal Antigens of Gynecologic Cancers

Tumors may express oncofetal antigens that are normally found in embryonic tissues but are not expressed in normal adult tissues. Oncofetal antigens associated with different gynecologic cancers include carcinoembryonic antigen (CEA), alpha-fetoprotein (AFP), human chorionic gonadotropin (hCG), and placental alkaline phosphatase (PLAP).

Carcinoembryonic Antigen

Carcinoembryonic antigen (CEA) is a protein that can be detected in low levels on normal adult colonic epithelium (64). CEA may be expressed and shed by adenocarcinomas originating at other sites, including ovary, cervix, breast, lung, bladder, and prostate. At a molecular level, CEA is related in structure to the immunoglobulins and may contribute to the adhesion of tumor cells to surrounding structures. **The incidence of CEA elevations in sera from patients with epithelial ovarian cancer is about 50%, but the serum levels usually are not sufficiently elevated to be of use for monitoring the clinical course of the disease** (65). Elevations of serum CEA more frequently are associated with advanced clinical stage, poorly differentiated neoplasms, and the mucinous histotype (65). In an immunohistologic study, CEA was found to be expressed in the majority of mucinous, endometrioid, or clear cell ovarian cancers, but in only 20% of serous cancers (65).

Alpha-fetoprotein

Alpha-fetoprotein (AFP) is a glycoprotein normally expressed by the fetus and reexpressed by hepatomas, testicular germ cell tumors, and certain ovarian germ cell tumors (66). AFP is a useful marker for monitoring germ cell tumors during therapy and often is expressed by embryonal tumors and endodermal sinus tumors. Fewer than 10% of epithelial ovarian cancers are AFP positive (67).

Human Chorionic Gonadotropin

The human chorionic gonadotropin (hCG) protein consists of two subunits, an α-chain that is shared with several other glycoprotein hormones and a β-chain that is unique to hCG (68). In addition to hydatidiform moles and choriocarcinomas, embryonal carcinomas with trophoblastic differentiation express hCG. Occasionally, hCG may be produced ectopically by squamous cervical cancers or by epithelial ovarian cancers (69).

Urinary Gonadotropin Peptide (UGP)

A 10 kd fragment of the hCG β-chain is expressed by most ovarian cancers and appears in the urine of 82% of patients with ovarian cancer. Complementarity with CA 125 has been reported (70).

Placental Alkaline Phosphatase

Another embryonic protein, *placental alkaline phosphatase (PLAP),* is expressed normally by the placenta and is found only in trace amounts in other normal tissues. Ectopic PLAP production has been reported in a variety of tumors, including cervical and epithelial ovarian carcinomas. With the use of sensitive monoclonal antibody–based radioimmunoassays, elevated serum PLAP levels have been detected in 30–60% of patients with ovarian cancer (71). In immunohistologic studies, anti-PLAP monoclonal antibodies have bound to most ovarian cancers (71). In normal ovaries, PLAP is found only in germinal cysts.

Antigens of Gynecologic Cancers

Antigens associated with gynecologic malignancies were first identified with *heteroantisera*, but more recent advances have depended on *monoclonal antibodies*.

TA-4

The *TA-4* (tumor-associated) antigen has been found in squamous cell carcinomas of the cervix. Immunohistologic studies also have detected small amounts of TA-4 on normal squamous epithelium (72). Elevated levels of TA-4 have been found in about 50% of patients with cervical cancer, and antigen levels have correlated with the clinical course of the disease (73).

CA 125

CA 125 was the first marker to be defined with a monoclonal antibody against epithelial ovarian cancer (74). The OC 125 monoclonal antibody that binds to the CA 125 antigen was produced by immunization of mice with a serous cystadenocarcinoma cell line. The CA 125 antigenic determinant is found on a high-molecular-weight mucinlike glycoprotein (75). **In immunohistologic studies, more than 80% of nonmucinous epithelial ovarian cancers express CA 125** (76). CA 125 antigen has been detected in amnion and in fetal tissues derived from coelomic epithelium, including müllerian duct, peritoneum, pleura, and pericardium (36). In normal adult tissues, epithelial cells of fallopian tubes, endometrium, and endocervix, as well as mesothelial cells lining the pleura, pericardium, and peritoneum express small amounts of CA 125. The surface epithelium of both the fetal and adult ovary appear to be negative (77).

CA 125 has been associated with molecules ranging from 200–1000 kd. The expression of multiple CA 125 determinants on each glycoprotein molecule has facilitated development of a radioimmunometric assay for quantitation of CA 125 antigen in serum and ascitic fluid (78–79). In the assay, a plastic bead coated with OC 125 antibody binds antigen in a patient's serum. Radiolabeled OC 125 antibody then is used to detect the bound antigen. Values in a patient's serum are compared with those obtained with a standard CA 125 preparation. **More than 80% of patients with ovarian cancer have CA 125 antigen levels > 35 units/ml compared with only 1% of normal persons** (78). Although antigen levels are highest in the sera of patients with ovarian cancer, they are not restricted to patients with this type of cancer. Elevated serum levels are found in a variety of gynecologic malignancies, including endometrial, fallopian tube, and endocervical carcinomas (80). In addition, 60% of patients with advanced pancreatic cancer have elevated serum CA 125 values, and a small fraction of patients with breast, lung, and colorectal cancer also can have elevated serum values (78). Consequently, CA 125 is not useful in distinguishing ovarian cancers from other neoplasms of unknown primary site.

When CA 125 antigen levels are determined before treatment and after treatment in patients with ovarian cancer, changes in antigen level have correlated with the course of the disease in about 90% of the patients (78, 81). Rising or persistently elevated CA 125 antigen levels provide 1–14 months' (median 3 months') lead time before recurrent ovarian cancer can be detected by noninvasive techniques (82). Elevated CA 125 levels at the time of a second-look surveillance operation predict the presence of persistent disease with 96% accuracy. The sensitivity of the test is limited in that CA 125 values < 35 units/ml are associated with persistent disease in 40–60% of cases, although the residual tumor nodules are usually < 1 cm in greatest diameter (83).

CA 125 has also proved useful in distinguishing malignant from benign pelvic masses (84-86). **A marked elevation of CA 125 (> 95 U/ml) is associated with a 96% positive predictive value in postmenopausal patients with an adnexal mass. The specificity of the test is lower in premenopausal patients, where elevation of CA 125 levels can occur in endometriosis, adenomyosis, uterine fibroids, salpingitis, first-trimester pregnancy, and apparently normal menstruation.** Elevations can also be observed with benign ascites, pancreatitis, liver disease, and renal failure.

Several observations suggest that the CA 125 assay may contribute to the early diagnosis of ovarian cancer. In a retrospective study of serum samples obtained from a patient before her clinical presentation with Stage III epithelial ovarian cancer, CA 125 antigen was elevated 10–12 months before diagnosis (87). A larger study using the Janus Serum Bank in Oslo, Norway, indicated that CA 125 was elevated in 50% of patients with ovarian cancer up to 18 months before diagnosis and in 25% up to 5 years before detection by conventional techniques (88). With regard to sensitivity, CA 125 can detect approximately 60% of patients with Stage I or II disease (81). A false-positive rate of 0.6% has been found in a population of postmenopausal nuns with a mean age similar to that found in patients with ovarian cancer (89). Greater specificity can be attained by combining CA 125 with ultrasound (90) or by following CA 125 over time (91). In screening studies in Sweden and the United Kingdom, CA 125 has been used to trigger transabdominal sonography (92, 93). A manageable number of elevated CA 125 values (> 30 U/ml) were observed in each study (2%), 14 cases of ovarian were detected among 27,000 women screened, and no more than four laparotomies were performed to diagnose each case. Recent advances in transvaginal sonography suggest that this modality may have > 95% sensitivity for early-stage disease, but some 10–15 laparotomies may be required to diagnose each case of malignancy when this technique of screening is applied. **Given the false-positive values with either CA 125 or transvaginal sonography, particularly in a premenopausal population, neither test should be used routinely to screen apparently healthy women for ovarian cancer.** Each modality may, however, contribute to a screening strategy that will prove feasible and cost-effective.

Other Antigens

Use of other antigenic markers in combination with CA 125 may increase the sensitivity of the test. Several other monoclonal antibodies have been generated against ovarian tumor–associated antigens, including NB/70K (94), HMFG2 (95), PLAP (95), and UGP (70). The use of CA 125 in combination with each of these assays has been reported to be slightly, but significantly, more sensitive than any single assay. Recent studies suggest that a combination of CA 125, macrophage colony stimulating factor (96), and OVX1 (97), a mucin determinant, can detect 98% of Stage I ovarian cancers with a false-positive rate of 12%. If these markers can detect preclinical disease, a combination of blood tests might be used to trigger transvaginal sonography, reducing the need for this modality and the consequent false-positive evaluations by an order of magnitude.

Immunohistochemical determination of estrogen receptors (ER) from endometrial cancers with the use of monoclonal antibodies has permitted studies of receptor expression by individual endometrial tumor cells (98). Immunocytochemical assays for EGFR (14), p185 [c-erbB-2] (25) and the *fms* gene product (26) have had prognostic significance in retrospective studies. Thus murine monoclonal antibodies have identified a number of tumor-associated antigens expressed by epithelial ovarian carcinomas. Virtually all of the antibodies that have been characterized recognize antigens not restricted to malignant cells.

Immunologic Interactions Between Tumor and Host

Cellular and Humoral Immunity

Lymphocytes are the primary regulators of the immune response. They are the only cell type that retains "immunologic memory" for prior exposure to foreign antigens.

On the basis of *phenotypic* and *functional* characteristics, lymphocytes can be divided into two main classes: *T cells* and *B cells*. All blood cells, including T and B lymphocytes, are derived from pluripotent stem cells in the bone marrow. T (or thymus-derived) lymphocytes differentiate under the influence of the thymus. In chickens, the bursa of Fabricius directs differentiation of B lymphocytes. In mammals, the organ that influences B cell differentiation is thought to be the bone marrow.

B Lymphocytes

B lymphocytes are the only cells that synthesize antibody. Plasma cells represent the final stage of B cell differentiation and are capable of secreting large quantities of immunoglobulin. Immunoglobulin is also found on the B cell surface, where it functions as an antigen receptor.

There are five classes of immunoglobulin that may be synthesized by B cells: IgM, IgG, IgA, IgD, and IgE (Table 3.3) (99). The basic immunoglobulin molecule consists of heavy and light polypeptide chains. The *heavy chains* (mu, gamma, alpha, delta, and epsilon) are unique to each immunoglobulin class, whereas the *light chains* (kappa and lambda) may be found in all classes (Fig. 3.7). However, a single immunoglobulin molecule will have light chains of only

Table 3.3   Selected Structural and Functional Properties of Human Immunoglobulins

Immunoglobulin	Heavy Chain	Light Chain	Molecular Weight ($\times 10^3$) (Daltons)	Serum Concentration (mg/ml)	Complement Activation (C1 Pathway)	Mediation of ADCC
IgG1	γ1	κ or λ	146	9	+ +	+
IgG2	γ2	κ or λ	146	3	+	−
IgG3	γ3	κ or λ	170	1	+ + +	+
IgG4	γ4	κ or λ	146	0.5	−	+ / −
IgM	μ	κ or λ	970	1.5	+ + +	−
IgA1	α1	κ or λ	160	3.0	−	−
IgA2	α2	κ or λ	160	0.5	−	−
IgD	δ	κ or λ	184	0.03	−	−
IgE	ϵ	κ or λ	188	0.00005	−	?

Adapted with permission of Grune and Stratton, Inc. From Turner MW: Immunoglobulins. In Holborow EJ, Reeves WG (eds): *Immunology in Medicine*, ed 2. London and New York, Academic Press, 1983.

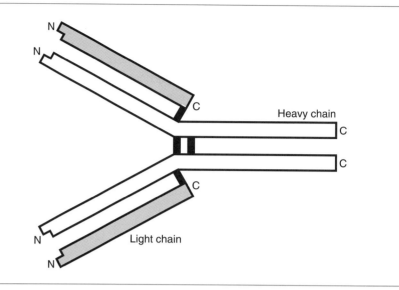

Figure 3.7. The basic immunoglobulin structure. The unit consists of two identical light polypeptide chains and two identical heavy polypeptide chains linked together by disulfide bonds (red). Note the position of the amino (*N*) and carboxyl (*C*) terminal ends of the peptide chains. (Redrawn, with permission, from Roitt I, et al: *Immunology.* St Louis, CV Mosby, 1985, p 5.1.)

one type, either kappa or lambda. Further subclasses of immunoglobulins (IgG1, IgG2, IgG3, IgG4, IgA1, and IgA2) are based on variations in the "constant" region of the heavy chain. *Constant regions* of the amino acid sequence are found near the carboxyl ends of both heavy and light chains. The constant regions of the heavy chains (*Fc region*) determine the biologic function of antibody molecules, including the ability to bind to complement and to *Fc receptors* on lymphoreticular cells. *Variable regions* of the amino acid sequence are found near the N terminal regions of both the heavy and light chains. These regions include three complementarity-determining regions (CDRs) that contribute to the antigen binding site.

As B cells mature, the genes encoding the variable and constant immunoglobulin regions for both the heavy and light chains are rearranged so that each B cell becomes committed to the production of immunoglobulin of a single specificity. It is estimated that more than 100,000 different antibody specificities can be produced. There are several mechanisms that generate antibody diversity during rearrangement of the immunoglobulin genes. The heavy-chain variable (V_H), diversity (D_H), joining (J_H), and constant (C_H) gene regions undergo somatic recombination to form a complete heavy-chain gene ($V_{HD\ HJ\ HC\ H}$). Similarly, somatic recombination of the light-chain variable (V_L), joining (J_L), and constant (C_L) regions produces a complete light-chain gene ($V_{LJ\ LC\ L}$). Variation in the site of recombination results in the addition of nucleotides (N regions) between joined segments in both heavy ($V_{HND\ HNJ\ HC\ H}$) and light ($V_{LNJ\ LNC\ L}$) chains. Different heavy and light chains can associate, generating new specificities. Finally, somatic mutation of CDRs also contributes to diversity. Mature B cells also express receptors for the Fc portion of immunoglobulin and the C3 component of complement. After exposure to specific antigen, B cells can differentiate further into plasma cells. Plasma cells produce memory B cells that can initiate an accelerated *anamnestic response* after a second exposure to the same antigen.

T Lymphocytes

T lymphocytes exhibit a characteristic cell surface phenotype and mediate cellular immunity (100). Development of a large number of monoclonal antibodies that recognize cell surface antigens has permitted the definition of subsets of T cells with distinct functional activities. The T cell receptor for foreign antigens is a molecule (Ti) that is associated with the CD3 cell surface determinant. Functional activities of T cells include proliferation in the presence of specific antigen, release of soluble mediators, and regulation of B cells, macrophages, and other T cells.

T cells can be divided into two major phenotypic subsets: _helper/inducer T cells (CD4)_ and _cytotoxic/suppressor T cells (CD8)._ They are acquired during maturation in the thymus. The CD4 subset contains T cells that provide "help" for the initiation of immunoglobulin synthesis by B cells, and they facilitate interactions with macrophages and other T cells. The CD8 molecule is expressed on cytotoxic T cells, which can bind and kill antigen-bearing target cells. CD8 also is expressed by suppressor T cells, which inhibit activities of other T cells and B cells. Helper/inducer T cells can be subdivided further into two functional subsets based on their production of different soluble factors. The _TH1 helper/inducer T cell subset_ releases interleukin-2 (IL-2) and gamma interferon (Γ-IF) and mediates delayed-type hypersensitivity reactions. The _TH2 helper/inducer T cell subset_ produces interleukin 4 (IL-4) or interleukin 5 (IL-5) and interacts with B lymphocytes to facilitate immunoglobulin synthesis (101).

Monocytes-Macrophages

Mononuclear cells of the monocyte-macrophage series are integrally involved in the generation of immune responses. Both blood monocytes and tissue macrophages express class II MHC antigens, complement receptors, and Fc receptors. Macrophages internalize antigen by phagocytosis, pinocytosis, or receptor-mediated endocytosis. After internalization, the antigen is partially degraded, producing antigenic fragments. The processed antigen is expressed in a highly immunogenic form on the macrophage surface in association with the class II MHC determinants. The appropriate antigen-specific T cell has the capacity to recognize a complex of antigen and the class II MHC antigens via its antigen receptor. The requirement of MHC antigens for appropriate recognition of apparently unrelated antigens has been termed _MHC restriction_ (43). The host's own MHC antigens are required because allogeneic macrophages are unable to mediate antigen presentation to T cells. T cells of the helper/inducer subset recognize antigen in the context of class II MHC molecules. The cytotoxic T cell, however, requires class I MHC determinants for recognition and subsequent killing of antigen-bearing target cells. In addition to their antigen-presenting function, macrophages have the capability to phagocytose and kill microorganisms. Macrophages can undergo differentiation to an activated state after exposure to mediators or to certain infectious agents and their products (102). Activated macrophages secrete additional cytokines and have heightened phagocytic and cytotoxic activities. In the activated state, macrophages are cytotoxic for tumor cells and can suppress lymphocyte proliferation.

Null Cells

Null cells are a subset of blood mononuclear cells that lack most cell surface markers characteristic of mature T cells, B cells, or monocytes. Fc receptors can, however, be expressed by null cells. This subset includes K cells, which mediate *antibody-dependent cell-mediated cytotoxicity (ADCC)*, a cytotoxic reaction in which IgG immunoglobulin binds an effector leukocyte to a target cell that bears an antigen recognized by the antibody. Large granular lymphocytes called *natural killer (NK) cells* mediate the killing of tumor cells and are also included among the null cells.

NK cells may express Fc receptors as well as certain T cell and monocyte/granulocyte markers, but NK cells do not belong to any of the classically defined T lymphocyte or monocyte subsets (103). The T cell receptor genes are not rearranged in NK cells. Most NK cells express the CD56 and CD57 cell surface markers. NK cells kill certain tumor cells without prior exposure to tumor cell antigens by a mechanism involving direct cell contact and release of NK granule contents. Because NK cells have Fc receptors, they can also function as ADCC effector cells in the presence of antibody-coated target cells. The human IgG3 isotype is the most effective immunoglobulin for mediating ADCC. Murine IgG2a and IgG3 are also capable of mediating ADCC with human effectors (104). A summary of four different types of cell binding in cell-mediated cytotoxicity is presented in Figure 3.8.

Figure 3.8. Cell-mediated cytotoxicity: four different types of cell binding in cell-mediated cytotoxicity. (1) Cytotoxic T cells (Tc) bind their target while recognizing antigen and MHC determinants. (2) NK cells recognize determinants expressed on neoplastic cells. (3) K cells recognize the Fc of IgG antibody bound to antigen on the target cell surface. (4) Experimentally, glycoproteins on the surface of effector and target can be cross-linked by lectins. (Redrawn, with permission, from Roitt I, et al: *Immunology.* St Louis, CV Mosby, 1985, p 11.5.)

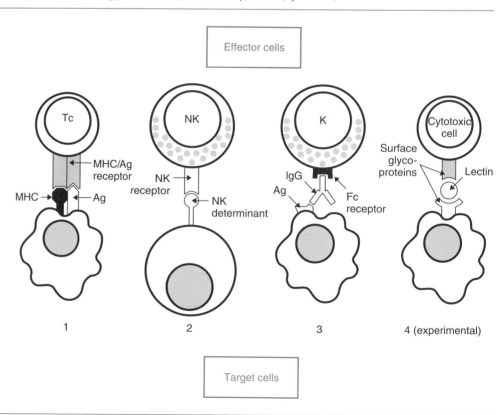

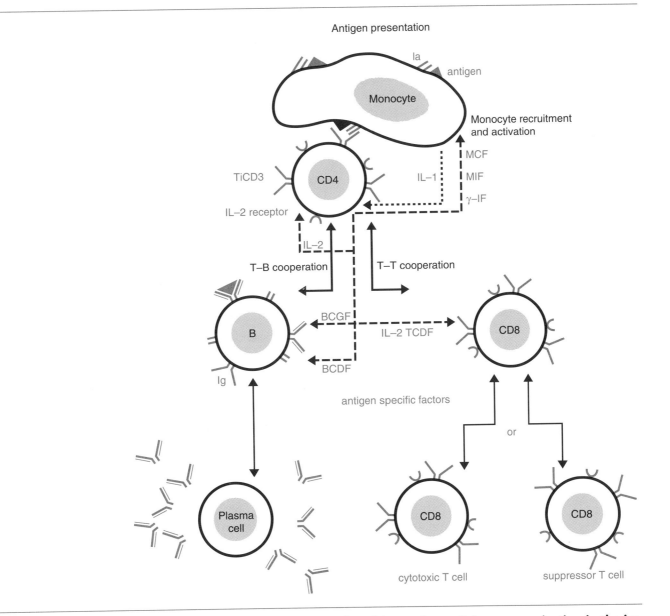

Antigen presentation

Figure 3.9. Scope of cell-mediated immunity: cellular communication in the immune response via interleukins. γ-*IFN*, gamma interferon; *IL-1*, interleukin-1; *IL-2*, interleukin-2; *IL-3*, interleukin-3; *IL-4*, interleukin-4; *IL-5*, interleukin-5; *IL-6*, interleukin-6; *IG*, immunoglobulin.

Cytokines

A variety of soluble mediators (cytokines) produced by lymphoreticular cells are responsible for cell-cell communication during immune responses (Fig. 3.9) (105). A number of cytokines with defined activities have been characterized biochemically. A summary of cell-mediated immunity and intercellular communication with cytokines is presented in Figure 3.9.

Interleukins

Macrophages produce *interleukin 1 (IL-1)* when the T cell antigen receptor interacts with antigen class II MHC complexes on the macrophage surface. The IL-1 molecule released by the macrophage induces the T lymphocyte to express a cell surface receptor for interleukin 2 (IL-2). These events lead to synthesis of *interleukin 2 (IL-2)*, a growth factor produced by T cells that drives the proliferation of T cells bearing IL-2 receptors, resulting in clonal expansion of the responding T cells. In addition to the IL-2 receptor, activated T cells express other cell-surface markers not found on resting T cells, including class II MHC molecules, transferrin receptor, and several antigens restricted to activated T cells. After activation, T cells of the helper/inducer subset produce a large number of mediators in addition to IL-2.

At least 13 different interleukins have now been described. Different interleukins affect T or B lymphocyte function and attract or activate different hematopoietic cells. *Interleukins 4, 5, and 6* were originally described on the basis of their effects on B lymphocyte proliferation and differentiation. Interleukins 4 and 6 also affect differentiation of T lymphocytes. *Interleukin 3 (IL-3)*, which is synthesized by activated T cells, stimulates differentiation of hematopoietic stem cells (106).

Interferons

Interferons are produced in response to viral infection and can protect previously uninfected cells. The *three major classes of interferons (alpha, beta, and gamma)* can be distinguished by molecular weight, cell source, and biologic activity (107). *Leukocyte interferon alpha* is encoded by as many as 12 different genes expressed by a variety of cell types. *Beta and gamma interferons* are produced by fibroblasts and activated T cells, respectively. One of the primary T cell mediators responsible for macrophage activation is gamma (or immune) interferon. Interferons can enhance expression of cell-surface MHC antigens. Increased MHC antigen expression may facilitate the antiviral immune response, as viral antigens are recognized in association with self-MHC antigens. Interferons also can enhance the cytotoxic activity of NK cells and inhibit the proliferation of some tumor cells *in vitro*. Inhibition of tumor growth by interferons has been observed less frequently *in vivo*.

Tumor Necrosis Factor and Lymphotoxin

Tumor necrosis factor (TNF-α) and *lymphotoxin (TNF-β)* are two additional cytokines that may have cytotoxic activity for tumor cells (108). TNF-β is produced by lectin-activated lymphocytes, whereas TNF-α is released by lipopolysaccharide-activated macrophages. TNF-α causes hemorrhagic necrosis of human and murine tumor grafts and is cytotoxic or cytostatic for certain tumor cell lines *in vitro*. Synergistic *in vitro* cytotoxicity for tumor cells has been observed with TNF and interferon.

Idiotype

Antigen-specific factors produced by activated T cells may have activities that either enhance or suppress immune responses to specific antigens. Immune responses involve complex pathways in which soluble mediators and lymphoreticular cells influence the level and duration of the response. The antigen receptors (immunoglobulin and Ti-CD3 complex) that initiate specific immune responses are themselves antigenic in that they express highly variable amino acid sequences in the antigen-binding region. These regions are referred to collectively as the *idiotype* of the antigen receptor, and each can induce specific cellular and humoral *anti-idiotypic immunity*. The *anti-idiotypic receptors* are likewise antigenic and similarly lead to induction of specifically reactive antibody and lymphocytes (109). In this way, an interacting network of anti-idiotypic receptors that can upregulate or downregulate specific immune responses is produced.

Mechanisms of Tumor Cell Killing

Tumor cells can be destroyed by several immune mechanisms, including cell-mediated cytotoxicity by T cells, macrophages, natural killer (NK), or lymphokine-activated killer (LAK) cells, and antibody-mediated cytotoxicity in the presence of complement components or Fc receptor-bearing effector cells.

Antibody-Mediated

Antibody-mediated mechanisms of tumor cell killing include both complement-dependent cytotoxicity and antibody-mediated cellular cytotoxicity (ADCC).

Complement (C') is a set of nine serum proteins (C1 to C9) that interact in a sequence to mediate tumor cell lysis. Antibody bound to a tumor cell can bind the first component of complement (C1) to the constant region of the immunoglobulin heavy chain. Human immunoglobulins of the IgM and some IgG classes are capable of binding C1. IgG1 and IgG3 human immunoglobulins can mediate ADCC, but IgM is ineffective.

For *ADCC*, antibodies facilitate interaction of effector leukocytes with tumor cells. Two types of ADCC have been described:

1. In the first, antibody binds to the tumor cell and subsequently binds to effector leukocytes that bear receptors for the Fc portion of the IgG heavy chains. A number of Fc receptor–positive cells may function as ADCC effectors, including macrophages, null cells, and granulocytes.

2. Alternatively, effectors may become "armed" by the binding of antibody to Fc receptors. Armed effectors can then bind to tumor cells through the antigen-combining site formed by the variable regions of the IgG heavy and light chains.

In either case, immunoglobulin serves as a bridge assuring close association between effectors and targets. Effector cells can also be activated by these interactions. Binding of activated effectors damages the tumor target-cell membrane. Antibody-mediated mechanisms of tumor cell destruction may be blocked by soluble tumor antigens that can bind antibody in plasma to form immune complexes, preventing unbound antibody from reaching antigens on the tumor cell surface. In addition, levels of ADCC effector cells may be reduced in the blood of cancer patients and at the tumor site.

T Lymphocyte–Mediated

Transfer of T lymphocytes can confer tumor-specific immunity in murine tumor models. Both helper/inducer and cytotoxic/suppressor T-cell subsets have been required to transfer immunity in some tumor systems, whereas helper/inducer T cells are sufficient in others (42). Mononuclear cells associated with ovarian cancers are primarily T lymphocytes, and both helper/inducer and cytotoxic/suppressor subsets are present (54). Helper/inducer T cells have been observed at the implantation site of invasive moles in a pattern similar to that observed during rejection of histoincompatible allografts (60). The mechanism of T cell killing requires direct contact with the target cells through specific receptors. Irreversible membrane damage and loss of osmotic integrity result from a process that has not been completely defined. Release of mediators such as TNF-β or porphyrin, direct membrane-membrane interaction, transmembrane signaling that triggers autodestruction, or the activity of phospholipase may be involved (110).

Natural Killer (NK) Cell–Mediated

Natural killer (NK) cells destroy tumor cells by non-MHC–restricted direct contact, which does not require sensitization to a specific tumor-associated antigen. Autologous, allogeneic, or xenogeneic tumor targets, as well as virus-infected cells, are NK sensitive. The recognition structure(s) that allows NK cells to distinguish tumor from most normal target cells has not yet been defined. NK cells are found primarily in the blood and spleen, but few have been observed in most human tumors. **NK cytotoxicity can be augmented with interferons and IL-2, which suggests that NK cells may mediate some of the antitumor activity produced by agents that induce interferon production.** Down-regulation of NK activity has been observed with cytoxan, corticosteroids, and prostaglandins. Recently NK cells have been shown to secrete a number of cytokines, including interleukins, interferons, natural killer cytotoxic factor, lymphotoxin, colony-stimulating factor, and B cell growth factor. A schematic presentation of the regulatory mechanisms that influence NK cell activity is presented in Figure 3.10.

Lymphokine-Activated Killer (LAK) Cell–Mediated

Exposure of peripheral blood mononuclear cells *in vitro* to certain lectins, alloantigens, or interleukin-2 (IL-2) induces a population of cytotoxic effectors called lymphokine-activated killer (LAK) cells (111). **LAK cells are cytotoxic**

Figure 3.10. Schematic representation of IL-2 (TCGF), IFN, and T cell regulatory mechanisms influencing NK cell activity. The proliferation of NK cells is under T cell control. IL-2 also may induce proliferation and stimulate the NK activity of proliferating NK cells. Interferon (IFN) induces expression of IL-2 receptors on the NK progenitor, enhancing proliferation; however, IFN also feeds back on T cells to reduce their activity. (Redrawn, with permission, from Roitt I, et al: *Immunology*. St Louis, CV Mosby, 1985, p 18.5.)

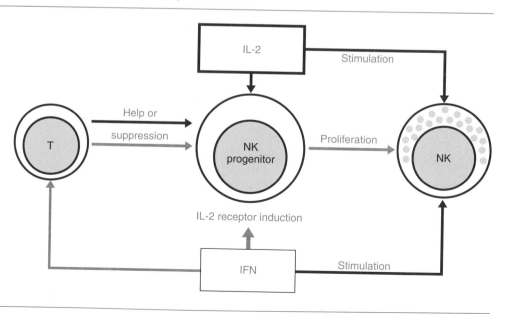

for a wide variety of fresh and cultured tumor cells but not for normal cells. By phenotypic and functional criteria, LAK cells are distinct from NK cells or cytotoxic T cells. LAK cells can lyse certain NK-resistant targets and express some T cell surface markers. Systemic administration of LAK cells and IL-2 can cause regression of murine tumors and metastases. Similar treatment in human patients has produced temporary regression of metastatic melanoma and renal cell carcinoma in 15–20% of patients.

Activated Macrophage–Mediated	Exposure of murine peritoneal macrophages to nonspecific immunostimulants such as *bacillus Calmette-Guerin (BCG)* or *Corynebacterium parvum (C. Parvum)* induces activated tumoricidal macrophages (102). Two signals are required to fully activate the tumoricidal function of macrophages. First, the nonspecific immunostimulants induce the release of endogenous gamma interferon that partially activates macrophages, which increases their ability to bind selectively to tumor cells. Subsequent exposure to a bacterial endotoxin (lipopolysaccharide) can provide a second signal that further increases the ability of macrophages to kill tumor cells. Activated macrophages secrete cytolytic proteases, which are thought to play a major role in tumoricidal activity. On the other hand, macrophages produce prostaglandins that inhibit many macrophage functions, as well as those of lymphocytes and NK cells.

The number of macrophages found in human tumors is highly variable, which may reflect variable amounts of chemotactic factors produced by lymphocytes or by tumor cells. Animal and human tumors may also produce factors that inhibit chemotaxis of macrophages, further limiting their accumulation. Therefore both the number of macrophages within tumors and their level of activation may be important in regulating tumor growth.

Immunocompetence of Patients With Gynecologic Cancer

Evaluation of the immunocompetence of patients with gynecologic cancer has been used to determine whether the tumor has compromised host immunity, to identify immune parameters that could supply prognostic information, and to provide a baseline for intervention with immunotherapy. Components of the immune response have been quantitated, and in some cases their function has been assessed. Peripheral blood leukocytes, lymphocyte subsets, and immunoglobulin levels have been measured. Functional assays performed *in vitro* have included *lymphocyte proliferation* triggered by antigens such as purified protein derivative (PPD) or mitogens such as phytohemagglutinin (PHA) and pokeweed mitogen (PWM). *In vivo* function of T cells and monocytes has been evaluated with delayed-hypersensitivity skin tests evoked by ubiquitous microbial antigens or contact allergens such as dinitrochlorobenzene (DNCB). Production of antibody after immunization with novel antigens such as keyhole-limpet hemocyanin (KLH) has been used to assess B cell function. Response to antigens derived from gynecologic cancers has been studied to determine whether these determinants are recognized by the host. Studies have been complicated by the complex nature of the antigens used and the difficulty of obtaining appropriate controls.

In addition to the tumor burden itself, the patient's age, nutritional status, and performance status may affect immunocompetence. If the patient with cancer has received prior therapy, the effect of therapy must also be considered in evaluating immune function. Chemotherapy, radiotherapy, and surgery may affect immunocompetence, although the selectivity for certain immune components and the duration of the effects vary, depending on the agent.

Nonspecific Immunocompetence

Increasing tumor burden has been associated with decreasing immunocompetence of cancer patients. Certain histologic tumor types have been associated with selective defects in T cells, B cells, monocytes, or granulocytes. *T cell and monocyte function* are impaired in patients with disseminated carcinoma, whereas leukemias have often been associated with granulocyte defects. *B cell function* is impaired in patients with untreated ovarian cancer (112). Proliferation to PWM and the primary antibody response to KLH are reduced as compared with responses by normal controls. In early-stage ovarian cancer, T cell function is often normal when measured by lymphocyte proliferation assays *in vitro* or by delayed cutaneous reactivity to recall microbial antigens *in vivo* (113). Delayed cutaneous responses to contact allergens such as DNCB are impaired in most patients with advanced ovarian, cervical, and endometrial cancers. Reactivity declines with advancing stage, and anergy is associated with a poor prognosis (113).

Given recent data that link human papillomavirus (HPV) with cervical cancer, the increased frequency of warts observed in immunosuppressed persons is of interest. An intense lymphoreticular cell infiltrate is associated with regressing HPV lesions, suggesting that the host response may be important in preventing progression of virus-induced tumors. Women who have genital papillomas with at least one intraepithelial or invasive lesion have fewer helper T cells, more cytotoxic/suppressor T cells, and a more modest T cell proliferative response than do women without those lesions (114). Patients with GTN have decreased numbers of both helper and cytotoxic/suppressor T cells when compared with normal persons (115), although fewer helper T cells are also found in normal pregnancy.

NK Activity

In vitro cell-mediated cytotoxicity assays have been used to characterize effector activities in mononuclear cells from gynecologic cancer patients (116–118). In most cases, cancer cell lines of various histologic origins have been used as targets. Mononuclear cells isolated from peripheral blood, ascitic fluid, and solid tumors of patients with ovarian cancer have lower levels of NK activity than do mononuclear cells isolated from normal peripheral blood (117). Although fresh ovarian tumor cells are relatively NK-resistant, effector lymphocytes treated with interferon have low levels of cytotoxic activity for autologous or allogeneic ovarian tumor cells (117–122).

ADCC Activity

ADCC activity in the peripheral blood of ovarian cancer patients is comparable to that found in normal peripheral blood. ADCC effector cells are present in ascitic fluid from most patients with ovarian cancer, but, depending on the target cell used, macrophages isolated from solid ovarian tumors may lack ADCC activity (123).

Monocytes/Macrophages   Blood monocytes and ascitic macrophages from patients with ovarian cancer have cytotoxic activities similar to normal blood monocytes or peritoneal macrophages from patients with benign gynecologic disease (124). Some ovarian tumor cells are not susceptible to *macrophage-mediated cytotoxicity*. Macrophage-derived factors can stimulate the growth of ovarian tumor cells *in vitro* (125). Tumor-derived soluble factors also affect macrophage activities. Two factors with counteracting activities have been described, sometimes coexisting in the same cancer-cell culture supernatants. P15E, a tumor-derived product related to the retroviral transmembrane protein, inhibits the chemotactic response of monocytes. Ovarian cancer cell lines and short-term cultures of ovarian tumor also produce a protein with chemotactic activity for macrophages (126). The number of macrophages found in tumors is highly variable and may be regulated by the interaction of both tumor-derived and host-derived factors.

Specific Immunocompetence   Gynecologic cancers may be infiltrated with lymphoreticular cells (54), but there is no direct evidence that lymphocytic infiltration represents a tumor-specific immune response that limits tumor growth. Alternatively, tumor-associated lymphoreticular cells may provide an environment conducive to enhanced tumor growth. T cells are the most prevalent mononuclear cells infiltrating ovarian, cervical, and endometrial carcinomas. Both the helper/inducer and cytotoxic/suppressor subsets are found within these tumors (53, 54). Helper/inducer T cells are predominant at the implantation site of invasive moles (59). In contrast, B cells outnumber T cells in cervical condylomas with or without cervical intra-epithelial neoplasia (127).

In early studies, lymphocytes from patients with ovarian or cervical cancer proved cytotoxic or cytostatic *in vitro* for allogeneic ovarian or cervical cancer cell lines. Patient serum or tumor-cell culture supernatants could block the antitumor activity exerted by a patient's lymphocytes. NK cells from a proportion of healthy persons are also toxic for tumor cell lines, but fresh autologous tumor cell targets are less sensitive to NK cytotoxicity. Peripheral blood or tumor-derived lymphocytes from patients with ovarian cancer have low or undetectable cytotoxicity for autologous tumor cells. Antigen-specific T cell cytotoxicity may be difficult to detect in peripheral blood or lymph node populations because of an admixture of low numbers of specific T cells with larger numbers of T cells exhibiting different specificity. The availability of IL-2 has permitted clonal expansion of individual T cell clones, making possible the evaluation of T cells present at low frequency. An average of 30% of T cell clones cultured in the presence of IL-2 from ovarian ascitic T cells have cytotoxic activity for autologous tumor cells (128). Some clones also have NK activity, but few are cytotoxic for fresh allogeneic ovarian tumor cells.

Several *in vivo* and *in vitro* assays have been used to determine lymphocyte reactivity in the presence of tumor cell extracts. Delayed cutaneous reactivity to autologous or allogeneic tumor extracts has been observed in a proportion of patients with ovarian and cervical carcinoma. Lymphocytes from patients with ovarian cancer in remission proliferate in culture when exposed to extracts of ovarian tumor or fetal ovary. Stimulation of lymphocytes from parous women provides further evidence of possible recognition of oncofetal antigens in proliferation assays (129).

Both *leukocyte migration inhibition (LMI)* and *leukocyte adherence inhibition (LAI)* assays are thought to be *in vitro* correlates of delayed cutaneous reactivity. Interpretation of the specificity of responses to complex mixtures of antigens in tumor extracts has been difficult. Use of purified antigens may help to define the specificity of the responding lymphocytes. The LMI assay measures the effect of migration-inhibition factor released by antigen-stimulated lymphocytes on the movement of leukocytes. Both autologous and allogeneic tumor extracts inhibit migration of leukocytes from patients with cervical and ovarian cancer in an organ site-specific pattern of reactivity (130, 131). In the LAI assay, lymphokine release by antigen-stimulated T cells causes leukocytes to lose glass adherence. The incubation of lymphocytes from patients with low-stage ovarian cancer with the purified NB/70K antigen results in a positive LAI assay in the majority of cases, whereas this is true in only 20% of patients with advanced ovarian cancer and 10% of normal persons (132).

Tumor-specific antibodies have been identified infrequently in sera from patients with ovarian or cervical cancer (133, 134). Incomplete characterization of these antibodies has prevented their classification as individually specific or histologic type specific.

Immune complexes have been identified in sera of patients with gynecologic cancer. Levels of immune complexes in sera from patients with ovarian and cervical cancer correlate with tumor burden (133). A transient increase in immune complexes has been associated with regression of gestational trophoblastic neoplasms (60). Tumor-associated antigens have been found in immune complexes from ovarian ascitic fluid (133). Paternal MHC antigens have been isolated from circulating immune complexes in gestational trophoblastic disease (60).

Immunotherapy

Two basic approaches have been applied to immunotherapy of human cancers. In *active immunotherapy*, attempts are made to stimulate the patient's own immune response to destroy tumor cells, an approach that presupposes some level of immunocompetence. In *passive immunotherapy*, immune cells or antibodies are transferred to cancer patients, which may circumvent deficits in immunocompetence.

Active Immunotherapy With Bacterial Products and Contact Allergens

Strategies for active immunotherapy have been based, in part, on tumor regression observed after injection of bacterial toxins into cancer patients nearly a century ago by Dr. William B. Coley. Subsequent experimentation in animals has indicated that bacterial immunostimulants such as *BCG* and *C. parvum* are most effective when there is direct contact between the microorganisms and tumor cells. Antitumor activity of bacterial immunostimulants may relate to activation of macrophages, attraction of NK cells, release of cytokines, or microvascular changes, as well as to the possible stimulation of specific immunity directed toward tumor-associated antigens.

Intratumoral injection of BCG in human melanoma has caused regression of cutaneous nodules. Sometimes noninjected cutaneous nodules also regress, but visceral or lymph node metastases rarely respond (135). Intravesical administration of BCG has produced convincing local antitumor activity (136).

Gynecologic tumors such as ovarian carcinoma often are confined to the peritoneal cavity and are reasonable targets for regional immunotherapy. Intracavitary immunotherapy in ovarian cancer patients with killed *C. parvum* has caused regression of ascites and pleural effusions (124, 137). In ovarian cancer patients with minimal residual disease, small tumor nodules also regress in about 30% of the cases (138, 139). Intraperitoneal *C. parvum* therapy increases leukocyte numbers in the peritoneal cavity as well as their ADCC and NK activity. Intratumoral *C. parvum* injection of cervical cancers before surgical removal has prolonged the time to relapse when compared with a control group treated by surgery alone (140).

Systemic administration of bacterial immunostimulants to patients with gynecologic cancer has been mostly ineffective (141, 142). Bacterial immunostimulants have been combined with autologous or allogeneic tumor cells and administered to patients with gynecologic cancer to stimulate responses to tumor-associated antigens (143, 144), but this approach also has been disappointing. Virus modification may enhance tumor cell immunogenicity. Extracts of virally infected tumor cells have augmented delayed skin test (145) and antibody responses (146) to tumor-associated antigens in patients with gynecologic cancer. The ultimate value of immunotherapy with virus-modified tumor cells in patients with vulvar and cervical carcinoma remains to be determined (147). Immunization with paternal lymphocytes has been associated with regression of metastatic choriocarcinoma in a single case (148). Although paternal lymphocytes are highly immunogenic, choriocarcinoma cells may not express paternal antigens.

Genes for certain tumor-associated proteins have been cloned with recombinant DNA technology. The isolated genes are incorporated into potentially immunogenic viruses, such as vaccinia virus, for use as vaccines (149). Genes for different cytokines also have been cloned. Transfer of cytokine genes such as IL-2 and gamma-IF into animal tumors has potentiated their immunogenicity in animal models. Similar approaches may augment immunogenicity of human tumors.

Active Immunotherapy With Purified Mediators

Local inflammatory responses induced by bacterial immunostimulants and contact allergens are associated with release of *cytokines* by infiltrating leukocytes, which may play a role in tumor cell destruction. Large amounts of highly purified recombinant cytokines are now available. Therapy with purified mediators may reduce toxicity seen with more complex agents such as bacterial immunostimulants.

Interferon

Interferons of alpha, beta, and gamma types have been produced in recombinant form. Systemic interferon therapy has been beneficial in relatively few malignancies, such as hairy cell leukemia, chronic myelogenous leukemia, nodular lymphoma, and myeloma. Genital warts, known to harbor papillomavirus, have also responded to interferon therapy. Alpha or beta interferon administered topically, intramuscularly, intralesionally, or systemically has produced tumor regression, although only a few studies have included placebo controls (150, 151). Possible application of local interferon treatment to cervical intraepithelial neoplasia (152) or cervical carcinoma (153) awaits completion of large, well-controlled studies with long-term follow-up.

Alpha interferon has inhibited the growth of ovarian ascitic tumor cells in clonogenic assays *in vitro*, although cells isolated from solid ovarian tumors are often less susceptible (154). In five separate studies (155–159), purified or recombinant alpha interferon has been administered systemically to patients with ovarian cancer, with a combined response rate of only 10%. Intraperitoneal administration of alpha or gamma interferon to treat minimal residual ($\leq$ 5 mm) ovarian cancer has produced a 38–45% temporary response rate (160–162). Intraperitoneal alpha interferon added to cisplatin may improve the response rate (163, 164). Intraperitoneal recombinant beta interferon has been tested in patients with larger tumor burdens, and no responses have been observed. (165).

Interleukin-2 and Tumor Necrosis Factor-α

Systemic administration of recombinant interleukin-2 in human cancer patients, primarily those with melanoma and renal cancer, has produced a response rate of less than 15% (166). Another cytokine with cytotoxic activity for tumor cells is tumor necrosis factor (TNF). Clinical trials of recombinant TNF-α (108) have demonstrated little antitumor activity. This may relate, in part, to observations that TNF-α can stimulate, rather than inhibit, growth of some neoplasms *ex vivo* (30).

Active specific immunotherapy with purified mediators is in an early stage and has been evaluated mostly in patients with advanced disease. Now that large amounts of purified mediators are available, much needs to be learned about the complex interactions between mediators, lymphoreticular cells, and tumor cells so that rational trials may be designed.

Passive Immunotherapy With Lymphoreticular Cells

Passive immunotherapy has used either transfer of immune effector cells or the transfer of antibodies. In one early study, immune lymphocytes from pigs treated with human tumors inhibited tumor growth in a small number of cancer patients. This approach was severely limited by the prompt host rejection of foreign cells. *Adoptive immunotherapy* with autologous lymphocytes has recently become possible because of the availability of large amounts of recombinant IL-2, which is required to support the proliferation and activation of human lymphocytes *ex vivo*. Initial trials in patients with advanced cancer have tested systemic administration of autologous LAK cells obtained by *in vitro* activation of peripheral leukocytes with mitogen or recombinant IL-2 (111). In more recent trials, autologous LAK cells have been administered intravenously in combination with IL-2. A combined response rate of 27% has been observed in 146 cancer patients treated in two separate studies (167, 168). Responses have been observed most often in patients with renal cell cancer and melanoma. One of two ovarian cancer patients has responded to LAK cells plus IL-2. LAK therapy has been associated with hypotension, oliguria, "third space" fluid shifts, and pulmonary edema. Constant infusion of IL-2 may reduce the severity of side effects associated with bolus IL-2 doses (167). In trials of intraperitoneal LAK cells with IL-2 in patients with ovarian cancer, partial responses have been observed in approximately 20% of the cases. In addition to systemic toxicity, IL-2 and LAK cells produced peritoneal inflammation associated with pain, adhesion formation, and fibrosis (168). LAK cells are apparently unable to distinguish among tumor cells from different persons. The stimulation and selective growth of specific lymphocytes responsive to gynecologic tumors may be possible if appropriate tumor-associated antigen targets can be identified. Specifically immune lymphocytes isolated from tumors may be more effective for adoptive immunotherapy (169). Tumor-infiltrating lymphocytes (TIL) include T cells that are capable of lysing autologous tumor cells and of homing to tumor sites.

Passive Immunotherapy With Antibodies

Heteroantisera

Serotherapy provides another approach to providing exogenous immunity. Early studies used heteroantisera raised in rabbits or other species. In a murine model of ovarian cancer, either active immunotherapy with intraperitoneal *C. parvum* or its biochemically dissociated fractions or passive immunotherapy with a specific rabbit heteroantiserum can cure mice previously injected with a lethal dose of tumor cells (170–172). Antitumor activity of *C. parvum* appears to be related to the activity of both granulocytes and activated macrophages that are attracted into the peritoneal cavity. Combination intraperitoneal therapy with both *C. parvum* and rabbit heteroantiserum is more effective than either agent alone in mice with larger tumor burdens. ADCC may have an important role in tumor-cell destruction in this model. *C. parvum* injection augments ADCC activity of peritoneal cells for mouse tumor cells *in vitro* (170) and potentiates rabbit heteroantiserum therapy *in vivo* under similar conditions. Clinical trials have indicated that *C. parvum* can augment the number and activity of human effectors within the peritoneal cavity (138, 139). Because of encouraging results in animal models, intraperitoneal administration of rabbit heteroantiserum has been combined with multiagent chemotherapy and radiotherapy in a randomized trial in patients with Stage III ovarian cancer (173).

Monoclonal Antibodies

The recent production of a variety of immune monoclonal antibodies reactive with tumor-associated antigens may provide new agents for serotherapy. Systemic serotherapy with unconjugated murine monoclonal antibodies has provided clinical benefit in only a few cases of nongynecologic cancer. In B cell lymphoma, serotherapy with anti-idiotypic monoclonal antibodies has produced a complete remission in one patient and partial remissions in a majority of others in a small series (174). A number of obstacles may limit the utility of serotherapy, including interference by circulating antigen, tumor cell heterogeneity, modulation of tumor-associated antigens, and host recognition and elimination of foreign mouse proteins. Many of the murine immunoglobulin isotypes do not fix human complement or mediate ADCC effectively with the small number of human effector cells found at tumor sites. Monoclonal antibodies conjugated to radioisotopes, drugs, or toxins would not be dependent on host cells or factors for cytotoxicity.

Radionuclide conjugates have been used more extensively for diagnostic than for therapeutic studies. Effective homing of conjugates to tumor, however, would be one requirement for effective serotherapy. Monoclonal antibodies that recognize tumor-associated antigens of gynecologic tumors and labeled with ^{123}I, ^{131}I, or ^{111}In have been used for radioimmunodetection of primary and metastatic tumor deposits. Both polyclonal and monoclonal antibodies to hCG have imaged tumor sites in gestational trophoblastic neoplasia in the presence of circulating antigen (175, 176). A monoclonal antibody reactive with a choriocarcinoma-associated antigen has imaged occult lung disease not recognized by computerized tomography (176). Polyclonal and monoclonal antibodies have been used for imaging epithelial ovarian cancer, including antibodies that recognize carcinoma- or sarcoma-associated antigens (177–182).

105

In the majority of patients with ovarian cancer studied, the radioimaging data correlated with clinical findings. Ovarian tumors as small as 0.8 cm have been imaged with a radioiodinated antibody (179). Specificity of imaging is not yet sufficient for diagnosis of ovarian cancer in patients with a pelvic mass. In a prospective study using ^{123}I-radiolabeled monoclonal antibody, 95% of the primary ovarian cancers were imaged, but there was a 50% false-positive rate in patients without ovarian cancer (178). It may be possible to reduce the high false-positive rate with the use of multiple antibody conjugates or antibody conjugates with greater specificity for ovarian cancer versus other carcinomas or benign tissues. Radionuclide imaging may be most useful in following disease status during therapy. Lymph nodes involved with cervical cancer have been imaged with intralymphatically injected ^{123}I-labeled antibody. However, high uptake of antibody conjugates is observed in patients with uninvolved nodes (183).

Intraperitoneal injection of conjugates may improve imaging of peritoneal tumor deposits by avoiding interference from circulating tumor antigen. Therapeutic doses of radionuclide conjugates have been administered into body cavities of patients with advanced ovarian cancer (184, 185), with regression of small tumor nodules in a small fraction of patients. Sequestering the radiolabeled conjugate in the body cavity also reduces exposure of normal and radiosensitive body tissues, although myelotoxicity has still proved dose limiting.

A number of monoclonal antibodies reactive with epithelial ovarian cancer have been conjugated to toxins such as *Pseudomonas* exotoxin or ricin A chain (186, 187). The antibody conjugates kill ovarian tumor cell lines *in vitro*. The toxin generally must enter the ribosomal compartment to mediate toxicity. The clinical usefulness of immunotoxins in human patients awaits further evaluation.

Recent developments in monoclonal antibody and gene cloning technology have provided large amounts of pure reagents for studying the biology and heterogeneity of tumor cells, as well as the intricacies of the immunologic interactions between tumor and host. This complex relationship has no doubt contributed to the lack of success seen with previous attempts at immunotherapy. Increased knowledge of tumor immunobiology and the availability of pure antibodies and cytokines should facilitate the design and implementation of new approaches to immunotherapy.

References

1. **Woodruff JD, Julian CG:** Multiple malignancies in the upper genital canal. *Am J Obstet Gynecol* 103:810, 1969.

2. **Jacobs IJ, Kohler MF, Wiseman R, et al:** The clonal origin of ovarian cancer: analysis by loss of heterozygosity, p53 mutation and X chromosome inactivation. *J Natl Cancer Inst* 84:1793, 1992.

3. **Mok CH, Tsao SW, Knapp RC, et al:** Unifocal origin of advanced human epithelial ovarian cancers. *Cancer Res* 52:5119, 1992.

4. **Cooper GM:** *Oncogenes.* Boston, Jones & Bartlett, 1990.

5. **Hunter T:** Cooperation between oncogenes. *Cell* 64:249, 1991.

6. **DiCioccio RA, Piver MS:** The genetics of ovarian cancer. *Cancer Invest* 10:135, 1992.

7. **Sato T, Saito H, Morita R, et al:** Allelotype of human ovarian cancer. *Cancer Res* 51:5118, 1991.

8. **Ehlen T, Dubeau L:** Loss of heterozygosity on chromosomal segments 3p, 6q and 11p in human ovarian carcinomas. *Oncogene* 5:219, 1990.

9. **Britton LC, Wilson TO, Gaffey TA, et al:** Flow cytometric DNA analysis of stage I endometrial carcinoma. *Gynecol Oncol* 34:317, 1989.

10. **Okamoto A, Sameshima Y, Yamada Y, et al:** Allelic loss on chromosome 17p and p53 mutations in human endometrial carcinoma of the uterus. *Cancer Res* 51:5632, 1991.

11. **Yokota J, Tsukada Y, Nakajima T, et al:** Loss of heterozygosity on the short arm of chromosome 3 in carcinoma of the uterine cervix. *Cancer Res* 49:3598, 1989.

12. **Rodriguez GC, Berchuck A, Whitaker RS, et al:** Epidermal growth factor receptor expression in normal ovarian epithelium and ovarian cancer. II. Relationship between receptor expression and response to epidermal growth factor. *Am J Obstet Gynecol* 164:745, 1991.

13. **Stromberg K, Collins TJ IV, Gordon AW, et al:** Transforming growth factor-α acts as an autocrine growth factor in ovarian carcinoma cell lines. *Cancer Res* 52:341, 1992.

14. **Berchuck A, Soisson AP, Olt GJ, et al:** Epidermal growth factor receptor expression in normal and malignant endometrium. *Am J Obstet Gynecol* 161:1247, 1989.

15. **Talavera F, Reynolds RK, Roberts JA, Menon KM:** Insulin-like growth factor I receptors in normal and neoplastic human endometrium. *Cancer Res* 50:3019, 1990.

16. **Reynolds RK, Talavera F, Roberts JA, et al:** Regulation of epidermal growth factor and insulin-like growth factor I receptors by estradiol and progesterone in normal and neoplastic endometrial cell cultures. *Gynecol Oncol* 38:396, 1990.

17. **Maruo T, Yamasaki M, Ladines-Llave CA, Mochizuki M:** Immunohistochemical demonstration of elevated expression of epidermal growth factor receptor in the neoplastic changes of cervical squamous epithelium. *Cancer* 69:1182, 1992.

18. **Berchuck A, Rodriguez G, Olt G, et al:** Regulation of growth of normal ovarian epithelial cells and ovarian cancer cell lines by transforming growth factor-β. *Am J Obstet Gynecol* 166:676, 1992.

19. **Boyd JA, Kaufman DG:** Expression of transforming growth factor β-1 by human endometrial carcinoma cell lines: inverse correlation with effects on growth rate and morphology. *Cancer Res* 50:3394, 1990.

20. **Berchuck A, Rodriguez GC, Kamel A, et al:** Epidermal growth factor receptor expression in normal ovarian epithelium and ovarian cancer. I. Correlation of receptor expression with prognostic factors in patients with ovarian cancer. *Am J Obstet Gynecol* 164:669, 1991.

21. **Slamon DJ, Godolphin W, Jones LA, et al:** Studies of the HER-2/*neu* proto-oncogene in human breast and ovarian cancer. *Science* 244:707, 1989.

22. **Berchuck A, Kamel A, Whitaker R, et al:** Overexpression of HER-2/*neu* is associated with poor survival in advanced epithelial ovarian cancer. *Cancer Res* 50:4087, 1990.

23. **Lupu R, Colomer R, Zugmaier G, et al:** Direct interaction of a ligand for the *erb*B2 oncogene with the EGF receptor and p185[c-erbB-2]. *Science* 249:1552, 1990.

24. **Lupu R, Colomer R, Kannan B, Lippman ME:** Characterization of a growth factor that binds exclusively to the *erb*B-2 receptor and induces cellular responses. *Proc Natl Acad Sci USA* 89:2287, 1992.

25. **Berchuck A, Rodriguez G, Kinney RB, et al:** Overexpression of HER-2/*neu* in endometrial cancer is associated with advanced stage disease. *Am J Obstet Gynecol* 164:15, 1991.

26. **Kacinski BM, Chambers SK, Stanley ER, et al:** The cytokine CSF-1 (M-CSF) expressed by endometrial carcinomas *in vivo* and *in vitro* may also be a circulating tumor marker of neoplastic disease activity in endometrial carcinoma patients. *J Radiat Oncol Biol Phys* 19:619, 1990.

27. **Kacinski BM, Carter D, Mittal K, et al:** Ovarian adenocarcinomas express *fms*-complementary transcripts and *fms* antigen, often with coexpression of CSF-1. *Am J Pathol* 137:135, 1990.

28. **Wu S, Rodabaugh K, Martínez-Maza O, et al:** Stimulation of ovarian tumor cell proliferation with monocyte products including interleukin-1, interleukin-6, and tumor necrosis factor-α. *Am J Obstet Gynecol* 166:997, 1992.

29. **Watson JM, Sensinstaffar JL, Berek JS, Martínez-Maza O:** Constitutive production of interleukin 6 by ovarian cancer cell lines and by primary ovarian tumor cultures. *Cancer Res* 50:6959, 1990.

30. **Wu S, Boyer CM, Whitaker RS, et al:** Tumor necrosis factor-alpha (TNF-α) as an autocrine and paracrine growth factor for ovarian cancer: monokine induction of tumor cell proliferation and TNF-α expression. *Cancer Res* 53:1939, 1993.

31. **Enomoto T, Inoue M, Perantoni AO, et al:** K-*ras* activation in premalignant and malignant epithelial lesions of the human uterus. *Cancer Res* 51:5308, 1991.

32. **Hayashi Y, Hachisuga T, Iwasaka T, et al:** Expression of *ras* oncogene product and EGF receptor in cervical squamous cell carcinomas and its relationship to lymph node involvement. *Gynecol Oncol* 40:147, 1991.

33. **Bast RC Jr, Jacobs I, Berchuck A:** Malignant transformation of ovarian epithelium. *J Natl Cancer Inst* 84:556, 1992.

34. **Riou GF, Bourhis J, Le MG:** The c-*myc* protooncogene in invasive carcinomas of the uterine cervix: clinical relevance of overexpression in early stages of the cancer. *Anticancer Res* 10:1225, 1990.

35. **Sasano H, Garrett CT, Wilkinson DS, et al:** Protooncogene amplification and tumor ploidy in human ovarian neoplasms. *Hum Pathol* 21:382, 1990.

36. **Howley PM, Munger K, Werness BA, et al:** Molecular mechanisms of transformation by the human papillomaviruses. *Int Symp Princess Takamatsu Cancer Res Fund* 20:199, 1989.

37. **Levine AJ, Momand J:** Tumor suppressor genes: the p53 and retinoblastoma sensitivity genes and gene products. *Biochem Biophys Acta* 1032:119, 1990.

38. **Dyson N, Howley PM, Munger K, Harlow E:** The human papilloma virus-16 E7 oncoprotein is able to bind to the retinoblastoma gene product. *Science* 243:934, 1989.

39. **Marks JR, Davidoff AM, Kerns BJ, et al:** Overexpression and mutation of p53 in epithelial ovarian cancer. *Cancer Res* 51:2979, 1991.

40. **Kohler MF, Kerns BJM, Soper JT, et al:** Mutation and overexpression of p53 in early-stage epithelial ovarian cancer. *Obstet Gynecol* 81:643, 1993.

41. **Kohler MF, Berchuck A, Davidoff AM, et al:** Overexpression and mutation of p53 in endometrial carcinoma. *Cancer Res* 52:1622, 1992.

42. **Rosenberg SA:** Adoptive immunotherapy of cancer: accomplishments and prospects. *Cancer Treat Rev* 68:233, 1984.

43. **Wagner H, Pfizenmaier K, Rollinghoff M:** The role of the major histocompatibility gene complex in murine cytotoxic T cell responses. *Adv Cancer Res* 31:77, 1980.

44. **Bernards R, Schrier PI, Houweling A, et al:** Tumorigenicity of cells transformed by adenovirus type 12 by evasion of T-cell immunity. *Nature* 305:776, 1983.

45. **Baldwin RW:** Specific antitumor immunity and its role in host resistance to tumors. In Herberman RB (ed): *Basic and Clinical Tumor Immunology*. Boston, Martinus Nijhoff, 1983, p 107.

46. **Hoover HC Jr, Surdyke M, Dangel RB, et al:** Delayed cutaneous hypersensitivity to autologous tumor cells in colorectal cancer patients immunized with an autologous tumor cell: bacillus Calmette-Guerin vaccine. *Cancer Res* 44:1671, 1984.

47. **Vanky FT, Stjernsward J:** Lymphocyte stimulation (by autologous tumor biopsy cells). In Herberman RB, McIntire KR (eds): *Immunodiagnosis of Cancer*. New York, Marcel Dekker, 1979, p 998.

48. **Vose BM, Howell A:** Cultured human antitumor T cells and their potential for therapy. In Herberman RB (ed): *Basic and Clinical Tumor Immunology*. Boston, Martinus Nijhoff, 1983, p 129.

49. **Grimm EA, Vose BM, Chu EW, et al:** The human mixed lymphocyte-tumor cell interaction test. I. Positive autologous lymphocyte proliferative responses can be stimulated by tumor cells as well as by cells from normal tissues. *Cancer Immunol Immunother* 17:83, 1984.

50. **Old LJ:** Cancer immunology: the search for specificity. *Cancer Res* 41:361, 1981.

51. **Yajima H, Noda T, Michele de Villiers E, et al:** Isolation of a new type of human papillomavirus (HPV52b) with a transforming activity from cervical cancer tissue. *Cancer Res* 48:7164, 1988.

52. **Feizi T:** Demonstration by monoclonal antibodies that carbohydrate structures of glycoproteins and glycolipids are oncodevelopmental antigens. *Nature* 314:53, 1985.

53. **Auffray C, Strominger JL:** Molecular genetics of the human major histocompatibility complex. *Adv Hum Genet* 15:197, 1986.

54. **Kabawat SE, Bast RC Jr, Welch WR, et al:** Expression of major histocompatibility antigens and nature of inflammatory cellular infiltrate in ovarian neoplasms. *Int J Cancer* 32:547, 1983.

55. **Ferguson A, Moore M, Fox H:** Expression of MHC products and leukocyte differentiation antigens in gynaecological neoplasms: an immunohistological analysis of the tumour cells and infiltrating leukocytes. *Br J Cancer* 52:551, 1985.

56. **Morris HB, Gatter KC, Pulford K, et al:** Cervical wart virus infection, intraepithelial neoplasia and carcinoma; an immunohistological study using a panel of monoclonal antibodies. *Br J Obstet Gynaecol* 90:1069, 1983.

57. **Sunderland CA, Redman CWG, Stirrat GM:** HLA A, B, C antigens are expressed on nonvillous trophoblast of the early human placenta. *J Immunol* 127:2614, 1981.

58. **Berkowitz RS, Anderson DJ, Hunter NJ, Goldstein DP:** Distribution of major histocompatibility (HLA) antigens in chorionic villi of molar pregnancy. *Am J Obstet Gynecol* 146:221, 1983.

59. **Berkowitz RS, Goldstein DP, Hoch EJ, Anderson DJ:** Immunobiology of molar pregnancy and gestational trophoblastic tumors. *J Reprod Med* 29:796, 1984.

60. **Lahey SJ, Steele G Jr, Berkowitz R, et al:** Identification of material with paternal HLA antigen immunoreactivity from purported circulating immune complexes in patients with gestational trophoblastic neoplasia. *J Natl Cancer Inst* 72:983, 1984.

61. **Rapp F:** Herpes simplex virus type 2 and cervical cancer. In Hickey RC (ed): *Current Problems in Cancer.* Chicago, Year Book, 1981, p 5.

62. **Vonka V, Kanka J, Hirsch I, et al:** Prospective study on the relationship between cervical neoplasia and herpes simplex type-2 virus. II. Herpes simplex type-2 antibody presence in sera taken at enrollment. *Int J Cancer* 33:61, 1984.

63. **Zur Hausen H:** Human genital cancer: synergism between two virus infections or synergism between a virus infection and initiating events? *Lancet* 2:1370, 1982.

64. **Shively JE, Beatty JD:** CEA-related antigens: molecular biology and clinical significance. *CRC Crit Rev Oncol Hematol* 2:355, 1985.

65. **Stall KE, Martin EW Jr:** Plasma carcinoembryonic antigen levels in ovarian cancer patients: a chart review and survey of published data. *J Reprod Med* 26:73, 1981.

66. **McIntire KR, Waldmann TA:** Measurement of alphafetoprotein. In Rose NR, Friedman H (eds): *Manual of Clinical Immunology,* ed 2. Washington, DC, American Society for Microbiology, 1980, p 936.

67. **Casper S, van Nagell JR Jr, Powell DF, et al:** Immunohistochemical localization of tumor markers in epithelial ovarian cancer. *Am J Obstet Gynecol* 149:154, 1984.

68. **Rustin GJS, Bagshawe KD:** Gestational trophoblastic tumors. *CRC Crit Rev Oncol Hematol* 3:103, 1985.

69. **Hussa RO, Fein HG, Pattillo RA, et al:** A distinctive form of human chorionic gonadotropin beta-subunit-like material produced by cervical carcinoma cells. *Cancer Res* 46:1948, 1986.

70. **Cole LA, Nam JH:** Urinary gonadotropin fragment (UGF) measurements in the diagnosis and management of ovarian cancer. *Yale J Biol Med* 62:367, 1989.

71. **Nouwen EJ, Pollet DE, Schelstraete JB, et al:** Human placental alkaline phosphatase in benign and malignant ovarian neoplasia. *Cancer Res* 45:892, 1985.

72. **Ueda G, Inoue Y, Yamasaki M, et al:** Immunohistochemical demonstration of tumor antigen TA-4 in gynecologic tumors. *Int J Gynecol Pathol* 3:291, 1984.

73. **Kato H, Miyauchi F, Morioka H, et al:** Tumor antigen of human cervical squamous cell carcinoma: correlation of circulating levels with disease progress. *Cancer* 43:585, 1979.

74. **Bast RC Jr, Feeney M, Lazarus H, et al:** Reactivity of a monoclonal antibody with human ovarian carcinoma. *J Clin Invest* 68:1331, 1981.

75. **Davis HM, Zurawski VR Jr, Bast RC Jr, Klug TL:** Characterization of the CA 125 antigen associated with human epithelial ovarian carcinomas. *Cancer Res* 46:6143, 1986.

76. **Kabawat SE, Bast RC, Welch WR, et al:** Immunopathologic characterization of a monoclonal antibody that recognizes common surface antigens of human ovarian tumors of serous, endometrioid, and clear cell types. *Am J Clin Pathol* 79:98, 1983.

77. **Kabawat SE, Bast RC Jr, Bhan AK, et al:** Tissue distribution of a coelomic-epithelium-related antigen recognized by the monoclonal antibody OC 125. *Int J Gynecol Pathol* 2:275, 1983.

78. **Bast RC Jr, Klug TL, St John E, et al:** A radioimmunoassay using a monoclonal antibody to monitor the course of epithelial ovarian cancer. *N Engl J Med* 309:883, 1983.

79. **Klug TL, Bast RC Jr, Niloff JM, et al:** Monoclonal antibody immunoradiometric assay for an antigenic determinant (CA 125) associated with human epithelial ovarian carcinomas. *Cancer Res* 44:1048, 1984.

80. **Niloff JM, Klug TL, Schaetzl E, et al:** Elevation of serum CA 125 in carcinomas of the fallopian tube, endometrium, and endocervix. *Am J Obstet Gynecol* 148:1057, 1984.

81. **Jacobs I, Bast RC Jr:** The CA 125 tumour-associated antigen: a review of the literature. *Hum Reprod* 4:1, 1989.

82. **Lavin PT, Knapp RC, Malkasian G, et al:** CA 125 for the monitoring of ovarian carcinoma during primary therapy. *Obstet Gynecol* 69:223, 1987.

83. **Berek JS, Knapp RC, Malkasian GD, et al:** CA 125 serum levels correlated with second-look operations among ovarian cancer patients. *Obstet Gynecol* 67:685, 1986.

84. **Malkasian GD Jr, Knapp RC, Lavin PT, et al:** Preoperative evaluation of serum CA 125 levels in premenopausal and postmenopausal patients with pelvic masses: discrimination of benign from malignant disease. *Am J Obstet Gynecol* 159:341, 1988.

85. **Einhorn N, Bast RC Jr, Knapp RC, et al:** Preoperative evaluation of serum CA 125 levels in patients with primary epithelial ovarian cancer. *Obstet Gynecol* 67:414, 1986.

86. **Soper JT, Hunter VJ, Daly L, et al:** Preoperative serum tumor associated antigen levels in women with pelvic masses. *Obstet Gynecol* 75:249, 1990.

87. **Bast RC Jr, Siegal FP, Runowicz C, et al:** Elevation of serum CA 125 prior to diagnosis of an epithelial ovarian carcinoma. *Gynecol Oncol* 22:115, 1985.

88. **Zurawski VR Jr, Orjaseter H, Andersen A, Jellum E:** Elevated serum CA 125 levels prior to diagnosis of ovarian neoplasia: relevance for early detection of ovarian cancer. *Br J Cancer* 42:677, 1988.

89. **Zurawski VR Jr, Broderick SF, Pickens P, et al:** Serum CA 125 levels in a large group of nonhospitalized women: relevance for the early detection of ovarian cancer. *Obstet Gynecol* 69:606, 1987.

90. **Jacobs I, Bridges J, Reynolds C, Stabile I, et al:** Multimodal approach to screening for ovarian cancer. *Lancet* 1:268, 1988.

91. **Zurawski VR Jr, Sjovall K, Schoenfeld DA, et al:** Prospective evaluation of serum CA 125 levels in a normal population. Phase I. The specificities of single and serial determinations in testing for ovarian cancer. *Gynecol Oncol* 36:299, 1990.

92. **Einhorn N, Sjovall K, Knapp RC, et al:** A prospective evaluation of serum CA 125 levels for early detection of ovarian cancer. *Obstet Gynecol* 80:14, 1992.

93. **Jacobs I, Prys Davies A, Oram D:** Role of CA 125 in screening for ovarian cancer. In Sharp F, Mason WP, Creasman W (eds): *Ovarian Cancer 2: Biology, Diagnosis and Management.* London, Chapman & Hall Medical, 1992, p 265.

94. **Knauf S, Kalwas J, Helmkamp BF, et al:** Monoclonal antibodies against human ovarian tumor associated antigen NB/70K: preparation and use in a radioimmunoassay for measuring NB/70K in serum. *Cancer Immunol Immunother* 21:217, 1986.

95. **Ward BG, Cruickshank DJ, Tucker DF, Love S:** Independent expression in serum of three tumour-associated antigens: CA 125, placental alkaline phosphatase and HMFG2 in ovarian carcinoma. *Br J Obstet Gynaecol* 94:696, 1987.

96. **Xu FJ, Ramakrishnan S, Daly L, et al:** Increased serum levels of macrophage colony-stimulating factor in ovarian cancer. *Am J Obstet Gynecol* 165:1356, 1991.

97. **Xu FJ, Yu YH, Daly L, et al:** The OVX1 radioimmunoassay (RIA) complements CA 125 for predicting the presence of residual disease at second look surgical surveillance procedures. *Proc Am Soc Clin Oncol* 11:94, 1992.

98. **Budwit-Novotny DA, McCarty KS, Cox EB, et al:** Immunohistochemical analyses of estrogen receptor in endometrial adeno-carcinoma using a monoclonal antibody. *Cancer Res* 46:5419, 1986.

99. **Turner MW:** Immunoglobulins. In Holborow EJ, Reeves WG (eds): *Immunology in Medicine ed 2*. London, Grune & Stratton, 1983, p 35.

100. **Foon KA, Todd RF III:** Immunologic classification of leukemia and lymphoma. *Blood* 68:1, 1986.

101. **Bottomly K:** A functional dichotomy of CD4 + T lymphocytes. *Immunol Today* 9:195, 1988.

102. **Adams DO, Hamilton TA:** The cell biology of macrophage activation. *Annu Rev Immunol* 2:283, 1984.

103. **Ortaldo JR, Herberman RB:** Heterogeneity of natural killer cells. *Annu Rev Immunol* 2:359, 1984.

104. **Steplewski Z, Herlyn D, Lubeck M, et al:** Mechanisms of tumor growth inhibition. *Hybridoma* 5:S59, 1986.

105. **Smith KA:** Lymphokine regulation of T cell and B cell function. In Paul WE (ed): *Fundamental Immunology*. New York, Raven Press, 1984, p 559.

106. **Schrader JW:** The panspecific hemopoietin of activated T lymphocytes (interleukin-3). *Annu Rev Immunol* 4:205, 1986.

107. **Borden EC:** Interferons and cancer: how the promise is being kept. In Gresser I (ed): *Interferon 1983*. London, Academic Press, 1983, p 43.

108. **Oettgen HF, Old LJ:** Tumor necrosis factor. In DeVita VT Jr, Hellman S, Rosenberg SA (eds): *Important Advances in Oncology*. Philadelphia, JB Lippincott, 1987, p 105.

109. **Schreiber H:** Idiotype network interactions in tumor immunity. *Adv Cancer Res* 41:291, 1984.

110. **Berke G:** Functions and mechanisms of lysis induced by cytotoxic T lymphocytes and natural killer cells. In Paul WE (ed): *Fundamental Immunology,* 2nd ed. New York, Raven Press, 1989, pp 735-764.

111. **Rosenberg SA:** Immunotherapy of cancer by systemic administration of lymphoid cells plus interleukin-2. *J Biol Response Mod* 3:501, 1984.

112. **Mandell GL, Fisher RI, Bostick F, Young RC:** Ovarian cancer: a solid tumor with evidence of normal cellular immune function but abnormal B cell function. *Am J Med* 66:621, 1979.

113. **Khoo SK, Mackay E, Daunter B:** Dinitrochlorobenzene reactivity of women with cancer of the ovary, cervix and corpus uteri. *Int J Gynaecol Obstet* 17:58, 1979.

114. **Carson LF, Twiggs LB, Fukushima M, et al:** Human genital papilloma infections: an evaluation of immunologic competence in the genital neoplasia-papilloma syndrome. *Am J Obstet Gynecol* 155:784, 1986.

115. **Ho P-C, Lawton JMW, Wong L-C, Ma H-K:** T-cell subsets and natural killer cell activity in patients with gestational trophoblastic neoplasia. *Am J Obstet Gynecol* 155:330, 1986.

116. **Berek JS, Bast RC Jr, Lichtenstein A, et al:** Lymphocyte cytotoxicity in the peritoneal cavity and blood of patients with ovarian cancer. *Obstet Gynecol* 64:708, 1984.

117. **Mantovani A, Allavena P, Sessa C, et al:** Natural killer activity of lymphoid cells isolated from human ascitic ovarian tumors. *Int J Cancer* 25:573, 1980.

118. **Introna M, Allavena P, Biondi A, et al:** Defective natural killer activity within human ovarian tumors: Low numbers of morphologically defined effectors present in situ. *J Natl Cancer Inst* 70:21, 1983.

119. **Allavena P, Introna M, Mangioni C, Mantovani A:** Inhibition of natural killer activity by tumor-associated lymphoid cells from ascites ovarian carcinomas. *J Natl Cancer Inst* 67:319, 1981.

120. **Oh S-K, Moolten FL:** Purification and characterization of an immunosuppressive factor from ovarian cancer ascites fluid. *Eur J Immunol* 11:780, 1981.

121. **Lichtenstein AK, Berek J, Zighelboim J:** Natural killer inhibitory substance produced by the peritoneal cells of patients with ovarian cancer. *J Natl Cancer Inst* 74:349, 1985.

122. **Allavena P, Zanaboni F, Rossini S, et al:** Lymphokine-activated killer activity of tumor-associated and peripheral blood lymphocytes isolated from patients with ascites ovarian tumors. *J Natl Cancer Inst* 77:863, 1986.

123. **Haskill S, Koren H, Becker S, et al:** Mononuclearcell infiltration in ovarian cancer. II. Immune function of tumour and ascites-derived inflammatory cells. *Br J Cancer* 45:737, 1982.

124. **Mantovani A, Sessa C, Peri G, et al:** Intraperitoneal administration of *Corynebacterium parvum* in patients with ascitic ovarian tumors resistant to chemotherapy: effects on cytotoxicity of tumor-associated macrophages and NK cells. *Int J Cancer* 27:437, 1981.

125. **Salmon SE, Hamburger AW:** Immunoproliferation and cancer: a common macrophage-derived promotor substance. *Lancet* 1:1289, 1978.

126. **Wang JM, Cianciolo GJ, Snyderman R, Mantovani A:** Coexistence of a chemotactic factor and a retroviral P15E-related chemotaxis inhibitor in human tumor cell culture supernatants. *J Immunol* 137:2726, 1986.

127. **Vayrynen M, Syrjanen K, Mantyjarvi R, et al:** Immunophenotypes of lymphocytes in prospectively followed up human papillomavirus lesions of the cervix. *Genitourin Med* 61:190, 1985.

128. **Ferrini S, Biassoni R, Moretta A, et al:** Clonal analysis of T lymphocytes isolated from ovarian carcinoma ascitic fluid: phenotypic and functional characterization of T-cell clones capable of lysing autologous carcinoma cells. *Int J Cancer* 36:337, 1985.

129. **Crowther ME, Poulton TA, Hudson CN:** The relationship between cellular responses of parous women and ovarian cancer patients to tumour extracts. *J Obstet Gynaecol* 1:263, 1981.

130. **Faiferman I, Gleicher N, Cohen CJ, Koffler D:** Leukocyte migration in ovarian carcinoma: comparison of inhibitory activity of tumor extracts. *J Natl Cancer Inst* 59:1593, 1977.

131. **Rivera ES, Hersh EM, Bowen JM, et al:** Leukocyte migration inhibition assay of tumor immunity in patients with cervical squamous cell carcinoma. *Cancer* 43:2297, 1979.

132. **Kotlar HKR, Knauf S, Beecham J, et al:** Detection of ovarian cancer by the humoral leukocyte adherence inhibition test using a purified tumor-associated antigen. *Eur J Cancer Clin Oncol* 21:483, 1985.

133. **van de Linde AW, Streefkerk M, Te Velde ER, et al:** Tumor-specific antibodies in sera from patients with squamous cell carcinoma of the uterine cervix: detection by a membrane immunofluorescence assay on cultured cervical carcinoma cells. *Cancer Immunol Immunother* 11:201, 1981.

134. **Dawson JR, Lutz PM, Shau H:** The humoral response to gynecologic malignancies and its role in the regulation of tumor growth: a review. *Am J Reprod Immunol* 3:12, 1983.

135. **Bast RC Jr, Zbar B, Borsos T, Rapp HJ:** BCG and cancer. *N Engl J Med* 290:1413, 1458, 1974.

136. **Lamm DL, Thor DE, Harris SC, et al:** Intravesical and percutaneous BCG immunotherapy of recurrent superficial bladder cancer. In Terry WD, Rosenberg SA (eds): *Immunotherapy of Human Cancer.* New York, Elsevier, 1982, p 315.

137. **Webb HE, Oaten SW, Pike CP:** Treatment of malignant ascitic and pleural effusions with *Corynebacterium parvum. Br Med J* 1:338, 1978.

138. **Bast RC Jr, Berek JS, Obrist R, et al:** Intraperitoneal immunotherapy of human ovarian carcinoma with *Corynebacterium parvum. Cancer Res* 43:1395, 1983.

139. **Berek JS, Knapp RC, Hacker NF, et al:** Intraperitoneal immunotherapy of epithelial ovarian carcinoma with *Corynebacterium parvum. Am J Obstet Gynecol* 152:1003, 1985.

140. **Mignot MH, Lens JW, Drexhage HA, et al:** Lower relapse rates after neighborhood injection of *Corynebacterium parvum* in operable cervix carcinoma. *Br J Cancer* 44:856, 1981.

141. **Alberts DS, Moon TE, Stephens RA, et al:** Randomized study of chemoimmunotherapy for advanced ovarian carcinoma: a preliminary report of a Southwest Oncology Group Study. *Cancer Treat Rev* 63:325, 1979.

142. **Barlow JJ, Piver MS, Lele SB:** High-dose methotrexate with "rescue" plus cyclophosphamide as initial chemotherapy in ovarian adenocarcinoma: a randomized trial with observations on the influence of *C parvum* immunotherapy. *Cancer* 46:1333, 1980.

143. **Hudson CN, Levin L, McHardy JE, et al:** Active specific immunotherapy for ovarian cancer. *Lancet* 2:877, 1976.

144. **Gusdon JP Jr, Homesley HD, Jobson VW, Muss HB:** Treatment of advanced ovarian malignancy with chemoimmunotherapy using autologous tumor and *Corynebacterium parvum. Obstet Gynecol* 62:728, 1983.

145. **Freedman RS, Bowen JM, Atkinson EN, et al:** Virusaugmented delayed hypersensitivity skin tests in gynecological malignancies. *Cancer Immunol Immunother* 17:142, 1984.

146. **Savage HE, Rossen RD, Hersh EM, et al:** Antibody development to viral and allogeneic tumor cell-associated antigens in patients with malignant melanoma and ovarian carcinoma treated with lysates of virus-infected tumor cells. *Cancer Res* 46:2127, 1986.

147. **Freedman RS, Bowen JM, Herson JH, et al:** Immunotherapy for vulvar carcinoma with virus-modified homologous extracts. *Obstet Gynecol* 62:707, 1983.

148. **Cinader B, Hayley MA, Rider WD, Warwick OH:** Immunotherapy of a patient with choriocarcinoma. *Can Med Assoc J* 84:306, 1961.

149. **Estin CD, Stevenson US, Plowman GD, et al:** Recombinant vaccinia virus vaccine against the human melanoma antigen p97 for use in immunotherapy. *Proc Natl Acad Sci USA* 85:1052, 1988.

150. **Vesterinen E, Meyer B, Purola E, Cantell K:** Treatment of vaginal flat condyloma with interferon cream. *Lancet* 1:157, 1984.

151. **Schonfeld A, Nitke S, Schattner A, et al:** Intramuscular human interferon-beta injections in treatment of condylomata acuminata. *Lancet* 1:1038, 1984.

152. **Choo YC, Seto WH, Hsu C, et al:** Cervical intraepithelial neoplasia treated by perilesional injection of interferon. *Br J Obstet Gynaecol* 93:372, 1986.

153. **Ikic D, Krusic J, Kirhmajer V, et al:** Application of human leucocyte interferon in patients with carcinoma of the uterine cervix. *Lancet* 1:1027, 1981.

154. **Epstein LB, Shen J-T, Abele JS, Reese CC:** Further experience in testing the sensitivity of human ovarian carcinoma cells to interferon in an in vitro semisolid agar culture system: comparison of solid and ascitic forms of the tumor. In Salmon S, (ed): *Cloning of Human Tumor Stem Cells.* New York, Alan R Liss, 1980, p 277.

155. **Einhorn N, Cantell K, Einhorn S, Strander H:** Human leukocyte interferon therapy for advanced ovarian carcinoma. *Am J Clin Oncol* 5:167, 1982.

156. **Freedman RS, Gutterman JU, Wharton JT, Rutledge FN:** Leukocyte interferon (IFN-a) in patients with epithelial ovarian carcinoma. *J Biol Response Mod* 2:133, 1983.

157. **Abdulhay G, DiSaia PJ, Blessing JA, Creasman WT:** Human lymphoblastoid interferon in the treatment of advanced epithelial ovarian malignancies: a Gynecologic Oncology Group study. *Am J Obstet Gynecol* 152:418, 1985.

158. **Niloff JM, Knapp RC, Jones G, et al:** Recombinant leukocyte alpha interferon in advanced ovarian carcinoma. *Cancer Treat Rev* 69:895, 1985.

159. **Ezaki K, Okabe K, Domyo M, et al:** Effect of human fibroblast interferon on the cytotoxic activity of natural killer cells and lymphocytes against autochthonous and allogeneic tumor cells. *Gann* 74:723, 1983.

160. **Berek JS, Hacker NF, Lichtenstein A, et al:** Intraperitoneal recombinant α-interferon for "salvage" immunotherapy in stage III epithelial ovarian cancer: a gynecologic Oncology Group study. *Cancer Res* 45:4447, 1985.

161. **Willemse PHB, De Vries EGE, Aalders JG, et al:** Intraperitoneal human recombinant interferon alpha-2b in minimal residual ovarian cancer. *Eur J Cancer* 26:353, 1990.

162. **Pujade-Lauraine E, Guastella JP, Colombo N, et al:** Intraperitoneal recombinant human interferon gamma (IFNg) in residual ovarian cancer: efficacy is independent of previous response to chemotherapy. *Proc Am Soc Clin Oncol* 713:225, 1991.

163. **Nardi M, Cognetti F, Pollera CF, et al:** Intraperitoneal recombinant alpha-2-interferon alternating with cisplatin as salvage therapy for minimal residual disease ovarian cancer a phase II study. *J Clin Oncol* 8:1036, 1990.

164. **Bezwoda WR, Golombick T, Dansey R, Keeping J:** Treatment of malignant ascites due to recurrent/refractory ovarian cancer: the use of interferon-alpha or interferon alpha plus chemotherapy: in vivo and in vitro observations. *Eur J Cancer* 27:1423, 1991.

165. **Rambaldi A, Introna M, Colotta F, et al:** Intraperitoneal administration of interferon beta in ovarian cancer patients. *Cancer* 56:294, 1985.

166. **Rosenberg SA, Lotze MT, Muul LM, et al:** A progress report on the treatment of 157 patients with advanced cancer using lymphokine-activated killer cells and interleukin-2 or high-dose interleukin-2 alone. *N Engl J Med* 316:889, 1987.

167. **West WH, Tauer KW, Yannelli JR, et al:** Constant-infusion recombinant interleukin-2 in adoptive immunotherapy of advanced cancer. *N Engl J Med* 316:898, 1987.

168. **Steis RG, Urba WJ, VanderMolen LA, et al:** Intraperitoneal lymphokine-activated killer cell and interleukin-2 therapy for malignancies limited to the peritoneal cavity. *J Clin Oncol* 8:1618, 1990.

169. **Durant JR:** Immunotherapy of cancer: the end of the beginning? *N Engl J Med* 316:939, 1987.

170. **Bast RC Jr, Knapp RC, Mitchell AK, et al:** Immunotherapy of a murine ovarian carcinoma with *Corynebacterium parvum* and specific heteroantiserum. I. Activation of peritoneal cells to mediate antibody-dependent cytotoxicity. *J Immunol* 123:1945, 1979.

171. **Berek JS, Cantrell JL, Lichtenstein AK, et al:** Immunotherapy with biochemically dissociated fractions of Proprionebacterium acnes in a murine ovarian cancer model. *Cancer Res* 44:1871, 1984.

172. **Berek JS, Lichtenstein AK, Knox RM, et al:** Synergistic effects of combination sequential immunotherapies in a murine ovarian cancer model. *Cancer Res* 45:4215, 1985.

173. **Pino y Torres JL, Bross DS, Hernandez E, et al:** Multimodality treatment of patients with advanced ovarian carcinoma. *Int J Radiat Oncol Biol Phys* 8:1671, 1982.

174. **Miller RA, Maloney DG, Warnke R, Levy R:** Treatment of B-cell lymphoma with monoclonal anti-idiotype antibody. *N Engl J Med* 306:517, 1982.

175. **Morrison RT, Lyster DM, Alcorn LN, et al:** Gamma scintigraphy using Tc-99m labeled antibody to human chorionic gonadotropin. *Clin Nucl Med* 9:20, 1984.

176. **Wahl RL, Khazaeli MB, LoBuglio AF, et al:** Radioimmunoscintigraphic detection of occult gestational choriocarcinoma. *Am J Obstet Gynecol* 156:108, 1987.

177. **van Nagell JR Jr, Kim E, Casper S, et al:** Radioimmunodetection of primary and metastatic ovarian cancer using radiolabeled antibodies to carcinoembryonic antigen. *Cancer Res* 40:502, 1980.

178. **Granowska M, Britton KE, Shepherd JH, et al:** A prospective study of ^{123}I-labeled monoclonal antibody imaging in ovarian cancer. *J Clin Oncol* 4:730, 1986.

179. **Epenetos AA, Shepherd J, Britton KE, et al:** [123]I radioiodinated antibody imaging of occult ovarian cancer. *Cancer* 55:984, 1985.

180. **Epenetos AA, Carr D, Johnson PM, et al:** Antibody-guided radiolocalisation of tumours in patients with testicular or ovarian cancer using two radioiodinated monoclonal antibodies to placental alkaline phosphatase. *Br J Radiol* 59:117, 1986.

181. **Davies JO, Davies ER, Howe K, et al:** Radionuclide imaging of ovarian tumours with ^{123}I-labelled monoclonal antibody (NDOG$_2$) directed against placental alkaline phosphatase. *Br J Obstet Gynaecol* 92:277, 1985.

182. **Symonds EM, Perkins AC, Pimm MV, et al:** Clinical implications for immunoscintigraphy in patients with ovarian malignancy: a preliminary study using monoclonal antibody 791T/36. *Br J Obstet Gynaecol* 92:270, 1985.

183. **Epenetos AA, for the Hammersmith Oncology Group (HOG) and the Imperial Cancer Research Fund (ICRF):** Antibody guided lymphangiography in the staging of cervical cancer. *Br J Cancer* 51:805, 1985.

184. **Hammersmith Oncology Group and the Imperial Cancer Research Fund:** Antibody-guided irradiation of malignant lesions: three cases illustrating a new method of treatment. *Lancet* 1:1441, 1984.

185. **Epenetos AA, Hooker G, Krausz T, et al:** Antibody-guided irradiation of malignant ascites in ovarian cancer: a new therapeutic method possessing specificity against cancer cells. *Obstet Gynecol* 68:71S, 1986.

186. **FitzGerald DJ, Willingham MC, Pastan I:** Antitumor effects of an immunotoxin made with Pseudomonas exotoxin in a nude mouse model of human ovarian cancer. *Proc Natl Acad Sci USA* 83:6627, 1986.

187. **Pirker R, FitzGerald DJP, Hamilton TC, et al:** Anti-transferrin receptor antibody linked to Pseudomonas exotoxin as a model immunotoxin in human ovarian carcinoma cell lines. *Cancer Res* 45:751, 1985.

4

Pathology

Yao S. Fu
J. Donald Woodruff

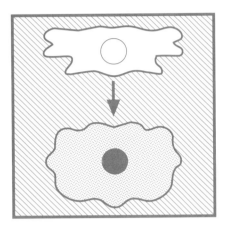

Despite the introduction of many new techniques for the investigation of the patient with suspected malignancy, histopathology is still the "gold standard" for the definitive diagnosis prior to the institution of therapy. Gynecologic pathology offers a special challenge, because physiologic alterations make interpretation of the tissue changes more complicated. The endometrium is a prime example of the problem with the intricate patterns associated with hyperplasias, polyps, and exogenous or endogenous hormones producing pseudomalignant alterations. Thus it is essential for the clinician to provide adequate information, including symptoms, the patient's age, menstrual history, current medications, gross findings, and prior therapy. If tissue has been examined previously in another laboratory, this should be noted and reviewed. No patient should be treated on the basis of a "report" from another laboratory without confirmation at the treating institution.

Cervix

Cervical epithelial changes represent a major problem in differential diagnosis among proliferative, inflammatory, and neoplastic lesions. During pregnancy, an associated decidual reaction may produce major diagnostic problems. The large, pale, sometimes bizarre, reactive decidual cells may suggest abnormal early invasive elements. An *Arias-Stella reaction* is occasionally noted in the endocervix and endometrium, in which hobnail cells with enlarged hyperchromatic nuclei line the crowded glands. This may be misconstrued as neoplasia. Furthermore, *microglandular hyperplasia* of the endocervical glands, as noted in women during pregnancy or in those taking oral contraceptives, produces closely apposed small glandular profiles suggestive of adenocarcinoma.

Mesonephric duct remnants and hyperplastic endocervical glands in the form of tunnel clusters or diffuse hyperplasia are common findings within the stroma of the cervix. Because they can lie deeper than 5 mm, these glands may be confused with well-differentiated adenocarcinoma and adenoma malignum.

117

Human papillomavirus (HPV) infections in the cervix produce the classic *koilocytotic atypia* (1) (Fig. 4.1). The nucleus is displaced to the border of the cell by the viral protein, producing the "hollow cell" appearance. In the endocervix the changes are less well defined, and the vacuolization in the cytoplasm is the important feature.

Cervical Intraepithelial Neoplasia (CIN)

The term "cervical intraepithelial neoplasia" (CIN), as proposed by Richart (2), refers to a lesion that may progress to invasive carcinoma. CIN is preferable to the term "dysplasia," which has been used to denote the same changes. However, dysplasia means "abnormal maturation" and, as a consequence, proliferating metaplasia without mitotic activity has erroneously been termed dysplasia of various degrees. Squamous metaplasia should not be diagnosed as dysplasia, because it does not progress to invasive cancer.

The criteria for the diagnosis of intraepithelial neoplasia may vary with the pathologist, but the significant features are cellular immaturity, cellular disorganization, nuclear abnormalities, and increased mitotic activity. The extent of the mitotic activity, immature cellular proliferation, and nuclear atypicality identifies the degree of neoplasia. If the mitoses and immature cells are present simply in the lower third of the epithelium, the lesion usually is designated as CIN 1. Involvement of the middle and upper thirds is diagnosed as CIN 2 and CIN 3, respectively (Fig. 4.2). Correlation of HPV type, morphology of CIN, and follow-up data suggest that HPV types 6 and 11 are associated with the acuminate form of condyloma; CIN 2 and CIN 3 are usually related to HPV types 16, 18, 31, 33, and 35 (3, 4).

Figure 4.1. CIN 1 with koilocytosis. The normal maturation process and differentiation from the basal and parabasal layers to the intermediate and superficial layers are maintained. In the upper layers, koilocytes are characterized by perinuclear halos, well-defined cell borders, and nuclear hyperchromasia, irregularity and enlargement.

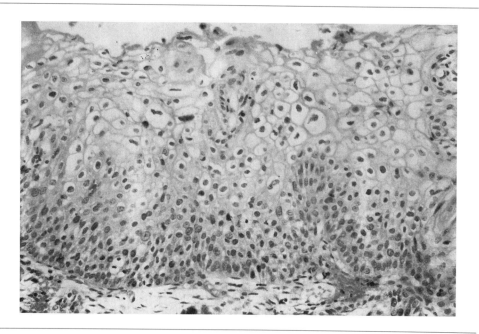

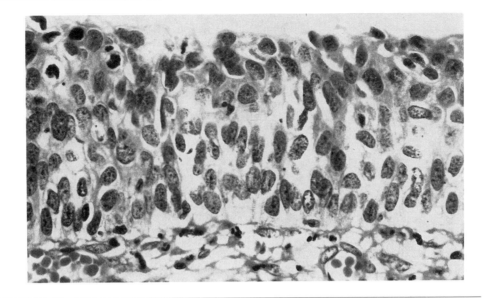

Figure 4.2.   **CIN 3** with the entire thickness of the epithelium replaced by abnormal cells that have large hyperchromatic, irregular nuclei. The normal maturation is lost. Mitotic figures are seen in the superficial layers (left upper corner).

Adenocarcinoma in situ (AIS)   In adenocarcinoma *in situ*, the endocervical glandular cells are replaced by tall columnar cells with nuclear stratification, hyperchromasia, irregularity, and increased mitotic activity. Cellular proliferation results in crowded, cribriform glands. However, the normal branching pattern of the endocervical glands is maintained. The majority of neoplastic cells resemble those of the endocervical mucinous epithelium (5). Endometrioid and intestinal cell types are less common. About 50% of women with cervical AIS also have squamous CIN. Thus some of the AIS lesions are incidental findings in specimens removed for squamous neoplasia. Because AIS is located near or above the transformation zone, conventional cervical smears may not sample AIS. Cytobrush specimens may improve detection of AIS. If the focus of AIS is small, cervical biopsy and endocervical curettage may give negative findings. A more comprehensive survey of the cervix in the form of conization is necessary for such cases. This type of specimen also allows exclusion of coexisting invasive adenocarcinoma. **The term "microinvasion" should not be used for adenocarcinomas.** Once the gland has invaded, there is no definable technique by which one can identify the true "depth of invasion" because the invasion may have originated from the mucosal surface or the periphery of the underlying glands. The "breakthrough" of the basement membrane cannot be truly described; thus the tumor is either adenocarcinoma *in situ* or invasive adenocarcinoma.

Microinvasive Cervical Squamous Carcinoma

Microinvasion requires a cervical conization to assess correctly the depth and the linear extent of involvement. The earliest invasion is characterized by a protrusion from the stromoepithelial junction. This focus consists of cells that appear better differentiated than the adjacent noninvasive cells and have abundant pink-staining cytoplasm, hyperchromatic nuclei, and small to medium-sized nucleoli (6). **These early invasive lesions in the form of tonguelike processes without measurable volume are classified as FIGO Stage Ia1.** With further

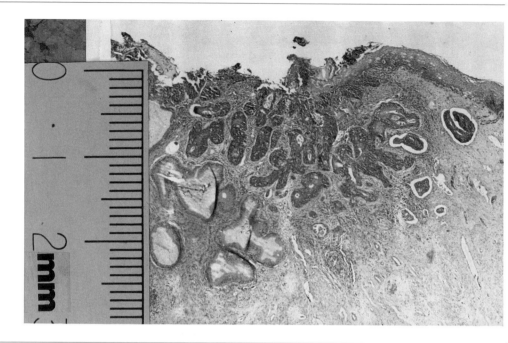

Figure 4.3. Microinvasive squamous carcinoma. Multiple irregular tonguelike processes and isolated nests of malignant cells are seen, some surrounded by clear spaces, simulating capillary lymphatic invasion. This is an artifact caused by tissue shrinkage. The depth of stromal invasion is measured from the basement membrane of the overlying CIN. In this case it is 1.5 mm.

Figure 4.4. Invasive squamous cell carcinoma, large cell nonkeratinizing type. Tumor cells form irregular nests and have abundant eosinophilic cytoplasm and distinct cell borders indicative of squamous differentiation.

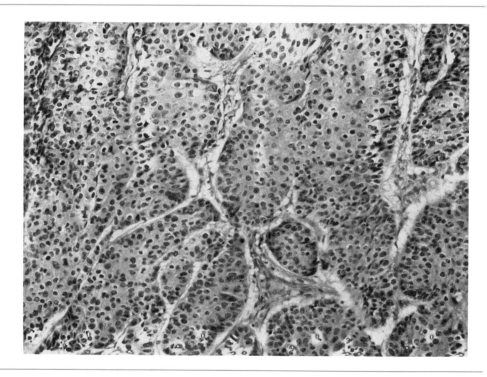

progression, more tonguelike processes and isolated cells occur in the stroma (Fig. 4.3). The latter responds by a proliferation of fibroblasts (desmoplasia) and a bandlike infiltration of chronic inflammatory cells. With increasing depth of invasion, invasion occurs at multiple sites, and the growth becomes measurable by depth and linear extent. **Those lesions ≤ 5 mm in depth and ≤ 7 mm in linear extent are classified as FIGO stage Ia2** (7). With increasing stromal invasion, the involvement of capillary-lymphatic spaces is increased. Foreign body multinucleated giant cells containing keratin debris and dilated capillaries and lymphatic spaces are commonly seen in the stroma.

The depth of invasion should be measured with the micrometer from the base of the epithelium to the deepest point of invasion. **The depth of invasion is significant for the development of pelvic lymph node metastasis and tumor recurrence. Although lesions that have invaded < 3 mm rarely metastasize, patients whose lesions invade 3–5 mm have positive pelvic lymph nodes in 5–8% of cases** (8). Although the significance of the cutoff at 3 mm has not been identified completely, it may be postulated that capillary lymphatic spaces are extremely small at this level, and whether or not they can carry tumor cells beyond the specific zone is unclear. Uneven shrinkage of tissue by fixative often creates space between the tumor nests and the surrounding fibrous stroma, simulating vascular lymphatic invasion (Fig. 4.3). **A suspected vascular involvement with invasion of < 3 mm should be interpreted with care.** A lack of endothelial lining indicates that the space is shrinkage artifact rather than true vascular invasion.

Invasive Cervical Cancer

Squamous Cell Carcinoma

Invasive squamous cell carcinoma is the most common variety in the cervix. Histologically, there are *large cell keratinizing, large cell nonkeratinizing,* and *small cell* types (9). Large cell keratinizing tumors are made up of tumor cells forming irregular infiltrative nests with laminated keratin pearls in the center. Large cell nonkeratinizing carcinomas reveal individual cell keratinization but do not form keratin pearls (Fig. 4.4). The category of small cell carcinoma includes *poorly differentiated squamous cell carcinoma* and *small cell anaplastic carcinoma.* If possible, these two tumors should be separated. The former contains cells that have small to medium-sized nuclei, open chromatin, small or large nucleoli, and more abundant cytoplasm than those of the latter. The designation of small cell anaplastic carcinoma should be reserved for that resembling oat cell carcinoma of the lung. It infiltrates diffusely and consists of tumor cells that have scanty cytoplasm, round to oval small nuclei, coarsely granular chromatin, and high mitotic activity. The nucleoli are absent or small. The small cell neuroendocrine tumors express neuroendocrine differentiation by immunohistochemistry or electron microscopy.

Patients with the large cell type, with or without keratinization, have a better prognosis than those with the small cell variant. Furthermore, small cell anaplastic carcinomas behave more aggressively than poorly differentiated squamous carcinomas that contain small cells. The prognosis is adversely affected by the presence of vascular lymphatic invasion, deep stromal invasion, infiltration of parametrial tissue, and pelvic lymph node metastasis.

Adenocarcinoma

In recent years there has been an increasing number of cervical adenocarcinoma affecting young women in their 20s and 30s. Adenocarcinoma *in situ* is believed to be the precursor of invasive adenocarcinoma, and it is not surprising that the two often coexist. In addition, squamous neoplasia, intraepithelial or invasive also occurs in 30–50% of cervical adenocarcinomas. Adenocarcinoma may be detected by cervical smears, but less reliably so than squamous carcinomas. A definitive diagnosis may require cervical conization.

Invasive adenocarcinoma may be pure (Fig. 4.5) or mixed with squamous cell carcinoma, the *adenosquamous carcinoma*. Within the category of pure adeno carcinoma, the tumors are quite heterogeneous (9) with a wide range of cell types growth patterns, and differentiation. About 80% of cervical adenocarcinomas are made up predominantly of cells of the endocervical type with mucin production The remaining tumors are populated by endometrioid cells, clear cells, intestinal cells, or a mixture of more than one cell type. By histologic examination alone some of these tumors are indistinguishable from those arising elsewhere in the endometrium or ovary.

Within each tumor type, the growth patterns and nuclear abnormalities vary according to the degree of differentiation. In well-differentiated tumors, tall co lumnar cells line the well-formed branching glands and papillary structures, while pleomorphic cells tend to form irregular nests and solid sheets in poorly differ entiated neoplasms. The latter may require mucicarmine and PAS stains to confirm their glandular differentiation.

Figure 4.5. Invasive adenocarcinoma of the cervix, well-differentiated. Irregular glands are lined with tall columnar cells with vacuolated mucinous cytoplasm re sembling endocervical cells. Nuclear stratification, mild nuclear atypism, and mitotic figures are evident.

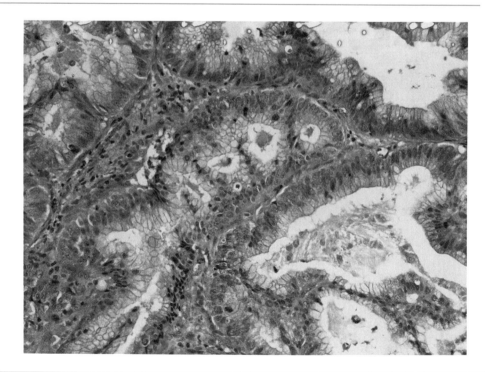

Several special variants of adenocarcinoma are indicated below. *Minimal deviation adenocarcinoma (adenoma malignum)* is an extremely well-differentiated form of adenocarcinoma in which the branching glandular pattern strongly simulates that of the normal endocervical glands. In addition, the lining cells have abundant mucinous cytoplasm and uniform nuclei (10, 11). Because of this, the tumor may not be recognized as malignant in small biopsy specimens, thereby causing considerable delay in diagnosis. Earlier studies reported a dismal outcome for women with this tumor, but more recent studies have found a favorable prognosis if the disease is detected early (12). Although rare, similar tumors have also been reported in association with endometrioid, clear, and mesonephric cell types (12).

An entity recently described by Young and Scully (13) as *villoglandular papillary adenocarcinoma* also deserves special attention. It primarily affects young women, some of whom are pregnant or users of oral contraceptives. Histologically, the tumors have smooth, well-defined borders, are well differentiated, and are either *in situ* or superficially invasive. The follow-up information is encouraging, none of these tumors having recurred after cervical conization or hysterectomy. Among women undergoing pelvic nodal dissection, no metastases have been detected. This tumor appears to have limited risk for spread beyond the uterus.

In mature *adenosquamous carcinomas,* the glandular and squamous carcinomas are readily identified on routine histologic sections and do not cause diagnostic problems. In poorly differentiated or immature adenosquamous carcinomas, however, glandular differentiation can be appreciated only after special stains, such as mucicarmine and periodic acid–Schiff (PAS). In the study by Benda et al. (14), 30% of squamous cell carcinomas demonstrated mucin secretion when stained with mucicarmine. These squamous cell carcinomas with mucin secretion have a higher incidence of pelvic lymph node metastases than squamous cell carcinomas without mucin secretion (14) and are similar to the signet-ring variant of adenosquamous carcinoma previously described by Glucksmann and Cherry (15).

Glucksmann and Cherry also recognized *glassy cell carcinoma* as a poorly differentiated form of adenosquamous carcinoma. Individual cells have abundant eosinophilic, granular, ground-glass cytoplasm, large round to oval nuclei, and prominent nucleoli. The stroma is infiltrated by numerous lymphocytes, plasma cells, and eosinophils. About half of these tumors contain glandular structures or stain positive for mucin. The poor prognosis of this tumor is linked to understaging and resistance to radiotherapy.

Other variants of adenosquamous carcinoma include *adenoid basal carcinoma* and *adenoid cystic carcinoma. Adenoid basal carcinoma* simulates the basal cell carcinoma of the skin (16). Nests of basaloid cells extend from the surface epithelium deep into the underlying tissue. Cells at the periphery of tumor nests form a distinct parallel nuclear arrangement, the so-called peripheral palisading. An "adenoid" pattern occasionally develops, with "hollowed-out" nests of cells. Mitoses are rare, and the tumor often extends deep into the cervical stroma.

Adenoid cystic carcinoma of the cervix behaves much like such lesions elsewhere in the body. The tendency is for the tumor to invade into the adjacent tissues and metastasize late: often 8–10 years after the primary tumor has been removed. Like other adenoid cystic tumors, they may metastasize directly to the lung. The pattern simulates that of the adenoid basal tumor, but there is a cystic component and the glands of the cervix are involved (16). Mitoses may be seen but are not numerous.

Sarcoma

The most important sarcoma of the cervix is the *embryonal rhabdomyosarcoma* which occurs in children and young adults. The tumor has grapelike polypoid nodules, the so-called *sarcoma botryoides*, and the diagnosis depends on the recognition of rhabdomyoblasts (9). Leiomyosarcomas and mixed mesodermal tumors involving the cervix may be primary but are more likely to be secondary to uterine tumors.

Malignant Melanoma

On rare occasions "melanosis" has been seen in the cervix. Thus malignant melanoma may arise *de novo* in this area. Histopathologically, it simulates melanoma elsewhere, and the prognosis depends on the depth of invasion into the cervical stroma.

Metastatic Cancer

The cervix is commonly involved in cancer of the endometrium and vagina. The latter is rare, and most lesions that involve the cervix and vagina are designated cervical primaries. Consequently, the clinical classification is that of cervical neoplasia extending to the vagina, rather than vice versa. Endometrial cancer may extend into the cervix by three modes: direct extension from the endometrium, submucosal involvement by lymph vascular extension, and multifocal disease. The latter is most unusual, but occasionally a focus of adenocarcinoma may be seen in the cervix, separate from the endometrium. This should not be diagnosed as a metastasis but, rather, as "multifocal disease." Malignancies involving the peritoneal cavity (e.g., ovarian cancer) may be found in the cul-de-sac and extend directly into the vagina and cervix. Carcinomas of the urinary bladder and colon occasionally extend into the cervix. Cervical involvement by lymphoma, leukemia, and carcinoma of the breast, stomach, and kidney is usually part of the systemic spread. However, an isolated metastasis to the cervix may be the first sign of a primary tumor elsewhere in the body.

Uterus

Endometrium

The endometrium is probably the most labile and complicated tissue in the female genital tract. It responds dramatically to the cyclic ovarian hormones and to local, systemic, and exogenous stimuli. These agents produce complicated and often varied patterns. Even the "normal cyclic" patterns may be confusing. Both the stroma and the glands are of the same embryologic origin and are estrogen- and progestin-dependent.

Bleeding and subsequent regeneration of the endometrium produce atypical patterns that may be misinterpreted as malignancy. Specifically, during bleeding, the degenerated and fragmented endometrium appears as closely apposed glands that simulate back-to-back glands in adenocarcinoma. The degenerated deciduoid stroma resembles squamous metaplasia. Thus the possibility of adenoacanthoma is strongly suggested. After the bleeding, the basalis endometrium reepithelializes the surface epithelium. Material from an endometrial biopsy or curettage performed at this time often contains double-contoured masses, characterized by an inner syncytium-like concentration of small deep stromal cells and an outer layer of pale-staining epithelial cells. These masses may simulate small cell carcinoma of the cervix or endometrial stromal sarcoma. Other artifacts caused by endometrial biopsy, curettage, or suction include isolated, crowded, back-to-back glands and invaginated, "telescoped" glands. These glandular profiles can be mistaken for hyperplasia.

During the late secretory phase, the *pseudo-Arias-Stella* phenomenon (hypersecretory pattern) may suggest atypical adenomatous hyperplasia. The presence of a decidual reaction and the active secretion suggests the appropriate diagnosis.

Arias-Stella Reaction The Arias-Stella reaction is a well-defined histopathologic entity and a feature noted in all endometria associated with viable trophoblasts. This reaction can be recognized in patients receiving progestin therapy, in those with a persistent corpus luteum (*Halban's syndrome*), in those with a progestin-secreting ovarian tumor, and rarely in patients on long-term oral contraceptives. The Arias-Stella reaction is identified histopathologically by irregular hypersecretory glands with individual hyperchromatic nuclei seen primarily at the luminal edge of the epithelial cell (Fig. 4.6).

Exaggerated Placental Site and Placental Site Trophoblastic Tumor At the implantation site, sheets of intermediate trophoblastic cells with large, atypical, hyperchromatic, sometimes multinucleated nuclei are mixed with chorionic villi and decidual cells. If the patient has been bleeding for several weeks, the villi may have disappeared, leaving only intermediate trophoblast in the myometrium. Nodules or plaques of intermediate trophoblast embedded in a hyalinized stroma

Figure 4.6. Arias-Stella reaction of the endometrium. The glands are closely packed and hypersecretory with large hyperchromatic nuclei suggesting malignancy.

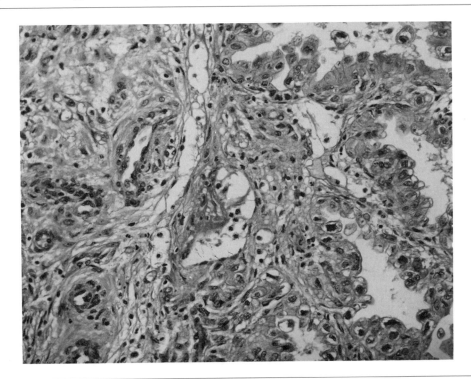

sometimes occur in the endometrium or myometrium at the implantation site (17). Rarely, neoplastic proliferation of intermediate trophoblast results in placental site trophoblastic tumor, which infiltrates the myometrium and vascular spaces. These intermediate trophoblastic cells have abundant amphophilic or eosinophilic cytoplasm, atypical nuclei, prominent nucleoli, and an average of two mitotic figures per 10 high-power fields (17). In contrast to choriocarcinoma, placental site trophoblastic tumor lacks the extensive hemorrhagic necrosis and the characteristic mixture of cytotrophoblast and syncytiotrophoblast.

Endometrial Hyperplasia

Hyperplasia, typical or atypical, is one of the most common diagnoses made on endometrial tissue removed from patients with abnormal bleeding. Endometrial hyperplasia has become an increasingly complex problem with its confusing array of terminologies and interpretations. Therefore the clinician and pathologist must discuss each case of hyperplasia and correlate the clinical with the pathologic features in order to treat the individual patient properly.

The diagnosis of endometrial hyperplasia is based on the abnormal architecture of glandular profiles and the nuclear features of glandular cells. As such, the specimen must consist of a reasonable quantity of intact endometrial tissue, and the abnormalities should occur in more than a few solitary foci. Because the endometrium does not respond as a unit and polyps are frequent, all areas of the endometrium must be evaluated accurately and the most aggressive patterns must be included in the diagnosis.

The terms *cystic, adenomatous,* and *atypical adenomatous* have been used to describe hyperplasias with increasing glandular crowding and complexity and a

Figure 4.7. Simple cystic hyperplasia of the endometrium. The normal tubular pattern is replaced by cystically dilated proliferative endometrial glands.

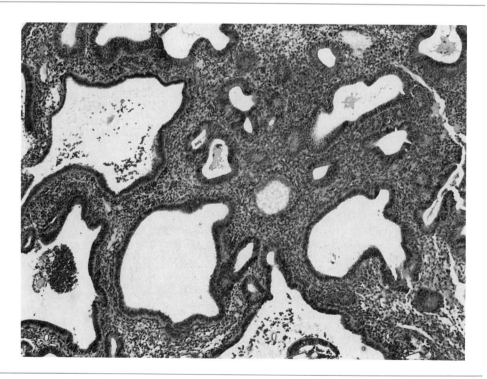

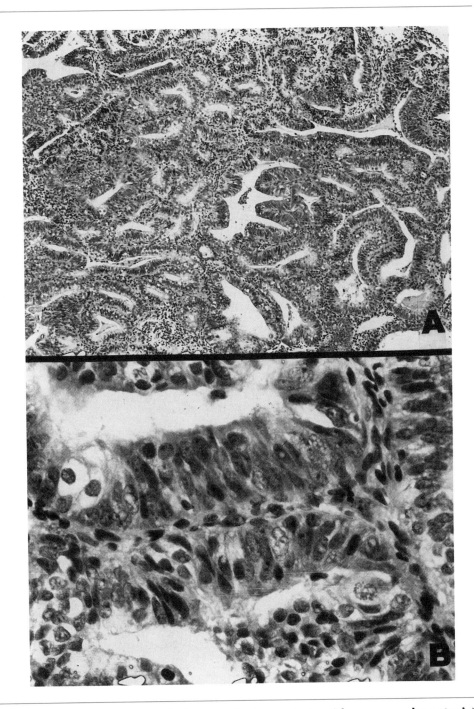

Figure 4.8.   Atypical hyperplasia (complex hyperplasia with severe nuclear atypia) of endometrium. A. The proliferative endometrial glands reveal considerable crowding and papillary infoldings. The endometrial stroma, although markedly diminished, can still be recognized between the glands. B. Higher magnification demonstrates disorderly nuclear arrangement and nuclear enlargement and irregularity. Some contain small nucleoli.

127

concurrent decrease in the amount of stroma. When the individual glandular cells resemble those of normal proliferative endometrium, the nuclear atypia is absent. "Nuclear atypia" refers to nuclear enlargement, rounding, and irregularity, an increased mitotic activity, and the formation of nucleoli (18).

The terminology of simple hyperplasia (Fig. 4.7), complex hyperplasia, and atypical hyperplasia has been recommended (19). *Simple hyperplasia* includes those with cystic and branching adenomatous patterns. *Complex hyperplasia* refers to the presence of overtly crowded, papillary, or closely apposed glands (Fig. 4.8A). Any hyperplasia associated with nuclear atypia is classified as *atypical hyperplasia* (Fig. 4.8B). Using these criteria, Kurman et al. (19) studied a group of 170 women with untreated hyperplasia and found that the frequency of regression, persistence, and progression to carcinoma for women with simple hyperplasia was 80%, 19%, and 1%, respectively. For complex hyperplasia the corresponding figures were 80%, 17%, and 3%, whereas for atypical hyperplasia the figures were 60%, 17%, and 23%, respectively. In a separate study of 96 women with hyperplasia untreated for 1 to 13 years, 3% of cases that lacked nuclear atypia progressed to carcinoma, compared with 24% of cases that demonstrated nuclear atypia (18). Thus, **nuclear atypia is a more reliable indicator of progression to carcinoma than architectural abnormality.**

Nuclear atypia in endometrial hyperplasia also correlates with response to oral medroxyprogesterone acetate therapy. With this therapy, 80% of cases of endometrial hyperplasia lacking atypia regressed, 20% persisted, and none progressed to carcinoma. In the presence of nuclear atypia, 25% of hyperplasias regressed, 50% persisted, and 25% progressed to carcinoma (20).

Grossly, the hyperplastic tissue is pale brownish red or reddish and velvety in appearance rather than grayish and friable, as seen in endometrial cancer. Frozen-section diagnosis is unreliable because there are too many variations from one area to another. Permanent tissue preparation is necessary to identify the variable and most significant changes.

Endometrial Response to Hormonal Therapy The atrophic endometrium in postmenopausal women who are placed on estrogen and progestin therapy converts to weakly proliferative endometrium, resembling that seen in chronic anovulation, or hyperplastic endometrium, depending on the dosage and duration of estrogen therapy. Progestin effects, including stromal edema, deciduoid reaction, and secretory glands, also develop.

Carcinoma of the Endometrium

Adenocarcinoma may occur as a focal lesion or as one that diffusely involves the endometrial cavity. Focal lesions occasionally are found in a polyp. Such lesions are usually firm and reddish brown with an occasional gray or hemorrhagic focus from infarction. Particularly in the perimenopausal and early postmenopausal patient, the lesion is found high in the fundus and may develop even in the presence of a corpus luteum in the ovary.

The similarity between well-differentiated adenocarcinoma (Fig. 4.9) and atypical hyperplasia may make absolute differentiation difficult. Kurman and Norris (21) proposed the following criteria for adenocarcinoma in endometrial biopsy and curettage specimens:

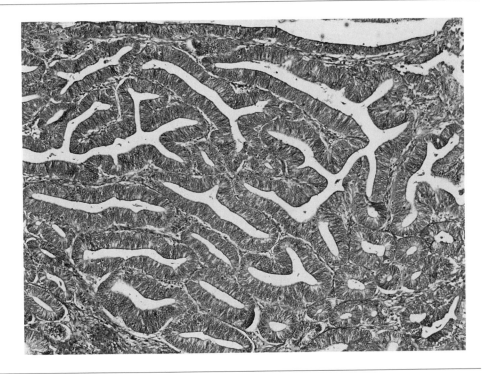

Figure 4.9.   Well-differentiated adenocarcinoma of endometrium. The glands and complex papillae are in direct contact with no intervening endometrial stroma, the so-called back-to-back pattern.

1. Neoplastic glands accompanied by desmoplastic reaction, or

2. Confluent glands with a cribriform pattern, complex papillary formation, or masses of squamous metaplasia.

The area of epithelial abnormality should be at least 2.1 mm in diameter (half of a low-power microscopic field). When the tissue fragments are small, there is a tendency toward underdiagnosis, because about 25% of atypical endometrial hyperplasias have a coexisting adenocarcinoma that may not have been sampled.

For Hendrickson et al., (22) a diagnosis of endometrial adenocarcinoma requires both marked architectural atypia and at least moderate cytologic abnormality. The architecture should be complex, papillary, or confluent. Nuclear atypism includes enlargement, chromatin clearing, prominent nucleoli, and mitotic figures.

About 20% of adenocarcinomas contain foci of endocervical mucinous metaplasia or ciliated cells. In addition to the classic adenocarcinoma, several types of neoplasms occur in the endometrium.

Adenocarcinoma With Squamous Differentiation   The squamous element may appear cytologically benign or malignant with local infiltration (Fig. 4.10). The former was previously referred to as adenoacanthoma, and the latter as adenosquamous carcinoma. Adenoacanthomas usually have well-differentiated or moderately differentiated glandular elements, whereas adenosquamous carcinomas tend to be associated with a poorly differentiated glandular component. The difference in glandular differentiation and a proclivity for deeper myometrial

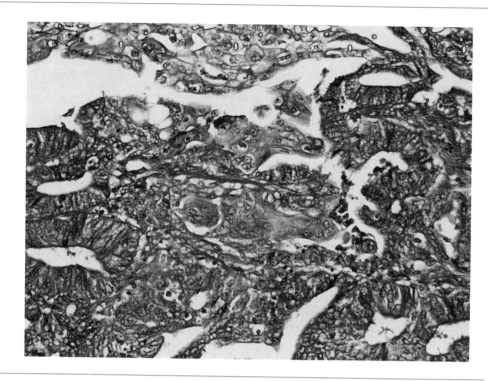

Figure 4.10. Adenocarcinoma with squamous differentiation of endometrium. This lesion is also classified as adenoacanthoma. Squamous cells with eosinophilic cytoplasm and distinct cell borders form solid clusters in the lumina of neoplastic glands.

invasion and vascular invasion explain why adenosquamous carcinomas are more aggressive than classic adenocarcinomas and adenoacanthomas (23).

Secretory Carcinoma Secretory carcinoma is an extremely rare variant of adenocarcinoma of the endometrium. In these lesions, epithelial cells are tall and pale with clear secretory cytoplasm. Staining demonstrates glycogen. The pure secretory cancer is probably the least aggressive of all endometrial lesions because invasion is seen rarely.

Papillary Serous Carcinoma This type is similar to a papillary serous lesion of the ovary. The complex papillae are lined with cuboidal or low columnar cells with severe nuclear anaplasia, prominent nucleoli, and high mitotic activity (Fig. 4.11). An aggressive behavior with peritoneal spread can occur with minimal myometrial invasion, presumably through transtubal spread.

Clear Cell Carcinoma The lesions of clear cell carcinoma are similar to those seen in the ovary and in the vagina of children exposed to diethylstilbestrol (DES) *in utero*. An association with DES has not been demonstrated with the endometrial lesion. The tumor appears to be another variant of the totipotent paramesonephric epithelium. The lesions are uncommon, accounting for 2–3% of all adenocarcinomas of the endometrium. They tend to be deeply invasive at the time of diagnosis.

Prognostic Factors

The most important histologic features that affect prognosis are cell type, histologic grade, depth of myometrial invasion, and endocervical involvement. Clear cell and papillary serous carcinomas are more aggressive than endometrioid endometrial adenocarcinomas.

Histologic Grade   Adenocarcinoma of the endometrium is graded by the architecture alone (GOG) or a combination of architecture and nuclear features (FIGO and WHO). Graded by using the FIGO method, the well-differentiated (grade 1) lesions contain 98% or more glandular or papillary formations, moderately differentiated (grade 2) tumors have 2–50% solid areas, and poorly differentiated (grade 3) neoplasms have more than 50% solid areas. In the presence of moderate or severe nuclear atypia, the grade is upgraded by 1 or 2 by the FIGO system of grading. For example, a papillary serous carcinoma with severe nuclear atypia is graded as 3, even though no solid areas are recognized. The GOG defines grade 1 tumors as having < 5% solid foci; grade 2, 5 to 50% solid; and grade 3, > 50% solid. Approximately 80–85% of adenocarcinomas are grade 1–2 lesions.

Endocervical Involvement   Identification of endocervical involvement may be made by curettage of the cervix before instrumentation of the endometrial cavity. **Because many of the large, diffuse malignancies shed tissues into the cervical canal, definite involvement of the endocervix can be diagnosed only if there is benign endocervical tissue associated with the cancer. Fragments of desquamated tissue are not an adequate demonstration of true endocervical involvement.**

Figure 4.11.   Papillary serous carcinoma of endometrium. Branching papillae are supported by delicate fibrovascular cores and lined with columnar cells with moderate nuclear atypism, multiple nucleoli, and mitotic figures.

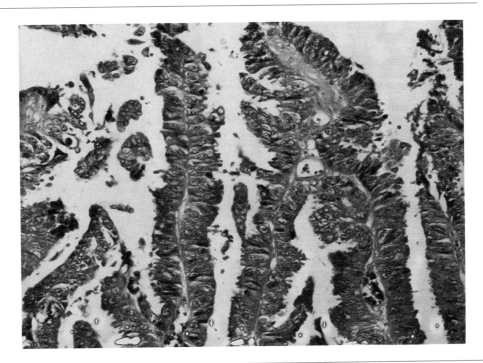

Myometrial Invasion Invasion into the underlying musculature is also of major prognostic importance. In a diffuse cancer, varying areas may show differing depths of myometrial invasion as well as differing degrees of histologic differentiation. One of the confusing features in defining early myometrial invasion is the irregularity of the basal layer. In the normal uterus, the irregularity of the endomyometrial junction is evident in every section.

Adenocarcinoma can extend into underlying adenomyosis. The prognosis in such cases is good, even though the tumor seemingly has involved the entire myometrium. Thus these cases represent a direct extension of adenomyosis rather than myometrial invasion. The presence of endometrial stromal cells between the tumor and the myometrium is a helpful sign of preexisting adenomyosis.

Squamous Cell Carcinoma

Squamous cell carcinoma is a rare lesion, which usually occurs in older women. The occurrence of squamous metaplasia has been noted with long-standing pelvic inflammatory disease, after radium application, with vitamin A deficiency, and with long-term use of an intrauterine device (IUD). Patches of squamous epithelium are not rare in the postmenopausal endometrium, and in extreme cases the entire endometrium may be replaced by stratified squamous epithelium (the so-called *ichthyosis uteri*) from which a squamous cancer can arise.

Sarcomas

Mesenchymal tumors of the uterus constitute only about 3% of uterine malignancies. Uterine sarcomas include *leiomyosarcomas*, *endometrial stromal sarcomas*, and *mixed mesodermal tumors*.

Leiomyosarcoma

Leiomyosarcomas account for 20–30% of uterine sarcomas. They may arise *de novo* from the smooth muscle of the uterus or result from malignant transformation of a benign leiomyoma. Microscopically, it is difficult to distinguish degenerative changes from true neoplasia. Symplastic giant cells are commonly found in areas of marked degeneration, and thus it is mandatory to find mitoses in order to make the diagnosis of sarcoma (24) (Fig. 4.12).

The number of mitoses in 10 high-powered fields (HPFs) is the criterion for the division between the benign and malignant lesions. If ≥ 10 mitoses per 10 HPFs are found, the tumor is considered malignant. Lesions with 5–9 mitoses per 10 HPFs and atypical nuclear cytology are also considered malignant, whereas those with a like number of mitoses and no atypia are of borderline malignancy (25). *Cellular leiomyomas* and *atypical leiomyomas* are benign lesions with < 5 mitoses per 10 HPFs. Although they have some mitotic activity, the cytologic pattern is not atypical.

Exceptions to the above rules are *mitotically active leiomyomas*, in which up to 15 mitoses per 10 HPFs may be found without nuclear atypia (26). These tumors are < 10 cm in size and well circumscribed. Not all leiomyosarcomas meet the mitotic activity criterion. For example, the mitotic activity in a *myxoid leiomyosarcoma* is usually < 2 per 10 HPFs. Thus the diagnosis of leiomyosarcoma sometimes has to rely on other signs of malignancy, such as local infiltration, vascular invasion, and extrauterine spread.

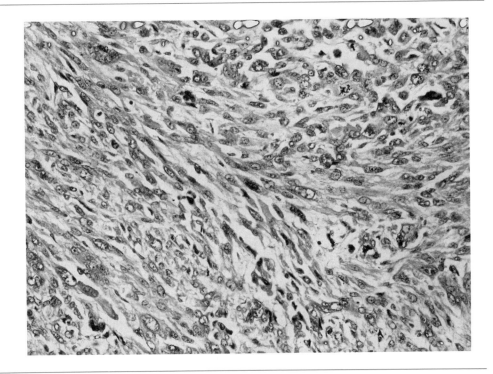

Figure 4.12.   Leiomyosarcoma of the uterus. Interlacing bundles of spindle cells have fibrillar cytoplasm, irregular and hyperchromatic nuclei, and multiple mitotic figures.

Conditions that must be differentiated from leiomyosarcomas are intravenous leiomyomatosis and benign metastasizing leiomyoma. *Intravenous leiomyomatosis* is a rare lesion that appears to arise from the muscle wall of the vessel and invades directly into the vascular channels. It can often be diagnosed at surgery by the demonstration of cordlike processes extending into the myometrial vessels and adjacent broad ligament. These tumors may occur at any age, and, although the gross appearance is ominous, the prognosis is excellent because only rare metastases have been reported.

The term "benign metastasizing leiomyoma" is a misnomer. In most instances, the patient has been treated by hysterectomy for a benign leiomyoma and subsequently has been found to have a similar lesion elsewhere in the body, most commonly the lung. The secondary tumors often appear 15–20 years after removal of the primary disease, and there is no histologic evidence of malignancy. Consequently, such tumors must be considered examples of lesions arising at multiple sites rather than benign "metastasizing" lesions.

A condition known as *leiomyomatosis peritonealis disseminata* is one in which subperitoneal nodules, often removed at the time of elective cesarean section, are scattered over the pelvic organs and throughout the peritoneal cavity. These have been confused with diffuse metastatic disease, but they represent a benign replacement of subperitoneal decidual nodules with fibrous tissue and subsequently smooth muscle (27).

Endometrial Stromal Sarcomas

Endometrial stromal sarcomas account for about 15–25% of uterine sarcomas. The three types are the *benign stromal nodule*, the *well-differentiated (low-grade) stromal sarcoma*, and the *poorly differentiated stromal sarcoma*. Benign stromal nodules have smooth, well-circumscribed borders and most often appear as benign submucosal leiomyomas. No nuclear atypia or mitoses are seen in these lesions.

Well-differentiated (low-grade) endometrial stromal sarcoma resembles proliferative endometrial stroma with distinct small arterioles in the background (28). The mitotic activity is low, usually < 3 mitoses per 10 HPFs. Those having even > 10 mitoses per 10 HPFs behave in the same manner. The clinical course is indolent, but local recurrence does occur. This lesion was formerly known as *endolymphatic stromal myosis*.

Poorly differentiated endometrial stromal sarcomas have high mitotic rates, lack small arterioles, exhibit extreme nuclear pleomorphism, and are highly aggressive. They perhaps are more appropriately classified as undifferentiated stromal sarcomas. Spread typically occurs through the pelvic vasculature and eventually reaches distant sites, usually the lungs.

Mixed Mesodermal Tumors

Three distinct groups of müllerian mixed mesodermal tumors exist. The benign category, *müllerian adenofibroma*, consists of benign endometrial or endocervical epithelium and somewhat hypercellular fibromuscular stroma. The second group, *müllerian adenosarcoma*, contains malignant homologous or heterologous stroma and branching glands lined with hyperplastic endometrial or, less commonly, endocervical cells. This is a low-grade malignant tumor with potential for local recurrence and occasionally metastasis. The third group, *malignant mixed mesodermal tumor*, is made up of malignant epithelial and stromal elements. This tumor most frequently affects women in their sixth to ninth decades and represents 2% of all uterine malignancies. Grossly, the tumor is polypoid (Fig. 4.13). Microscopically, the lesions are composed of "malignant" stroma and epithelium

Figure 4.13. Polypoid mixed mesodermal tumor of the uterus.

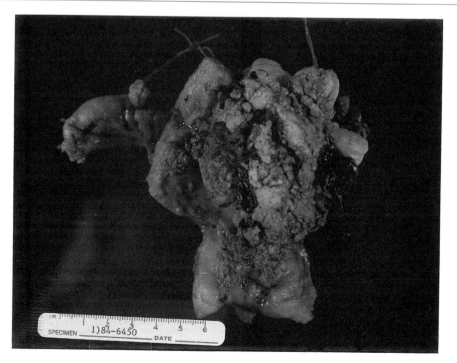

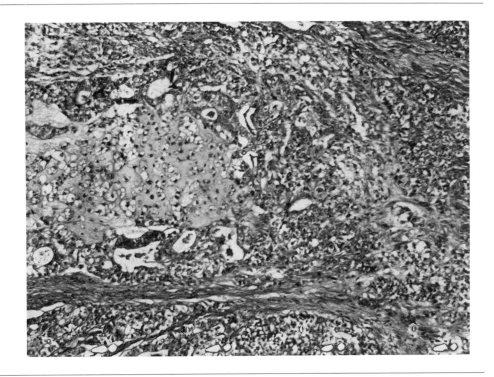

Figure 4.14.   Mixed mesodermal sarcoma of uterus. This lesion consists of poorly differentiated adenocarcinoma with rare glandular lumina (right half of figure) and chondrosarcoma (left half of figure).

(Fig. 4.14). The latter is usually representative of adenocarcinoma with varying degrees of anaplasia and often foci of adenosquamous neoplasia. The stroma is abnormally proliferative and is characterized by varying types of neoplastic alterations, many of which are foreign to the uterus (e.g., cartilage and bone). The most malignant element in the stroma is the rhabdomyoblast. Tumors containing any or all of these "foreign" tissues have been classified as *heterologous* tumors, in contrast to the *homologous* lesions that contain only endometrial stroma or smooth muscle. The prognosis for these two types is the same.

Ovary

The anlage of the gonad, either ovary or testis, appears very early in fetal development as an aggregation of cells on the anterior aspect of the *wolffian body*, covered with the primitive mesothelium or coelomic epithelium. The development of the gonad is dependent on the migration of germ cells from their original site in the wall of the yolk sac into the gonadal area. The important embryologic factors that aid in the understanding of ovarian neoplasia include the following:

1. During the undifferentiated stage of development the primitive gonads have the potential to develop into either a testis or an ovary. The ovary is a cortical structure without a capsule, whereas the testis has a capsule at 8–10 weeks of embryonic life.

2. The ovarian stroma and epithelium are of the same mesodermal origin. The peritoneum is of similar origin. The epithelium lining the ovary and the peritoneum is similar to the coelomic epithelium that gives rise to the fallopian tube, uterus, and cervix, the müllerian duct.

Histology

Coelomic Epithelium Covering the ovary is the coelomic or peritoneal epithelium (*mesothelium*). The term "germinal epithelium" is no longer acceptable, because there is no evidence that germ cells are formed in or by this epithelium. The mesothelium is perishable and is uncommonly identified on the surface of the adult ovary, although it is often well preserved in the ovaries of young children. Originally, it consists of a single layer of cuboidal or "flat" peglike epithelial cells. In the common epithelial inclusions routinely present in the ovarian cortex of the ovulating woman, differentiation of the included mesothelium into a tubal, endometrial, or endocervical variety of epithelium is identifiable. This surface epithelium is of mesodermal origin and, by invagination at 5.5–6 weeks of embryonic life, forms the paramesonephric duct. Consequently, there is a similarity in lesions arising in the genital canal, the ovary, and the adjacent peritoneum.

Germ Cell The germ cell arrives at the gonadal ridge as early as 4 weeks after ovulation. Originally, it lies directly beneath the surface epithelium and may become encapsulated and progress toward the hilum. Conversely, many germ cells do not become encapsulated by primitive granulosa cells but appear as aggregates that superficially simulate the dysgerminoma. Mitoses may be seen until encapsulation is complete, usually at 7 months of embryonic life. At completion of the differentiative processes, usually at birth, 2 million primordial follicles are present. At menarche, 300,000–400,000 have survived the attrition that can be recognized in the early gonad by foci of calcification.

Cortex and Medulla The ovary is divisible into a "cortex" and a medulla. During reproductive life, the "cortex" is broad, constituting from one-half to two-thirds of the depth of the ovary. Thus the ovary, in contrast to the testis, is primarily a cortical structure. The ovarian medulla consists primarily of a matrix surrounding the major ovarian blood vessels and lymphatics. It also contains such structures as the rete ovarii and hilar cells, which are the residua of the male-directed elements and thus are potentially androgenic.

Epithelial Ovarian Neoplasia

Epithelial neoplasia arising in or on the ovary represents the second most common malignancy in the female genital canal. Approximately 75% of all primary ovarian neoplasms arise from the coelomic epithelium. The "epithelial" tumors contain varying amounts and activities of the gonadal mesenchyme (Table 4.1). The latter, commonly known as ovarian stroma, contains two elements, both of mesodermal origin (i.e., the potentially functioning theca and the supporting connective tissue). Therefore all ovarian tumors are potentially hormone producing, because an integral element of each lesion is the basic gonadal stroma.

Epithelial ovarian tumors are classified according to cell type and behavior:

1. Benign

2. Borderline malignant or low malignant potential

3. Malignant

In benign tumors, the epithelium is made up of a single layer of cells without nuclear stratification and atypism. The criteria for the diagnosis of borderline malignant tumors (Fig. 4.15) are (29):

Table 4.1   Epithelial Ovarian Tumors

Histologic Type	*Cellular Type*
I. Serous A. Benign B. Borderline C. Malignant	Endosalpingeal
II. Mucinous A. Benign B. Borderline C. Malignant	Endocervical
III. Endometrioid A. Benign B. Borderline C. Malignant	Endometrial
IV. Clear Cell "Mesonephroid" A. Benign B. Borderline C. Malignant	Müllerian
V. Brenner A. Benign B. Borderline ("proliferating") C. Malignant	Transitional
VI. Mixed epithelial A. Benign B. Borderline C. Malignant	Mixed
VII. Undiffererentiated	Anaplastic
VIII. Unclassified	Mesothelioma, etc

Adapted, with permission, from Serov SF, Scully RE, Sobin LH: International histological classification of tumours no. 9. Histological typing of ovarian tumours. Geneva: World Health Organization, 1973.

1. Epithelial proliferation with papillary formation and pseudostratification

2. Nuclear atypia and increased mitotic activity

3. Absence of true stromal invasion (i.e., without tissue destruction)

It should be emphasized that about 20–25% of borderline malignant tumors have spread beyond the ovary. The peritoneal implants may not be distinguished from those secondary to a well-differentiated carcinoma. Thus, the diagnosis of borderline malignant versus malignant ovarian tumor must be based on the histologic features of the primary tumor. In the malignant tumors, stromal invasion is present. Rare examples of microinvasion have been reported in borderline malignant tumors (29).

The major cell types include

1. Serous

2. Mucinous

3. Endometrioid

4. Clear cell

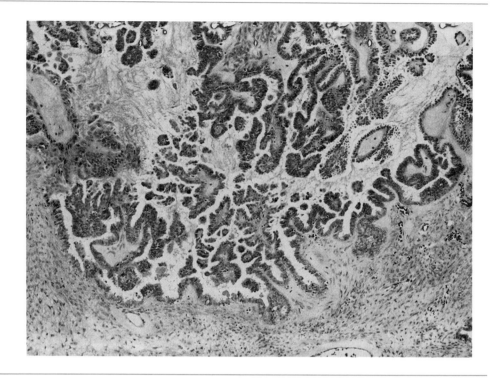

Figure 4.15. Borderline malignant serous tumor of the ovary. Complex papillary fronds are lined with pseudostratified columnar cells. The epithelium and the stroma are clearly separated by a basement membrane, indicating no stromal invasion.

5. Transitional

6. Undifferentiated

Serous Tumors

The largest group of ovarian cystomas of the epithelial variety have been classified as serous. The serous tumors develop by invagination of the surface ovarian epithelium and are so classified because they secrete serous fluid (as do tubal secretory cells). *Psammoma bodies*, more correctly foci of foreign material, frequently are associated with these invaginations and may be a response to irritative agents that produce adhesion formation and the entrapment of the surface epithelium. In the wall of the mesothelial invaginations, papillary ingrowths are common, representing the early stages of development of a papillary serous cystadenoma. There are many variations in the proliferation of these mesothelial inclusions. Several foci may be lined with flattened inactive epithelium; in adjacent cavities, papillary excrescences are present, often resulting from local irritants.

Benign Serous Tumors The simplest variety of ovarian cyst is a unilocular structure, usually lined with a layer of flattened or cuboidal epithelium. The larger serous cysts usually are lobulated and multilocular and contain watery fluid. When the serous cyst is opened, discrete papillary outgrowths from the lining may be found in one or more of the compartments, the so-called *papillary adenofibroma*. In this tumor, the papillary growths result from excessive proliferation of the stroma rather than the epithelium. **It is impossible to distinguish grossly between benign and malignant proliferations; thus frozen section is important, particularly in the young woman desirous of maintaining fertility.** Fortunately, the cellular alterations in the papillary serous tumors usually remain constant from one area to the next.

The epithelium, both on the surface and in the invaginations, is similar to that of the fallopian tube with both the ciliated and nonciliated secretory elements. Occasionally other epithelial or mesothelial elements may be present. In the benign tumor, the epithelium has a single cell layer, although an appearance of stratification may be given by tangential sectioning through the exuberant papillae. Most significantly, mitoses are absent.

Borderline Malignant Serous Tumors   **Approximately 10% of all ovarian serous tumors fall into the category of a "tumor of low malignant potential" or "borderline malignant" tumor, and 50% occur before the age of 40 years**.

Up to 40% of women with ovarian serous borderline malignant tumors have extraovarian implants, and up to 40% of these women eventually die of disease (29). Although multiple foci of disease have been documented in the abdominal cavity with secondary deposits in the pelvis, omentum, and adjacent tissues, including lymph nodes, metastases outside the abdominal cavity are exceptional. Death can occur as the result of intestinal obstruction (30).

The implants are divided histologically into invasive and noninvasive groups. In the *noninvasive group*, papillary proliferations of atypical cells involve the peritoneal surface and form smooth invaginations. The degree of nuclear atypia is similar to that of the primary tumor. A desmoplastic stromal reaction, characterized by dense layers of fibroblasts and infiltration with acute and chronic inflammatory cells, can occur in association with some of the implants. Atypical cells, single or in clusters, may be associated with psammoma bodies, necrosis, cholesterol clefts, or hemorrhage (31).

The *invasive implants* resemble well-differentiated serous carcinoma and are characterized by atypical cells forming irregular glands with sharp borders. The interface between the epithelium and stroma is ill defined or obliterated. Marked cytologic atypia is usually present. Single cells may be found in both invasive and noninvasive implants.

Bell et al. (31) have reported that only 3 of 50 women with noninvasive implants died, while 4 of 6 women with invasive implants died. In the series of McCaughey, 2 of 13 with noninvasive implants and all 5 with invasive implants died (32). Others have noted no differences in prognosis (33, 34).

Rare examples of borderline malignant serous tumors with foci of microinvasion have been reported by Bell and Scully (35). These foci can be recognized by single cells, cribriform glands, or papillary clusters extending into the stroma, often with empty spaces between the epithelium and the stroma. Invasion of lymphatic spaces may be seen. Most patients are young, FIGO Stage I, and sometimes pregnant. Only one of 30 such patients died of disease. This patient had Stage III disease and died 1 month after surgery (35).

Malignant Serous Tumors   The grade of the tumor should be identified. In well-differentiated serous adenocarcinoma, papillary and glandular structures predominate. The nuclei are uniformly round to oval with 0–2 mitoses per HPF (Fig. 4.16). Poorly differentiated neoplasms are characterized by solid sheets of cells, nuclear pleomorphism, and high mitotic activity, usually 2–3 mitoses per HPF (Fig. 4.17). A moderately differentiated tumor is intermediate between the well-

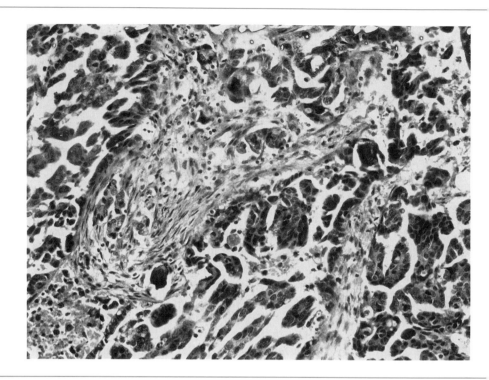

Figure 4.16. Well-differentiated serous papillary adenocarcinoma of ovary. Clusters and papillae of malignant cells are in direct contact with fibrous stroma indicative of stromal invasion.

Figure 4.17. Poorly differentiated carcinoma of ovary. There are predominantly solid sheets with rare ill-defined spaces suggestive of glandular differentiation. Individual cells have large nuclei and prominent nucleoli.

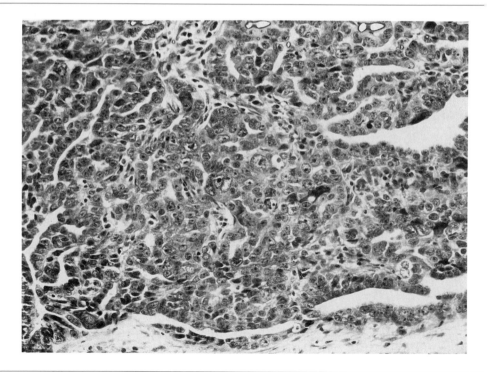

differentiated and poorly differentiated groups. Laminated, calcified psammoma bodies are found in 80% of serous carcinomas.

Mucinous Tumors

These cystic tumors with locules lined with mucin-secreting epithelium comprise approximately 8–10% of primary epithelial ovarian tumors. They may reach an enormous size, filling the entire abdominal cavity.

Benign Mucinous Tumors   Mucinous tumors are commonly intraovarian, multilocular, and rarely papillary. The tumors are bilateral in 8–10% of cases. They are characteristically lobulated, with a smooth outer surface. Adhesions are uncommon unless the cyst has leaked, degenerated, or become malignant. The wall of the cyst is usually thin, often translucent, and whitish or blue-white. The most distinctive histologic feature is the characteristic tall columnar epithelial cell with its clear, refractile cytoplasm and basally placed nucleus resembling an endocervical cell. Breakdown of the septa that separate the locules may result in extravasation of mucoid material into the stroma. A pseudostratified appearance may be seen in some foci, which results from the characteristic undulation of the epithelium. The ability of the ovarian stroma to respond to the proliferating epithelium or its secretion is dramatic in certain cases (e.g., during pregnancy the host may be masculinized).

Borderline Malignant Mucinous Tumors   The mucinous "tumor of low malignant potential" is an enigma. Mucinous tumors are made up largely of endocervical mucus-secreting cells and may reveal areas in which intestinal, serous, or endometrioid epithelia seem to suggest immaturity. Such foci do not change the prognosis but are simply demonstrations of the multipotentiality of the surface epithelium. Tumors with more than four stratified layers or cytologically malignant cells are best classified as well-differentiated mucinous carcinoma. Although it is common to find a rather uniform pattern from section to section in the borderline malignant serous lesions, this is not true in the mucinous tumors. Frequently, well-differentiated mucinous epithelium may be seen immediately adjacent to a poorly differentiated focus. Therefore it is important to take multiple sections from many areas in the mucinous tumor in order to identify the most significant anaplastic alteration.

Malignant Mucinous Tumors   Although papillary proliferations are much less common in the mucinous tumors than in the serous tumors, such alterations are basic evidence of atypical proliferation, and it is in these foci that the true mitotic activity of the mucinous carcinoma can be most accurately identified (Fig. 4.18). **Bilateral tumors occur in 8–10% of cases.** The mucinous lesions are intraovarian in 95–98% of cases. Malignancy develops in 5–10% of benign mucinous cysts. Because the majority of ovarian mucinous carcinomas contain intestinal type cells, they cannot be distinguished from metastatic carcinoma of the gastrointestinal tract on the basis of histology alone. Primary ovarian neoplasms rarely metastasize to the mucosa of the bowel, although they commonly involve the serosa, whereas gastrointestinal lesions frequently involve the ovary by direct extension or vascular lymphatic spread.

Pseudomyxoma Peritonei   In pseudomyxoma peritonei, the neoplastic epithelium secretes large amounts of gelatinous mucinous material. It is most commonly secondary to an ovarian mucinous carcinoma, a mucocele of the appendix, or a well-differentiated colon carcinoma.

141

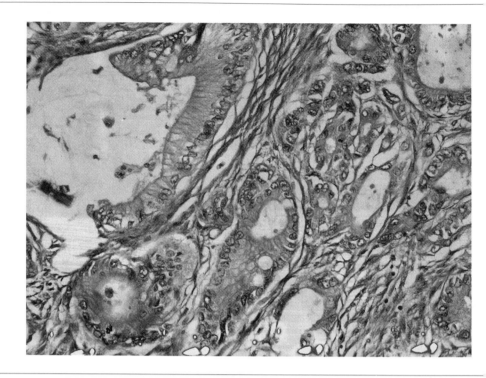

Figure 4.18. Mucinous adenocarcinoma of the ovary. Irregular glandular spaces are lined with a layer of tall columnar cells with abundant mucinous cytoplasm resembling endocervical cells. The nuclei are mildly atypical.

Endometrioid Tumors

Endometrioid lesions constitute 6–8% of epithelial tumors. Endometrioid neoplasia includes all the benign demonstrations of endometriosis.

In 1925 Sampson (36) suggested that certain cases of adenocarcinoma of the ovary probably arose in areas of endometriosis. His criteria were so strict that few cases were reported in the literature until 1960, because he required that typical benign endometriosis be found in association with adenocarcinoma and that a transition between the two be identified. The adenocarcinomas were similar to those seen in the uterine cavity, and approximately 50% contained squamous elements. Tumors that met these criteria were associated with an excellent prognosis.

The malignant potential of endometriosis is very low, although a transition from benign to malignant epithelium may be demonstrated (Fig. 4.19). Malignancies arising in endometriosis may show the hemorrhagic foci characteristic of benign lesions. The neoplasms that develop *de novo* from the mesothelium are not distinctive. Most are not as large as the mucinous tumors or as papillary as the serous tumors.

Borderline Malignant Endometrioid Tumors

The endometrioid tumor of low malignant potential has a wide morphologic spectrum. Tumors may resemble an endometrial polyp or complex endometrial hyperplasia with crowding of glands. When there are back-to-back glands with no intervening stroma, the tumor is classified as a well-differentiated endometrioid carcinoma. Some borderline malignant tumors have a prominent fibromatous component. In such cases, the word "adenofibroma" is used.

142

Malignant Endometrioid Tumors   Endometrioid tumors are characterized by an adenomatous pattern with all the potential variations of epithelia found in the uterus. Adenocarcinoma with benign-appearing squamous metaplasia has an excellent prognosis. Conversely, patients with mixed adenosquamous carcinomas have a very low survival rate. In poorly differentiated ovarian malignancies, there are frequently "adenoid" foci, but these areas are not sufficient to allow classification of these lesions as "endometrioid."

Multifocal Disease   The "endometrial" and/or endometrioid tumors afford the greatest opportunity to evaluate "multifocal disease." **Endometrioid tumors of the ovary are often associated with similar lesions in the endometrium**. Identification of multifocal disease is important, because patients with disease metastatic from the uterus to the ovaries have a 30–40% 5-year survival, whereas those with synchronous multifocal disease have a 75–80% 5-year survival (37). When the histologic appearance of endometrial and ovarian tumors is different, the two tumors most likely represent two separate primary lesions. When they appear similar, the endometrial tumor can be considered a separate primary tumor if it is well-differentiated and only superficially invasive.

Clear Cell (Mesonephroid) Tumors

The incidence of clear cell carcinoma among all ovarian tumors is difficult to assess, although it is 3% at The Johns Hopkins Hospital. A more accurate figure is lacking because of the high frequency with which clear cells coexist with other cell types. Clinically, these tumors are the most common ovarian neoplasms associated with hypercalcemia and/or hyperpyrexia, and most such cases are associated with metastatic disease. They are commonly unilateral with a smooth surface unless the malignancy has extended beyond the confines of the ovary. Cystic and solid components are commonly associated.

Figure 4.19.   Endometrioid cancer arising in adjacent endometriosis.

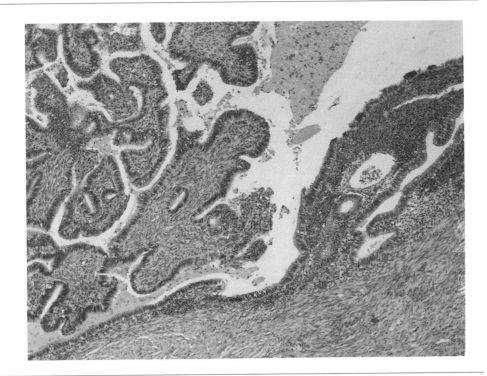

Borderline Clear Cell Tumors Although this category of tumor of low malignant potential is included in the classification of clear cell tumors, there are no clearly defined histologic criteria for this lesion.

Malignant Clear Cell Tumors Several basic histologic patterns are present in the clear cell adenocarcinoma (i.e., tubulocystic, papillary, and solid). The tumors are made up of *clear cells* and *hobnail cells*. The tall clear cells have abundant clear or vacuolated cytoplasm, hyperchromatic, irregular nuclei and nucleoli of various sizes. Hobnail cells project their nuclei to the apical cytoplasm (Fig. 4.20). Other tumor cells have densely eosinophilic cytoplasm. Focal areas of endometriosis and endometrioid carcinoma sometimes occur. The clear cell carcinoma seen in the ovary is histologically identical to that seen in the uterus or vagina of the young patient who has been exposed to DES *in utero*.

Brenner Tumors

Benign Brenner Tumors Brenner tumors grossly simulate the ovarian fibroma in that they are solid and white or yellow-white, with a smooth capsule. On cut section, the stroma is proliferative, particularly around the nests of epithelial cells. These nests may be cystic or solid, resembling transitional epithelium of the urinary tract (Fig. 4.21). The nuclei have a grooved, coffee-bean appearance. Endocervical mucinous cells occur in about 25% of cases. The majority of Brenner tumors are found incidentally at the time of hysterectomy for benign disease.

Borderline Brenner Tumors Borderline or "proliferating" Brenner tumors have been described. In such cases, the epithelium does not invade the stroma. Some investigators subclassify those tumors that resemble low-grade papillary transi-

Figure 4.20. Clear cell "mesonephroid" carcinoma of the ovary. Note the solid variant of clear cell carcinoma with sheets of cells that have clear cytoplasm ("hobnail" cells).

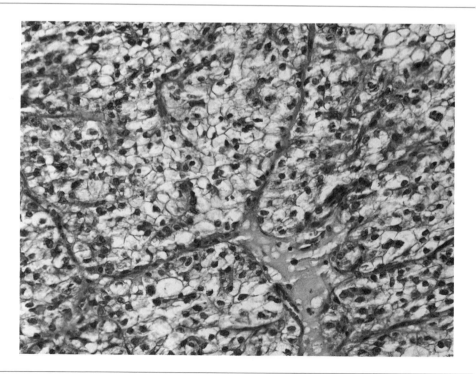

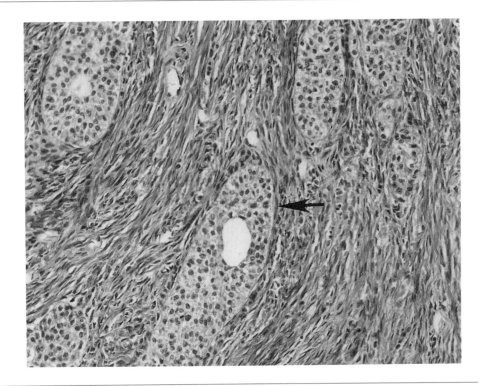

Figure 4.21.   Benign Brenner tumor of the ovary. Note the nests of transitional metaplasia *(arrow)* found within the fibrotic stroma.

tional cell carcinoma of the urinary bladder as proliferating tumors and those with a higher grade of transitional cell carcinoma *in situ* as borderline malignant Brenner tumors (38). Complete surgical removal usually results in cure.

Malignant Brenner Tumors   These are rare and are defined as benign Brenner tumors coexisting with invasive transitional cell and/or another type of carcinoma. The tumor infiltrates the tissue with associated destruction.

Transitional Cell Tumors (TCC)   The designation *transitional cell tumor* refers to a primary ovarian carcinoma resembling transitional cell carcinoma of the urinary bladder without a recognizable Brenner tumor. An important finding is that those ovarian carcinomas that contain more than 50% of TCC are more sensitive to chemotherapy and have a more favorable prognosis than other poorly differentiated ovarian carcinomas of comparable stage (39, 40). Transitional cell tumors differ from malignant Brenner tumors in that they are more frequently diagnosed in an advanced stage and, therefore, are associated with a poorer survival rate (41).

Undifferentiated Carcinoma

The undifferentiated carcinomas include large and small cell types. In the former, cells with large round to oval nuclei, prominent nucleoli, a moderate amount of cytoplasm, and high mitotic activity are arranged in solid sheets without glandular or squamous differentiation. In the small cell carcinoma, the cells have small, hyperchromatic nuclei, scanty cytoplasm, and high mitotic activity. This neoplasm occurs mainly in young women, who may present with hypercalcemia. Immunohistochemical stains are helpful to differentiate this tumor from a lymphoma leukemia, or sarcoma.

Endosalpingiosis, Peritoneal Serous Borderline Tumors, and Peritoneal Surface Serous Carcinomas

Primary peritoneal tumors indistinguishable from primary ovarian serous tumors are well documented. In the case of borderline serous peritoneal tumors and serous peritoneal carcinomas, the ovaries are normal or minimally involved and the tumors affect predominantly the uterosacral ligaments, pelvic peritoneum or omentum. The overall prognosis for borderline serous peritoneal tumors is excellent and comparable to that of ovarian borderline serous tumors (42–44). In the review of 38 cases of peritoneal borderline serous tumors from the literature 32 women had no persistent disease, 4 were well after resection of recurrence, 1 developed an invasive serous carcinoma, and 1 died of tumor (42).

Peritoneal serous carcinomas have the appearance of a moderately to poorly differentiated serous ovarian carcinoma. Primary peritoneal endometrioid carcinoma is less common.

Mesotheliomas

Peritoneal malignant mesotheliomas fall into four categories (45):

1. Fibrosarcomatous

2. Tubopapillary (papillary-alveolar)

3. Carcinomatous

4. Mixed

These lesions appear as multiple intraperitoneal masses and can develop after hysterectomy and bilateral salpingo-oophorectomy for benign disease. Malignant mesotheliomas should be distinguished from ovarian tumor implants and primary peritoneal müllerian neoplasms.

Germ Cell Tumors

Dysgerminoma (Germinoma)

Dysgerminomas are found in both sexes and may arise in gonadal or extragonadal sites. The latter include the midline structures from the pineal gland to the mediastinum and the retroperitoneum. Histologically, they represent abnormal proliferations of the basic germ cell. In the ovary, the germ cells are encapsulated at birth (the primordial follicle), and the unencapsulated or free cells die. If either of the latter processes fails, it is conceivable that the germ cell could free itself of its normal control and multiply indiscriminately.

The size of dysgerminomas varies widely, but they are usually 5–15 cm in diameter (46). The capsule is slightly bosselated, and the consistency of the cut surface is spongy and gray-brown in color. Bilaterality is found grossly in about 5–8% of cases, but microscopic involvement of the contralateral gonad is recognized in 10–15%. Occult disease can be detected intraoperatively by frozen sections on the bisected contralateral ovary.

The histologic characteristics of the dysgerminoma are very distinctive. The large round, ovoid, or polygonal cells have abundant, clear, very pale-staining cyto-

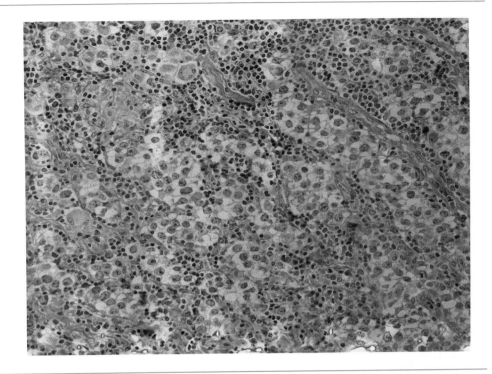

Figure 4.22.   Dysgerminoma of ovary. Primitive germ cells are divided into clusters and lobules by fibrous septa rich in lymphocytes. Rare multinucleated giant cells are present in the left upper corner.

plasm, large and irregular nuclei, and prominent nucleoli (Fig. 4.22). Mitotic figures are seen in varying numbers, although they are not usually numerous. Another characteristic feature is the arrangement of the elements in lobules and nests separated by fibrous septa, which are often extensively infiltrated with lymphocytes, plasma cells, and granulomas with epithelioid cells and multinucleated giant cells. When necrosis is extensive, the lesion may be confused with tuberculosis. Occasional dysgerminomas may contain syncytiotrophoblastic giant cells and be associated with precocious puberty or virilization. The presence of these cells does not appear to alter the behavior of the tumor (47).

Associated Teratoid Elements   Because the dysgerminoma is a germ cell tumor and parthenogenesis (stimulation of the basic germ cell to atypical division) is the most commonly accepted genesis for the more immature teratomas, it is logical that these two tumors may coexist. Choriocarcinoma, endodermal sinus tumor, and other extraembryonal lesions are also commonly associated with the dysgerminoma.

Gonadoblastoma

Scully introduced the term "gonadoblastoma" to describe a gonad with sex-cord cells arranged in tubules, unencapsulated germ cells, and calcified "bodies" (48). Although not a true "tumor," such gonads are a prime source of germ cell tumors, principally dysgerminomas. These lesions commonly appear in a person with a Y chromosome in the genotype. In a review of 74 cases of gonadoblastoma, most arose in gonads of an "unknown" karyotype (48). The hormonal effect was generally androgenic, and chromatin-negative nuclei were present in 90%. The largest lesion was 8 cm, and the lesions were benign, although a dysgerminoma may be superimposed. Talerman (49) has noted combined dysgerminoma and

147

gonadoblastoma in siblings with dysgenetic gonads. All combinations of germ cell tumors may occur.

Teratomas

The teratoma (Greek: *teratos*, "monster," and *onkoma*, "swelling") is one of the most fascinating neoplasms of the body. These lesions are compound tumors, composed of cells from more than one germ layer. This definition emphasizes the origin of teratomas from cells retaining totipotency (i.e., the ability to differentiate into any or all of the three germ cell layers and into embryonal and extraembryonal tissues).

Teratomas have a peak incidence in the reproductive years. Most appear in the first two decades of life. Approximately 85–90% of all teratomas are benign and are made up of mature adult tissue, the so-called *mature cystic teratoma* or *dermoid cyst*. Fifteen to 20% of benign lesions are bilateral. The remaining 10–15% are immature. A simplified teratoma consists of one germ cell layer. For example, a dermoid cyst consists entirely of skin and appendages, a carcinoid tumor consists of gut endocrine cells, and struma ovarii consists of thyroid tissue. If found postmenopausally, they may have been present for years. Malignant degeneration occurs in about 1–2% of mature teratomas, usually after the fifth decade of life.

Grossly, these lesions are characterized by a smooth, tense capsule overlying the primary cystic component. The size varies from microscopic to gross tumors that fill the lower abdomen and weigh up to 15 pounds. The predominant content of the cyst is sebaceous material, usually mixed with hair. Occasionally, the contents of the cyst may be clear, because neural tissue and its excretory element, the choroid plexus, are common components of the mature teratoma. Most dermoid cysts are unifocal, although as many as nine individual tumors have been found in one gonad. The lesion often contains a solid prominence, *Rokitansky's protuberance*, which is usually located at the point of contact with the residual ovarian tissue. Teeth and bone are commonly found in Rokitansky's protuberance. Many sections of this area should be obtained, because this is where the greatest variation in the cellular elements exists.

Microscopic examination reveals that, although the ectodermal derivatives are prevalent, tissues of mesodermal and endodermal origin are found in almost all cases. The most prominent elements are stratified squamous epithelium and its appendages. Respiratory epithelium and the associated peribronchial glands and cartilage can be demonstrated in 50–75% of the tumors. Neural elements and endodermal epithelium are recognized in 10–15% of the cases.

Struma Ovarii   Adult teratomas contain thyroid tissue in 12–15% of cases, but such an occurrence does not justify a diagnosis of struma ovarii. The latter should be made only if the thyroid tissue is dominant or if there is evidence of either neoplasia or hormonal function. The neoplastic alterations in struma may be confusing, and in certain instances a carcinoid pattern has been associated with the struma. Furthermore, the adenocarcinoma arising in a struma has been misinterpreted as "papillary serous tumor."

The struma is grayish brown and spongy in gross appearance. Most such lesions are recognized in the fifth and sixth decades of life. Large cystic areas may be present, either as a part of the struma or as an associated teratoid structure such as a mucinous cyst. The microscopic appearance is usually that of normal thyroid tissue. A variety of abnormal features, including thyroiditis, fetal adenoma, and classic varieties of malignancy, have been described. Metastases have been reported and occasionally may demonstrate more maturity than the original lesion.

Carcinoid Primary ovarian carcinoid has been accepted as a demonstration of unilateral development in a teratoma. These neoplasms have been associated with struma as well as with other teratoid elements. Ovarian carcinoids may be metastases from an intestinal primary lesion, in which case they are commonly bilateral. This tumor has been mistaken histologically for either a granulosa cell tumor or an arrhenoblastoma because of the cordlike or tubular arrangement of the cells. The use of argentophilic stains may be helpful in identifying the cells of origin because the carcinoid arises from neural crest elements. Both trabecular and insular patterns have been appreciated in ovarian carcinoids (50). **The carcinoid arising in the gastrointestinal tract has not been associated with the classic carcinoid syndrome unless the liver has been involved with metastatic disease. Conversely, there have been several cases of ovarian carcinoid in which the characteristic symptoms have been present without metastasis.** The difference in the venous drainage of the ovary may account for these variations in symptoms.

Immature Teratoma

Of fundamental importance in the understanding of the teratoma is a recognition of the maturation of the various elements. If maturation continues along normal lines, the mature or adult teratoma results, and the prognosis is excellent. Conversely, abnormal maturation of these elements produces undisciplined growth that can be fatal. Teratomas containing immature elements, although relatively rare, have been recognized more commonly in the past two decades (Fig. 4.23).

Among the tumors with embryonal elements, those containing neural tissues demonstrate most clearly the importance of the ability to mature. *Gliomatosis peritonei* is the most dramatic demonstration of the significance of maturation, because a majority of these patients have survived, even with this disseminated disease. **A determination of the amount of undifferentiated neural tissue is of prognostic importance. A grade 1 tumor is one in which < 1 low-power microscopic field (LPF) contains immature neural elements, a grade 2 tumor has 1–3 LPFs with immature elements, and a grade 3 tumor has > 3 LPFs with these elements. The prognosis can be correlated with the grade of these immature neural elements, i.e., with a higher grade, there is a poorer prognosis**.

Previously, the majority of "malignant teratomas" have been classified as secondary neoplasms developing in a primarily benign teratoma. In the last decade, lesions composed primarily of immature embryonal or extraembryonal elements have become more prevalent, and the basic demonstration of malignancy is the inability of the tissue to mature rather than the presence of individual cell anaplasia; i.e., the mitotic activity may be low. This unique aspect is demonstrated by an absence of aneuploidy in the few cases that have been studied.

Malignant change in benign cystic teratomas has been recorded as occurring in 1–2% of cases, usually after the age of 40 years (50). The most common malignancy developing in the initially benign teratoma is squamous cell carcinoma. Other neoplasms have been reported (e.g., melanomas, which may arise from the skin or retinal anlage, and sarcomas, including leiomyosarcomas and

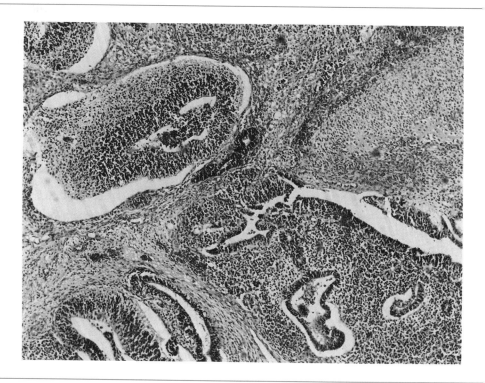

Figure 4.23. Ovarian teratoma. This tumor contains both mature and immature neural elements with a neural tubelike structure near its center.

mixed mesodermal tumors). Carcinomas may arise from any of the epithelial elements.

Endodermal Sinus Tumors The classic example of the extraembryonal lesion is the endodermal sinus tumor (EST) or "yolk sac" tumor described by Teilum (51). Classically, they occur in young females, the average age being 16–17 years. The gross picture is that of a soft grayish brown tumor. Cystic areas caused by degeneration are present in these rapidly growing lesions. The capsule is intact in a majority of cases (Stage Ia).

The tumor is unilateral in 100% of the cases; thus biopsy of the opposite ovary in such young patients is contraindicated. The association of such lesions with gonadal dysgenesis must be appreciated, and chromosomal analysis should be performed preoperatively in premenarchal patients.

Microscopically, the characteristic feature is the endodermal sinus, or *Schiller-Duval body* (Fig. 4.24). The cystic space is lined with a layer of flattened or irregular endothelium into which projects a glomerulus-like tuft with a central vascular core. These structures vary throughout the tumor, and the reticular, myxoid elements represent undifferentiated mesoblast. The lining of the papillary infolding and the cavity is irregular, with an occasional cell containing clear, glassy cytoplasm, simulating the hobnail appearance of the epithelium in clear cell tumors. The association of EST with dysgerminoma must be emphasized if diagnosis and therapy are to be optimal. Alpha-fetoprotein (AFP) can be demonstrated in the tumor by means of the immunoperoxidase technique.

Embryonal Carcinoma

Recently, the term *embryonal carcinoma* has been reintroduced into the classification of ovarian tumors (52). The tumor is composed of embryonal elements of epithelial appearance. Both hCG and AFP can be elevated, suggesting that these elements are related to trophoblastic and other extraembryonal tissues. The yolk sac vesicles seen in endodermal sinus tumors are not found in this tumor.

Choriocarcinoma

Included among the extraembryonal tumors is the choriocarcinoma. The cell by which trophoblast can be distinguished is the syncytial or mature element, because undifferentiated cytotrophoblast may be difficult to distinguish from cells of embryonal carcinoma. Thus, in some instances, a large ovarian tumor may be associated with a positive pregnancy test and yet histologically demonstrate none of the more mature and diagnostic trophoblastic elements.

The tumor marker in such cases is human chorionic gonadotrophin (hCG) and, as with AFP, can be demonstrated by immunoperoxidase staining. AFP may also be positive in these tumors, suggesting the presence of other elements such as endodermal sinus tumor. However, both AFP and hCG may be found in association with tumors in which there are no definable extraembryonal elements.

Gonadal Stromal Tumors

An understanding of the embryology of the ovary is essential to explain the histogenesis of functioning gonadal stromal tumors. From the common mesenchymal stem cell arise various epithelial (*granulosa*) and connective tissue (*theca*) elements, and various admixtures are present in most feminizing tumors. The

Figure 4.24.   Endodermal sinus tumor of the ovary. Note the classic "Schiller-Duval body" with its central vessel and mantle of endoderm *(arrow)*.

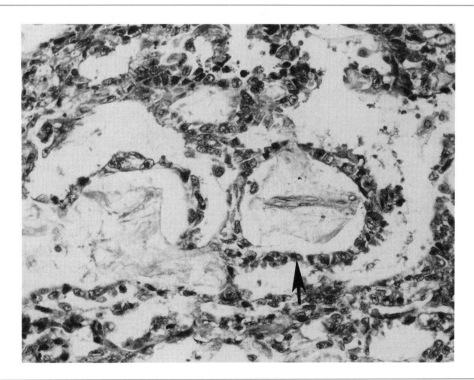

ovarian stromal cell may be stimulated to tumorigenesis and steroid function by diverse local or systemic agents.

These lesions have often been included under the general term of "sex cord stromal tumors." The combination of granulosa cells and gonadal stroma would justify this general designation.

Granulosa Cell Tumor

Granulosa cell tumors range from a few millimeters to 20 cm or more in diameter. The tumors are rarely bilateral, and they have a smooth, lobulated surface. The solid portions of the tumor are granular, frequently trabeculated, and are commonly yellow or gray-yellow in color. The granulosa-theca cell tumor is probably the most inaccurately diagnosed lesion of the female gonad. Of 477 ovarian tumors from the Emil Novak Ovarian Tumor Registry diagnosed initially as granulosa-theca cell tumors, almost 15% were reclassified after histologic review. Lesions misdiagnosed as granulosa cell tumors included metastatic carcinomas, teratoid tumors, and poorly differentiated mesothelial tumors (45).

The classic granulosa cell is round or ovoid with scant cytoplasm. The nucleus contains compact, finely granular cytoplasm suggesting hyperchromatism. "Coffee-bean" grooved nuclei are common, as are mitoses, thus simulating the corresponding elements in the normal, mature follicle. Conversely, if the "epithelial elements" are bizarre with atypical mitoses, the lesion should not be categorized as a "poorly differentiated granulosa cell tumor" but, rather, as an undifferentiated mesothelial neoplasm. In the most common variety, the granulosa cells show a tendency to arrange themselves in small clusters or rosettes around a central cavity, so there is a resemblance to primordial follicles (i.e., *Call-Exner bodies,* (Fig. 4.25). The stroma is similar to the theca and may be luteinized. Several histologic patterns have been described: (*a*) folliculoid, (*b*) diffuse, (*c*) cylindroid, (*d*) pseudoadenomatous, and (*e*) mixed (53). In children and adolescents, the granular cell tumors are often cystic, contain luteinized cells, and are associated with precocious puberty.

Thecoma

Most thecomas are composed of the fibrous ovarian stroma and a luteinized thecal component (e.g., the fibrothecoma). The stroma is commonly functional. Grossly, thecomas are firm and fibrous with smooth lobulated surfaces, and cystic areas may result from degeneration. The tumors are generally gray-white, although a yellowish hue is imparted to the areas that contain active theca. Stains for lipid on the frozen (not fixed) material are often positive. The lesions are usually unilateral and found in the fifth and sixth decades of life.

Microscopically, the thecoma or fibrothecoma is distinguished by the presence of spindle cells that occasionally may become rounded and take on an epithelioid appearance. These cells are distributed in an irregular interlacing manner throughout the tumor and are separated by connective stromal tissue, often with foci of hyaline change. Thecomas are similar to fibromas except for the round appearance of the cells and the presence of lipid in the cytoplasm.

In the thecoma, there are often foci of granulosa cells. A strict division between the granulosa and theca cell tumors is not appropriate because of their similar endocrinologic effects. Furthermore, diverse patterns may be found in different

152

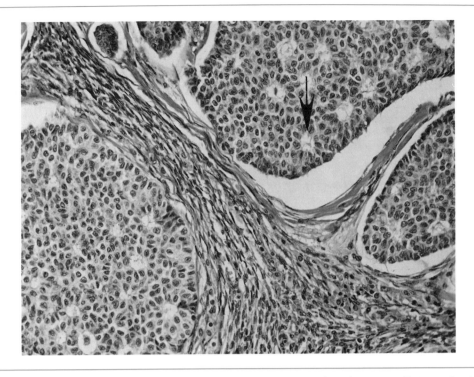

Figure 4.25.   Granulosa cell tumor of the ovary. Note the classic "Call-Exner bodies" *(arrow)* with a minimal stromal component in this tumor of folliculoid pattern.

parts of the same tumor, and the mingling of epithelial and connective tissue elements is frequent, lending support to the concept of a common origin from the ovarian mesenchyme. The sclerosing stromal tumor, as described by Chalvardjian and Scully (54), refers to the nodular proliferation of stromal cells with a rich vascular network and fibrosis.

Diffuse Thecosis   Diffuse or focal thecosis is commonly seen in the ovary during pregnancy and is related to stimulation by hCG. The most dramatic demonstration is the *luteoma of pregnancy* (Fig. 4.26), a solid tumor associated with fetal and maternal virilization that regresses spontaneously postpartum (55). In the postmenopausal ovary, such foci are noted frequently throughout the cortex and have been labeled *thecosis, thecomatosis*, or *hyperthecosis*. In these situations, the "luteinized cells" are related to the elevated pituitary gonadotropins recognized in the first decade of postmenopausal life. Estrogen can be produced by the stimulated stromal cells and may be associated with endometrial proliferations ranging from hyperplasia to cancer. If a thecoma is present in one ovary, there is often diffuse thecomatosis (or stromal hyperplasia) in the contralateral ovary.

The stromal cell may be activated to produce various steroids by a number of known and unknown stimuli. **An estrogenic, androgenic, and on occasion even a progestogenic effect may be noted in association with a stromal tumor (luteinized or nonluteinized). The histologic appearance of the cell does not correlate with its functional activity.**

Fibroma

The fibroma is a tumor that probably is more common than has been identified clinically. A small nodule of gonadal stroma can be found frequently

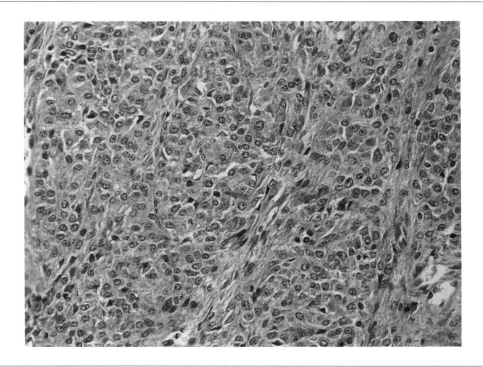

Figure 4.26. Luteoma of pregnancy. This lesion has large, regular cells with clear cytoplasm.

just beneath the surface epithelium of many ovaries removed at hysterectomy and bilateral salpingo-oophorectomy. The component cells resemble cortical stromal cells and may contain fat droplets, but they do not secrete active hormones. Rarely, malignancy may develop in this gonadal stroma, producing a *stromal sarcoma*.

Virilizing Ovarian Tumors

Virilizing ovarian tumors are found in all age groups, ranging from 2 to 80 years (56). The designation *arrhenoblastoma* was coined by Meyer for the group of tumors that had been thought to originate in certain male-directed cells persisting in the ovary from fetal life. A great variety of lesions are associated with clinical evidence of masculinization, including the Sertoli-Leydig cell (arrhenoblastoma), stromal, and metastatic neoplasms. About 5% of "granulosa cell" tumors produce virilization. Thus the hormonal activity is the significant clinical feature, while histopathologic findings identify the tumor type and guide the prognosis.

The size of virilizing tumors is variable, and they are occasionally only microscopic entities. However, most such tumors are 10–20 cm in greatest dimension and have been reported to weigh more than 25 pounds. In 95% of the cases, they are unilateral. The surface is smooth, and the cut surface is grayish yellow to orange. The consistency is generally firm, but cystic degeneration and focal areas of hemorrhage are common.

Histologically, masculinizing tumors include a variety of patterns. The well-differentiated Sertoli cell tumor of the classic form is characterized by tubules lined with well-differentiated columnar cells. In other lesions, only imperfect attempts at tubule formation or irregular columns of cells without definable lumina may be seen. Interstitial (Leydig) cells, with their lipoid content, are the most definable element, and their presence determines the extent of hormonal function of the tumor. Reinke crystalloids may be demonstrated.

The undifferentiated tumor may look like a sarcoma. In the majority of cases, however, a thorough examination will identify either a cordlike arrangement of cells, imperfect tubule formation, or lipid-containing cell elements. Metastatic lesions may be associated with masculinization. In these cases, the clinical history is of great value to the pathologist. About 15% of Sertoli-Leydig cell tumors have a retiform pattern resembling endometrioid tumors and may require special stains for definitive diagnosis (57).

Lipoidal Cell Tumors (Steroid Cell Tumors)   Lipoidal cell tumors are subdivided into stromal luteomas (25%), Leydig cell tumors including hilus cell tumors (15%), and steroid cell tumors of not otherwise specified types (60%). The cells within this group of tumors have abundant eosinophilic, granular cytoplasms and lipid droplets and thus resemble adrenal cortical cells, hilar cells, and luteinized cells. Depending on the enzymes present in the tumor cells, the hormonal products may be estrogen, androgen, progesterone, adrenal cortical hormones, and ACTH causing Cushing's syndrome.

Hilar or Leydig Cell Tumors   A small proportion of virilizing tumors of the ovary arise from the hilar cells. In the early postmenopausal years, these cells are "luteinized" and Reinke crystalloids are found both intracellularly and extracellularly. Luteinization is probably the result of elevated pituitary gonadotropins. These cells are located near the nerves, and there may be a neurohormonal relationship.

Classically, the hilar cell tumor occurs in the late fifth or early sixth decade of life, when the hilar cell is most commonly seen in the perineural region of the ovarian hilus. The tumors are routinely small (< 5 cm), unilateral, and uniformly benign in spite of incomplete surgical removal. Despite clinical virilism, the endometrium often demonstrates an estrogenic effect, such as hyperplasia.

Stromal luteomas and Leydig cell tumors are generally benign. However, 25–40% of steroid cell tumors of otherwise not specified type are clinically malignant with extraovarian spread. Pathologic features that suggest malignant potential include > 2 mitoses per 10 HPFs, necrosis, a tumor size > 7 cm, hemorrhage, and moderate or severe nuclear atypism. Thus careful histologic examination and classification are helpful in determining clinical outcome, although there are rare steroid cell tumors that appear histologically benign but behave in a malignant manner (57).

Massive Edema of the Ovary   Massive edema of the ovary is characterized by massive edema of the gonad, in the cortex of which are large pale cells, occurring singly or in small nests (56). The stroma is edematous and essentially hypocellular. Such alterations were described initially in the masculinized female and may be related to chronic torsion of the large polycystic ovary. However, similar changes may be seen with a variety of ovarian neoplasms, and the endocrinologic alterations may be masculinizing or femininizing. Thus histology does not define the hormonal function of this benign lesion.

Metastatic Tumors to the Ovaries

Metastatic ovarian cancer comprises approximately 5–8% of all ovarian malignancies and presents some of the most challenging and controversial clinical and pathologic appearances (58). Ovarian metastases may arise from genital or extragenital primary tumors.

Genital Primary

Carcinoma of the endometrium is the genital tumor that most commonly metastasizes to the ovary. Of primary importance is the differentiation of metastasis from multifocal neoplasia. The prognosis for multifocal disease is better than that for a true metastatic lesion. Typically, the "multifocal lesions" are found in the cortex of the ovary rather than in the lymphatics and simulate the pattern of an endometrial lesion.

Carcinoma of the lower genital canal rarely metastasizes to the ovary, but, if it does happen, it usually spreads by direct extension. Other tumors arising in the adjacent pelvic structures (e.g., retroperitoneal sarcomas and teratomas) may also invade the ovary directly.

Extragenital Primary

Four possible routes exist for dissemination from extragenital primary malignancies to the ovary:

1. Peritoneal implantation of cancer cells on the ovarian surface

2. Lymphatic metastasis

3. Hematogenous spread

4. Extension by direct continuity from an adherent intestinal cancer

Lymphatic extension has been the most widely accepted thesis for cancer dissemination, but there has been no convincing demonstration of the spread of cancer cells from the stomach via the retroperitoneal lymph nodes to the ovarian lymphatics.

Most metastases to the ovaries are from the breast or the stomach. Grossly, the tumors are solid, freely mobile, and bosselated. Cystic areas are the result of degeneration. Bilateral involvement is present in 70–80% of the cases.

A variety of microscopic patterns may be seen in the ovary of the patient with a primary malignancy in the gastrointestinal tract. Of major significance is the lesion that replicates an ovarian mucin-secreting tumor. Furthermore, both primary and secondary mucinous lesions may produce a stromal reaction with subsequent hormone production. Thus when a patient has a diffuse mucin-secreting ovarian adenocarcinoma, a thorough study of the gastrointestinal tract must be made regardless of the histologic nature of the ovarian neoplasm. Metastatic colonic carcinoma can sometimes closely simulate endometrioid carcinoma.

The most common microscopic appearance of metastatic breast cancer is that characterized by small columns of anaplastic cells filtering "Indian file" into the cortex of the ovary. They may be missed, particularly if they are encased in the dense ovarian stroma (Fig. 4.27). Metastases from a primary kidney tumor may simulate a clear cell tumor of the ovary.

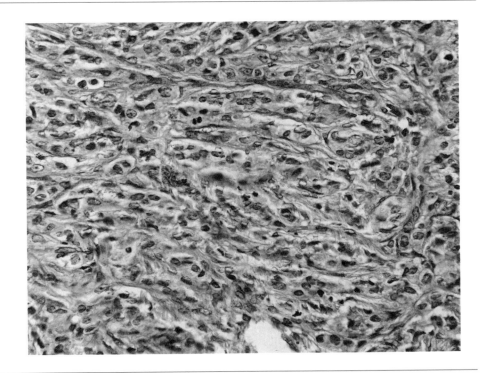

Figure 4.27. Metastatic carcinoma in the ovary. Note the "Indian file" pattern found in this metastatic breast carcinoma.

Krukenberg Tumors The use of the term *Krukenberg tumor* should be limited to the pathologic entity described by Krukenberg. Most Krukenberg tumors are metastatic from the gastrointestinal tract, but primary ovarian Krukenberg tumors exist. Grossly, the Krukenberg tumors are solid and almost always bilateral, and they retain the general shape of the ovary. The external surface is smooth, with a well-developed capsule, similar to most metastatic ovarian malignancies. On section, the cut surface is usually whitish gray and quite firm. The stroma of the Krukenberg tumor is variable, composed of compact and edematous foci. The pathognomonic feature is the presence of "signet-ring" cells, which may be arranged in acini or appear as individual cells. The nucleus is flattened against the cell wall by the accumulated mucoid secretion within the cell (Fig. 4.28). Stains for mucin or mucopolysaccharide, such as mucicarmine and periodic acid-Schiff (PAS), are positive. Krukenberg tumors may be associated with hormonal function. As is true of primary mucin-secreting tumors of the ovary, the gonadal stroma, not the malignant element, is the site of hormone production. These tumors can produce both a maternal and a fetal masculinizing effect.

Lymphomas Lymphomas of the ovary are usually metastatic and bilateral. Burkitt's lymphoma preferentially affects children and young adults. Lymphomas may be confused with dysgerminomas, arrhenoblastomas, or small cell carcinoma.

Fallopian Tube

Primary tubal neoplasms are rare. Conversely, secondary involvement of the tube from lesions arising in adjacent organs is common.

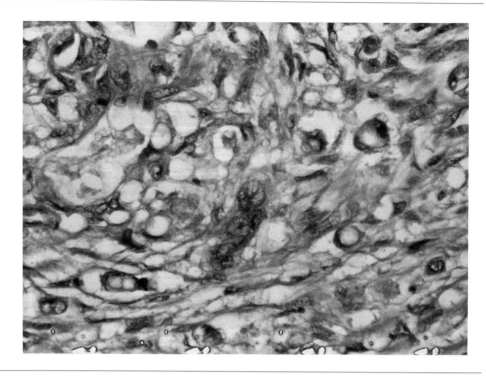

Figure 4.28.   Krukenberg tumor of the ovary metastatic from a gastric carcinoma. Malignant cells have discrete vacuoles that push nuclei eccentrically, giving a signet-ring appearance. Mucicarmine stain demonstrates the cytoplasmic vacuoles to be mucin.

The *adenomatoid tumors* are the most common and confusing of the benign tubal neoplasms. They are found in the broad ligament, the fundus, and the ovary. These tumors are of mesothelial origin. Grossly, they are rarely more than 1–2 cm in diameter, and multiple foci are common. Microscopically, the tumor is made up of confluent acini lined with a low cuboidal epithelium. The marked adenomatous appearance and disturbance of the tubal architecture suggest malignancy, but the lesions produce no destruction in the adjacent tissue and do not metastasize.

Carcinoma *in situ* has been reported and the microscopic diagnosis is based on the presence of mitoses. These lesions have not been associated with metastasis. Atypical tubal epithelial proliferations are common in association with inflammatory disease, particularly of the granulomatous variety, as well as with excessive estrogen stimulation. They are not neoplastic.

Carcinoma of the Fallopian Tube

In a typical case of tubal cancer, the tube is enlarged and sausage-shaped and gives the impression of a large pyosalpinx. Unlike the latter, adhesions to surrounding structures are rare. The external surface is usually smooth. The fimbriated ends are patent or occluded in approximately equal numbers of cases.

Tubal carcinomas are generally *papillary* or *papillary alveolar*, characteristic of the basic structure of the tube. The papillary alveolar pattern is the result of the fusion of adjoining papillae (Fig. 4.29). The microscopic appearance of the common papillary malignancy is characterized by papillae covered with a multilayered atypical epithelium. Mitoses are frequent but not bizarre.

Tubal carcinomas may spread transtubally, by direct extension, or by vascular lymphatic invasion. Thus, even with limited stromal invasion, the tumor may be widespread (59). Bilateral involvement is present in about half the cases. In many cases, the ovary is also involved. When there is a typical gross appearance combined with the characteristic alveolar papillary architecture, the diagnosis of a primary tubal tumor must be considered.

Sarcomas

Primary tubal sarcoma is an extremely rare and highly malignant tumor. The lesions are usually diagnosed as *leiomyosarcomas. Malignant mixed mesodermal tumors* have also been reported in the tube. They have the same microscopic patterns as those from the uterus or ovary. The papillary alveolar epithelial component is commonly undifferentiated, and the stromal component is disorganized. Mesodermal tissue, most frequently cartilaginous and rhabdomyoblastic, is often recognized. In the metastases, one or both components may be present.

Vulva

Embryologically, the vulva is ectoderm and, although the histopathologic appearance may simulate that of the vagina and cervix, the clinical significance of the alterations is frequently different. The gross appearance of the vulva can be abnormal because of local trauma and irritants to which the external genitalia are exposed constantly. Most dermatologic lesions described elsewhere on skin surfaces have been recognized on the vulva.

Figure 4.29.   Carcinoma of the fallopian tube. This is the mixed papillary and the papillary alveolar pattern.

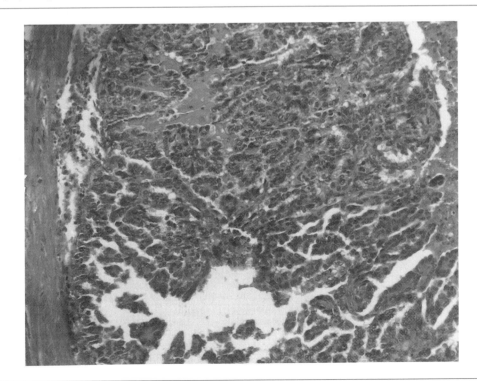

Many benign tumors, similar to those seen elsewhere on the body, are found on the vulva (60). Any discolored, elevated, or chronically irritative lesion must be diagnosed correctly. Biopsies of confluent warts, suspicious pigmented lesions, ulcerations, and chronic erythematous foci should be obtained for histology. Any of these could represent a basal cell carcinoma, carcinoma *in situ*, or invasive malignancy. **Failure to perform a biopsy of a visible lesion is a common cause of delayed diagnosis of vulvar cancer.**

Epithelial Disorders of the Vulva

In 1990 the International Society for the Study of Vulvar Disease (ISSVD) introduced a new classification for epithelial disorders of the vulva (61) to replace the older "dystrophy" terminology (62). This new classification is shown in Table 4.2. Lesions with nuclear atypia are now classified as *vulvar intraepithelial neoplasia* (VIN).

Lichen Sclerosus Lichen sclerosus is common on the vulva and is seen in all age groups (63). Biopsy is mandatory in all but the prepubertal girl.

The classic histopathologic finding associated with lichen sclerosus is thinning of the epithelium with homogenization of the dermis and a chronic inflammatory infiltrate. Keratin "plugging" of the hair follicles is a common finding. Although lichen sclerosus is irritating, particularly to the postmenopausal patient, there is little, if any, evidence to suggest that it is a premalignant lesion. Lichen sclerosus frequently is found adjacent to vulvar cancer, but the condition is associative and not causal.

Squamous Cell Hyperplasia In squamous cell hyperplasia the epithelium is hyperkeratotic, thickened, and hyperplastic, as manifested by elongation and widening of the rete pegs. There is a mild to moderate inflammatory infiltrate in the dermis. The histologic changes are nonspecific and require appropriate special stains to rule out an infectious process, such as candidal vulvitis. During the course of lichen sclerosus, the epithelium sometimes undergoes hyperplasia, which may be a response to a chronic irritant (e.g., scratching).

Vulvar Intraepithelial Neoplasia

The incidence of VIN has increased dramatically during the past 40 years. The average age is the late fourth decade of life, but ages range from the teens to 90 (64–66).

Table 4.2   Classification of Epithelial Disorders of the Vulva

Nonneoplastic Epithelial Disorders of the Skin and Mucosa
Lichen sclerosus (lichen sclerosus et atrophicus)
Squamous cell hyperplasia (formerly hyperplastic dystrophy)
Other dermatoses

Classification of Vulvar Intraepithelial Neoplasia
VIN1—Mild dysplasia (formerly mild atypia)
VIN2—Moderate dysplasia (formerly moderate atypia)
VIN3—Severe dysplasia (formerly severe atypia)
        —Carcinoma in situ

Reproduced, with permission, from Ridley CM, Frankman O, Jones ISC, et al: New nomenclature for vulvar disease: report of the Committee on Terminology of the International Society for the Study of Vulvar Disease. J Reprod Med 35:483, 1990.

VINs are graded as 1 (mild dysplasia), 2 (moderate dysplasia), or 3 (severe dysplasia or carcinoma *in situ*) on the basis of cellular immaturity, nuclear abnormalities, maturation disturbance, and mitotic activity. In VIN 1, immature cells, cellular disorganization, and mitotic activity occur predominantly in the lower third of the epithelium, whereas in VIN 3, immature cells with scanty cytoplasm and severe chromatinic alterations occupy most of the epithelium. Dyskeratotic cells and mitotic figures occur in the superficial layer (Fig. 4.30). VIN 2 has an appearance intermediate between those of VIN 1 and VIN 3. Additional cytopathic changes of human papillomavirus infection, such as perinuclear halos with displacement of the nuclei by the intracytoplasmic viral protein, thickened cell borders, binucleation, and multinucleation, are common in the superficial layers of VIN, especially in grades 1 and 2. These viral changes are not definitive evidence of neoplasia but, rather, are indicative of viral exposure. Most vulvar condylomas are associated with HPV types 6 and 11, whereas HPV type 16 is detected in more than 80% of VINs by molecular techniques.

Bowenoid papulosis (bowenoid dysplasia) is a diagnosis made by correlation of clinicopathologic findings. Biopsies of these lesions reveal VIN ranging from grade 1 to grade 3. Clinically, patients with bowenoid papulosis present with multiple small, pigmented papules (40% of cases), usually < 5 mm in diameter (67). Most women are in their 20s, and some are pregnant. After childbirth, the lesions may regress spontaneously. A conservative local excision or laser therapy is recommended when the lesions fail to regress. Progression to invasive carcinoma is rare (68). The term "Bowenoid papulosis" is no longer recommended by the ISSVD.

Figure 4.30. Carcinoma *in situ* of the vulva (VIN 3). Immature atypical cells are seen throughout epithelium.

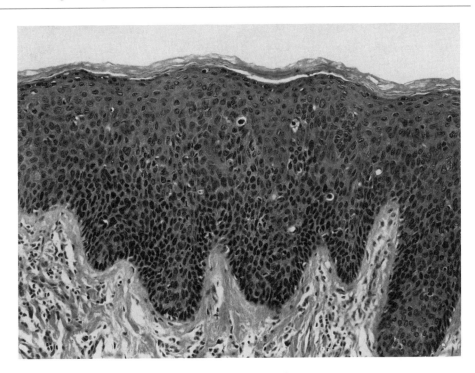

Paget's Disease

Paget's disease of the vulva usually occurs in the sixth through the eighth decades of life (9, 60). Grossly, the lesion is red with white epithelial islands, and the perianal area is commonly involved. The lesion may be widespread and has been known to involve the vagina, cervix, urethra, bladder, and even the ureters. Regardless of this "invasion," if the lesion is initially *in situ* or intraepithelial, it usually remains so (9) (Fig. 4.31).

The majority of cases of vulvar Paget's disease are intraepithelial, with an underlying malignancy occurring in approximately 25% of the cases. Because these lesions demonstrate apocrine differentiation, the malignant cells are believed to arise from the undifferentiated basal cells, which convert into an appendage type of cell during the carcinogenesis. The "transformed cells" spread intraepithelially throughout the squamous epithelium and may extend into the appendages. In the minority of patients with an underlying invasive carcinoma of the apocrine sweat gland, Bartholin gland, or anorectum, the malignant cells are believed to migrate through the dermal ductal structures and reach the epidermis. In such cases, metastasis to the regional lymph nodes and other sites can occur.

Paget's disease must be distinguished from superficial spreading melanoma. All sections should be studied thoroughly with differential staining, particularly the use of *periodic acid-Schiff* (PAS) and *mucicarmine* stains. Mucicarmine is routinely positive in the cells of Paget's disease and negative in a melanotic lesion.

Figure 4.31. Paget's disease of vulva. The epidermis is permeated by abnormal cells with vacuolated cytoplasm and atypical nuclei. This heavy concentration of abnormal cells in the parabasal layers is typical of Paget's disease.

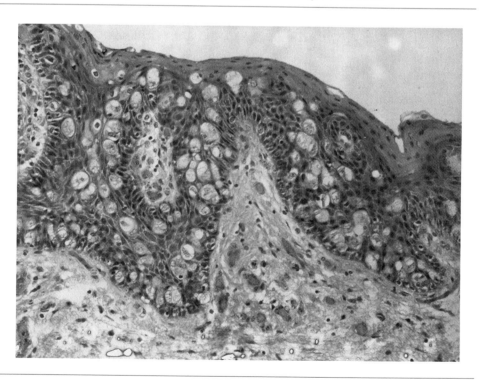

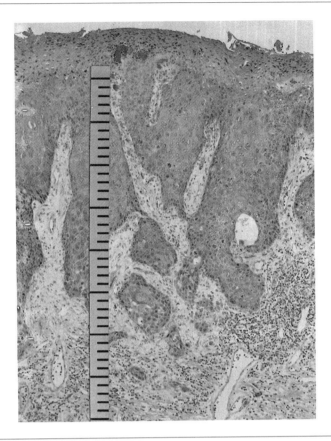

Figure 4.32.   Early invasive carcinoma of vulva originating from VIN. Multiple irregular nests of malignant cells extend from the base of rete pegs. Desmoplastic stromal reaction and chronic inflammation are useful diagnostic signs of stromal invasion. The depth of stromal invasion is measured from the base of the most superficial dermal papilla vertically to the deepest tumor cells. In this tumor it is 3.6 mm in depth.

Microinvasive Carcinoma of the Vulva	Microinvasive carcinoma of the vulva is poorly characterized. Attempts have been made to use the same criteria as those used to define microinvasive carcinoma of the cervix (i.e., identifying the depth of invasion from the adjacent basement membrane), but this has proved to be difficult and confusing (69). For example, when measured from the adjacent basement membrane, an elongated rete peg of 6 mm may be misconstrued as invasive cancer. Consequently, at present, the term "microinvasive carcinoma of the vulva" should be used with caution. Although the cervix routinely shows the presence of *in situ* changes adjacent to invasive cancer, the same is not true for the vulva. On the vulva, the transition from normal tissue to invasive cancer may be abrupt without intervening histopathologic abnormalities. **The International Society of Gynecologic Pathologists recommended that the depth of stromal invasion be measured vertically from the most superficial basement membrane to the deepest tumor (Fig. 4.32). Tumor thickness is the distance between the granular layer of epidermis and the deepest tumor. When the tumor is < 1 mm in depth or thickness, metastasis to the inguinal lymph nodes is extremely rare among reported series (see Chaper 11). However, when invasion is > 1 mm, there**

is a significant risk of inguinal lymph node metastasis. There remains a lack of uniformity in the measurement of stromal invasion, and strict criteria for the diagnosis of microinvasive carcinoma of the vulva remain to be defined.

Invasive Cancer of the Vulva

The varieties of invasive vulvar cancer are shown in Table 4.3.

Squamous Cell Carcinoma

Approximately 90–92% of all invasive vulvar cancers are of the squamous cell type. In these malignancies, mitoses are noted, but atypical keratinization is the histologic hallmark of invasive vulvar cancer (69). The majority of vulvar squamous carcinomas reveal keratinization (Fig. 4.33). *Anaplastic carcinoma* may consist of large immature cells, spindle sarcomatoid cells, or small cells. The latter may simulate small cell anaplastic carcinoma of the lung or *Merkel cell tumor*. Histologic features that correlate with the occurrence of inguinal lymph node metastasis, in the order of importance, are vascular invasion, tumor thickness, depth of stromal invasion, and increased amount of keratin (70).

Verrucous Carcinoma

The large, exuberant, locally invasive lesions of verrucous carcinoma are seen in the fifth and sixth decades of life. The tumors are frequently huge and extend deeply into the adjacent ischiorectal fossa, urethra, and rectum. Although locally invasive, lymph node metastases are essentially unknown (71). Microscopically, the lesion has a papillary, exophytic appearance. In addition, bulky smooth-bordered rete pegs extend deeply into the dermis. The tumor cells retain the normal maturation process and demonstrate only minimal nuclear atypia (Fig. 4.34). Most important, there are no isolated irregular nests of cells destroying the underlying tissue, as commonly seen in the conventional squamous cell carcinoma. To reach a correct diagnosis, it is essential to provide pertinent clinical information, especially the appearance, size, and local extent, and a biopsy specimen that includes the dermis and the base of the lesion. Superficial biopsy specimens often lead to the underdiagnosis of a verrucous carcinoma as a squamous papilloma or condyloma.

Basal Cell Carcinoma

Grossly, basal cell carcinomas are ulcerative with slightly rolled, raised edges. They are known as *rodent ulcers*. Microscopically, the masses of small, dark basal cells spread serpiginously into the underlying dermis but may maintain

Table 4.3   Types of Vulvar Cancer

Type	%
Squamous	90%
Melanoma	2–4%
Basal cell	2–3%
Bartholin gland (adenocarcinoma, squamous cell, transitional cell, adenoid cystic)	1%
Metastatic	1%
Verrucous	<1%
Sarcoma	<1%
Appendage (e.g., hidradenocarcinoma)	rare

164

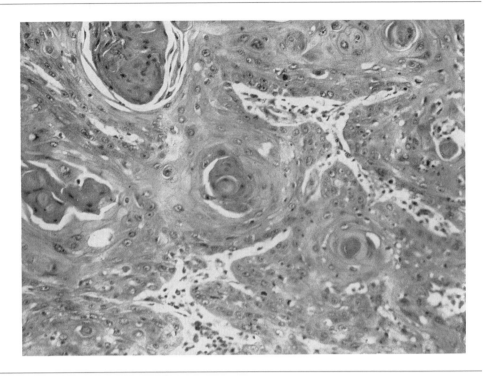

Figure 4.33.   Squamous cell carcinoma of the vulva, keratinizing type. The multiple pearl formations consist of laminated keratin.

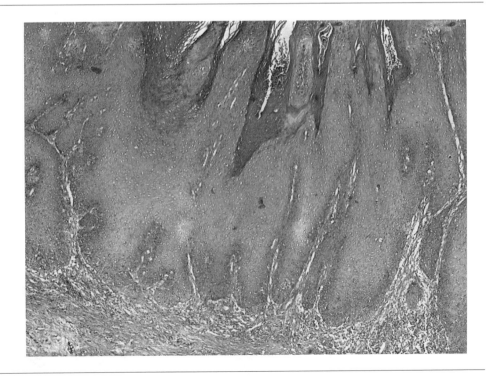

Figure 4.34.   Verrucous carcinoma of the vulva. Note the exophytic hyperkeratotic papillary fronds and endophytic bulky rete pegs with smooth borders.

continuity with the surface epithelium. The regular palisading of the peripheral basal cells identifies the lesion. Metastasis to the regional nodes is rare (9).

Merkel Cell Tumor

The *Merkel cell tumor* is believed to arise from touch-sensitive receptor cells normally found in the basal layer of the epidermis. The tumor cells have small, hyperchromatic nuclei, scanty cytoplasm, and high mitotic activity. Squamous differentiation sometimes occurs. The diagnosis can be confirmed by the presence of neuroendocrine markers by immunohistochemistry or neurosecretory granules by electron microscopy (9).

Bartholin Gland Carcinoma

Several varieties of malignancy have been described as arising from the Bartholin gland. The most common is an *adenocarcinoma*, and this is followed by *squamous cell carcinoma, transitional carcinoma* arising from the duct and indistinguishable histologically from that arising in the bladder, and *adenoid cystic carcinoma* (Fig. 4.35). Rarely, an undifferentiated carcinoma simulating melanoma or sarcoma may occur. Thus the diagnosis of Bartholin gland carcinoma is made by a combination of histologic findings and clinical manifestations consistent with the anatomic location of the Bartholin gland. The lesion behaves aggressively. Regional nodes are involved in 50% of the patients.

Malignant Melanoma

Malignant melanoma represents approximately 2–4% of all primary vulvar malignancies and 2–3% of all melanomas arising in the female. More than 400 cases have been reported to date (72). The ages of 48 patients reported from the Mayo Clinic in 1983 ranged from 25 to 85 years. The youngest patient at

Figure 4.35. Adenoid cystic tumor of the Bartholin gland. Basaloid cells form cribiform, sieve-like spaces containing mucinous material. The hyaline stroma is another distinct feature of this tumor.

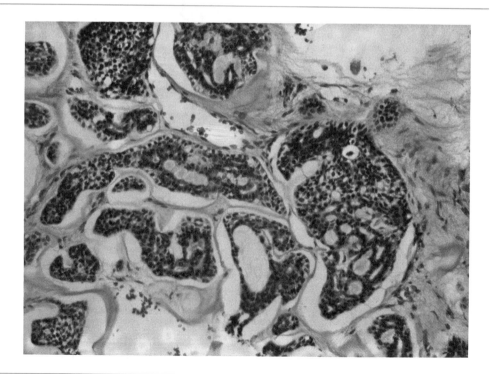

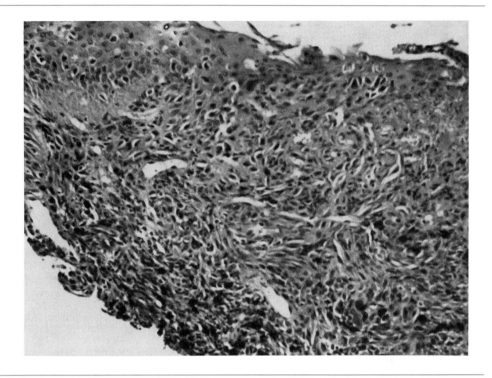

Figure 4.36.   Vulvar melanoma. Spindle-shaped melanoma cells form interlacing bundles, and some contain melanin pigment (left lower corner). Epidermal invasion is evident in the form of Pagetoid migration (left upper corner).

The Johns Hopkins Hospital was 20 years of age. Melanomas usually arise in the labia minora but have been reported at all sites, including the perianal area. As in other areas, malignant melanoma on the vulva may be of the superficial spreading or nodular variety, the latter being the more aggressive. Diagnosis is made by biopsy of any suspicious lesion, pigmented or nonpigmented, particularly if there is a perilesional halo, nodularity, or induration (Fig. 4.36).

Biopsy of all pigmented lesions that have not been present and unchanged for several years is mandatory, and the biopsy specimen should be taken from the center of the lesion. The suggestion that the margins are more important is erroneous, because the pathologist must evaluate the most aggressive focus. There is no evidence to suggest that biopsy "spreads the tumor."

Histopathologically, melanomas usually demonstrate junctional activity because the melanocytes are normally located in the basal layer. The neoplastic melanocytes proliferate in single forms or in clusters and migrate through the epidermis, resembling Paget's cells. The cellular activity and irregularity at the basal layer without involvement of the underlying tissues are characteristic of the so-called melanoma *in situ* or *atypical melanocytic hyperplasia*. Later, the melanin-containing cells with mitotic activity appear to "drop off" into the underlying tissue. The prognosis of malignant melanoma is worsened by increasing depth of dermal invasion, that is, the papillary dermis (*Clark's level II*), the reticular dermis (*Clark's level III*), the deep dermis (*Clark's level IV*), and the underlying adipose tissue (*Clark's level V*). Such histologic markers are not evident in all regions of the vulva, but Breslow's thickness, measured from the epidermal granular layer to the deepest tumor, also provides important information about the risk of metastases, tumor recurrence, and mortality (73, 74).

Sarcoma

Sarcomas are extremely uncommon, the incidence being less than 1% of all primary vulvar malignancies. The gross lesions are either hard and nodular or ulcerative. *Leiomyosarcomas* and *fibrosarcomas* have been reported. The histopathologic appearance is similar to that of such lesions occurring elsewhere. *Rhabdomyosarcoma* of the vulva generally occurs in the young female during the first two decades. The lesion is rapidly progressive and is in the category of an embryonal or alveolar type. The neoplasm spreads to the regional and retroperitoneal nodes. Histopathologically, the lesion may suggest a lymphoma, but, with immunohistochemical stains, muscle differentiation is expressed by immunoreactivity with smooth muscle–specific actin, desmin, and myoglobin. Electron microscopy may demonstrate cytoplasmic thin and thick microfilaments consistent with skeletal muscle differentiation. The rare *epithelioid sarcoma* is locally invasive and is characterized by local recurrences and rarely by distant metastasis.

Secondary Malignant Tumors

Metastases in the vulva most commonly arise from malignancies of the endometrium, cervix, vagina, urinary bladder, or rectum by direct extension or vascular-lymphatic spread.

Vagina

The vagina is of mesodermal (not endodermal) origin. Embryologic abnormalities such as *adenosis* contribute to the development of clear cell adenocarcinoma. Although glandular structures in the vagina are "rare," Sandberg (75) demonstrated that 40% of females have adenosis if routine sections are taken through the vagina at autopsy. In the 1970s, attention was directed to the frequency with which adenosis may be found in the vagina of the young female exposed to DES *in utero*. About 90% of children whose mothers received this medication during the first 8 weeks of pregnancy will have adenosis demonstrable by biopsy. Conversely, fewer than 10% have adenosis if DES was administered after the 16th week of gestation.

Squamous metaplasia is common in foci of adenosis and must be differentiated from true neoplasia. Squamous atypia (dysplasia) may develop in adenosis, suggesting that condyloma and *in situ* neoplasia similar to that seen at the cervical transformation zone may occur (76). However, there is no evidence that there is an increased incidence of invasive squamous cancer in these patients.

Vaginal Intraepithelial Neoplasia (VAIN)

Carcinoma *in situ* of the vagina has been described as developing *de novo* as well as after surgical and radiation therapy for cervical cancer. Such *in situ* disease demonstrates multifocal intraepithelial neoplasia, which is so common in the cervix, vagina, and vulva and is often associated with human papillomavirus infection. Histologically, vaginal intraepithelial neoplasia resembles cervical intraepithelial neoplasia, with the classic full-thickness alterations of the epithelium or precursory variations from mild to marked *in situ* neoplasia. Rarely, the lesion is keratinizing.

Invasive Vaginal Cancer

Primary invasive malignancies of the vagina comprise only 1.5–2% of all malignancies arising in the female genital tract (77). Secondary malignancy is much more common because cervical cancer often extends first to the vagina and because vulvar, endometrial, and ovarian malignancies often invade or metastasize to the vagina. Rare cases, such as malignancy arising in a neovagina, have been reported.

Squamous Cell Carcinoma

The majority of primary invasive malignancies of the vagina are of the squamous type. The most common locations for invasive squamous cancer are the proximal halves of the anterior or posterior walls of the vagina. As the lesion enlarges, there is increasing induration, ulceration, and subsequent involvement of the adjacent bladder or rectum. Microscopically, the pearl-forming variety of squamous carcinoma is more common in the vagina than in the cervix.

Adenocarcinoma

Benign and malignant adenomatous tumors arising in the cervix and vagina, lined with cells varying from the irregular hobnail epithelium to a clear secretory cell, simulate the clear cell adenocarcinoma of the kidney. However, the majority are of paramesonephric, rather than mesonephric, origin. Endometrioid carcinomas may arise in foci of endometriosis.

Herbst (78, 79) has described a specific variety of adenocarcinoma, a "clear cell" carcinoma, that arises in the vagina of young women whose mothers received diethystilbestrol (DES) during pregnancy (Fig. 4.37). Approximately 500 cases have been reported, primarily during the second and third decades of life, the youngest patient being 6 years and the oldest 34 years of age (79). Most cases have been found on initial examination, but at least eight cases have been discovered in patients during follow-up of "benign adenosis," and at least three of

Figure 4.37. Vaginal clear cell carcinoma. Note the formation of tubules with hobnail cells lining the lumen. These cells are characterized by nuclear protrusion into the apical cytoplasm.

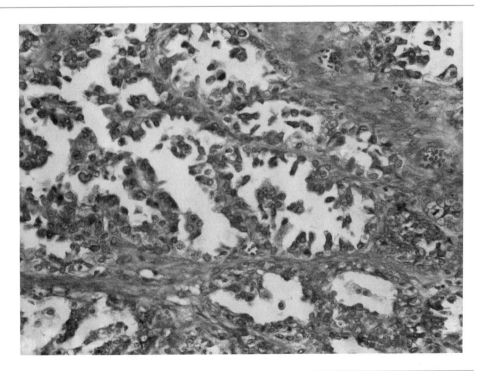

the latter were multifocal. Microscopically, the tumors are classified as clear cell or tubopapillary, the latter being the most aggressive.

Rare Tumors

Fibroepithelial Polyp Fibroepithelial polyps sometimes contain large, irregular stromal cells with hyperchromatic nuclei, which may lead to an erroneous interpretation of malignancy (80). However, the stroma lacks the hypercellularity of the cambium layer beneath the mucosa that is seen in embryonal rhabdomyosarcoma.

Fibrosarcoma and Leiomyosarcoma Sarcomas rarely occur in the vagina. Nuclear atypism, increased mitotic activity, and local infiltration are signs of malignancy.

Embryonal Rhabdomyosarcoma Embryonal rhabdomyosarcoma, a rare tumor found in the vagina during the first 5 years of life, arises from the growing tip of the müllerian (paramesonephric) duct with its very active stroma. The multicystic grapelike form is referred to as *sarcoma botryoides*. Grossly, the disease is characterized by a mass of edematous grayish red polyps that fill and frequently extrude from the vagina. Extension to the uterus, parametrium, and regional nodes is common. Distant metastases are late developments (Fig. 4.38). This malignant tumor has an innocuous histologic appearance. Because of extensive edema, the first appearance suggests acellularity, and an erroneous diagnosis of benign vaginal polyp may be made. Individual details of the cells in the more concentrated areas must be studied carefully to identify the malignant features, including the presence of rhabdomyoblasts (9).

Figure 4.38. Embryonal rhabdomyosarcoma of the vagina (sarcoma botryoides). This lesion consists of primitive mesenchymal cells and rhabdomyoblasts, which have abundant eosinophilic cytoplasm. With further differentiation, cross striations may become evident.

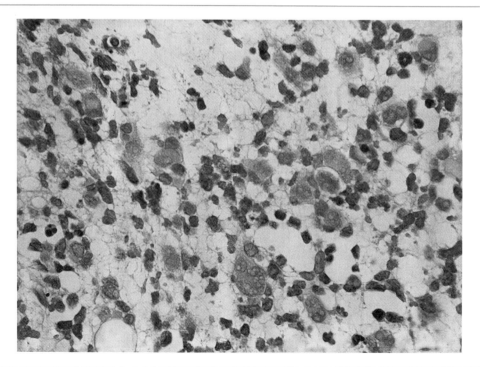

Malignant Melanoma Melanosis is an uncommon finding in the vagina. These changes reveal the relationship of stratified squamous epithelium to neural crest elements. Although primary malignant melanoma is a rare lesion, a sufficient number of cases have been reported for their authenticity to be accepted. The classic junctional activity is similar to that noted elsewhere on the skin.

Verrucous Carcinoma As on the vulva, verrucous carcinomas may occur in the vagina. Grossly, the lesions appear massive and suggest extensive invasive cancer. Microscopically, there is usually no extension beyond the local area.

Lymphoma Lymphomas are very rare. Although primary vaginal lymphomas have been reported, they are usually secondary. Immunohistochemical stains are helpful to differentiate these lesions from sarcomas and squamous cancers.

Endodermal Sinus Tumor Endodermal sinus tumor is a germ cell tumor that may arise *de novo* in the vagina. Most commonly appearing during the first decade of life, the lesion grossly simulates sarcoma botryoides. As in the ovary, this neoplasm grows rapidly. Histopathologically, it is identical to that seen in the ovary, and it must be differentiated from a mesonephroid lesion and sarcoma botryoides (81).

Mucinous Carcinoma A rare primary mucin-secreting carcinoma of the vagina has been identified (82). Such lesions arise from embryologic remnants that result from incomplete separation of the cloaca by the urorectal fold, thus leaving remnants of the mucin-secreting rectal epithelium in the vagina and/or urethra. They must be differentiated from a mucin-secreting carcinoma of the bowel extending directly into the vagina.

References

1. **zur Hausen H:** Condylomata acuminata and human genital cancer. *Cancer Res* 36:794, 1976.

2. **Richart RM:** Cervical intraepithelial neoplasia. *Pathology Annual.* vol 8. East Norwalk, Connecticut, Appleton-Century-Crofts, 1973, p 301.

3. **Crum CP, Ikenberg H, Richart RM, Gissman L:** Human papillomavirus type 16 and early cervical neoplasia. *N Engl J Med* 310:880, 1984.

4. **Fu YS, Huang I, Beaudenon S, et al:** Correlative study of human papillomavirus DNA, histopathology and morphometry in cervical condyloma and intraepithelial neoplasia. *Int J Gynecol Pathol* 7:297, 1988.

5. **Fu YS, Berek JS, Hilborne LH:** Diagnostic problems of cervical in situ and invasive adenocarcinoma. *Appl Pathol* 5:47, 1987.

6. **Fu YS, Berek JS:** Minimal cervical cancer: definition and histology. In Grundmann E, and Beck L (eds). *Minimal Neoplasia—Diagnosis and Therapy. Recent Results in Cancer Research.* Vol. 106, Berlin, Springer-Verlag, 1988, pp 47–56.

7. **Burghardt E, Girardi F, Lahousen M, et al:** Microinvasive carcinoma of the uterine cervix (International Federation of Gynecology and Obstetrics Stage IA). *Cancer* 67:1037, 1991.

8. **Fu YS, Reagan, JW:** Pathology of the uterine cervix, vagina and vulva. Philadelphia, WB Saunders, 1989.

9. **Robert ME, Fu YS:** Squamous cell carcinoma of the uterine cervix: a review with emphasis on prognostic factors and unusual variants. *Semin Diagn Pathol* 7:173, 1990.

10. **Kaku T, Enjoji M:** Extremely well-differentiated adenocarcinoma ("adenoma malignum"). *Int J Gynecol Pathol* 2:28, 1983.

11. **Gilks CB, Young R, Aguirre P, et al:** Adenoma malignum (minimal deviation adenocarcinoma) of the uterine cervix. *Am J Surg Pathol* 13:719, 1989.

12. **Kaminski PF, Norris HJ:** Minimal deviation carcinoma (adenoma malignum) of the cervix. *Int J Gynecol Pathol* 2:141, 1983.

13. **Young RH, Scully RE:** Villoglandular papillary adenocarcinoma of the uterine cervix a clinicopathologic analysis of 13 cases. *Cancer* 63:1773, 1989.

14. **Benda JA, Platz CE, Buchsbaum H, et al:** Mucin production in defining mixed carcinoma of the uterine cervix: a clinicopathologic study. *Int J Gynecol Pathol* 4:314, 1985

15. **Glucksmann A, Cherry CP:** Incidence, histology and response to radiation of mixed carcinomas (adenoacanthomas) of the uterine cervix. *Cancer* 9:971, 1956.

16. **Ferry JA, Scully RE:** "Adenoid cystic" carcinoma and adenoid basal carcinoma of the uterine cervix: a study of 28 cases. *Am J Surg Pathol* 12:134, 1988.

17. **Kurman RJ:** The morphology, biology, and pathology of intermediate trophoblast: a look back to the present. *Hum Pathol* 9:847, 1991.

18. **Huang SJ, Amparo E, Fu YS:** Histologic classification and behavior of endometrial hyperplasia. *Surg Pathol* 1:215, 1988.

19. **Kurman RJ, Kaminski PF, Norris HJ:** The behavior of endometrial hyperplasia: a long-term study of "untreated" hyperplasia in 170 patients. *Cancer* 56:403, 1985.

20. **Ferenczy A, Gelfand M:** The biologic significance of cytologic atypia in progesterogen treated endometrial hyperplasia. *Am J Obstet Gynecol* 160:126, 1989.

21. **Kurman RJ, Norris HJ:** Evaluation of criteria for distinguishing atypical endometrial hyperplasia from well-differentiated carcinoma. *Cancer* 49:2547, 1982.

22. **Hendrickson MR, Ross JC, Kempson RL:** Toward the development of morphologic criteria for well-differentiated adenocarcinoma of the endometrium. *Am J Surg Pathol* 7:819, 1983.

23. **Zaino RJ, Kurman RJ:** Squamous differentiation in carcinoma of the endometrium: a critical appraisal of adenoacanthoma and adenosquamous carcinoma. *Semin Diagn Pathol* 5:154, 1988.

24. **Kempson RL, Hendrickson MR:** Pure mesenchymal neoplasms of the uterine corpus selected problems. *Semin Diagn Pathol* 5:172, 1988.

25. **Zaloudek CJ, Norris HJ:** Mesenchymal tumors of the uterus. In Fengolio C, Wolff M (eds): *Progress in Surgical Pathology.* New York, Masson Publishing USA, 1981, pp 1–35.

26. **Perrone T, Dehner LP:** Prognostically favorable "mitotically active" smooth-muscle tumors of the uterus: a clinicopathologic study of 10 cases. *Am J Surg Pathol* 12:2, 1988.

27. **Parmley TH, Woodruff JD, Winn K:** The histogenesis of leiomyomatosis peritonealis disseminata. *Obstet Gynecol* 46:511, 1975.

28. **Chang KL, Crabtree GS, Lim-Tan SK, et al:** Primary uterine endometrial stroma neoplasms: a clinicopathologic study of 117 cases. *Am J Surg Pathol* 14:415, 1990.

29. **Bell DA:** Ovarian surface epithelial-stromal tumors. *Hum Pathol* 22:750, 1991.

30. **Genadry R, Poliakoff S, Rotmensch J, et al:** Papillary intraperitoneal proliferation often referred to as a papillary serous tumor of low malignant potential. *Obstet Gynecol* 58:730, 1981.

31. **Bell DA, Weinstock MA, Scully RE:** Peritoneal implants of ovarian serous borderline tumors: histologic features and prognosis. *Cancer* 62:2212, 1988.

32. **McCaughey WTE, Kirk ME, Lester W, et al:** Peritoneal epithelial lesions associated with proliferative serous tumours of the ovary. *Histopathology* 8:195, 1984.

33. **Michael H, Roth LM:** Invasive and noninvasive implants in ovarian serous tumors of low malignant potential. *Cancer* 57:1240, 1986.

34. **Gershenson DM, Silva EG:** Serous ovarian tumors of low malignant potential with peritoneal implants. *Cancer* 65:578, 1990.

35. **Bell DA, Scully RE:** Ovarian serous borderline tumors with stromal microinvasion: a report of 21 cases. *Hum Pathol* 21:397, 1990.

36. **Sampson JA:** Endometrial carcinoma of the ovary. *Arch Surg* 10:1, 1925.

37. **Kurman RJ, Craig JM:** Endometrioid and clear cell carcinomas of the ovary. *Cancer* 29:1653, 1972.

38. **Roth LM, Dallenbach-Hellweg G, Czernobilsky B:** Ovarian Brenner tumors. I. Metaplastic, proliferating and of low grade potential. *Cancer* 56:582, 1985.

39. **Robey SS, Silva EG, Gershenson DM, et al:** Transitional cell carcinoma in high-grade stage ovarian carcinoma: an indicator of favorable response to chemotherapy. *Cancer* 63:839, 1989.

40. **Silva EG, Robey-Cafferty SS, Smith TL, et al:** Ovarian carcinomas with transitional cell carcinoma pattern. *Am J Clin Pathol* 93:457, 1990.

41. **Austin RM, Norris HJ:** Malignant Brenner tumor and transitional cell carcinoma of the ovary: a comparison. *Int J Gynecol Pathol* 6:29, 1987.

42. **Bell DA, Scully RE:** Serous borderline tumors of the peritoneum. *Am J Surg Pathol* 14:230, 1990.

43. **Fromm G-L, Gershenson DM, Silva EG:** Papillary serous carcinoma of the peritoneum. *Obstet Gynecol* 75:89, 1990.

44. **Truong LD, Maccato ML, Awalt H, et al:** Serous surface carcinoma of the peritoneum: a clinicopathology study of 22 cases. *Hum Pathol* 21:99, 1990.

45. **Thor AD, Young RH, Clement PB:** Pathology of the fallopian tube, broad ligament, peritoneum, and pelvic soft tissue. *Hum Pathol* 9:856, 1991.

46. **Gordon A, Lipton D, Woodruff JD:** Dysgerminoma: a review of 158 cases from the Emil Novak Ovarian Tumor Registry. *Obstet Gynecol* 58:497, 1981.

47. **Zaloudek C, Tavassoli FA, Norris HJ:** Dysgerminoma with syncytiotrophoblastic giant cells: a histologically and clinically distinctive subtype of dysgerminoma. *Am J Surg Pathol* 5:361, 1981.

48. **Scully RE:** Gonadoblastoma: a review of 74 cases. *Cancer* 25:1340, 1970.

49. **Talerman A:** Gonadoblastoma and dysgerminoma in two siblings with dysgenetic gonads. *Obstet Gynecol* 38:416, 1971.

50. **Woodruff JD, Protos P, Peterson WF:** Ovarian teratomas: relationship of histologic and ontogenic factors to prognosis. *Am J Obstet Gynecol* 102:702, 1968.

51. **Teilum G:** Classification of endodermal sinus tumor and so-called embryonal carcinoma of the ovary. *Acta Pathol Microbiol Scand* 64:407, 1965.

52. **Kurman RJ, Norris HJ:** Embryonal carcinoma of the ovary: a clinicopathologic entity distinct from endodermal sinus tumor resembling embryonal carcinoma in the adult testis. *Cancer* 38:2420, 1976.

53. **Novak ER, Kutchmeshgi J, Mupas RS, Woodruff JD:** Feminizing gonadal stromal tumors: analysis of the granulosa-theca cell tumors of the ovarian tumor registry. *Obstet Gynecol* 38:701, 1971.

54. **Chalvardjian A, Scully RE:** Sclerosing stromal tumors of the ovary. *Cancer* 31:664, 1973.

55. **Garcia-Bunuel R, Berek JS, Woodruff JD:** Luteomas of pregnancy. *Obstet Gynecol* 45:407, 1975.

56. **Ireland K, Woodruff JD:** Masculinizing ovarian tumors. *Obstet Gynecol Surv* 31:83, 1975.

57. **Young RH:** Ovarian tumors other than those of surface epithelial-stromal type. *Hum Pathol* 22:763, 1991.

58. **Lash RH, Hart WR:** Intestinal adenocarcinomas metastatic to the ovaries: a clinicopathological evaluation of 22 cases. *Am J Surg Pathol* 11:114, 1987.

59. **Sedlis A:** Carcinoma of the fallopian tube. *Surg Clin North Am* 58:121, 1978.

60. **Woodruff JD, Mattingly RF (eds):** Surgical conditions of the vulva. In *Operative Gynecology*. Philadelphia, JB Lippincott, 1978, pp 629–640.

61. **Ridley CM, Frankman O, Jones ISC, et al:** New nomenclature for vulvar disease: report of the Committee on Terminology of the International Society for the Study of Vulvar Disease. *J Reprod Med* 35:483, 1990.

62. **Wilkinson EJ, Kneale B, Lynch PJ:** Report of the ISSVD Terminology Committee. *J Reprod Med* 31:973, 1986.

63. **Gardner HL, Kaufman RH:** Benign diseases of the vulva and vagina. 2nd ed. Boston, GK Hall, 1981.

64. **Zacur HA, Genadry R, Woodruff JD:** The patient at-risk for development of vulvar cancer. *Gynecol Oncol* 9:199, 1980.

65. **Buscema J, Stern J, Woodruff JD:** The significance of the histologic alterations adjacent to invasive vulvar carcinoma. *Am J Obstet Gynecol* 137:902, 1980.

66. **Friedrich EG Jr, Wilkinson EJ, Fu YS:** Carcinoma-in-situ of the vulva: a continuing challenge. *Am J Obstet Gynecol* 136:830, 1980.

67. **Ulbright TM, Stehman FB, Roth LM, et al:** Bowenoid dysplasia of the vulva. *Cancer* 50:2910, 1982.

68. **Bergeron C, Negashfar Z, Canaan C, et al:** Human papillomavirus type 16 in intra-epithelial neoplasias (bowenoid papulosis) and coexistent invasive carcinoma of the vulva. *Int J Gynecol Pathol* 6:1, 1987.

69. **Woodruff JD:** Early invasive carcinoma of the vulva. *Clin Oncol* 1:349, 1982.

70. **Binder SW, Huang I, Fu YS, et al:** Risk factors for the development of lymph node metastasis in vulvar squamous cell carcinoma. *Gynecol Oncol* 37:9, 1990.

71. **Japaze H, van Dinh T, Woodruff JD:** Verrucous carcinoma of the vulva: study of 24 cases. *Obstet Gynecol* 60:462, 1982.

72. **Chung AF, Woodruff JM, Lewis JL:** Malignant melanoma of the vulva: a report of 44 cases. *Obstet Gynecol* 45:638, 1975.

73. **Brand E, Fu YS, Lagasse LD, Berek JS:** Vulvovaginal melanoma: report of seven cases and literature review. *Gynecol Oncol* 33:54, 1989.

74. **Breslow A, Macht SD:** Optimal size of resection margin for thin cutaneous melanoma. *Surg Gynecol Obstet* 145:691, 1977.

75. **Sandberg ED:** The incidence and distribution of occult vaginal adenosis. *Am J Obstet Gynecol* 101:322, 1968.

76. **Stafl A, Mattingly RF:** Vaginal adenosis: a precancerous lesion? *Am J Obstet Gynecol* 120:666, 1974.

77. **Pride GL, Schultz AE, Chuprevich TW, Buchler DA:** Primary invasive squamous carcinoma of the vagina. *Obstet Gynecol* 53:218, 1979.

78. **Herbst A, Scully RE:** Adenocarcinoma of the vagina in adolescence. *Cancer* 25:745, 1970.

79. **Herbst A, Green TH Jr, Ulfelder H:** Primary carcinoma of the vagina: an analysis of 68 cases. *Am J Obstet Gynecol* 106:210, 1970.

80. **Chirayil SJ, Tobon H:** Polyps of the vagina: a clinicopathologic study of 18 cases. *Cancer* 47:2904, 1981.

81. **Rezaizadeh MM, Woodruff JD:** Endodermal sinus tumor of the vagina. *Gynecol Oncol* 6:459, 1978.

82. **Askin FB, Muhlendorf K, Walz BJ:** Mucinous carcinoma of anal duct origin presenting clinically as a vaginal cyst. *Cancer* 42:566, 1978.

5 Epidemiology and Biostatistics

Daniel W. Cramer

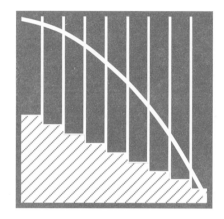

Epidemiologic and biostatistical principles have wide application in gynecologic oncology. They are used to define occurrence and survival, to determine causative factors, and to devise strategies for treatment or prevention. Principles of descriptive statistics, epidemiologic evidence for cancer etiology, validity, and statistical inference are reviewed. Risk factors and methods of prevention for gynecologic cancers are discussed.

Descriptive Statistics

Cancer Occurrence

Cancer is described in populations by statistics related to its occurrence and to survival from it.

Incidence

The incidence rate (IR) is defined as the number of new cases of disease per population per time.

$$IR = \text{new cases/person-time}$$

The fact that time is a component of the denominator should help the clinician to avoid the misapplication of this term to other measures of disease occurrence.

Cancer Incidence **Cancer incidence is generally stated as cases per 100,000 population per year or as cases per 100,000 person-years.** The incidence rate must be measured in a specific population over a specific period. For example, cancer registries count the number of new cancer cases diagnosed over a year in a defined geographic region and divide that figure by the total population in tha region. Estimates of population are provided by the Census Bureau.

Crude Incidence   **The crude incidence is simply the number of new case: that occur over a specified time per population without regard to age.**

Age-Specific Incidence Rate   **The age-specific incidence rate is the numbe of new cancers within a particular age group that develop in a populatio of that same age range over a specified time.** Age-specific incidence rates fo the common gynecologic cancers in the United States based on all females in th Surveillance, Epidemiology, and End Results Survey (SEER) area, 1984 to 1988 are shown in Figure 5.1.

1. *Invasive cervical cancer* rates show a gradual rise and plateau after th age of 50 at about 20 cases per 100,000 woman-years.

2. *Endometrial cancer* rates show a sharp increase in the perimenopausa years, with a peak incidence between the ages of 65 and 75 at abou 110 cases per 100,000 woman-years.

Figure 5.1   Age-specific incidence curves for the gynecologic cancers in wome in the United States (SEER data). (Redrawn with permission from Cramer DW Epidemiologic and Statistical Aspects of Gynecologic Oncology. In Knapp RC, Ber kowitz RS (eds): *Gynecologic Oncology*, ed 2, New York, MacMillan, 1993, p 139–150).

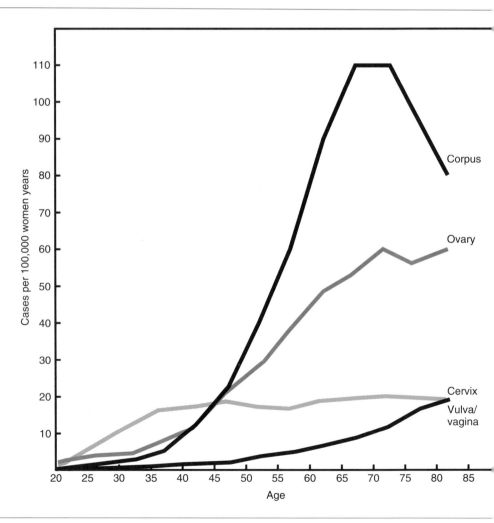

3. *Ovarian cancer* also increases in the perimenopausal years and peaks between the ages of 70 and 80 at about 60 cases per 100,000 woman-years.

4. *Vulvar cancers* occur about three times more frequently than vaginal cancers. Vulvar and vaginal cancers display similar age-incidence patterns and therefore are combined in Figure 5.1. Vulvovaginal cancers gradually increase during life, with a peak occurrence after age 80.

Age-Specific Mortality Rates   Age-specific mortality rates based on the SEER data (1) for the gynecologic cancers in the United States are shown in Figure 5.2. Mortality rates are incidence rates in which "new deaths" are counted instead of "new cases." A different perspective on the relative importance of the gynecologic cancers is presented in Figure 5.2. Mortality rates for ovarian cancer are higher than those for cervical or endometrial cancer. Indeed, deaths from ovarian cancer currently exceed the total number of uterine cancer deaths (endometrial and cervical combined) in the United States.

Figure 5.2   Age-specific mortality curves for the gynecologic cancers in women in the United States (SEER data). (Redrawn with permission from Cramer DW: Epidemiologic and Statistical Aspects of Gynecologic Oncology. In Knapp RC, Berkowitz RS (eds): *Gynecologic Oncology*, ed 2, New York, MacMillan, 1993, pp 139–150).

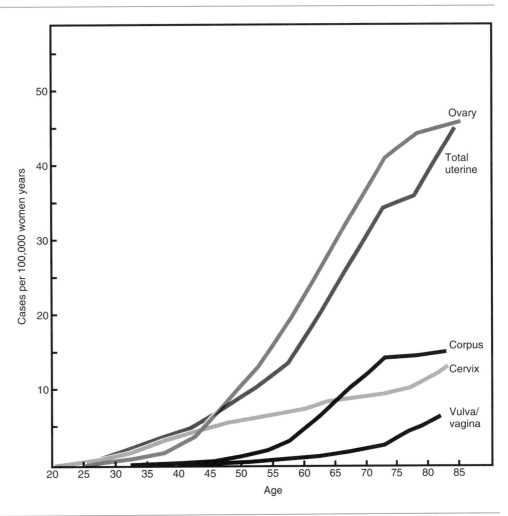

Age-specific incidence or mortality rates are the best way to describe the occurrence of cancer in a population. However, age-specific rates may be cumbersome when one is attempting to compare cancer occurrence among many populations. This requires a summary measure of occurrence. Crude incidence rates could be used but may give misleading information. For example, an "old" population would have a higher crude incidence of endometrial cancer and a lower crude incidence of carcinoma *in situ* of the cervix than a "young" population, even though both populations may have an identical age-specific incidence for each disease.

Age-Adjusted Incidence Rates **Age-adjusted incidence (AAI) rates may be obtained by multiplying the incidence rate for each age stratum by the proportion of individuals in that stratum in a standard population.** These "weighted" age-specific incidence rates are summed as follows:

$$AAI = \frac{\Sigma\, IR_i W_i}{\Sigma\, W_i}$$

where IR_i is the incidence rate in the "i" age stratum, and W_i is the number of people in the "i" stratum in the standard population. The actual age-adjusted rate will vary, depending on the standard chosen but will give a correct impression about cancer occurrence among populations that may differ in age structure.

Cumulative Incidence **The cumulative incidence may be thought of as the proportion of people who develop disease (or die from it) during some period of observation.** Cumulative "incidence" is technically a misnomer, because it does not contain time in the denominator but, rather, is expressed as a percentage from 0 to 100. Commonly, the *cumulative incidence rate* (CIR) is calculated from age-specific incidence rates:

$$CIR = IR_i\,(\Delta T_i)$$

Where IR_i is the age-specific rate for the "i" age stratum and ΔT_i is the size of the age interval of the "i" stratum (usually $\leq$ 5 years).

When cumulative incidence is summed over the age range 0 to 75, it yields the *"lifetime risk"* for cancer occurrence or death.

Cumulative incidence or lifetime risks, like age-adjusted rates, may be used to compare racial and geographic variation in cancer rates. Lifetime risks for the major gynecologic cancers for selected geographic areas (2) are compared in Table 5.1.

Table 5.1   Lifetime Risk for Diagnosis of the Major Gynecologic Cancers by Geographic Area around 1980

	Cervix Invasive (%)	Endometrium (%)	Ovary (%)
Scandinavia (Sweden)	1.01	1.58	1.73
South America (Colombia)	5.31	0.67	0.87
United States (Los Angeles-White)	0.83	3.05	1.53
(Los Angeles-Black)	1.37	1.34	0.89
Israel	0.43	1.22	1.37
Japan (Osaka)	1.83	0.27	0.47
U.K. (Birmingham)	1.27	1.10	1.25
Southern Europe (Italy)	1.09	1.50	1.11
India (Bombay)	2.22	0.24	0.75
Australia (Queensland)	1.21	1.30	0.97

Data from Muir C, Waterhouse J, Mack T, et al: *Cancer Incidence in Five Continents*, vol 5, International Agency for Research on Cancer, 1987.

Lifetime Risk

Cervical Cancer   Lifetime risks for cervical cancer range from 0.4% in Israel to 5.3% in Cali, Colombia, where cervical cancer is the most common malignancy in women. In general, the incidence of cervical cancer is more common in underdeveloped countries and less frequent in Western and industrialized countries and among white women.

Endometrial Cancer   Lifetime risks of endometrial cancer vary from a low of 0.2% in India to a high of 3% among white females in California. In general, the incidence of endometrial cancer is lower in third world countries and higher in Western and industrialized countries. Black and Asian women have a lower incidence of endometrial cancer than white women.

Ovarian Cancer   Lifetime risks of ovarian cancer vary from 0.5% in Japan to 1.7% in Sweden. Similar to endometrial cancer, the risk is generally lower in third world countries and in black and Asian populations and higher in industrialized countries and in white populations.

Prevalence

The last measure of cancer occurrence to be discussed is prevalence. **Prevalence is the proportion of people who have a particular disease or condition at a specified time.** Prevalence is related to incidence according to the following well-known association.

$$\text{Prevalence} = \text{incidence} \times \text{average duration of disease}$$

Two examples of studies that yield prevalence data are those based on autopsy findings and screening tests. The frequency of occult cancers identified in a series of autopsies yields prevalence data. The first application of a screening test in a previously unscreened population will yield the prevalence of preclinical disease.

Cancer Survival

The probability of survival of cancer patients over time often fits an exponential function. An exponential function will yield a curve similar in shape to that shown in Figure 5.3 when the proportion of cancer patients surviving is plotted against time. Summary measures of this curve commonly include median survival time (the point at which 50% of the patients died: 2 years in the figure) and the probability of survival at 1, 2, and 5 years (85%, 50%, and 15%, respectively, in the figure).

To say that survival is exponential means that the rate of death is constant over time. This can also be demonstrated by plotting the logarithm of the probability of survival against time and demonstrating a straight line. Alternatively, a line that bends downward indicates decreasing survival over time.

Figure 5.3   Idealized plot of exponential survival curve. One-year survival, median survival, and 5-year survival points are illustrated. (Redrawn with permission from Cramer DW: Epidemiologic and Statistical Aspects of Gynecologic Oncology. In Knapp RC, Berkowitz RS (eds): *Gynecologic Oncology*, New York, MacMillan, 1986, pp 201–222).

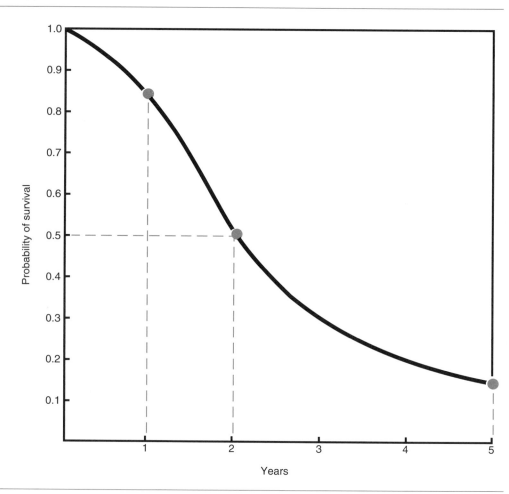

**Table 5.2   Five-Year Survival Rates for the Major Gynecologic Cancers
in the United States**

Site/Stage	5-Year Relative Rates (%)	
	Whites	*Black*
Cervix		
All stages (except *in situ*)	68	59
Stage I	86	80
Stage II	61	44
Stage III	37	34
Stage IV	15	13
Unknown	74	61
Endometrium		
All stages	85	54
Stage I	93	73
Stage II	76	27
Stage III	55	17
Stage IV	23	13
Unknown	76	61
Ovary		
All stages	37	37
Stage I	85	86
Stage II	58	72
Stages III and IV	20	20
Unknown	29	38

Data from Sondik EJ, Young JL, Horm JW, Gloeckler LA: *Annual Cancer Statistics Review.* NIH Publication 86–2789, 1985.

Relative survival is defined as the ratio of the observed survival rate for the patient group to the survival rate expected for a population with similar demographic characteristics. Relative survival rates are a modification of the survival curve and are most useful in examining long-term survival.

Five-Year Relative Survival Rates

Five-year relative survival rates are frequently cited as the proportion of cancer patients who are potentially cured. Five-year relative survival rates for white and black females in the United States from the SEER data (3) are shown in Table 5.2 by type and stage of gynecologic cancer.

Etiologic Studies and Statistical Inference

Studies of cancer occurrence or survival are descriptive in nature. Such studies are useful in helping public health officials to allocate resources and to establish broad hypotheses about the causes of cancer. They are limited in the latter respect, however, because a complete understanding of the role of chance or other statistical biases is often not possible in descriptive studies.

In the past 50 years a field of medical investigation, epidemiology, has developed to identify more precisely the causes of disease in human beings. Because it is unethical and impossible to purposely expose human beings to potential carcinogens, epidemiology takes advantage of "natural experiments" in which persons are exposed inadvertently to possible carcinogens as a result of their occupation, lifestyle, or prior medical therapy. The tools of the epidemiologist are the cohort and the case-control studies (4).

Types of Studies

Cohort Study

In a cohort study, the groups to be studied (the cohorts) are defined by characteristics (or exposures) that occur before the disease or outcome of interest, and the study groups are observed over time to determine the frequency of disease that develops in the cohorts. Cohort studies are most feasible for rare exposures and common outcomes when general population rates of disease can be used for the nonexposed rate of disease.

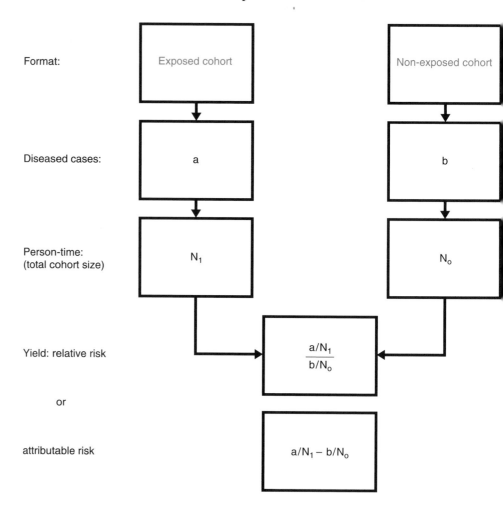

Format:

Exposed cohort   Non-exposed cohort

Diseased cases: a   b

Person-time:
(total cohort size) N_1 N_o

Yield: relative risk $\dfrac{a/N_1}{b/N_o}$

or

attributable risk $a/N_1 - b/N_o$

Retrospective Cohort Study In a retrospective cohort study, the exposures and outcomes have already occurred when the study is begun. For example, many studies of radiation and female cancer are based on records of women irradiated for cervical cancer 10 to 30 years previously and use medical records and death certificates to determine those who subsequently died of a particular disease.

Prospective Cohort Study In a prospective cohort study, the relevant exposure may or may not have occurred when the study is begun, but the outcome has not yet occurred. After the cohort is selected, the investigator must wait for the disease or outcome to appear in the cohort members.

Clinical Trial

An experimental study or clinical trial is a special type of prospective cohort study in which the investigator can assign the exposure to minimize the

possibility that bias accounts for differences in the exposed and nonexposed cohorts. Clinical trials are ideal to determine the effect of different cancer therapies (the "exposure") on disease recurrence or death (the "outcome"). In these trials, control over confounding is achieved by *randomization;* i.e., subjects are assigned to the therapy or experimental conditions in a random fashion. This generally assures an equal distribution of known and unknown confounding factors in the study groups being compared.

In either retrospective or prospective cohort studies, the frequency of disease among those who have been exposed is compared with the frequency of disease among the nonexposed as a ratio or a difference.

Relative Risk   **The relative risk is the ratio of disease frequency in the exposed population divided by disease frequency in the nonexposed population.** A number greater than 1 may indicate that exposure increases the risk of disease.

Attributable Risk   **The attributable risk is the difference in the disease frequency among the exposed and nonexposed populations.** A number greater than 0 may indicate that exposure increases the risk of disease.

Case-Control Study

In the case-control study, groups are selected according to whether or not they have disease. These groups are compared with respect to existing or past characteristics (exposures) that are possibly relevant to the cause of the disease.

Case-Control Design   The odds of exposure among the diseased cases (a,b) is compared with the odds of exposure among the controls (c,d). The resulting term (ad/bc) is the exposure odds ratio.

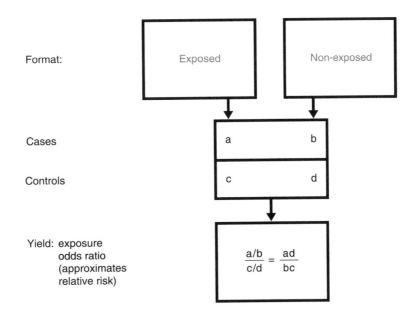

If an entire population could be characterized by its exposure and disease status, the exposure odds ratio would be identical to the relative risk obtained in a cohort study. Although this is not feasible, as long as the cases and controls actually sampled have not been preferentially selected on the basis of their exposure status,

183

the exposure odds ratio in the sampled population will approximate the relative risk.

Attributable risk is not directly obtainable in a case-control study. Case-control studies are most feasible for examining the association between a relatively common exposure and a relatively rare disease. The design must control carefully for biases.

Interpretation of Data

The clinician is confronted constantly by epidemiologic studies claiming that some new exposure is associated with cancer. Whether or not the conclusion of a particular cancer study is believable is determined primarily by its freedom from bias and its statistical significance. Other criteria that can help the physician decide whether the conclusion of a study is credible relative to the *dose response*, *consistency*, and *biologic credibility*.

Validity

Validity means freedom from bias. Bias refers to a systemic error in the design, conduct, or analysis of a study that results in a mistaken conclusion. An understanding of the major types of bias and how to control them is necessary to distinguish the valid from the invalid study.

Observation Bias Observation bias or misclassification means that subjects have been classified incorrectly with respect to exposure or disease. This may occur if the criteria for exposure or disease are not defined clearly or if records are incomplete. Besides adequate criteria and complete records, one method to achieve control over observation bias is "blindness" of observation. The investigator who is to record whether disease occurred among subjects in a cohort study should not know whether the subjects are in the exposed or the nonexposed cohort. Ideally, the investigator who is to record exposure status of subjects in a case-control study should not know whether they are case or control subjects, although this is often not possible. At the very least, the investigator must be certain that case and control subjects have not been questioned in a different manner about their exposure status, which could lead to preferential recall of the exposure in case subjects.

Selection Bias Selection bias means that case and control subjects have been selected on a correlate of the exposure. It is less likely to occur in cohort studies than in case-control studies. In general, the larger the study, the less likely the occurrence of selection bias. Alternatively, studies based entirely on a population from a single hospital could be subject to a selection bias.

Confounding Confounding means that some other factor not considered in the design or analysis accounts for an association because the factor is correlated with both exposure and disease. Obvious confounders for any cancer study are age, race, and socioeconomic status, as we have indicated previously how cancer risk can vary with these characteristics. Confounding may be controlled for during the design of a study by selection or matching or by randomization in the case of a clinical trial. If confounders are not controlled for during the study design, they can be controlled for during the analysis by stratification or by multivariate analysis. *Stratifying* means examining the association of interest only within groups that are similar with respect to a potential confounder (5). *Multivariate analysis* is a statistical technique used during analysis that controls for a

184

number of confounders simultaneously and is commonly used in epidemiologic studies (6).

Statistical Inference

Statistical inference is the process by which the investigator uses a sample population to draw conclusions about a "universe" population (i.e., a large population to which the investigator would like the results to be generalized). Assuming that the investigator has selected the subjects to be studied and has collected observations in a valid manner, there remains the question of whether the findings are merely a chance result.

The process of statistical inference involves the following steps:

1. A series of observations is obtained from a sample and summarized by some statistical parameter (e.g., a mean, a proportion, a rate ratio).

2. A value for the parameter of interest is specified under the *null hypothesis*.

3. A statistical test is chosen that is based on the nature of the parameter and the null hypothesis.

4. Significance testing is performed to assess the strength of the conflict between what is found in the sample and what is predicted by the null hypothesis.

5. A confidence interval on the parameter of interest may be constructed on the basis of the statistical test, which defines the range in which the "true value" of the parameter is expected to fall.

Type I Error = *P* Value

The degree of conflict between the sample results and the null hypothesis is summarized by the *P value, alpha,* or *type I error,* which indicates the probability that one is declaring the null hypothesis to be false on the basis of the sample, when in reality the null hypothesis is true for a universe population. P values $< 5\%$ generally are declared to be "significant." The lower the P value, the greater the confidence that the observed result is not a chance result. If a P value $> 5\%$ is obtained, the null hypothesis cannot be rejected, but this does not necessarily imply that the null hypothesis is true.

Type II Error

The probability of declaring the null hypothesis to be true on basis of the sample, when in reality the null hypothesis for the universe population is false, is described as a *type II or beta error.* To calculate a beta error, an "alternate hypothesis" must be stated. In planning cancer studies, an investigator often is asked to calculate the power (1 minus the beta error) that a study will have to detect an association, given a certain study size and certain assumptions about the nature of the association. Study power should be kept in mind in small clinical trials that find no significant difference among therapies. Such studies may be cited as evidence of "no effect of therapy," when in fact the sample size was inadequate to detect modest differences in response rates.

185

Statistical Distributions and Tests

The "*t* distribution" and the "*t* test" are used to determine whether the means of two groups differ. The "*F* distribution" and the "*F* test" are used to determine whether variances differ. Proportions may be compared in two or more groups by reference to chi-square, binomial, poisson, or hypergeometric distributions. The statistical test for significance chosen depends on the nature of the parameters and the null hypothesis. A complete description of these tests is found in basic textbooks and will not be reviewed in this chapter (7).

Dose Response

Dose response means that an increase in risk of disease (or other outcome) is observed with an increase in the amount of exposure. Examples of a dose response include increasing risk of endometrial cancer with increasing estrogen dose or increasing duration of use (8).

Consistency

Issues of consistency and credibility require the researcher to look beyond his or her own data to review other relevant studies. Agreement among different investigators, especially if they have used different study methods, is reassuring evidence of a true association. For example, virtually all the studies on the association between menopausal estrogens and endometrial cancer found an association (9–12).

Biologic Credibility

Biologic credibility means that an association is plausible that takes into consideration all aspects of what is known of the natural history or demographics of the disease or what has been observed in relevant experimental models. An association that has biologic credibility is supported by a framework of diverse observations. The search for biologic credibility often yields a greater understanding of disease pathogenesis and is a process that is easier to illustrate than to explain.

Continuing on the theme of menopausal estrogens and endometrial cancer, does this association have biologic credibility? The following facts are known:

1. Continuous administration of estrogen can cause endometrial hyperplasia (13).

2. Women with excessive endogenous estrogen from granulosa tumors may develop endometrial cancer (14).

3. Women with decreased degradation of estrogen secondary to liver failure may develop endometrial cancer (15).

4. Women who are obese have excessive peripheral conversion of androstenedione to active estrogen and are at increased risk of endometrial cancer (16–18).

5. The perimenopausal period is characterized by anovulatory cycles with unopposed estrogen, and this is the same age group in which the age-specific incidence of endometrial cancer is increasing rapidly.

This general framework of epidemiologic and biologic observations not only supports the validity of an association between menopausal estrogen and endometrial cancer, but it also suggests that the risk of endometrial cancer is mediated largely through states that lead to an excess of estrogen relative to progesterone.

Risk Factors for Gynecologic Cancers

In the previous section, a "framework" for viewing epidemiologic associations was discussed. Even though the pathogenetic models for the gynecologic cancers are far from clear, that process of ordering diverse epidemiologic observations will be emphasized in this section on specific risk factors for the major gynecologic cancers (Table 5.3).

Cervical Cancer   The framework for viewing squamous cell carcinoma of the cervix is that it is the end stage of cervical intraepithelial neoplasia (CIN), progressing from dysplasia, to carcinoma *in situ*, to invasive disease. Thus risk factors for cervical cancer will be those that relate to the initiation of atypical transformation and those that relate to the progression of dysplasia.

Factors related to the initiation of cervical cancer are overwhelmingly associated with sexual history and include (19–23):

1. Early age at first intercourse

Table 5.3   Risk Factors for Gynecologic Cancers

Factor	*Cervix*	*Endometrium*	*Ovary*
Marriage and sexual	Increased risk associated with coitus at an early age, multiple partners, or "high-risk males"	Increased risk in women who have never married	Increased risk in women who have never married
Contraception	Barrier methods protective; oral contraceptives may increase risk	Nonsequential oral contraceptives protective	Oral contraceptives protective
Reproductive experiences	Increasing risk with increasing parity	Decreasing risk with increasing parity	Decreasing risk with increasing parity
Age at menopause	No apparent association	Late menopause increases risk	Early menopause may increase risk
Menopausal hormones	No apparent association	Greatly increased risk from "unopposed estrogen"	Weak increased risk with "unopposed estrogen"
Family history	Weak evidence of familial tendency	Weak evidence of familial tendency	Ovarian cancer among first-degree relatives a strong risk factor
Body habitus/diet	Carotene, vitamin C, and folic acid potentially protective	Obesity a strong risk factor; ingestion of animal fat increases risk	Ingestion of foods high in dairy sugar may increase risk
Smoking	Increased risk	Decreased risk	Conflicting evidence
Other exposures	Douching may increase risk	Association with estrogen-producing tumors of the ovary, liver disease	Foreign bodies (talc) per vagina may increase risk

2. Intercourse with multiple sexual partners

3. "High-risk" males

Early age at first intercourse may be important because adolescence is a period of heightened squamous metaplasia, and intercourse during such times may increase the likelihood of atypical transformation (24). The woman who has had intercourse with multiple partners increases her likelihood of exposure to sexually transmitted diseases that may be the specific agents that cause atypical transformation. The "high-risk" male is one who has himself had contact with multiple partners as indicated by marital "clusters" of cervical cancer (25). High risk of cervical neoplasia occurs in women who have had contact with males with penile condylomata acuminata (26).

The list of possible sexually transmitted pathogens that might cause cervical intraepithelial neoplasia (CIN) includes trichomonas (27), cytomegalovirus (28), and herpes simplex virus (HSV), type 2 (29). However, infection with the human papillomavirus (HPV), especially types 16 and 18, is emerging as the most likely causative agent in cervical cancer (30, 31). There is also the possibility that significant interactions may occur between the infectious agents, especially HPV and HSV type II (32, 33).

Regardless of which specific sexually transmitted diseases are found eventually to be associated with atypical transformation, a woman can decrease her risk of cervical cancer by safe sexual practices. Ethnic or religious groups that encourage monogamy have low rates of cervical cancer (20). Use of barrier methods of contraception, especially those that combine both mechanical and chemical (i.e., spermicidal) protection, decrease the risk of cervical cancer (34).

Some consideration should be given to the possibility that noncoital factors may have a role in disease initiation. Douching with coal tar substances, as occurred earlier in this century, was a strong risk factor for cervical cancer and demonstrated that chemical carcinogenesis of the cervix can occur (35). Even though coal tar douches are no longer used, douching should be discouraged among adolescents at the stage of active squamous metaplasia. Smoking also has been associated with cervical cancer. Even after adjustment for a number of potentially confounding factors, such as number of partners and age at first intercourse, smoking has been found to significantly increase the risk of cervical cancer in a dose-response fashion (36). This association has biologic credibility since potentially mutagenic substances are secreted in the cervical mucus of smokers (37).

A factor indisputably related to the progress of CIN is the woman's use of cervical cytology. Population studies have demonstrated a correlation between the use of cytology and declining mortality from cervical cancer (38). **Case-control studies demonstrate that women who have had Pap smears at least every 3 years have one-tenth the risk of invasive disease of women who have never had a Pap test** (39). Other factors that relate to disease progression may include oral contraceptive use and diet. Oral contraceptive use (especially long-term use) has been reported to increase the risk of high-grade intraepithelial lesions and invasive cervical cancer (40, 41). A link to adenocarcinomas of the cervix has also been postulated (42). Butterworth *et al.* attributed the potential harmful effects of oral contraceptives on the cervix to folate deficiency and recommended supplementation (43). Other case-control studies based on dietary histories and plasma levels suggest the importance of beta-carotene and vitamin C (44, 45). Thus any supplementation regimen should include these vitamins as well.

It is clear that future epidemiologic studies of cervical cancer will need to take into consideration a broad array of information regarding sexual history and contraceptive practices, smoking, and dietary factors to assess their possible interactions.

Endometrial Cancer

The framework for viewing the epidemiology of adenocarcinoma of the endometrium is that risk is mediated through states that lead to an excess of estrogen over progesterone. Thus factors that lead to the increased production of estrogen, decreased degradation of estrogen, or exogenous intake of estrogens are risk factors for the disease.

Factors that lead to increased production of estrogen include such tumors as granulosa cell and thecoma tumors of the ovary (14). A common and strong factor related to increased production is obesity via the peripheral conversion mechanism mentioned previously (16). Hypertension and adult-onset diabetes are risk factors for endometrial cancer, largely because of their association with obesity. Alternatively, factors that protect against endometrial cancer are those associated with decreased estrogen production. Surgical castration at an early age with retention of the uterus is a strong protective factor (46). Lean body mass, exercise, and smoking are associated with lower estrogen levels and are protective against endometrial cancer (47, 48), although smoking cannot be encouraged as a preventive measure. Endometrial cancer as a consequence of decreased degradation of estrogen is illustrated in case reports of endometrial cancer in women with cirrhosis of the liver (15).

Exogenous intake of estrogen is a factor that affects risk of endometrial cancer in a direct dose-response fashion (12). This intake may occur through menopausal estrogen taken without progestins or through the use of oral contraceptives of the sequential type that are estrogen-dominant (49). Alternatively, menopausal estrogen taken with a progestin and the use of combination birth control pills decrease the risk of endometrial cancer (13, 50). Future epidemiologic studies should aim to clarify the exact balance of estrogen and progestin that is required to protect the endometrium.

Ovarian Cancer

The "framework" for viewing the epidemiology of ovarian cancer is less clear, with several models proposed: *incessant ovulation, foreign body carcinogenesis,* and *hypergonadotropic hypogonadism.*

Incessant Ovulation   A popular theory is that trauma from repeated ovulation predisposes to ovarian cancer (51). Under this model, factors that produce "ovulatory rest" will be protective; indeed, risk of ovarian cancer decreases with increasing numbers of live births (52) or with increasing duration of oral contraceptive use (53). However, there are several features of ovarian cancer epidemiology that are not readily explained by this model. Peak incidence of ovarian cancer is after the age of 70—well beyond the cessation of ovulation. Native Japanese women have a low incidence of ovarian cancer; yet they also have very low birth rates and virtually no use of OCs. Gonadal radiation that induces

189

menopause should decrease the risk, according to the ovulation theory, but it actually increases the risk. Thus, although it accommodates some features of ovarian cancer epidemiology, incessant ovulation does not allow a complete ordering of the epidemiologic data.

Foreign Body Carcinogenesis Parmley and Woodruff (54) proposed that epithelial ovarian cancers might actually be ovarian mesotheliomas that arise from transformation of the surface lining of the ovary exposed to tubal effluents containing menstrual products or foreign contaminants. Intraperitoneal injections of magnesium silicates, such as asbestos and talc, produce proliferative changes in ovarian surface epithelium in animals (55, 56). This has led investigators to speculate that the use of talc in genital hygiene is a risk factor for ovarian cancer (57, 58). A recent paper observed that the risk appeared to be greatest in those women who used talc as a dusting powder to the genital area on a daily basis for many years, especially at times when they were likely to have been ovulating (59). Such use might allow the talc to become more deeply embedded in the substance of the ovary. However, genital talc exposure can probably account for only a small proportion of ovarian cancers, and this model also falls short of explaining the epidemiology of ovarian cancer.

Hypergonadotropic Hypogonadism Extrapolating from animal models, Gardner (60) suggested that ovarian cancer results from high gonadotropin levels consequent to ovaries that are incapable of exerting feedback control on the pituitary. The models were mostly based on ovarian failure (hypogonadism) as a precursor state, either occurring in strains susceptible to congenital deficiency of oocytes (61) or induced by gonadal radiation (62) or oocyte toxins such as polycyclic hydrocarbons (63). That gonadotropin stimulation was a necessary component (hypergonadotropic hypogonadism) was inferred from the ability of pituitary ablation (64) or deficiency of gonadotropin-releasing hormone (65) to block tumor development.

The relevance of the animal models to human beings has been doubted because the types of tumors in animals did not match the types that occur in human beings. However, the histology of human ovaries differs from that of rodent ovaries in that much greater stromal-epithelial admixture occurs in human ovaries—perhaps because the repeated ovulation produces inclusion cysts (66). In vitro studies have shown the importance of stromal-epithelial interaction in both epithelial differentiation and proliferation (67), suggesting that the same stimuli that cause stromal tumors in animals (which lack inclusion cysts) might cause epithelial tumors in human beings.

Thus it is reasonable to look for pathways in human beings that are equivalent to those of the animal models. Directly relevant to the radiation model are cohort studies that demonstrate that ovarian cancer occurs after radiation for cervical cancer (68) or among survivors of the atomic bomb (69). Potential chemical oocyte toxins in human beings might include tobacco smoke (70), caffeine (71), and tannic acid (72). The mumps virus is a biologic agent capable of producing oocyte loss, and mumps oophoritis has been proposed as a risk factor for ovarian cancer (73) through the mechanism of oocyte depletion.

A dietary component that may be a key factor in the etiology of ovarian cancer is milk sugar or galactose, which human beings commonly ingest in its double-sugar form, lactose (74–77). Evidence that galactose may be an ooctye toxin and related to ovarian cancer comes from animal studies, ecologic studies, and a case-control study. Rodents fed a 50% galactose diet show evidence of oocyte destruction and produce offspring with depleted oocytes when fed the same diet during pregnancy (74, 75). Internationally, there is a strong positive correlation between ovarian cancer rates and per capita milk consumption (76). In a case-control study (77), women with ovarian cancer consumed more lactose and more fermented dairy products, such as yogurt, in which the galactose component is more readily digested. In addition, women with ovarian cancer had lower activity of a principal enzyme involved in the metabolism of galactose, galactose-1-phosphate uridyl transferase (transferase), a deficiency of which is known to cause hypergonadotropic hypogonadism (78). When galactose consumption was viewed in relation to transferase activity, there was a highly significant tendency for women with ovarian cancer to have consumed more galactose than control subjects relative to their ability to metabolize it (77).

In the final set of animal models to be considered, rodents born with a congenital deficiency of oocytes have been shown to be at increased risk of developing ovarian tumors (63). This suggests that heredity or other intrauterine factors affecting oocyte numbers at birth may be risk factors for the disease. This is one possible explanation for the two- to fivefold increase in risk of ovarian cancer faced by women who have a primary relative with the disease (52).

Another feature of the animal models that may be relevant to human ovarian cancer is that conditions that lower gonadotropins are capable of blocking the tumorigenic effect of the oocyte toxin. This may suggest that oral contraceptives exert their protective effect principally by lowering gonadotropins. Similarly, case reports of ovarian tumors in patients receiving Pergonal or clomiphene suggest that agents that stimulate gonadotropins may increase the risk (79).

To summarize, although some features of ovarian cancer epidemiology are explained by incessant ovulation and foreign body contamination, the model probably most consistent with the epidemiologic findings is the hypergonadotropic hypogonadal model.

Vaginal and Vulvar Neoplasms

Other than clear cell adenocarcinomas of the vagina associated with maternal use of diethylstilbestrol (DES) (80), vaginal carcinoma is primarily a disease of women over 50, with an age incidence distribution nearly identical to that of vulvar carcinoma. Like cervical neoplasms, vulvar and vaginal carcinomas may be preceded at an earlier age by an *in situ* phase, but the natural history of these lesions is debated. Vulvar and vaginal cancers frequently occur in the same patient and in association with epithelial neoplasms of other anogenital sites, including the cervix, the anus, and even the urethra and bladder (81–84).

From the standpoint of developing a framework for pathogenesis, the "cloacal field theory" of a common origin of anogenital neoplasms is appealing. Thus risk factors known to exist for cervical neoplasms have also been shown to be pertinent for vulvar and vaginal neoplasms, especially the sexually transmitted diseases, herpes (85) and condylomata (86). Another possibly pertinent risk factor for vulvar neoplasms is smoking (87). Further study of dietary factors, especially the carotenoids, would be worthwhile.

191

Gestational Trophoblastic Neoplasia

Neoplasms of the trophoblast include complete and partial hydatidiform moles, invasive moles, and choriocarcinoma. The epidemiology of hydatidiform mole is probably better understood than that of other trophoblastic diseases, but it is likely to be relevant because of the association between molar pregnancy and subsequent invasive mole or choriocarcinoma. The prevalence of molar pregnancy varies from less than 1 per 100 deliveries in Asia, Indonesia, and other third world countries to 1 per 1000–1500 in the United States (88). Clearly, the risk of having a molar pregnancy increases with maternal age (89, 90), but it is less certain that adolescents are also at increased risk (91). Possible obstetric risk factors include miscarriage (92) and prior or subsequent twin pregnancies (93). The peculiar cytogenetic patterns of complete and partial hydatidiform moles are discussed in Chapter 13 and may indicate the importance of aberrant germ cells in the origin of these disorders.

Berkowitz et al. (94) suggested that deficiency of the vitamin A precursor, carotene, or of animal fats necessary for its absorption might be a factor in the cause of this disease. Vitamin A deficiency causes fetal wastage and aberrances of epithelial development in female animals and degeneration of seminiferous epithelium with poor gamete development in male animals (95–97). In addition, regions where molar pregnancy is common have a high incidence of night blindness (98).

CANCER PREVENTION AND SCREENING

Primary Prevention

The prevention of cancer is of utmost importance. Methods of primary prevention (i.e., identifying and eliminating the causes of cancer) are by no means certain, but some possible avenues are discussed:

1. *For cervical cancer,* avoidance of tobacco, use of barrier methods of contraception in early sexual life, and a diet high in folates, beta-carotene, and vitamin C would likely be beneficial.

2. *For endometrial cancer,* maintenance of ideal body weight, avoidance of a high-fat diet, and avoidance of unopposed estrogen therapy during menopause would likely be beneficial.

3. *For ovarian cancer,* use of oral contraceptives if not medically contraindicated may be beneficial.

Although controversial, reducing the amount of galactose in the diet and avoidance of talc in genital hygiene may be helpful. Women with more than one primary relative with ovarian cancer should consider prophylactic oophorectomy after they have completed childbearing.

Secondary Prevention

By screening, the clinician may also prevent cancer deaths by detecting cancer at a stage when it is more curable. The secondary prevention of cervical cancer has been successful, and screening programs for the other gynecologic cancers eventually may be devised. Therefore, the clinician should understand some principles of screening.

To be successful, a screening program must be directed at a "suitable" disease with a "suitable" screening test (99). A suitable disease must be one that has serious consequences, as most cancers do. Treatment must be available so that when such therapy is applied to screen-detected (preclinical) disease, it will be more effective than when applied after symptoms of the disease have appeared. Also, the preclinical phase of the disease must be long enough that the chances are good that a person will be screened. There must also be a suitable screening test that implies simplicity, acceptability to patients, low cost, and high validity, as defined in Table 5.4.

Sensitivity	**The sensitivity of a test is defined as the proportion of persons with a true positive result out of all those who have the disease.**
Specificity	**The specificity of a test is defined as the proportion of persons with a true negative result out of all those who do not have the disease.**
Predictive Value	**The predictive value of a positive test is a function of sensitivity, specificity, and disease prevalence.** This function implies that a positive screening test is more likely to indicate disease in a high-risk population than in a low-risk population (Table 5.4).
Screening Strategy	For cervical cancer, the 1982 Canadian Task Force report (100) suggested that as women accumulated a history of negative annual Pap smears, the interval may be safely lengthened to 3 years. In 1988 the American College of Obstetricians and Gynecologists issued a consensus report with the American College of Surgeons and the United States National Cancer Institute (101), which recommended annual Pap smears for sexually active women until three normal smears had been obtained. However, annual physical examinations, including breast examinations, were recommended for all women, once they became sexually active. While some

Table 5.4   Measures of Validity for a Screening Procedure

Status Determined by Screening	True Disease Status		
	Positive	*Negative*	*Total*
Positive	a (true positives)	b (false-positives)	a + b (all screened positive)
Negative	c (false-negatives)	d (true negatives)	c + d (all screened negative)
Total	a + c (all diseased)	b + d (all nondiseased)	N (all subjects)

Measure	Definition	Formula
Sensitivity	True positives / All diseased	$\dfrac{a}{a + c}$
Specificity	True negatives / All nondiseased	$\dfrac{d}{b + d}$
Predictive value of a positive screen	True positives / All screened positive	$\dfrac{a}{a + b}$

discretion is permitted in low-risk patients, such as those that are monogamous, the risk of cervical cancer relates to the sexual behavior of both sexual partners. Therefore, to be at low risk, the female must not only be monogamous; she must also have a monogamous partner. A full discussion of these recommendations is presented in Chapter 6.

Endometrial biopsies in perimenopausal women are appropriate for those at risk of endometrial cancer (obesity, nulliparity, estrogen use). At present, no effective screening strategy exists for ovarian cancer.

References

1. **Ries LAG, Hankey BF, Miller BA, et al:** *Cancer Statistics Review* 1973–1988. National Cancer Institute. NIH Pub. No. 91:2789, 1991.

2. **Muir C, Waterhouse J, Mack T, et al:** *Cancer Incidence in Five Continents*, vol 5, International Agency for Research on Cancer, 1987.

3. **Sondik EJ, Young JL, Horm JW, Gloeckler LA:** *Annual Cancer Statistics Review.* NIH Publication 86–2789, 1985.

4. **Rothman KJ:** *Modern Epidemiology.* Boston, Little Brown, & Co, 1986.

5. **Mantel N, Haenszel W:** Statistical aspects of the analyses of data from retrospective studies of disease. *J Natl Cancer Inst* 22:719, 1959.

6. **Breslow NE, Day NE:** *Statistical Methods in Cancer Research*, vol 1. International Agency for Research on Cancer, 1980.

7. **Armitage P:** *Statistical Methods in Medical Research*, New York, John Wiley & Sons, 1977.

8. **Cramer DW, Knapp RC:** Review of epidemiologic studies of endometrial cancer and exogenous estrogen. *Obstet Gynecol* 54:521, 1979.

9. **Smith DC, Prentice R, Thompson DJ, Herrmann WL:** Association of exogenous estrogens and endometrial carcinoma. *N Engl J Med* 293:1164, 1975.

10. **Ziel HK, Finkle WD:** Increased risk of endometrial carcinoma among users of conjugated estrogens. *N Engl J Med* 293:1167, 1975.

11. **Mack TM, Pike MC, Henderson BE, et al:** Estrogens and endometrial cancer in a retirement community. *N Engl J Med* 294:1262, 1976.

12. **Shapiro S, Kaufman DW, Slone D, et al:** Recent and past use of conjugated estrogens in relation to adenocarcinoma of the endometrium. *N Engl J Med* 303:485, 1980.

13. **Whitehead MI, Townsend PT, Pryse-Davies J, et al:** Effects of estrogens and progestins on the biochemistry and morphology of the postmenopausal endometrium. *N Engl J Med* 305:1599, 1980.

14. **Salerno W:** Feminizing mesenchymomas of the ovary: an analysis of 28 granulosa-theca cell tumors and their relationship to co-existent carcinoma. *Am J Obstet Gyncecol* 84:731, 1962.

15. **Spert H:** Endometrial cancer and hepatic cirrhosis. *Cancer* 2:597, 1949.

16. **MacDonald PC, Siiteri PK:** The relationship between the extraglandular production of estrone and the occurrence of endometrial neoplasia. *Gynecol Oncol* 2:259, 1974.

17. **Wynder EL, Escher GC, Mantel N:** An epidemiological investigation of cancer of the endometrium. *Cancer* 19:489, 1966.

18. **Gambrell RD Jr:** Prevention of endometrial cancer with progestogens. *Maturitas* 8:159, 1986.

19. **Terris M, Wilson F, Smith H, et al:** The epidemiology of cancer of the cervix. V. The relationship of coitus to carcinoma of the cervix. *Am J Public Health* 57:840, 1967.

20. **Martin CE:** The epidemiology of cancer of the cervix. II. Marital and coital factors in cervical cancer. *Am J Public Health* 57:815, 1967.

21. **Rotkin ID:** The epidemiology of cancer of the cervix. III. Sexual characteristics of a cervical cancer population. *Am J Public Health* 57:815, 1967.

22. **Skegg DCG, Corwin PA, Paul C:** Importance of the male factor in cancer of the cervix. *Lancet* 2:581, 1982.

23. **Herrero R, Brinton LA, Reeves WC, et al:** Sexual behavior, venereal diseases, hygiene practices, and invasive cervical cancer in a high risk population. *Cancer* 65:380, 1990.

24. **Singer A:** The cervical epithelium during puberty and adolescence. In Jordan JA, Singer A (eds): *The Cervix,* London, WB Saunders, 1976.

25. **Kessler I:** Human cervical cancer as a venereal disease. *Cancer Res* 36:783, 1976.

26. **Campton MJ, Singer A, Clarkson PK, McCance DJ:** Increased risk of cervical neoplasia in consorts of men with penile condylomata acuminata. *Lancet* 1:943, 1985.

27. **Patten SF, Hughes CP, Reagan JW:** An experimental study of the relationship between trichomonas vaginalis and dysplasia in the uterine cervix. *Acta Cytol (Baltimore)* 7:187, 1963.

28. **Melnick JL, Lewis R, Wimberly I, et al:** Association of cytomegalovirus (CMV) infection with cervical cancer: isolation of CMV from cell cultures derived from cervical biopsies. *Intervirology* 10:115, 1978.

29. **Aurelian L, Manak MM, McKinlay M, et al:** "The herpes hypotheses"—are Koch's postulates satisfied. *Gynecol Oncol* 12:556, 1981.

30. **Kurman RJ, Jenson AB, Lancaster WD:** Papillomavirus infections of the cervix, II. Relationship to intraepithelial neoplasia based on the presence of specific viral structural proteins. *Am J Surg Pathol* 7:39, 1983.

31. **Reeves WC, Brinton LA, Garcia M, et al:** Human papillomavirus infection and cervical cancer in Latin America. *N Engl J Med* 320:1437, 1989.

32. **zur Hausen H:** Human genital cancer: synergism between two virus infections or synergism between a virus infection and initiating events? *Lancet* 2:1 370, 1982.

33. **Hildesheim A, Mann V, Brinton LA, et al:** Herpes simplex virus type 2: a possible interaction with human papillomavirus types 16/18 in the development of invasive cervical cancer. *Int J Cancer* 49:335, 1991.

34. **Hildesheim A, Brinton LA, Mallin K, et al:** Barrier and spermicidal contraceptive methods and risk of invasive cervical cancer. *Epidemiology* 1:266, 1990.

35. **Smith FR:** Etiologic factors in carcinoma of the cervix. *Am J Obstet Gynecol* 21:18, 1931.

36. **Brinton LA, Schairer C, Haenszel W, et al:** Cigarette smoking and invasive cervical cancer. *JAMA* 255:3265, 1986.

37. **Schiffman MH, Haley NJ, Felton JS, et al:** Biochemical epidemiology of cervical neoplasia: measuring cigarette smoke constituents in the cervix. *Cancer Res* 47:3886, 1987.

38. **Miller AB, Lindsay J, Hill GB:** Mortality from cancer of the uterus in Canada and its relationship screening for cancer of the cervix. *Int J Cancer* 17:602, 1976.

39. **La Vecchia C, Decarli A, Gentile A, et al:** Pap smear and the risk of cervical neoplasia: quantitative estimates from a case control study. *Lancet* 11:779, 1984.

40. **Negrini BP, Schiffman MH, Kurman RJ, et al:** Oral contraceptive use, human papillomavirus infection, and risk of early cytological abnormalities of the cervix. *Cancer Res* 50:4670, 1990.

41. **Vessey MP, McPherson K, Lawlers M, Yeates D:** Neoplasia of the cervix uteri and contraception: a possible adverse effect of the pill. *Lancet* 2:930, 1983.

42. **Brinton LA, Tashima KT, Lehman HF, et al:** Epidemiology of cervical cancer by cell type. *Cancer Res* 47:1706, 1987.

43. **Butterworth CE, Hatch KD, Gore H, et al:** Improvement in cervical dysplasia associated with folic acid therapy in users of oral contraceptives. *Am J Clin Nutr* 39:73, 1982.

44. **Herrero R, Potischman N, Brinton LA, et al:** A case-control study of nutrient status and invasive cervical cancer. I. Dietary indicators. *Am J Epidemiol* 134:1335, 1991.

45. **Potischman N, Herrero R, Brinton LA, et al:** A case-control study of nutrient status and invasive cervical cancer. II. Serologic indicators. *Am J Epidemiol* 134:1347, 1991.

46. **Jansen D, Ostergaard E:** Clinical studies concerning the relationship of estrogens to the development of cancer of the corpus uteri. *Am J Obstet Gynecol* 67:1094, 1954.

47. **Frisch RE, Wyshak G, Albright NL, et al:** Lower prevalence of breast cancer and cancers of the reproductive system among former college athletes compared to non-athletes. *Br J Cancer* 52:885, 1985.

48. **Lesko MS, Rosenberg L, Kaufman DW, et al:** Cigarette smoking and the risk of endometrial cancer. *N Engl J Med* 313:593, 1985.

49. **Silverberg SG, Makowski EL:** Endometrial carcinoma in young women taking oral contraceptive agents. *Obstet Gynecol* 45:503, 1975.

50. **Weiss NS, Sayvet TA:** Incidence of endometrial cancer in relation to the use of oral contraceptives. *N Engl J Med* 302:551, 1980.

51. **Fathalla MF:** Incessant ovulation—a factor in ovarian neoplasia? *Lancet* 71:717, 1983.

52. **Cramer DW, Welch WR, Hutchison GB, et al:** Determinants of ovarian cancer risk. I. Reproductive experiences and family history. *J Natl Cancer Inst* 71:711, 1983.

52. **Centers for Disease Control Cancer and Steroid Hormone Study:** Oral contraceptives and the risk of ovarian cancer. *JAMA* 249:1596, 1983.

54. **Parmley TH, Woodruff JD:** The ovarian mesothelioma. *Am J Obstet Gynecol* 120:234, 1974.

55. **Graham J, Graham R:** Ovarian cancer and asbestos. *Environ Res* 1:115, 1967.

56. **Hamilton TC, Fox H, Buckley CH, et al:** Effects of talc on the rat ovary. *Br J Exp Pathol* 65:101, 1984.

57. **Longo DL, Young RC:** Cosmetic talc and ovarian cancer. *Lancet* 2:349, 1979.

58. **Cramer DW, Welch WR, Scully RE, Wojciechowski CA:** Ovarian cancer and talc: a case control study. *Cancer* 50:372, 1982.

59. **Harlow BL, Cramer DW, Bell DA, Welch WR:** Perineal exposure to talc and ovarian cancer risk. *Obstet Gynecol* 80:19, 1992.

60. **Gardner WU:** Hormonal imbalances to tumorigenesis. *Cancer Res* 8:397, 1948.

61. **Murphy ED, Russell ES:** Ovarian tumorigenesis following genic deletion of germ cells in hybrid mice. *Acta Un Int Cancer* 19:779, 1963.

62. **Furth J, Butterworth JS:** Neoplastic diseases occurring among mice subjected to general irradiation with x-rays. *Am J Cancer* 28:66, 1936.

63. **Howell JS, Marchant J, Orr JW:** The induction of ovarian tumors in mice with 9-10 dimethyl 1:2-benzanthracene. *Br J Cancer* 8:635, 1954.

64. **Marchant J:** The effect of hypophysectomy on the development of ovarian tumours in mice treated with demethylbenzanthracene. *Br J Cancer* 15:821, 1961.

65. **Tennent BJ, Beamer WG:** Ovarian tumors not induced by irradiation and gonadotropins in hypogonadal (hpg) mice. *Biol Reprod* 34:751, 1986.

66. **Radisavljevic SV:** The pathogenesis of ovarian inclusion cysts and cystomas. *Obstet Gynecol* 49:424, 1977.

67. **Cunha GR, Bigsby RM, Cooke PS, Sugimura Y:** Stromal-epithelial interaction in adult organs. *Cell Differ* 17:137, 1985.

68. **Boice JD, Day NE, Andersen A, et al:** Second cancers following radiation treatment for cervical cancer: an international collaboration among cancer registries. *J Natl Cancer Inst* 74:955, 1985.

69. **Darby SC, Nakashima E, Kato H:** A parallel analysis of cancer mortality among atomic bomb survivors and patients with ankylosing spondylitis given X-ray therapy. *Radiation Effects Research Foundation*, Technical Report 4-84, Hiroshima.

70. **Doll R, Gray R, Hafner B, et al:** Mortality in relation to smoking: 22 years observation on female British doctors. *Br Med J* 1:967, 1980.

71. **LaVecchia C, Francheschi S, Decarli A, et al:** Coffee drinking and the risk of epithelial ovarian cancer. *Int J Cancer* 33:559, 1984.

72. **Peaslee MH, Einhellig FA:** Reduced fecundity in mice on tannic acid diet. *Comp Gen Pharmac* 4:393, 1973.

73. **Cramer DW, Welch WR, Cassells S, Scully RE:** Mumps, menarche, menopause, and ovarian cancer. *Am J Obstet Gynecol* 147:1, 1983.

74. **Chen VT, Mattison DR, Feigenbaum L, et al:** Reduction in oocyte number following prenatal exposure to a diet high in galactose. *Science* 214:1145, 1981.

75. **Swartz WJ, Mattison DR:** Galactose inhibition of ovulation in mice. *Fertil Steril* 49:522; 1988.

76. **Cramer DW:** Lactase persistence and milk consumption as determinants of ovarian cancer risk. *Am J Epidemiol* 130:904, 1989.

77. **Cramer DW, Harlow BL, Willett WC, et al:** Galactose consumption and metabolism in relation to the risk of ovarian cancer. *Lancet* 2:66, 1989.

78. **Kaufman FR, Kogut MD, Donnell GN, et al:** Hypergonadotropic hypogonadism in female patients with galactosemia. *N Engl J Med* 304:994, 1981.

79. **Atlas M, Menczer J:** Massive hyperstimulation and borderline carcinoma of the ovary. *Acta Obstet Gynecol Scand* 61:261, 1982.

80. **Herbst AL, Kwiman RJ, Scully RE, Poskanzer DC:** Clear cell adenocarcinoma of the genital tract in young females. *N Engl J Med* 287:1259, 1972.

81. **Newman W, Cromer JK:** The multicentric origin of carcinomas of the female anogenital tract. *Surg Gynecol Obstet* 108:272, 1959.

82. **Marcus SL:** Multiple squamous carcinomas involving the cervix, vagina, and vulva: the theory of multicentric origin. *Am J Obstet Gynecol* 80:802, 1960.

83. **Stern BD, Kaplan L:** Multicentric foci of carcinomas arising in structures of cloacal origin. *Am J Obstet Gynecol* 104:255, 1969.

84. **Jones RW, McLean MR:** Carcinoma in situ of the vulva: a review of 31 treated and 5 untreated cases. *Obstet Gynecol* 68:499, 1986.

85. **Kaufman RH, Dreesman GR, Burek J, et al:** Herpes virus-induced antigens in squamous cell carcinoma in situ of the vulva. *N Engl J Med* 305:483, 1981.

86. **Crum CP, Fu YS, Levine RU, et al:** Intraepithelial squamous lesions of the vulva: biologic and histologic criteria for the distinction of condylomas from vulvar intraepithelial neoplasia. *Am J Obstet Gynecol* 144:77, 1982.

87. **Newcomb PA, Weiss NS, Daling JR:** Incidence of vulvar carcinoma in relation to menstrual, reproductive, and medical factors. *J Natl Cancer Inst* 73:391, 1984.

88. **Bagshawe KD, Lawler SD:** Choriocarcinoma. In: Schottenfeld DF, Frauemini JF (eds). *Cancer Epidemiology and Prevention*. Philadelphia, WB Saunders, 1982, pp 909–924.

89. **Stone M, Bagshawe KD:** An analysis of the influence of maternal age, gestational age, contraceptive method, and the primary mode of treatment of patients with hydatidiform mole and the incidence of subsequent chemotherapy. *Br J Obstet Gynaecol* 86:782, 1979.

90. **Hayashi H, Bracken MB, Freeman DH, et al:** Hydatidiform mole in the United States (1970–1977): a statistical and theoretical analysis. *Am J Epidemiol* 115:1238, 1982.

91. **Jacobs PA, Hunt PA, Matsuura J, et al:** Complete and partial hydatidiform mole in Hawaii: cytogenetics, morphology and epidemiology. *Br J Obstet Gynaecol* 89:258, 1982.

92. **Insler V, Meizner I, Kahane A, et al:** Long term follow-up in 109 women with gestational trophoblastic disease. *Excerpta Med Int Cong Sci* 551:405, 1981.

93. **DeGeorge FV:** Hydatidiform moles in other pregnancies of mothers of twins. *Am J Obstet Gynecol* 108:369, 1970.

197

94. **Berkowitz RS, Cramer DW, Bernstein MR, et al:** Risk factors for complete molar pregnancy from a case-control study. *Am J Obstet Gynecol* 152:1016, 1985.

95. **O'Toole BA, Fradkin R, Warkay J, et al:** Vitamin A deficiency and reproduction in rhesus monkeys. *J Nutr* 104:1513, 1974.

96. **Evans HM, Lepkovsky S, Murphy EA:** Vital need of the body for certain unsaturated fatty acids. VI. Male sterility on fat-free diets. *J Biol Chem* 106:445, 1934.

97. **Kim HL, Picciano MF, O'Brien W:** Influence of maternal dietary protein and fat levels on fetal growth in mice. *Growth* 45:8, 1981.

98. **McLaren DS:** Present knowledge of the role of vitamin A in health and disease. *Trans Roy Soc Trop Med Hyg* 60:436, 1966.

99. **Cole P, Morrison A:** Basic issues in population screening for cancer. *J Natl Cancer Inst* 64:1263, 1980.

100. **Canadian Task Force on Screening:** Cervical Cancer Screening Programs: Summary of the 1982 Canadian Task Force Report. *Can Med Assoc J* 127:581, 1982.

101. **Pearse WH:** Consensus report on frequency of Pap smear testing, American College of Obstetricians and Gynecologists, *Newsletter* 32:3, 1988.

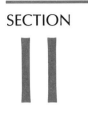
PRIMARY
DISEASE
SITES

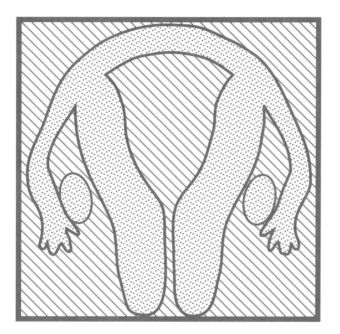

6

Preinvasive Disease

Richard Reid

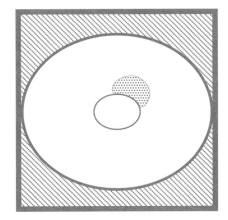

Cervix

Origins of Cervical Cancer

Although cancer can arise at any site within the lower genital tract, the metaplastic epithelium at the *squamocolumnar junction* has the greatest propensity for malignant transformation. Even in women who develop multifocal anogenital malignancies, the disease generally arises within the *transformation zone* (1, 2).

Epidemiologic studies over more than a century have shown that genital neoplasia is initiated by sexually transmitted carcinogens (3). Two decades of intense study have not uncovered any convincing evidence of a causal link between herpes and genital cancer (4). In contrast, over the last 5 years there has been a rapid accumulation of epidemiologic, virologic, and clinical evidence implicating the human papillomavirus as a major factor in the etiology of cervical (5–8), vulvar (8–9), and penile (10) neoplasia. The pathogenesis of cervical neoplasia can be viewed as the interaction of "seed and soil," the "seed" being the papillomavirus and the "soil" being metaplastic epithelium.

Transformation Zone

The upper and middle thirds of the cervical canal are lined with columnar epithelium, continuous with the endometrium proximally. The peripheral portion of the ectocervix is covered with squamous epithelium, continuous with the vulvar skin caudally. The boundary between this ectodermal squamous epithelium and the mucin-secreting columnar epithelium of the upper müllerian tract persists into adult life as a field of *squamous metaplasia* (11, 12). Colposcopic examination shows that this field of metaplasia (called the transformation zone) is a doughnut-shaped area with a radius of about 1–3 cm.

Epithelial Boundaries

There are six epithelial boundaries (Fig. 6.1) within the lower genital tract, which are discernible from about the 24th week of fetal development and persist throughout adult life (2).

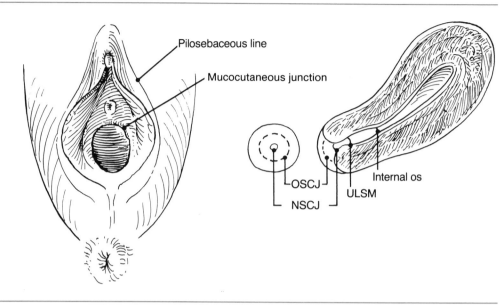

Figure 6.1   The six epithelial boundaries within the lower genital tract.

Pilosebaceous Line   The external vulva reveals a demarcation between the hair-bearing skin of the labium majus and the keratinized nonhairy skin of the interlabial sulcus and labium minus.

Mucocutaneous Junction   Painting the introitus with Lugol's iodine will reveal a sharp line that represents the junction between the glycogenated vaginal epithelium and the keratinized skin of the vulva. Epithelium on the proximal side stains mahogany brown, whereas distal epithelium has a slight yellowish discoloration.

Original Squamocolumnar Junction   The fetal junction between the glycogenated squamous epithelium of the vagina and the mucin-producing columnar epithelium of the endocervix is variable, lying within the cervical canal in 30%, on the cervical portio in 66%, and on the vaginal fornices in 4% of subjects (1).

New Squamocolumnar Junction   The original linear junction between squamous and columnar epithelium is replaced by a broad zone of metaplasia, in which there will be foci of epithelium at differing stages of maturation. The colposcopic demarcation between the squamous-appearing epithelium and the red, villus tissue is usually a junction between mature and immature squamous metaplasia (13). In women who have not undergone previous therapy, this junction denotes the upper extent of any histologically definable dysplasia (14), but it does not define the upper limit of squamous metaplasia. Thus the new squamocolumnar junction (SCJ) is the upper limit of squamous intraepithelial neoplasia but the lower limit of any adenocarcinoma *in situ*. When a cryosurgical or laser ablation of the transformation zone is performed, the oncogen-exposed squamous metaplasia within the distal third of the cervical canal must also be included within the area of destruction (8, 15).

Upper Limit of Squamous Metaplasia   In patients with satisfactory colposcopic examination findings, squamous metaplasia generally extends up the canal about 10–12 mm above the external os.

Histologic Internal Os   The mucin-secreting columnar epithelium of the endocervical canal merges with the cuboidal cells of the endometrium at a line termed the histologic internal os.

Dynamic Events in the Metaplastic Process

The exposure of an epithelium lined with a single layer of mucin-producing cells to an acidic environment (pH about 4–5) results in chemical denaturation of the columnar epithelium at the villus tips (1), which initiates a reparative process from which mature squamous epithelium eventually will develop. Metaplasia begins with the proliferation of activated reserve cells and culminates with the development of a mature squamous epithelium (16). This process can be simplified into two fundamental events:

1. The obliteration of the original columnar cells by the proliferation of activated squamous reserve cells.

2. The eventual maturation of this immature metaplastic epithelium into a mature squamous epithelium.

The presence of white blood cells in biopsy specimens of immature squamous metaplasia may lead pathologists to misinterpret the tissue as showing "chronic cervicitis." However, inflammatory cells are present as part of the metaplastic process and in no way denote a response to any infectious agent. *Chronic cervicitis* is a misleading term for immature squamous metaplasia and should never be accepted as a satisfactory explanation for a suspected abnormality.

Squamous metaplasia is encouraged by acidity and retarded by the buffering action of alkaline cervical mucus. The conversion of columnar to squamous epithelium is permanent, the trend with time being toward replacement of columnar epithelium with immature metaplasia and subsequent maturation to form a glycogenated epithelium. However, the process is not a continuous one. Rather, it usually occurs in "spurts," with the greatest activity occurring during fetal life, at adolescence, and during the first pregnancy.

Human Papillomavirus

Human papillomaviruses (HPVs) are site-specific DNA viruses that produce characteristic proliferations on epidermal and mucosal surfaces (17–19). Papillomavirus infection of the genital tract is common among sexually active women. Because clinically detectable condylomata acuminata are seldom seen on the cervix, it was thought that HPV infections were limited to the vulva, anus, and lower vagina. However, cervical HPV infections have been overlooked in the past because the lesions are usually macroscopically flat and invisible without the aid of acetic acid (20).

Several laboratories have established that more than 90% of cervical condylomas, all grades of cervical intraepithelial neoplasia (CIN), and invasive cancers contain HPV DNA. The association is strong (5, 6, 21–26) and type-specific, different HPV types having significantly different pathologic associations. Papillomavirus types 6, 11, 42, 43, and 44 are seldom found in *bona fide* neoplasms, whereas types 16, 18, 31, 33, 35, 45, 51, 52, 56, and 58 are most commonly seen in cancers and definite premalignancies (5). The progressive potential of precursor lesions is largely defined by the HPV type (27).

Transfection with oncogenic HPV DNAs can immortalize human keratinocytes in cell culture, and further growth of these immortalized cells on collagen rafts or in nude mice can produce histologic patterns essentially identical to CIN 3 (28, 29). **Therefore there is now substantial evidence to suggest that most intraepithelial neoplasia is initiated by oncogenic HPV infection.** Also, there have been reports of HPV-immortalized cells acquiring invasive properties simply by continued growth *in vitro* for 2–4 years (30–32). The HPV genome is consistently transcribed (33). Invasive cancer cells show increased levels of E6 and E7 viral transforming gene expression, but no detectable late gene expression. The E6 and E7 proteins encoded by the oncogenic HPV types antagonize the host tumor suppressor proteins, p53 and pRB, thereby deregulating cell growth (34). Integration of HPV genetic sequences into the host genome usually occurs just as the cell develops invasive properties (26). **In spite of these *in vitro* observations, the role of HPV in promoting progression of precursor lesions to invasive cancer remains uncertain. Chronic latent infections in otherwise healthy persons and low rates of progression of untreated high-grade intraepithelial lesions indicate that other important factors also must be operative.**

Pap Smear Screening

The Papanicolaou smear has been a most effective cancer-screening technique, resulting in a significant reduction in mortality from cervical cancer in screened populations (35–39). In an effort to further standardize the reporting of cervical cytology, the Bethesda System was introduced recently in the United States (40, 41). This system has been devised to supplant the Papanicolaou classification and is presented in Table 6.1. **The Bethesda System introduced the cytologic terms "low-grade" and "high-grade" squamous intraepithelial lesions (LSIL and HSIL). LSILs include condylomata and CIN 1, and HSILs include CIN 2 and 3. The new cytologic classification is not meant to replace the histologic terms "dysplasia" and "CIN."**

The optimal interval for cancer screening with the Pap smear is controversial. Annual screening data from British Columbia in the 1960s highlighted a sharp decrease in the prevalence of abnormal cytology in the screened population (36). Prevalence fell from 5.5/1000 first examinations to 0.7/1000 among women with two negative smears. This led the Canadian task force to conclude that tailoring the frequency of examination to the average risk (as determined by individual sexual behavior) would use health resources most efficiently (37). Subsequently, the American Cancer Society (39) issued similar advice, including the suggestion that "low-risk" women need smears only every 3 years. However, the majority of women would fit the American Cancer Society's definition of "high risk" (meaning any woman who began coitus before the age of 20 or anyone who has had more than two sexual partners during her lifetime). Moreover, categorization of a woman as being at "low risk" or "high risk" of a sexually transmitted disease without reference to the sexual behavior of her male partners is unrealistic.

In a recent Australian study of the Pap smear history of 237 patients with invasive cervical cancer, 35% of the patients reported never having had a Pap smear, and a further 19.4% had not had a smear for at least 4 years (42). Fifty-one patients (21.5%) reported having had a normal smear within the last 2 years. Closer analysis of these 51 patients revealed that the two most important causes of a history of a normal smear within 2 years of invasive cancer were poor patient recall of the date of the last smear and false-negative smear reporting.

Table 6.1   Comparison of Cytology Classification Systems

Bethesda System	Dysplasia/CIN System		Papanicolaou System
Within normal limits	Normal		I
Infection (organism should be specified)	Inflammatory atypia (organism)		II
Reactive and reparative changes			
Squamous cell abnormalities			
Atypical squamous cells of undetermined significance	Squamous atypia		IIR
Low-grade squamous intraepithelial lesion (LSIL)	HPV atypia		
	Mild dysplasia	CIN 1	
High-grade squamous intraepithelial lesion (HSIL)	Moderate dysplasia	CIN 2	III
	Severe dysplasia	CIN 3	
	Carcinoma in situ		IV
Squamous cell carcinoma	Squamous cell carcinoma		V

CIN = cervical intraepithelial neoplasia.

False-negative rates for cervical cytology have been 20–30% for squamous lesions and as high as 40% for adenocarcinomas (43). In the presence of invasive cancer, ulceration and infection are commonly present, and false-negative rates may be as high as 50%.

The current recommendation of the American College of Obstetricians and Gynecologists (44) is that "all women who are or have been sexually active or who have reached the age of 18 years should have an annual Pap test and pelvic examination. After a woman has had three or more satisfactory normal annual examinations, the Pap test may be performed at the discretion of her physician." The American College still recommends "an annual physical and pelvic examination and an annual Pap smear in the high-risk patient or when in doubt." Furthermore, the use of an annual Pap smear encourages other preventive health measures, such as a blood pressure measurement and a breast examination.

Triage of an Abnormal Papanicolaou Smear

Squamous metaplasia, benign HPV infections, and the various grades of cervical intraepithelial neoplasia all manifest colposcopically as acetowhite epithelium, with or without abnormal capillary patterns. Confusion between acetowhite areas of pathologic epithelium and acetowhite areas of immature squamous metaplasia can be minimized by not using the colposcope as a screening device (36). However, differentiation between warty proliferation and dysplasia can be a difficult problem.

There appear to be different mechanisms of acetowhitening for lesions of different severity. Acetowhite lesions associated with severe dysplasia (Fig. 6.2) probably occur because osmotic dehydration accentuates the high content of optically dense chromatin, whereas those of mild lesions are probably attributable to a transient reaction between acetic acid and abnormal envelope proteins in papillomavirus-infected keratinocytes (Fig. 6.3). Acetowhitening of middle-grade lesions appears to reflect a combination of both events (45). A skilled colposcopist usually can differentiate mild from severe dysplasia (46, 47). However, such distinction de-

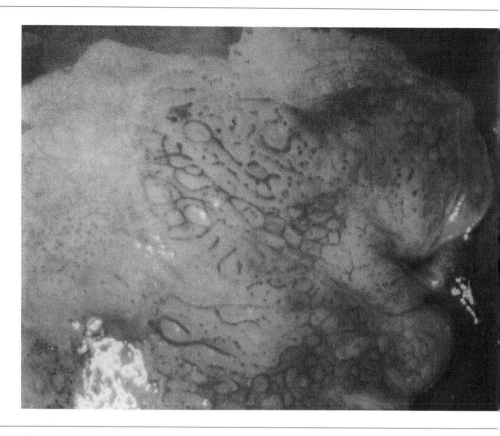

Figure 6.2 CIN 3, showing a straight peripheral margin, a dull white color, and coarse mosaicism.

pends on the use of objective colposcopic criteria. Grading based on the "degree of whiteness" or the "prominence" of any vascular atypia has not been reliable.

Colposcopic Index for Improved Accuracy

Colposcopic Criteria

Predictive accuracy depends on the use of exact colposcopic criteria. Four such criteria should be employed:

1. The sharpness of the peripheral margin

2. The color of acetowhitening

3. The type of vascular patterns

4. The iodine staining reaction

These criteria have been developed and tested by prospective computerized analyses (46, 47). The value of these individual colposcopic signs can be maximized by combining them into a weighted scoring system. Scores of 0, 1, or 2 are assigned for each criterion as described in Table 6.2.

1. Scores of 0 to 2 are predictive of flat condylomas or CIN 1.

2. Scores of 6 to 8 generally denote CIN 2–3.

3. Scores of 3 to 5 represent an area of overlap between low-grade and high-grade intraepithelial neoplasia.

The overall predictive accuracy of the combined colposcopic index is higher than 95%. Furthermore, generating a colposcopic score is simple. A diagram that defines the colposcopic appearance is drawn, points are scored for each of the individual criteria, and then points are added to give the colposcopic index (Table 6.2).

Systematic Method of Colposcopy

The initial clinical workup should be as follows:

1. The colposcopist should perform a complete medical history and a general physical examination.

2. Because squamous neoplasia of the lower genital tract is often multicentric, a careful inspection should be made of the vulva and the anus. If red, white, or discolored patches are seen, vulvar colposcopy and

Figure 6.3 CIN 1, mild dysplasia associated with papillomaviral infection of the cervix, showing a shiny, snow white color and a micropapillary surface contour.

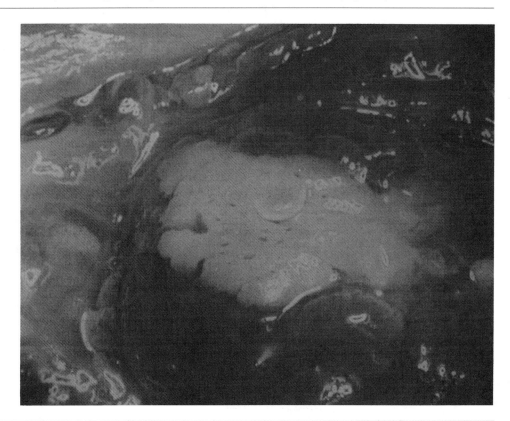

Table 6.2 Scoring System for Deriving the Colposcopic Index

Colposcopic Sign	Score		
	Zero Points	**One Point**	**Two Points**
Margin	Exophytic condylomas; areas showing a micropapillary contour. Lesions with distinct edges. Feathered, scalloped edges. Lesions with an angular, jagged shape. "Satellite" areas and aceto-whitening distal to the original SCJ.	Lesions with a regular (circular or semicircular) shape, show-ing smooth, straight edges.	Rolled, peeling edges. Any internal demarcation be-tween areas of differing col-poscopic appearance.
Color	Shiny, snow-white color. Areas of faint (semitransparent) whitening.	Intermediate shade (Shiny, but gray-white)	Dull reflectance with oyster-white color.
Vessels	Fine-caliber vessels, poorly formed patterns.	No surface vessels.	Definite, coarse punctation or mosaic.
Iodine	Any lesion staining mahogany brown. Mustard yellow stain-ing by a minor lesion (by first 3 criteria).	Partial iodine staining (mottled pattern).	Mustard yellow staining of a significant lesion (an aceto-white area scoring 3 or more points by the first three crite-ria).

directed biopsy are mandatory. However, physicians must not mistake the micropapillae labialis and nonspecific acetowhitening for *bona fide* condylomatous disease.

3. Before the application of acetic acid, speculum examination of the vagina and cervix should be performed with a good light (e.g., through the colposcope), to check on the nature of any vaginal discharge and to look for any preexisting areas of white epithelium.

4. A thorough bimanual and rectal examination should be performed at the completion of the colposcopy, because occasional patients will have negative colposcopic findings but will have a palpable cancer within the endocervix, vaginal walls, lower bowel, or adnexae.

A second cytologic specimen need not be obtained. Scraping with a spatula may precipitate bleeding that will complicate the colposcopic examination.

Locating the Source of the Abnormal Cells

The first objective of the colposcopic examination is to locate the source of the abnormal cells. Many times the cause will be immediately apparent. However if a gross cervical lesion is not seen, adherence to the following plan usually will identify the reason for the abnormal cytology:

1. The cervix is washed with 3% acetic acid. After 60–90 seconds, the cervix and vaginal fornices are inspected with the colposcope.

2. An additional maneuver that may assist in the visualization involves the application of Lugol's iodine. Quarter-strength Lugol's iodine is applied

and all areas are inspected again. High-grade lesions within less mature areas are identified by their mustard yellow staining reaction.

3. The lower vaginal walls should be inspected carefully as the speculum is withdrawn.

4. If an explanation for the abnormal smear is not yet apparent, the possibility of exfoliation from other sites must be considered (e.g., endometrial, ovarian, fallopian tube, or metastatic breast cancer). The possibility of cellular contamination from a vulvar or urinary tract lesion also should be considered.

5. When a HSIL smear is not explained after examination by an experienced colposcopist, the smear itself should be sent for expert review. If the presence of a high-grade cytologic abnormality is confirmed, diagnostic conization is mandatory.

Delineating the Margins of the Lesion

Distal Margin

An occasional patient (especially a DES-exposed patient) has an extension of the transformation zone onto the vaginal fornices or neoplastic transformation of vaginal condylomas. Occasionally, a vaginal lesion will have a higher grade than any abnormality within the metaplastic epithelium. The main safeguard against such an error is the use of Lugol's iodine.

Proximal Margin

Although the new squamocolumnar junction seen at colposcopy does not correspond with the upper limit of squamous metaplasia, visualization of this junction does establish the examination as satisfactory. The new squamocolumnar junction may be at any level from the cervical portio to the internal os.

Endocervical Curettage (ECC)

Experts vary in their opinions as to when ECC should be performed. Some advocate routine ECC to safeguard against missing an occult cancer within the canal (48, 49). With the increasing incidence of adenocarcinoma and adenosquamous carcinoma of the cervix, many of which are associated with CIN lesions, ECC provides a safeguard against missing such lesions (50). Others reserve the ECC for women who have recurrent cytologic atypia after previous therapy (15). When the entire new SCJ can be visualized in previously untreated patients and there is a concentric ring of unaltered columnar epithelium within the lower canal, it seems reasonable to omit a routine ECC. Moreover, even when collection of an endocervical sample is specifically indicated, taking a canal smear with a cytobrush offers an easy, painless alternative of comparable accuracy (51).

Triage Strategies

Experience from the mid-1960s showed that colposcopically directed punch biopsies could provide a histologic diagnosis with the same accuracy as a cervical cone biopsy. Therefore a group of "triage rules" were formulated (Table 6.3) as a basis for ablative therapy in satisfactory cases (52). Now that cervical excision biopsies can be easily performed in an office setting, some have advocated a "see

---

Table 6.3 Indications for Cervical Conization

1. Inability to visualize the new squamocolumnar junction.

2. CIN 2–3 on ECC.

3. Colposcopic suspicion of occult invasion, even if target biopsies show only CIN 3.

4. Significant discrepancy (2 grades) between the cytology and the histology.

5. Cytologic suspicion of adenocarcinoma *in situ*.

6. Microinvasion on the punch biopsy.

---

and treat" protocol with the loop electrosurgical excision procedure (LEEP) (53, 54). The rationale for immediate LEEP excision of the transformation zone at the first visit can be both diagnostic and therapeutic. The weakness of this strategy is that the indication for surgery is now based on an abnormal Papanicolaou smear, rather than on a careful diagnostic evaluation. In specific settings (e.g., in clinics for indigent women), benefits outweigh disadvantages. However, within a typical private practice setting, where less-experienced colposcopists are evaluating mainly low-grade abnormalities in young and compliant women, the "see and treat" philosophy will lead to substantial overtreatment, as well as additional morbidity and cost.

Colposcopically Directed Biopsies

The most prominent areas of colposcopic change do not necessarily coincide with the areas of greatest histologic abnormality. Therefore there is a risk of not selecting the most abnormal sites for target biopsy (27, 47). Specifically peripheral areas of prominent acetowhite lesions are often overinterpreted, whereas the subtle acetowhite areas of CIN 2–3 near the canal are easily overlooked.

The method of ensuring the accuracy of target biopsy is to grade the lesion by using the four criteria outlined to derive a *colposcopic score*. Representative biopsy specimens then should be taken from all significant acetowhite areas to include the most prominent area of epithelial opacity and the most prominent area of vascular atypia. In addition, any area suspected of occult invasion must be sampled carefully. Each biopsy specimen should be submitted as a separate sample.

Recording the Colposcopic Findings

After a colposcopic appraisal, it is important to draw an accurate diagram of the findings to summarize the appearance of the cervix just examined. Biopsy sites should be recorded so that any past or future histology reports can be related to the colposcopic diagram.

Optimal documentation of colposcopic findings includes photographs showing an acetic acid view of the ectocervix, a view through the endocervical speculum, and a view after iodine staining. For physicians who have already purchased a nonphotographic colposcope, purchase of a separate cervicography camera will allow easy photographic documentation (55).

Evolution of Modern Therapy

The relationship between cervical premalignancy and invasive cancer is less direct than initially supposed, because the prevalence of morphologic disorders of cervical epithelium greatly exceeds the eventual incidence of invasive cancer (56–58). Lesions destined to undergo malignant transformation cannot be separated from the rest of the precursor pool by histology (59, 60), and the rate of malignant progression can range from months to decades (61, 62). In the past, carcinoma *in situ* (CIS) was seen as a definite malignancy that was not yet invasive, and a full measure of anticancer therapy (even including radiation) was sanctioned. In the 1950s and 1960s, hysterectomy was the treatment of choice for most patients with CIS (63–69). In contrast, dysplasia was conceived as a nonspecific epithelial alteration that needed no special treatment or follow-up. Cone biopsy initially was regarded as diagnostic rather than therapeutic in order to differentiate CIS from invasive cancer.

It was not until the mid 1960s that it was shown that, by attention to the margins of resection, the protection against eventual invasive cancer afforded by therapeutic conization was comparable to that afforded by hysterectomy (64). Follow-up data have demonstrated that cone biopsy is as effective as hysterectomy in preventing malignant progression of CIS (65, 66). Also, it has been demonstrated that dysplasia and CIS represent different phases of the same disease spectrum (70, 71). Richart (72) popularized the term *cervical intraepithelial neoplasia* (CIN) to emphasize that the entire population of screening disorders should be regarded as a single disease entity.

Experience soon confirmed that colposcopically directed punch biopsies provided an accurate, noninjurious method of obtaining a histologic diagnosis in patients with an abnormal Papanicolaou smear (73). As an extension of the trend to treat CIS by excisional cone biopsy instead of hysterectomy, small localized lesions were managed by physical destruction of the abnormal transformation zone with cryosurgery (74), electrocoagulation diathermy (75), or the carbon dioxide laser (76). The use of these modalities has been found to be safe if a strict protocol is followed.

Evaluation Before Conservative Therapy

Before the initiation of ablative therapy for CIN, invasive cancer must be excluded. This requires careful inspection of the cervix for ulceration or surface irregularities and careful palpation to detect expansion or undue firmness. Colposcopists must be sure of their ability to recognize any areas of occult invasive cancer present within the visible portion of the transformation zone.

Provided that the colposcopic new SCJ is visible, the canal has been adequately assessed, and the histologic findings are compatible with the cytologic diagnosis, the histologic findings from an adequate number of colposcopically directed biopsies can be accepted as the definitive diagnosis. Diagnostic conization should be performed if specifically indicated (Table 6.3).

Treatment is planned according to lesion topography rather than histologic grade. Therapy for CIS is the same as that for CIN 1, with the majority of lesions being treated by transformation zone excision or superficial ablative destruction under colposcopic control.

The protection afforded by transformation zone ablation or conization is comparable to that provided by hysterectomy (77, 78). Any new cancer is likely to arise in the reservoir of HPV-infected epithelium on the vaginal vault, vulva, or anus. Therefore, removal of the upper canal and uterus, assuming the treatment margins are clear, adds nothing to the cancer prophylaxis provided by transformation zone ablation.

Invasive Cancer after Previous Therapy

Of particular concern are the reports of invasive cancer occurring in women who have had ablative therapies (49, 79, 80). Unlike cancers after previous conization or hysterectomy, two-thirds of these tumors appear within 12 months, and more than 90% are diagnosed within 2 years, suggesting that an invasive cancer was missed during the initial triage.

Analysis of clinical details has shown that the majority of mishaps are attributable to major breaches of the evaluation protocol. Most glaringly, 45 of the 99 cases reported by Townsend and Richart (49) had cryosurgery or hot cautery for "chronic cervicitis," without colposcopic examination and biopsy. Of 66 women who did undergo colposcopic examination (49, 79), major triage errors included:

1. Treatment without prior biopsy

2. Failure to adequately assess the endocervical canal

3. Failure to evaluate a positive ECC

4. Failure to act upon a colposcopic suspicion of possible invasion

Invasive cancer after previous therapy may occur in one of three ways:

1. *Failure to detect occult invasion at initial triage.* The colposcopic appearance of an overt invasive cancer reveals an ulcerated or exophytic tumor covered with necrotic epithelium and punctuated by abnormal tumor vessels. Warning signs that can safeguard against overlooking invasive cancer are listed in Table 6.4.

2. *Invasion within persistent CIN.* Invasive cancer may arise within foci of intraepithelial neoplasia not eradicated by the initial therapy. Any treatment that leaves a residual focus of CIN within the depths of a cervical crypt could predispose to the subsequent occurrence of an invasive cancer. In addition, failure to destroy the oncogen-exposed immature metaplasia immediately proximal to the new SCJ might permit potentially neoplastic epithelium to remain viable within the cervical canal (15). Therefore the entire transformation zone must be treated (81, 82).

3. *Malignant progression in adjacent vaginal epithelium.* About one-third of the invasive cancers that have developed after therapy for cervical intraepithelial neoplasia have occurred in the original squamous epithelium of the vaginal vault (78). Hysterectomy does not offer complete protection against subsequent cancer and may complicate matters by burying islands of HPV-infected squamous epithelium beneath the vaginal scar.

Treatment Philosophy

No one should die of invasive cancer as a consequence of inappropriate conservatism in diagnosis or treatment. Paradoxically, in those patients in whom cervical

Table 6.4   Warning Signs to Safeguard against Overlooking Invasive Cancer

1. Yellowish epithelium, especially areas that bleed when touched.

2. Colposcopically significant areas (index score ≥6 points) with an irregular surface.

3. Surface ulceration (particularly when bordered by acetowhite epithelium).

4. Atypical vessels (horizontal surface capillaries displaying a "tadpole" or "comma" shape; coarse subepithelial vessels showing an irregular caliber and a long, unbranched course).

5. Extremely coarse mosaicism or punctation, especially if there are wide, irregular intercapillary distances.

6. Large complex lesions (dull, "oyster-white" epithelium occupying 3 or 4 cervical quadrants and showing a mixture of high-grade colposcopic patterns).

7. High-grade colposcopic lesions extending >5 mm into the cervical canal.

8. CIN 2 or 3 on a tangentially sectioned punch biopsy in which the basement membrane cannot be defined adequately.

9. Cytologic evidence of possible squamous carcinoma (CIS cells in large syncytial sheets, prominent nucleoli, bizarre cells, or a "dirty background").

10. Cytologic evidence of adenocarcinoma *in situ*.

11. Recurrent abnormal cytology in a patient previously treated for CIN 3 (e.g., by cryosurgery, cone biopsy, or hysterectomy).

12. A Pap smear suggestive of HSIL in a postmenopausal woman or previously irradiated women.

cancer develops, malignant progression can take as little as 12–18 months or as long as 20 years (61, 62) and can occur in patients who initially had only CIN 1 (49, 79). If untreated, 36% of the patients with CIS will have an invasive malignancy within 20 years (83). For the last 20 years, the grading of cervical intraepithelial neoplasia and the exclusion of any occult invasion have depended on colposcopy and directed biopsy. Although this approach has been highly successful, invasive cervical cancer or adenocarcinoma *in situ* is occasionally misdiagnosed as a squamous intraepithelial lesion, and therefore treated inappropriately. Such misclassification occurs in 0.1–1% of all patients evaluated because of abnormal Pap smears (84). Historically, the error rate of colposcopically directed triage protocols was considered too low to justify routine excision and complete histologic examination of the abnormal transformation zone. However, the advent of the LEEP procedure has greatly simplified excision of the distal 1 cm of the cervical canal.

Ploidy Analysis and HPV Typing

Both ploidy analysis (85) and HPV typing (5) can subdivide screening disorders into groups that display markedly different biologic behavior (Tables 6.5 and 6.6). This behavior suggests that one can subdivide premalignant lesions into a simple grouping of *high-grade (CIN 2 to 3)* versus *low-grade (CIN 1 and flat condyloma)* (5, 40, 41, 86). High-grade lesions are a homologous population of genetically mutated cells, most of which are induced by oncogenic HPVs. Expert gynecologic pathologists can reliably identify such epithelia as *bona fide* precursors. Conversely, low-grade lesions represent a heterologous mixture of genuine precursors, benign HPV infections, and nonspecific reparative changes. Although it has been suggested that low-grade lesions can be recognized by the presence

Table 6.5   Relationship between Cell Ploidy and Subsequent Biologic Behavior

Cell Ploidy	Subsequent Biologic Behavior			Total
	Regressed	Unchanged	Progressed	
Diploidy & Polyploidy	29 (91%)	3 (9%)	0	32 (100%)
Aneuploidy	5 (7%)	55 (81%)	8 (12%)	68 (100%)
Total	**34 (34%)**	**58 (58%)**	**8 (8%)**	**100 (100%)**

Modified, with permission, from Fu YS, Reagan JW, Richart RM: Definition of precursors. *Gynecol Oncol* 12:S220, 1981.

Table 6.6   Relationship between HPV Type and Cervical Pathology

Viral Type	Cervical Diagnosis				Total
	Normal Mild Atypia	Low-Grade SIL	High-Grade SIL	Cancer	
HPV negative	1671 (91.0%)	115 (30.5%)	33 (12.6%)	16 (10.5%)	1835 (69.8%)
HPV 6, 11, 42, 43, 44 2 unclassified types	80 (4.4%)	111 (29.4%)	26 (10.0%)	8 (5.2%)	225 (8.6%)
HPV 16, 18, 31, 33, 35, 45 51, 52, 56, 58	85 (4.6%)	151 (40.1%)	202 (77.4%)	129 (84.3%)	567 (21.6%)
Total	**1836 (100%)**	**377 (100%)**	**261 (100%)**	**153 (100%)**	**2627 (100%)**

Modified with permission from Lorincz AJ, Reid R, Jenson AB, et al: Human papillomavirus infection of the cervix: relative risk associations of 15 common anogenital types. *Obstet Gynecol* 79:328, 1992.
SIL = squamous intraepithelial lesion.

of atypical mitotic figures, this has not been our experience. In addition, it may not be possible to cytologically differentiate "condyloma" from "CIN 1." Until the late 1970s, all low-grade lesions were generally regarded as mild dysplasia and therefore treated as such (45). In a retrospective review of his previous biopsy material, Meisels (86) reclassified 70% of "mild dysplasias" as condylomas. Applying these criteria to a group of viral lesions, Willett et al. (87) found that 10% of "flat condylomas" contained oncogenic HPVs, and Mitchell et al. (88) observed that 4% of the women followed up for cytologic evidence of benign HPV infection had carcinoma *in situ* within 5 years. Nasiell et al. (89) and Campion et al. (62) have followed up women with condylomata or CIN 1 on biopsy and reported progression to CIN 3 in about one-fourth of the cases.

Clinicians must be especially cautious about dismissing low-grade lesions on the basis of histologic criteria only. For example, Koss et al. (59) followed up 93 women with cervical screening disorders (67 with CIN 3 and 26 with CIN 1 or 2) for as much as 13 years. During the period of observation, invasive cancer developed in nine of the CIN 3 group (14%) and in one patient (4%) with CIN 1 (Table 6.7).

Historically, the most cost-effective approach has been empiric destruction of the transformation zone, irrespective of whether the lesion was graded as "CIN 1" or "flat condyloma." However, the rising prevalence of cervical HPV infection and changes in cytologic reporting practices have led to a situation in which 5–10% of all Pap smears are interpreted as showing at least minor-grade squamous atypia. Reevaluation of all patients with minor squamous atypia has resulted in substantial overutilization of colposcopic triage and transformation zone destruction. A potentially practical solution lies with individualizing the evaluation of those patients with cytologic atypia by performing colposcopy only on the minority of women in whom there is demonstrable high-risk HPV DNA (5, 7, 90–94). The application of this approach to date has been limited by the complexity, high cost, and relative insensitivity of the prototypic testing methods (Vira Pap, Viratype, and Viratype in situ). New technology has significantly expanded the number of type-specific HPV DNA probes and has replaced cumbersome expensive radiolabeling with an efficient chemiluminescent detection system (95). All major laboratories will soon have access to cheap, rapid, and highly accurate HPV tests. Nevertheless, the clinical application of this technology will await data to support its cost-effectiveness.

Treatment Modalities

Treatment modalities include hysterectomy, cone biopsy, and superficial ablative techniques, such as electrocoagulation diathermy, cryosurgery, or CO_2 laser. Patients with squamous lesions are suitable for superficial ablative therapies, provided that:

1. The entire transformation can be visualized colposcopically.

2. The biopsy is consistent with the Pap smear.

3. The ECC is negative.

4. There is no cytologic or colposcopic suspicion of occult invasion.

Excisional Conization

Formal conization remains mandatory in specific clinical circumstances (Table 6.3). Complications, including hemorrhage, sepsis, stenosis, infertility, and cervical incompetence, occur in about 2–12% of patients, depending on the vertical height and geometry of the excised specimen (96–98). When conization is performed, the width and length should be tailored to the indication and lesion topography in order to perform the least injurious excision that provides clear surgical margins (Fig. 6.4).

Conization Geometry

Traditional Broad, Deep Cone   Excision of a cone-shaped specimen with a diameter and depth of 2–3 cm has the disadvantage of removing a large portion of the fibromuscular cervix, thereby carrying a relatively high complication rate and predisposing the patient to a deformed, incompetent cervix (96, 98). Therefore

Table 6.7   Results of a 13-Year Observational Study of the Natural History of CIN 1 and 3

Histologic Grade	Disappeared	Persisted	Progressed	Total
CIN 3	17 (25%)	41 (61%)	9 (14%)	67 (100%)
CIN 1	10 (38%)	15 (58%)	1 (4%)	26 (100%)

Reproduced, with permission, from Koss LG, Stewart FW, Foote FW, et al: Some histological aspects of behavior of epidermoid carcinoma *in situ* and related lesions of the uterine cervix. *Cancer* 16:1160, 1963.

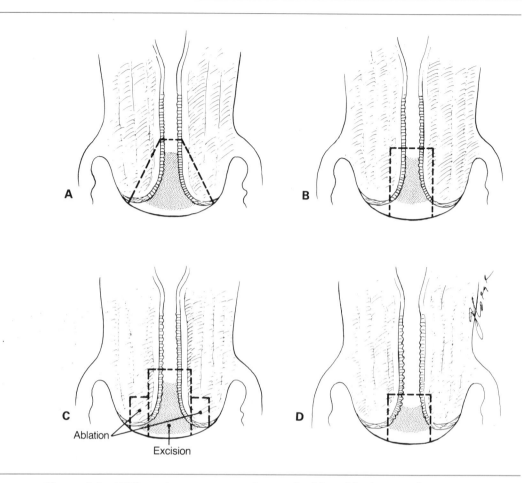

Ablation

Excision

Figure 6.4   Different cone geometries attainable with the CO₂ laser.

such cones should be reserved for uncommon situations in which there is strong clinical suspicion of occult invasion. Performing such cones with the CO_2 laser rather than the sharp knife might reduce scarring (97) (Fig. 6.4A).

Long Cylindrical Cone   If the lesion does not extend onto the peripheral portio, excision of a long central cylinder with a base of 1.5–2 cm and a vertical depth of 2–3 cm will provide full histologic assessment of the cervical canal while causing minimal damage to the fibromuscular cervix. Long cylindrical cones are much easier to excise with the CO_2 laser than with the cold knife (98) (Fig. 6.4B).

Combination Excisional and Ablative Cone   The most common indication for conization is a broad-based lesion that extends out of range within the cervical canal. Occult invasion within the ectocervical extension can be safely excluded by colposcopically directed biopsy. A combination of peripheral laser ablation and central laser excision might avoid undertreatment while minimizing complications (99, 100) (Fig. 6.4C).

"Mini-Cone"   In patients in whom there is little suspicion of a significant canal lesion but in whom the criteria for ablation of the transformation zone have not been met, an outpatient CO_2 laser excision of a small cylinder under local anesthesia can be performed (Fig. 6.4D). A cylinder with a vertical height of 10–

15 mm can be removed easily with a microscopically adapted laser, working through a Graves speculum (101). The risks of acute complications or scarring after "miniconization" are no greater than those of transformation zone ablation.

Surgical Techniques for Conization

Excisional conization of the cervix can be performed either with a cold knife or with the CO_2 laser.

Cold-Knife Conization   Cold-knife conization should be performed in the following manner:

1. Lateral sutures may be placed at 3 and 9 o'clock for traction and hemostasis.

2. The cervix should be infiltrated with a vasopressor to prevent bleeding.

3. A sound can be used in the endocervix to help guide the depth of the resection.

4. The specimen should be resected *in toto*, and only the stroma should be handled to avoid destroying the epithelial surface.

5. After excision, the specimen should be tagged at the 12 o'clock position and sent fresh to the pathology laboratory.

6. A dilatation and curettage (D & C) should be performed to exclude squamous intraepithelial neoplasia in the upper endocervical canal (or, rarely, in the endometrium).

7. Hemostatic sutures may be placed. An anterior and a posterior U suture are usually sufficient to control bleeding, and they do not bury the remaining ectocervical epithelium.

Laser Conization   A tightly focused beam of superpulsed CO_2 laser energy will make a sterile, bloodless incision, leaving less than 100 mm of coagulation necrosis at the cut margin. Hence, used skillfully, the CO_2 laser confers several major advantages over the cold knife.

1. The mechanics of beam delivery allow great flexibility in the geometry of the excised specimen. Choice of a cylindrical (rather than conical) shape avoids the need to sacrifice a significant proportion of the cervical fibromuscularis (Fig. 6.4). Thus the risks of cervical deformity or cervical incompetence are minimal, even with the need to resect a 20–25 mm cylinder of diseased canal.

2. Choice of a cylindrical geometry obviates the risk of cutting across diseased cervical crypts at the apex of the specimen.

3. Provided that lateral heat conduction is minimized by skillful technique, healing is rapid and predictable. The excised cylinder of diseased tissue is replaced by a downgrowth of submucosa and columnar epithelium from the midcanal, producing a pliable cervix with no net tissue loss. The risk of cervical stenosis is minimal.

4. Avoidance of a significant eschar and the prophylactic application of Monsel's solution to the conization bed reduces the risk of secondary hemorrhage to less than 1%.

Unfortunately, despite two decades of laser usage, many gynecologists continue to break some of the basic physical principles governing CO_2 laser surgery. Excessive thermal artifact within laser conization specimens is completely avoidable. Physicians who do not have access to adequate instrumentation (a super or ultrapulsed laser emitting a > 20 watt beam that can be focused to a 0.5 mm spot) will do better to use the cold knife rather than allow excessive lateral heat conduction through a suboptimal laser technique.

Provided the larger cervical arterioles are vasoconstricted by prior infiltration with epinephrine or Pitressin in solution, excisional conization with the CO_2 laser should result in negligible blood loss. The operation can be performed with either a handpiece or an operating microscope, depending on the laxity of the cervical ligaments. In patients who have a narrow vagina and cervix with minimal descent (e.g., nulliparous postmenopausal females), difficult exposure can be overcome by using the remote control afforded by the operating microscope.

Electrocoagulation Diathermy

Mode of Action Electrocoagulation diathermy is a surgical effect obtained by passing high-voltage electricity through the target tissue. It destroys tissue through two qualitatively different effects: fulguration and electrocoagulation. *Fulguration* is produced by holding the electrode just above the surface so that a spark of electricity arcs from the energy source (the electrosurgical machine) to ground (the patient). Local heating is so intense that tissue at the site of sparking undergoes rapid desiccation and charring. *Electrocoagulation* (or desiccation) is produced by inserting the electrode below the epithelial surface and allowing a current to dissect along the planes of electrical conductivity, causing heat denaturation and enzymatic degradation of structural proteins within a large volume of tissue.

It is important to differentiate between electrocoagulation diathermy and radial electrocautery of the surface epithelium with a red-hot wire. Electrocautery works by producing a simple conduction burn, which does not destroy the epithelium of the cervical crypts, and should not be used to treat cervical dysplasia.

Efficacy Treatment of CIN by electrocoagulation diathermy under general anesthesia was first reported in 1966. This method has been used extensively in Australia, although it is not commonly used in the United States. The Dysplasia Clinic at the Royal Women's Hospital in Melbourne, Australia, has consistently achieved the highest cure rates reported in the literature (75, 102). Of the 1864 patients treated by electrocoagulation diathermy from 1967–1982, 699 (37%) had CIN 1 or 2, and the remaining 1165 (63%) had CIN 3.

Success rates were unrelated to the histologic grade of the lesion, but they did correlate with the surface area of abnormal epithelium. During the first 7 years (1966–1972), the technique was used for patients in whom the entire new SCJ was visible without the use of an endocervical speculum (102). Over the next decade (1973–1981), Chanen and Rome (102) selected a greater proportion of patients for destructive therapy. The additional coagulation of the immature squamous metaplasia or columnar epithelium of the distal canal produced even higher success rates despite the inclusion of seemingly more difficult cases (Table 6.8).

218

Table 6.8   Treatment of CIN by Electrocoagulation Diathermy (ECD)

Treatment of CIN by Time Period	Patients Treated by ECD	Residual Disease
1966–1972	332	19 (5.7%)
1973–1981*	1,532	28 (1.8%)
Total	**1,864**	**47 (2.5%)**

Reproduced, with permission, from Chanen W, Rome RM: Electrocoagulation diathermy for cervical dysplasia and carcinoma *in situ*: A 15-year survey. *Obstet Gynecol* 61:673, 1983.
*From 1973 and thereafter, a special endocervical speculum was used to assess lesions extending into the canal. More extensive and more severe grades of CIN were treated with a significant increase in the proportion of patients with CIN 3 being treated with ECD. However, the basic technique of ECD was not altered.

However, fulguration with standard electrosurgical machines produces temperatures of $> 700°C$, making the technique too painful for use in nonanesthetized patients, even when a paracervical block is used.

Technique   The aim is to destroy the extent and depth of the abnormal transformation zone and adjacent columnar epithelium with the use of both needle and ball electrodes. Inadequate diathermy may fail to destroy the deeper crypts. The risks of underdestruction of tissue are worse than those of overdestruction. The technique is as follows:

1. With the patient under general anesthesia, the cervix is dilated to provide adequate exposure of the distal canal.

2. The portio is stained with Lugol's iodine to demarcate the geographic extent of the abnormal epithelium.

3. With an adequate coagulation current (e.g., a Valleylab model SSE-2 set at 3.5–4, or a Bovie model SV-X set at 40–45), the epithelium in the crypts and the distal canal is coagulated by numerous insertions of the needle electrode to a depth of about 1 cm in the long axis of the cervix. Multiple punctures (15 to 25) are made, the number depending on the area and extent of the lesion. Each insertion of the needle should last for at least 1–2 seconds. Insertion and withdrawal of the needle are facilitated by keeping current flowing throughout the procedure.

4. The ball electrode then is used to fulgurate and coagulate the epithelial surface until mucus stops bubbling up from the treated area. Continuous current with movement of the ball tends to produce more fulguration, whereas slower movement and direct contact with the tissue will produce deeper coagulation.

5. Constant mopping of the cervix with dry gauze facilitates a better contact, and the ball should be cleansed periodically of adherent tissue.

Cryosurgery

Mode of Action   Hypothermia is produced by the evaporation of liquid refrigerants and by allowing compressed gases to expand through a small jet (86). Heat exchange occurs at the surface of a metal probe placed on the surface of the tissue to be frozen. Only instruments that incorporate large, rapidly replenished gas reservoirs result in a uniform and predictable zone of cryonecrosis. Machines that depend on small, unheated N_2O cylinders cool tissues so slowly that ice formation is limited to the extracellular space. Cryonecrosis tends to be patchy and is accompanied by a wide zone of sublethal injury to adjacent tissues. Thawing results in the release of histamines and other vasoactive peptides, thereby producing local edema. Use of a *freeze-thaw-refreeze cycle* will increase the reliability of cell death, particularly when machines that produce suboptimal rates of cooling are used. Creasman et al. (103) reduced their failure rate from 29% to 7% by abandoning the single-freeze technique. The second freeze must not commence until the tissue is visibly thawed from the first treatment. For more effective heat transfer (and therefore a deeper zone of cryonecrosis), the probe should be coated with a water-soluble lubricant.

Efficacy Cryosurgery was first used in the treatment of CIN in 1968. It is a true outpatient modality that is cost-effective and well tolerated by patients. The extent of the lesion and the volume of tissue that must be destroyed are important variables associated with success (15). Series (104–108) reporting the results of cryosurgery in the treatment of CIN 3 reveal a primary success rate of 84% among 995 patients (Table 6.9). The higher rate for CO_2 laser ablation reported by some may reflect differences in the extent of tissue destruction rather than any intrinsic differences between the methods themselves (15).

Twenty years ago, pioneers of the various destructive methods had to decide where to place the upper margin of transformation zone ablation (15). In the United States, early advocates of cryosurgery decided that destruction of the metaplastic epithelium in the lower canal would lead to cervical stenosis (74). Therefore they selected flat probes and advised against freezing the columnar epithelium adjacent to the external os. At the same time, pioneers of diathermy observed that both initial failures and late recurrences were reduced when the therapeutic margins were extended to include all the metaplastic epithelium and not just that part of the transformation zone distal to the new SCJ (15). Fears that the destruction of the lower centimeter of the canal would produce cervical stenosis or infertility have proved groundless (109). Therefore, regardless of the modality used to treat the CIN, the ablation of the transformation zone should be in a "cowboy hat" configuration, rather than a flat cylinder (Fig. 6.5).

Technique Cryosurgery is performed without anesthesia. Premedication with nonsteroidal anti-inflammatory drugs may be useful to block the unpleasant symptoms caused by prostaglandin release from dying cells. The technique is as follows:

Table 6.9   Success Rates for Cryosurgical Destruction of CIN 3

Series	Patients	Successful Initial Treatment	Initial Success Rate
Ostergard (86)	250	210	84%
Kaufman (87)	126	103	82%
Popkin (88)	75	70	93%
Benedet (89)	365	316	87%
Hatch (90)	179	138	77%
Total	**995**	**837**	**84%**

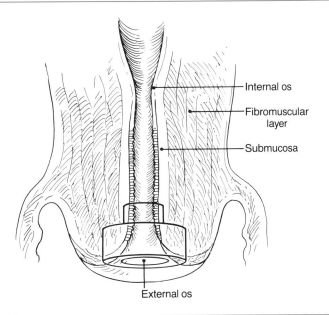

Internal os

Fibromuscular layer

Submucosa

External os

Figure 6.5   Destruction of the transformation zone in a "cowboy hat" configuration. The diameter of the peripheral disc corresponds to the peripheral margin of the lesion being treated, whereas the diameter of the central cylinder reflects the depth of the endocervical crypts.

1. After exposure of the cervix with a Grave's speculum, the topography of the abnormal epithelium is rechecked by repeat colposcopy.

2. The probe that best approximates the configuration of the lesion is then attached and the surface is covered with a water-soluble lubricant.

3. The probe tip, at room temperature, is positioned onto the tissues, with care taken to assure that the entire lesion is covered with the metal tip. Large lesions must be subdivided, with each part being frozen individually, while care is taken to ensure that the edges of the different ice balls overlap one another.

4. The refrigerant is circulated. Crystallization first occurs on the back of the probe tip and within 15 seconds spreads laterally from the edge of the probe onto the tissues. It is unnecessary to time the duration of freezing. Rather, freezing is continued until there is an ice ball about 5 mm beyond the edge of the probe.

5. If a portion of the vagina becomes attached to the probe during freezing, the probe should be defrosted and reapplied to the cervix.

6. When the probe is defrosted and disengaged from the cervix, a final inspection is made to ensure that the frost formation extends 5–6 mm beyond the edge of the lesion and that all ice balls overlap.

Rapid ice ball formation is an indication that the depth of cryonecrosis will correspond to the freeze margin beyond the probe. In contrast, with slow ice ball formation, the depth of cryonecrosis will be substantially less.

221

CO₂ Laser Ablation

Laser stands for *Light Amplification by Stimulated Emission of Radiation*. A laser beam is generated by the absorption of kinetic energy that produces the emission of *photons*, that is, packets of electromagnetic radiation (110–115). This process stimulates the emission of additional photons in the same phase and propagated in the same direction. Placing the laser medium in a cavity bounded at either end by mirrors that have a common axis rapidly amplifies the energy propagating back and forth through an "avalanche" process. When one of the mirrors is made partially transmissive, a portion of this energy is emitted as a laser beam. The emitted radiation has a defined wave length.

Physical Principles   Lasers must be used with an understanding of their physical principles (114–116). The choice of an appropriate wavelength is accomplished by choosing the proper machine. The CO_2 laser is the ideal choice for vaporizing sharply localized tissue volumes to a shallow depth, whereas the Nd:YAG (neodymium: yttrium aluminum garnet) laser functions mainly as an instrument for coagulating large volumes of tissue to a relatively deep level (117).

To achieve optimal vaporization with minimal surrounding tissue destruction, the CO_2 laser should be used with high power outputs (> 25 watts, preferably > 60 watts). The cautious but inappropriate use of low power outputs is the most damaging error (116, 118, 119).

In addition to the principle of using the highest controllable power output, thermal spread can be further decreased by selection of one of the superpulsed machines (111, 112, 116). The rapid superpulse and ultrapulse are major technologic advances and are better than older, continuous-mode machines. Energy is delivered in a series of high-energy pulses with power 5–7 times higher than the output attainable in continuous mode. The rapid superpulse keeps pulse duration shorter than the time needed to initiate lateral heat conduction, thus permitting a sufficient interpulse interval for the laser crater to cool to body temperature before the next energy pulse is delivered. If the rate of energy delivery can be maintained above the critical threshold, wet tissue will undergo instantaneous sublimation, creating the opportunity for char-free surgery. Conversely, if tissue is heated incrementally, desiccation and carbonization (and at least some degree of lateral heat conduction) are inevitable. Therefore it is important to deliver the required energy dose in the shortest possible time, as thermal injury is directly proportional to exposure time and crater temperature.

The choice of the appropriate power density depends on the use. When the objective is ablation of a wide field of epithelium to a shallow depth, average power density must be kept within the 750–2000 W/cm² range. Power density should not be allowed to fall below 750 W/cm² because excessive carbonization will occur (116). The power density for incision requires 50,000–250,000 W/cm², depending on the density of the tissue to be incised.

Beam geometry must be chosen to suit specific surgical objectives, incisions being performed with sharply focused beams and ablations with partially defocused spots (116). Because the quality of the treatment outcome is directly proportional to the speed of energy delivery, the power should not be decreased in situations requiring good control. The beam should be delivered in short bursts

(1/10 to 1/20 second) delivered at the same power level, which allows the maintenance of an optimal rate of energy delivery (116).

Technique   Although laser destruction of ectocervical epithelium is relatively painless, vaporization within the cervical canal requires effective pain relief (47). Because paracervical block does not always provide complete anesthesia, it is easier and more reliable to infiltrate just beneath the cervical mucosa with a dental syringe and a 27-gauge needle. The operation is performed as follows (113):

1. The cervix is stained with 50% Lugol's iodine, and the peripheral margin is outlined with the laser before the iodine stain fades.

2. The peripheral portion of the transformation zone is ablated to a depth approximating 7 mm.

3. The central button surrounding the external os is then destroyed for a distance of about 12 mm along the axis of the cervical canal.

To avoid inadvertent burns at the introitus, the Graves speculum blades should be extended vertically as far as is comfortable, and the axis of the vaginal canal should be kept parallel with that of the laser beam (119).

Loop Electrosurgical Excision Procedure

Electrosurgical loop electrodes have been used to perform cone biopsies since the 1920s. However, early techniques had several major problems: intense local heat production, galvanic uterine contractions, and thermal artifact within the excised specimen. In the 1980s these problems were eliminated by advances in electrosurgical generators and by the development of larger wire loops with insulated bases. Therefore this technology allowed excision of the transformation zone and distal canal with a single pass of the electrosurgical loop, with the patient under local anesthesia. In many centers, LEEP excision has become the preferred treatment for CIN lesions that lie within range of satisfactory colposcopic assessment (53, 54, 84, 120–129).

Mode of Action   Electricity produces three qualitatively different tissue effects, depending on voltage, current, and resistance:

1. *Fulguration*, which is produced by holding the electrode just above the surface, so that a spark of electricity arcs briefly from the energy source (the electrosurgical machine) to ground (the patient). Local heating is so intense that tissue at the site of sparking undergoes rapid desiccation and charring.

2. *Electrocoagulation*, which is produced by inserting the electrode below the epithelial surface and allowing a current to dissect along the planes of electrical conductivity, causing heat denaturation and enzymatic degradation of structural proteins within a large volume of tissue.

3. *Cutting*, which is produced by establishing and sustaining an electrical arc that supplies current in sufficient density to create explosive vaporization. The electrode can then float within a steam envelope, yielding a cut that resembles a continuous-mode laser incision.

Table 6.10 Failure Rates after LEEP (Recurrence Within One Year)

Author	Patients	Failure after LEEP* (%)	Maximum Follow-up (Months)
Murdoch et al. (84)	600	2.6	3
Prendiville et al. (123)	102	2.0	12
Bigrigg et al. (124)	1000	4.1	21
Luesley et al. (125)	616	4.4	6
Whiteley and Oláh (126)	80	5.1	6
Murdoch et al. (127)	1143	9.0	12
Wright et al. (129)	40	6.0	6

*Failure defined as either abnormal cytology and/or colposcopy or positive histology

Efficacy A number of large clinical series have reported success rates of > 90% (Table 6.10) (84, 123–129). Such success rates are comparable with results obtained by other methods of transformation zone destruction. However, LEEP has the significant advantages of being easy to learn and quick to perform, requiring only modest capital outlay and providing a tissue specimen that is generally of sufficient quality for histologic exclusion of occult invasion.

Complications The standard surgical complications of LEEP are similar to those of continuous-wave laser ablation and include:

1. Intraoperative and postoperative bleeding, the reported incidence ranging from 1–8% (128, 129). The risks of intraoperative bleeding are reduced by not excising deeper than 1 cm (especially laterally at the 3 and 9 o'clock positions), by pretreating any chlamydial cervicitis or bacterial vaginosis, and by not scheduling surgery until at least 3 months post partum. Postoperative bleeding occurs because of bacterial invasion of the eschar covering the cervical defect. Prophylactic application of Monsel's solution (ferric subsulfate) greatly reduces the frequency of this complication. Postoperative bleeding can be severe but generally amounts to no more than persistent spotting or the passage of dark blood clot. Colposcopy typically shows an organizing clot within the LEEP crater, and hemostasis usually can be achieved by application of Monsel's paste or by gentle fulguration. Because of the potential for prostaglandin-mediated symptoms such as uterine cramping, vomiting, diarrhea, and fainting, patients must be premedicated with nonsteroidal anti-inflammatory drugs before the secondary hemorrhage is treated.

2. Postoperative pelvic cellulitis or adnexal abscess formation, which is a rare but potentially serious complication. Within high-risk populations, it is prudent to exclude gonococcal or chlamydial cervicitis before surgery is performed.

3. Cervical stenosis, which complicates about 1% of LEEP treatments. Factors associated with heightened risk are incipient scarring from previous surgery, very wide (> 2 cm) or very high (> 2 cm) excisions, relative estrogen deficiency (in perimenopausal and lactating women), and intrauterine exposure to DES.

4. Cervical deformity and possible midtrimester abortion, which is particularly likely with excessive tissue removal. The use of shallow electrodes (0.8 cm) makes it impossible to cut to an unwise depth in one pass. However, excess tissue removal in the horizontal plane is an ever present danger, especially in the hands of an unwary operator.

Inappropriate use is an issue of great concern, especially in light of the "see and treat" protocols advocated by some gynecologists in the United Kingdom (121, 122). Because LEEP is a simple technique, obvious savings in time and money can be produced by attempting diagnosis and treatment in the same setting, rather than by following the traditional triage rules. However, delivery of health care in the United Kingdom is very different from that within the United States. In the English National Health System, patients with low-grade SIL smears are generally triaged to repeat cytology, rather than to referral for colposcopic biopsy. Patients who go to clinics in England are typically older (35–45 years) and have been called in for the evaluation of high-grade SIL smears. Given the greater specificity of high-grade cytologic patterns and the high volume and the centralized organization of English colposcopy services, the benefits of "see and treat" probably outweigh the disadvantages. Conversely, in the United States, the majority of women undergoing colposcopy are younger (18–25 years), have low-grade SIL or minor atypical smears, and are seen in private offices rather than regional clinics. Even though the LEEP complication rates are low, it would be inappropriate to excise the transformation zone in all of these women. Moreover, because LEEP is not an adequate alternative to formal excisional conization, the subsequent treatment of the few patients who have disease within the cervical canal will likely be complicated by blind shallow excision (130).

Technique   LEEP excision is performed through an insulated bivalve speculum, with the use of submucosal local anesthetic infiltration.

1. An electrode of appropriate size and shape (usually 2.0 × 0.8 cm) is pushed to a depth of 5–6 mm at the lateral lesional margin, pulled across and down through the transformation zone to a depth of 7–8 mm at the canal, and then out through the other lateral margin. This produces a doughnut-shaped piece of tissue with the endocervical os in the center.

2. To conform to a "cowboy hat"–shaped destruction, a second 5 mm cylinder should be removed with a 1 cm diameter electrode.

3. Hemostasis is completed by fulguration or desiccation of any specific bleeding points by means of the ball electrode. However, routine fulguration of a dry crater is counterproductive.

4. As prophylaxis against secondary hemorrhage, the crater base is lightly coated with Monsel's paste.

The Role of Hysterectomy

Hysterectomy in cases of preinvasive neoplasia is indicated only if there are associated gynecologic conditions that would be well treated by hysterectomy. In these circumstances, invasive cancer must be excluded before hysterectomy.

In the past, hysterectomy for CIN was often justified on the grounds of patient unreliability or cancerophobia. Reservations about the use of ablative therapies in unreliable patients are understandable. **However, in a review of the literature, Coppleson (78) noted 5442 reported patients treated with conization or cervical amputation. Only 18 of these women subsequently had invasive carcinoma, an incidence of 0.3%. By comparison, 38 cases of invasive carcinoma were reported among 8998 hysterectomies performed because of CIN, an incidence of 0.4%.**

Vagina, Vulva, and Anus

The lower anogenital tract encompasses large areas of stratified squamous epithelium and specialized hair-bearing skin. These epithelia are of cloacal origin, and all are exposed to similar environmental carcinogens (11). Therefore, it is not surprising that squamous neoplasia is often *multicentric* (involving several distinct anatomic sites within the lower tract) and *multifocal* (originating at several discrete foci within each anatomic site). Careful colposcopic examination of women with *cervical intraepithelial neoplasia (CIN)* 3 will show associated preinvasive disease at other sites in about 10% of the patients, *vaginal intraepithelial neoplasia (VAIN)* 3 in 3%, and *vulvar intraepithelial neoplasia (VIN)* 2 or 3 in 7% (131). Conversely, about 60% of women with VAIN 3 and about 30% of those with VIN 3 will be found to have preexisting or synchronous cervical neoplasia, either preinvasive or invasive (132, 133). Although CIN 3 and cervical cancer harbor a variety of papillomavirus types (6, 133), the great majority of multicentric neoplasias contain only HPV 16 (134–136).

Therapeutic Principles

In spite of the etiologic relationship between HPV infection and neoplasia within the lower genital tract, the occurrence of carcinomas is both rare and predictable. Although oncogenic HPVs generally induce a "field infection," neoplastic sequelae within the stable squamous epithelia of the vagina and vulva are much less common than in the cervix.

Benign Condylomata

Treatment of vulvar and vaginal condylomas should take account of the phases in the natural history of papillomavirus infection. Contact tracing studies suggest that, during an incubation period of 6 weeks to 8 months, latent viral infection becomes widely established within the lower genital tract (137). Thereafter rapid epithelial and capillary proliferation often results in focal papilloma formation. For patients seen early in the active phase, the clinician should understand that much of the apparent "spread" of disease really represents differing rates of evolution from latent to active infection at different sites. After about 3 months, lesion growth generally slows, presumably as a result of the host immune response (17).

Although essentially all condylomas are surrounded by diffuse areas of subclinical infection, repeated destruction of just the exophytic lesions will lead to stable remission in about 85% of women (138). However, the 15% of women with papillomavirus infections that are refractory to conventional office therapy constitute management problems. Given the chronicity of papillomavirus infections and the ease with which latent viral DNA can be detected in adjacent tissues, the major mechanism of treatment failure is probably reexposure of the healing area to a viral reservoir within the "normal" epithelium (8). Whether untreated

226

male partners also contribute to this viral reservoir remains an open question (139).

Despite the benefits of the CO_2 laser, use of this instrument as a "spot welder" does nothing to solve the problem of the surrounding subclinical infection. A randomized trial comparing laser with electrodiathermy reported control of only 9 of 21 patients in the laser group and 8 of 22 in the diathermy group (140). In contrast, use of the laser to destroy all areas of colposcopically detectable papillomavirus infection produced remission in 31 of 32 (97%) patients with refractory or very extensive disease (138). Therefore, once the decision to use the laser has been made, the approach should be to destroy all acetowhite areas of colposcopically suspected HPV infection (141).

Provided that this technique is not applied to simpler cases, the morbidity and expense of this approach are justifiable in selected cases. The great strength of extended ablation is that, skillfully used, the CO_2 laser can vaporize any disease volume, at any lower tract location, to a precise depth (142). Destruction of the colposcopically apparent subclinical infection may help to forestall recurrent disease. However, latent viral infection (i.e., the low-level, dormant reservoir of HPV DNA within colposcopically and histologically normal epithelium) cannot be eradicated.

Under difficult clinical circumstances, mechanical destruction should be combined with an antiviral drug regimen. Historically, refractory condylomas and intraepithelial neoplasias were managed by prolonged courses of topical 5-fluorouracil (5-FU) cream in doses that produced widespread cytotoxicity and consequent epithelial sloughing (143). However, such regimens were extremely painful and had low patient compliance. Since the mid-1980s, topical 5-FU has been used in doses below the cytotoxic threshold, in an attempt to mitigate selectively the growth of HPV-infected epithelium (144, 145). In patients with renal allografts or other immune deficiencies, Sillman et al. (143) showed that the use of maintenance low-dose 5-FU is required for disease control.

Documented therapeutic efficacy (88% vs 50%) for low-dose 5-FU regimens is restricted to patients with two or more of the following risk factors: impaired host immunity (overt immunosuppression, insulin-dependent diabetes, or connective tissue disease); cigarette smoking; oncogenic HPVs (especially HPV 16); multicentric foci of intraepithelial neoplasia; continued active growth for more than 9 months; and unsuccessful previous extended laser ablation (143). In "low-risk" patients, low-dose 5-FU adds almost nothing to the efficacy of laser therapy alone (93% vs 87%).

Interferons have documented efficacy against HPV infection *in vitro,* but evidence of clinical value has been difficult to establish. Intralesional interferon avoids most systemic side effects and can definitely produce regression of injected warts (50% active vs 20% placebo) (146). However, the practicality of such regimens is doubtful for several reasons: only a few papillomas can be injected during one course of treatment; there is no effect on either uninjected lesions or the subclinical reservoir; and at least one-third of patients with initial "successes" will develop new warts in adjacent areas. Also, this intralesional regimen has been tested on only small-volume and minimally refractory condylomas that could resolve with less expensive and simpler therapies.

227

Gall et al. (147, 148) investigated high-dose systemic interferon in patients with extensive and refractory warts. Their response rates were significant, but not good enough to justify the toxicity of such high interferon dosages.

In a randomized trial of extended laser plus self-administered subcutaneous interferon versus extended laser alone, adjuvant low-dose interferon reduced the failure rate by two-thirds (18% vs 55%) (149). Moreover, at least 50% of the patients who had recurrences at the adjuvant dose (1 million IU three times per week for 10 weeks) responded to crossover to a dosage within the usual therapeutic range (e.g., 3 million IU three times per week for 10 weeks). Since incorporation of adjuvant interferon into our protocol for extended laser ablation, the need for repeat surgery has fallen from 48% to 4% (145).

Vaginal Intraepithelial Neoplasia

Etiology

The prevalence of *vaginal intraepithelial neoplasia (VAIN)* is increasing, and the mean age at diagnosis is decreasing (150). However, the relative rarity of primary vaginal squamous carcinoma suggests that the malignant potential of VAIN may be quite low. Nonetheless, progression to invasion does occur (151, 152). About one-third of the invasive cancers after therapy for CIN occur at the vaginal vault. It is possible that the current epidemic of VAIN in young women will present a greater threat during the next two decades as this cohort ages.

Hybridization studies have shown that HPV 16 can be isolated from about 70% of VAIN lesions (135), often representing part of a field effect. Malignant conversion of vaginal condylomas has been documented (153), and there is a definite morphologic spectrum linking subclinical papillomavirus infection to vaginal cancer (131).

Clinical Features

Whether it occurs as a primary focus or as a distal extension of a cervical lesion, VAIN generally involves the upper third of the vagina. VAIN in the lower vagina is rare and usually is seen as an incidental finding in women with extensive multicentric intraepithelial neoplasia (133).

In premenopausal women, VAIN is identified easily through the colposcope, provided that care is taken to visualize the vaginal walls as the speculum is withdrawn. Two clinical patterns can be distinguished (133):

1. Keratotic, surface-roughened plaques, often visible to the naked eye, but best appreciated through the colposcope. Some of these lesions are sessile HPV 6– or HPV 11–induced condylomata, whereas others represent foci of HPV 16–induced VAIN.

2. Patches of flat acetowhite epithelium that are completely invisible before vinegar soaking. Coarse vascular patterns are often present, punctation being much more common than mosaicism. Most such lesions show significant histologic atypia, and HPV 16 is usually detectable.

During vaginal colposcopy, staining with quarter-strength Lugol's iodine is an essential safeguard against overlooking lesions in areas that are difficult to visualize, such as behind the speculum blades or within rugose folds.

In postmenopausal women who are not on adequate hormonal replacement, acetowhitening may be very faint. Therefore, it is often necessary to repeat the colposcopic examination after 3 weeks of estrogen therapy.

Management

VAIN is difficult to treat, especially when the vaginal lesions occur as part of a "field effect." Historically, surgical excision or vaginal irradiation was favored. Over the last decade, laser photovaporization and topical 5-FU therapy have emerged as better methods. Requirements for conservative therapy of VAIN are as follows:

1. The treating physician must be an expert colposcopist.

2. Target biopsies must explain the abnormality seen on the Pap smear.

3. There must be *no* cytologic, colposcopic, or histologic suspicion of occult invasion.

In a series of 98 cases of VAIN treated by photovaporization (151), an initial failure rate of only 11% was reported in women with unicentric disease, compared with 28% in patients with multicentric disease. Therefore patients with more difficult disease patterns need individualized management.

Unicentric VAIN with Uterus in Situ   Good results are attainable by either of two methods:

1. Laser photovaporization to the level of the lamina propria.

2. Topical 5-FU therapy (e.g. the instillation of one-third of a vaginal applicator of 5% cream on alternate nights for 4–6 weeks) (145), using appropriate precautions to safeguard against unintended chemical burns to the introitus and vulva (46, 47).

Multicentric VAIN with Uterus in Situ   Multicentric genital neoplasia is much more difficult to cure, perhaps because such patients have a diffuse vaginal reservoir of HPV infection and an associated active viral expression (136). Eventual success rates of about 90% can be obtained by repeatedly re-treating initial failures (150). After initial photovaporization, low-dose maintenance 5-FU therapy can be used (144). The usual regimen is to instill about 2 g of 5-FU weekly for about 6 months. Two grams of 5-FU is delivered by filling one-third of a 10 ml Ortho applicator with the 5% cream and inserting it deeply into the vagina at bedtime. Any residual cream must be carefully washed from the vulva upon waking to prevent chemical vulvitis. The patient should not have coitus while the 5-FU cream is in place and must not become pregnant while using the cream.

Recurrent VAIN after Pelvic Irradiation   Ruling out occult cancer in women with recurrent VAIN after prior radiation therapy mandates expert consultation. Therapy is also difficult, requiring both skilled local destruction and possibly 5-FU cream.

VAIN of the Vault Posthysterectomy   Whereas the CO_2 laser is ideal for treating vaginal lesions when the uterus remains *in situ*, VAIN after hysterectomy often requires excision of the vault scar (154). In a series of 23 British women

229

managed by laser vaporization of recurrent VAIN, Woodman et al. (152) report that only six patients were still free of disease after 30 months' follow-up. Of the 21 women in whom the VAIN involved the vault scar, three later had invasive cancer in islands of buried vaginal epithelium. Therefore, laser ablation should be reserved for foci of VAIN that can be visualized completely.

Vulvar Intraepithelial Neoplasia

Etiology

Over the last decade, there has been a substantial increase in the prevalence of *vulvar intraepithelial neoplasia (VIN)*, particularly of the multifocal variety in young women (131). Invasive carcinoma of the vulva is often associated with preinvasive disease. Although progression from VIN to invasive cancer has been observed most frequently in immunosuppressed and elderly women (155), the premalignant nature of a minority of VIN lesions is well established. VIN and invasive cancer are both aneuploid (156), and both lesions are associated with high-risk HPV infection (8, 131).

There is a strong association (20–60%) between VIN and other sexually transmitted diseases (156). The association with HPV infections is especially strong. Apart from a remote risk of verrucous carcinoma (131), vulvar condylomata associated with HPV types 6 or 11 have no neoplastic potential. However, some 7% of histologically benign condylomata do contain HPV 16 or 18. Therefore reports of occasional progression from "benign condyloma" to invasive cancer are not surprising (157). In addition, many lesions that appear to the naked eye to be unremarkable papillomas will show histologic evidence of VIN 2 or 3 on biopsy.

In a recent study of 36 women with vulvar intraepithelial neoplasia, including six in whom the lesions progressed to invasive cancer, Park et al. (158) described two dominant histological patterns: a bowenoid (warty) VIN, characterized by dyskaryotic acanthotic cells showing partial but disordered maturation, and a basaloid VIN, characterized by an epithelium composed completely of atypical immature parabasal cells (reminiscent of a classic carcinoma *in situ* of the cervix). Within this retrospective cohort study, the bowenoid variety was associated with a higher frequency of HPV 16 detection (16/23 vs 5/13) and a lower incidence of invasive carcinoma (3/23 vs 3/13).

Clinical Features

VIN is commonly multifocal. The hairless skin of the interlabial grooves, posterior fourchette, and perineum are most frequently affected (Fig. 6.6). More extensive disease is often confluent, involving the labia majora and minora and the perianal skin.

Lesions may be macular or papular, often presenting a keratotic, roughened surface. Discoloration is usual, with *white* lesions reflecting epithelial thickening and hyperkeratosis, *red* lesions reflecting hypervascularity and parakeratosis, and *gray* or *brown* lesions reflecting melanocytic overactivity and pigment incontinence (melanin deposits within macrophages, resulting from the inability of premalignant keratinocytes to retain pigment) (156).

Management

Treatment of VIN is controversial, with recommendations ranging from wide excision to superficial "skinning" vulvectomy. Although the treatment originally

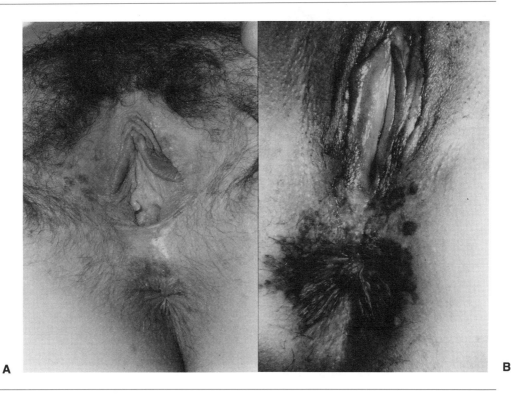

A

B

Figure 6.6 *A,* A multifocal VIN 3 lesion with multiple small hyperpigmented lesions on the labia major. *B,* VIN 3 with more confluent hyperpigmented areas on the posterior fourchette with extensive perianal involvement.

proposed for "carcinoma *in situ*" of the vulva was wide local excision, fears that the disease was preinvasive led to the widespread use of simple vulvectomy. In young patients, however, the risk of malignant progression is insufficient to justify such mutilating surgery.

Wide excision of small foci produces excellent results, but multifocal or extensive lesions are difficult to treat by this method. Therefore, in the past, the only reasonable alternative was a superficial vulvectomy with grafting (159). Although a definite improvement over conventional vulvectomy, cosmetic and functional results are unpredictable. The CO_2 laser offers an alternative by providing an effective but nonmultilating treatment for the bowenoid (warty) variety of VIN 3 (158). Because occult invasion > 1 mm carries a risk of lymph node metastasis, there is little room for error. The rate of invasive vulvar cancer associated with VIN is about 8%, although four-fifths of these are superficially invasive (< 1 mm) (160). When triage is restricted to physicians experienced in vulvar disease, however, the consensus view is that occult invasion can be excluded by careful colposcopy and liberal use of excisional biopsy (131, 142, 149, 160–162).

In contrast to the management of bowenoid VIN 3, the basaloid (undifferentiated) variety has a different natural history (158). Premalignant foci occurring in association with lichen sclerosus or lichen simplex chronicus always require excision.

231

Perianal Neoplasia

Etiology

Squamous carcinoma of the anus is an uncommon tumor that accounts for approximately 2% of cancers of the large bowel (164). It typically occurs in the elderly and previously was seen more frequently in women. However, there has been a striking increase in anorectal cancer in young, never married American men. The disease now occurs about 50 times more often in homosexuals than in heterosexual controls (165). Both histologic and viral analyses confirm an association with papillomavirus infection, HPV 16 being the type most frequently isolated (135, 165). Local trauma, human immunodeficiency virus (HIV), and depressed immune function are all potential cofactors (166).

Precursor lesions for invasive carcinoma of the anus have been considered very uncommon, generally being detected as a chance finding during histologic examination of tissue excised for benign anorectal disease (164). However, careful colposcopic examination of this region in women with multicentric squamous neoplasia will reveal *perianal intraepithelial neoplasia ("PAIN")* in almost one-third of cases (131).

Clinical Features

Perianal intraepithelial neoplasia occurs in two clinical forms:

1. As neoplastic transformation of macroscopic condylomata acuminata, frequently unsuspected before histologic examination of representative lesions.

2. As plaques of thickened, keratotic, often discolored perianal skin. Although such lesions are generally visible to the unaided eye, they are much better appreciated through the colposcope, after soaking with 5% acetic acid.

Proctoscopic examination of the anal canal and lower rectum will commonly reveal extensive acetowhite areas, some of which will also show significant histologic atypia. Men who have anal intercourse often develop large areas of squamous metaplasia between the dentate line and the proximal rectum. Somewhat analagous to the cervical transformation zone, this squamous metaplasia is very susceptible to infection by high-risk papillomaviruses (131).

Management

Treatment is essentially the same as for VIN, except that conservation of the normal tissues is even more vital. Although full-thickness excision with split-skin grafting can produce excellent cosmetic results, disruption of the nerve fibers within the lamina propria can lead to anal incontinence.

CO_2 Laser Therapy

Surgical Principles

When the CO_2 laser is used for treatment of vulvar, vaginal, or perianal lesions, care must be taken to achieve the correct depth of ablation. To accomplish this, the appropriate beam-delivery system must be selected.

For energy of a given wavelength, both spot size and depth of field are directly proportional to the focal length of the objective lens. Operating microscopes are preferred because they generally use 300–400 mm objectives, producing relatively large focal spots with an excellent depth of field. In contrast, handheld probes incorporate lenses of short focal length as a means of attaining very narrow spot diameters and correspondingly high power densities, and produce a series of nonuniform, poorly localized cuts.

There will always be some heat conduction to adjacent tissues, and the amount of lateral heat propagation when the laser is used as a thermal knife is low. During vulvar laser ablation, however, thermal spread can be limited by chilling the tissues with laparotomy packs soaked in iced saline solution before the initial laser impact and at frequent intervals during the operation. This will diminish postoperative pain and swelling and contribute to a significant reduction in healing time (116).

Most intraoperative bleeding arises from a laser puncture of the side of a small vessel. Therefore re-treating the bleeding point with a high-powered beam for about 2–3 seconds usually will secure hemostasis by sealing the perforated vessel. If this is not successful, the bleeding point should be tamponaded and coagulated with a low power density, or sutured.

Exposure on external surfaces is generally simple, but on internal surfaces it depends on the use of the correct instruments (e.g., a pediatric nasal speculum for the urethra, a speculum for the vagina, and an adequately sized anoscope for the anus). The angle of laser impact may be improved further by traction, lateral pressure with a cotton swab, or the use of a handheld mirror to reflect the beam into difficult areas.

Failure to recognize the true extent of disease will adversely affect success rates (167). Strategies for setting operative margins within the lower genital tract vary according to anatomic site: in patients with exophytic condylomata or VIN, soaking with 3–6% acetic acid will usually produce prominent acetowhitening of skin that appeared normal on examination with the naked eye (46, 47, 138).

The depths of destruction during vulvar surgery is too shallow to control by measurement. The depth must be controlled according to the visual characteristics at the site of impact (141).

Surgical Planes

From the surgical standpoint, tissue destruction occurs through two distinct mechanisms: immediate photovaporization and delayed coagulation necrosis (116). Tissue within the zone of coagulation necrosis will look normal at the time of surgery, separating only as an eschar after activation of the host inflammatory response. Any structures visible within the crater base already will have suffered irreversible thermal coagulation and will slough by the succeeding week. Therefore, the crater depth created must be such that the zone of thermal necrosis (rather than the zone of photovaporization) lies at the intended depth of penetration. Four characteristic surgical planes are identifiable (Table 6.11) (141, 168).

First Plane   Destruction to the first plane removes the surface epithelium to the level of the basement membrane. This plane is reached by placing the laser crater within the prickle cell layer. Penetration to the proper depth is accomplished by rapid oscillation of the micromanipulator, so that the spot describes a roughly parallel series of lines and each pass of the laser beam reveals bubbles beneath the charred surface squamous cells.

233

Table 6.11 The Four Surgical Planes Used for Accurate Control of Depth during Carbon Dioxide Laser Operation

	Surgical Plane			
Parameter	**First**	**Second**	**Third**	**Fourth**
Target tissue	Surface epithelium	Dermal papillae	Pilosebaceous ducts	Pilosebaceous glands
Zone of vaporization	Proliferating layer	Superficial papillary dermis	Upper reticular	Midreticular dermis
Zone of necrosis	Basement membrane	Deep papillary	Midreticular	Deep reticular
Type of healing	Rapid, cosmetic	Rapid, cosmetic	Usually cosmetic, may hypertrophy	Atrophic or hypertrophic, needs grafting
Visual landmark	Opalescent cell debris	Scorched basement membrane	Coarse collagen fibers	"Sand grains" (skin appendages)

Reproduced, with permission, from Reid R: Superficial laser vulvectomy. A new surgical technique for appendage-conserving ablation of refractory condylomas and vulvar intraepithelial neoplasia. *Am J Obstet Gynecol* 152:504, 1985.

Second Plane Ablation of the second plane removes the epidermis and the loose network of fine collagen and elastin fibers that constitute the papillary dermis. This plane is reached by rapid oscillations, with the beam moved quickly so that the laser scorches rather than craters the exposed corium. When done correctly, the scorched surface should show a finely roughened contour and a yellowish color. The zone of coagulation necrosis will lie within the papillary dermis with only minimal thermal injury to the underlying reticular dermis. The second plane is the preferred level of ablation for extensive condylomata, because these wounds heal rapidly and produce a result indistinguishable from normal skin.

Third Plane Destruction to the third plane removes the epidermis, the upper portions of the pilosebaceous ducts, and a part of the reticular dermis. Ablation to the midreticular layer uncovers coarse collagen bundles that can be seen through the operating microscope as gray-white fibers. This plane is reached with slower, more deliberate movements of the laser beam. Limiting destruction to the third surgical plane allows reepithelialization from the skin appendages. Although VIN often extends into the pilosebaceous ducts, involvement usually is limited to the superficial portions of the ducts, making laser ablation to the midreticular level appropriate (141). Depth of destruction should be individualized by examining representative histologic sections, and extension into pilosebaceous ducts is an indication for surgical excision.

Fourth Plane Production of a deliberate third-degree burn in order to destroy abnormal keratinocytes within the hair follicles or sweat glands is not desirable.

References

1. **Richart RM:** Causes and management of cervical intraepithelial neoplasia. *Cancer* 60:1951, 1987.

2. **Coppleson M, Pixley E, Reid BL:** *Colposcopy—A Scientific Approach to the Cervix Uteri in Health and Disease*, ed 3. Springfield, Illinois, Charles C Thomas, 1986.

3. **Rotkin ID:** A comparison review of key epidemiological studies in cervical cancer related to current searches for transmissable agents. *Cancer Res* 33:1353, 1973.

4. **Dreesman GR, Burek J, Adam EA, et al:** Expression of herpes-virus-induced antigens in human cervical cancer. *Nature* 283:591, 1980.

5. **Lorincz AJ, Reid R, Jenson AB, et al:** Human papillomavirus infection of the cervix: relative risk associations of 15 common anogenital types. *Obstet Gynecol* 79:328, 1992.

6. **Lorinz A, Reid R:** Association of human papillomavirus with gynecologic cancer. *Curr Opin Oncol* 1:123, 1989.

7. **Munoz N, Bosch FX, Shah KV, Meheus A:** The epidemiology of HPV and cervical cancer. *International Agency for Research on Cancer,* Oxford University Press, New York, 1992.

8. **Reid R, Greenberg M, Jenson AB, et al:** Sexually transmitted papillomaviral infections. I. The anatomic distribution and pathologic grade of neoplastic lesions associated with different viral types. *Am J Obstet Gynecol* 156:212, 1986.

9. **Park JS, Jones RW, McLean MR, et al:** A possible etiologic heterogeneity of vulvar intraepithelial neoplasia. *Cancer* 67:1599, 1991.

10. **Gross G, Ikenberg H, Gissman L, Hagedorn M:** Papillomavirus infection of the anogenital region: Correlation between histology, clinical picture and virus type. *J Invest Dermatol* 85:147, 1985.

11. **Langley FA, Crompton AC:** Epithelial abnormalities of the cervix uteri. In *Recent Results in Cancer Research.* New York, Springer Verlag, 1973, pp 2–5, 141–143.

12. **Pixley E:** Morphology of the fetal and prepubertal cervicovaginal epithelium. In Jordan JR and Singer A (eds): *The Cervix.* London, WB Saunders, 1976, p 75.

13. **Coppleson M:** Colposcopic features of papillomaviral infection and premalignancy on the lower genital tract. *Obstet Gynecol Clin North Am* 14:471, 1987.

14. **Stafl A, Mattingly RF:** Colposcopic diagnosis of cervical neoplasia. *Obstet Gynecol* 41:168, 1973.

15. **Reid R, Atkinson K, Chanen W, et al:** Symposium on cervical neoplasia. VI. Differing views. *Colpo Gynecol Laser Surg* 1:299, 1984.

16. **Reid BL, Singer A, Coppleson M:** The process of cervical regeneration after electrocauterisation. *Aust NZ J Obstet Gynecol* 7:125, 1967.

17. **Pfister H:** Biology and biochemistry of papillomaviruses. *Rev Physiol Biochem Pharmacol* 99:111, 1983.

18. **Gissman L:** Papillomaviruses and their association with cancer in animals and in man. *Cancer Surv* 3:161, 1984.

19. **Broker TR:** Structure and genetic expression of human papillomaviruses. *Obstet Gynecol Clin North Am* 14:329, 1987.

20. **Reid R, Laverty CR, Coppleson M, et al:** Noncondylomatous cervical wart virus infection. *Obstet Gynecol* 55:476, 1980.

21. **Lorincz AT, Temple GF, Kurman RJ, et al:** Oncogenic association of specific human papillomavirus types with cervical neoplasia. *J Natl Cancer Inst* 79:671, 1987.

22. **Manos NM, Ting Y, Wright DK, et al:** Use of polymerase chain reaction amplification for the detection of genital human papillomavirus. *Cancer Cells* 7:209, 1989.

23. **Schiffman MH, Bauer HM, Lorincz AT, et al:** A comparison of Southern blot hybridization and polymerase chain reaction methods for the detection of human papillomavirus DNA. *J Clin Microbiol* 29:573, 1991.

24. **Temple GF:** Temporal association of human papillomavirus infection with cervical cytologic abnormalities. *Am J Obstet Gynecol* 162:645, 1990.

25. **Reid R, Greenberg M, Lorincz AT, et al:** Should cervical cytology be augmented by cervicography or HPV DNA detection? *Am J Obstet Gynecol* 164:1461, 1991.

26. **Cullen AP, Reid R, Campion MJ, Lorincz AT:** Analysis of the physical state of different human papillomavirus DNAs in intraepithelial and invasive cervical neoplasms. *J Virol* 65:606, 1991.

27. **Campion MJ, McCance DJ, Cuzick J, Singer A:** Progressive potential of mild cervical atypia: prospective cytological and virological study. *Lancet* 2:8501:237, 1986.

28. **Woodworth CD, Waggoner S, Barnes W, et al:** Human cervical and foreskin epithelial cells immortalized by human papillomavirus DNA exhibit dysplastic differentiation in vivo. *Cancer Res* 50:3709, 1990.

29. **McCance DJ, Kopan R, Fuchs E, Lamains LA:** Human papillomavirus type 16 alters human epithelial cell differentiation in vitro. *Proc Natl Acad Sci USA* 85:7169, 1988.

30. **Ray AF, Peabody DS, Cooper JL, et al:** SV40 T antigen alone drives karyotype instability that precedes neoplastic transformation of human diploid fibroblasts. *J Cell Biochem* 42:13, 1990.

31. **Schramayr S, Caporossi D, Mak I, et al:** Chromosomal damage induced by human adenovirus type 12 requires expression of the E1B 55-kilodalton viral protein. *J Virol* 64:2090, 1990.

32. **Hurlin PJ, Kaur P, Smith PP, et al:** Progression of human papillomavirus type 18 immortalized human keratinocytes to a malignant phenotype. *Proc Natl Acad Sci USA* 88:570, 1991.

33. **Stoler MH, Rhodes CR, Whitbeck A, et al:** Gene expression of HPV types 16 and 18 in cervical neoplasia. *UCLA Symp Mol Cell Biol New Ser* 124:1, 1990.

34. **Werness BA, Levine AJ, Howley PM:** Association of human papillomavirus types 16 and 18 E6 proteins with p53. *Science* 248:76, 1990.

35. **Papanicolaou G, Traut HF:** *The Diagnosis of Uterine Cancer by the Vaginal Smear.* New York, Commonwealth Fund, 1943.

36. **Fidler HK, Boyes DA, Worth AJ:** Cervical cancer detection in British Columbia: a progress report. *J Obstet Br Comm* 75:392, 1968.

37. **Canadian Task Force Report:** *Can Med Assoc J* 114:1003, 1976.

38. **Johannesson G, Geitsson G, Day N:** The effect of mass screening in Iceland, 1965–1974, on the incidence and mortality of cervical cancer. *Int J Cancer* 21:418, 1978.

39. **Eddy DM:** Appropriateness of cervical cancer screening. *Gynecol Oncol* 12:168, 1981.

40. **National Cancer Institute Workshop:** The 1988 Bethesda system for reporting cervical/vaginal cytologic diagnoses. *J Am Med Assoc* 262:931, 1989.

41. The Bethesda system for reporting cervical/vaginal cytologic diagnoses—report of the 1991 Bethesda Workshop. *J Am Med Assoc* 267:1892, 1992.

42. **Wain GV, Farnsworth A, Hacker NF:** The Papanicolaou smear histories of 237 patients with cervical cancer. *Med J Aust* 157:14, 1992.

43. **Hurt GW, Silverberg SG, Fable WJ, et al:** Adenocarcinoma of the cervix: histopathologic and clinical features. *Am J Obstet Gynecol* 129:304, 1977.

44. **Pearse WH:** Consensus report on frequency of Pap smear testing. American College of Obstetricians and Gynecologists, *Newsletter* 32:3, 1988.

45. **Reid R, Herschman BR, Crum CP, et al:** Genital warts and cervical cancer. V. The tissue basis of colposcopic change. *Am J Obstet Gynecol* 149:293, 1984.

46. **Reid R, Stanhope CR, Herschman BR, et al:** Genital warts and cervical cancer. IV. A colposcopic index for differentiating subclinical papillomaviral infection from cervical intraepithelial neoplasia. *Am J Obstet Gynecol* 149:815, 1984.

47. **Reid R, Scalzi P:** Genital warts and cervical cancer. VII. An improved colposcopic index for differentiating benign papillomaviral infections from high-grade cervical intraepithelial neoplasia. *Am J Obstet Gynecol* 153:611, 1985.

48. **Benedet JL, Anderson GH, Boyes DA:** Colposcopic accuracy in the diagnosis of microinvasive and occult invasive carcinoma of the cervix. *Obstet Gynecol* 65:557, 1985.

49. **Townsend DE, Richart RM:** Diagnostic errors in colposcopy. *Gynecol Oncol* 12:S259, 1981.

50. **Urcuyo R, Rome RM, Nelson JH:** Some observations on the value of endocervical curettage performed as an integral part of colposcopic examination of patients with abnormal cervical cytology. *Am J Obstet Gynecol* 128:787, 1977.

51. **Weitzman GA, Korhonen MO, Reeves KO, et al:** Endocervical brush cytology: an alternative to endocervical curettage? *J Reprod Med* 33:677, 1988.

52. **Lorincz A, Reid R:** Association of human papillomavirus with gynecologic cancer. *Curr Opin Oncol* 1:123, 1989.

53. **Phipps JM, Gunasekera PC, Lewis BV:** Occult cervical carcinoma revealed by large loop diathermy. *Lancet* 2:453, 1989.

54. **Howe DT, Vincenti AC:** Is large loop excision of the transformation zone (LLETZ) more accurate than colposcopically directed punch biopsy in the diagnosis of cervical intraepithelial neoplasia? *Br J Obstet Gynaecol* 98:588, 1991.

55. **Stafl A:** Cervicography. *Clin Obstet Gynecol* 26:1007, 1983.

56. **Henson D, Tarone R:** An epidemiologic study of cancer of the cervix, vagina and vulva based on the Third National Cancer Survey in the United States. *Am J Obstet Gynecol* 129:525, 1977.

57. **Bibbo M, Keebler CM, Wied GL:** Prevalence and incidence rates of cervical atypia. *J Reprod Med* 6:79, 1971.

58. **Miller AB:** Control of carcinoma of cervix cancer by exfoliative cytology screening. In Coppleson M (ed): *Gynecologic Oncology: Fundamental Principles and Clinical Practice.* Edinburgh, Churchill Livingstone, 1981, p 38.

59. **Koss LG, Stewart FW, Foote FW, et al:** Some histological aspects of behavior of epidermoid carcinoma in situ and related lesions of the uterine cervix. *Cancer* 16:1160, 1963.

60. **Koss LG:** Dyplasia: a real concept or a misnomer? *Obstet Gynecol* 51:374, 1978.

61. **Barron BA, Richart RM:** Screening protocols for cervical neoplastic disease. *Gynecol Oncol* 12:S156, 1981.

62. **Campion MJ, McCance DJ, Cezick J, Suggen A:** Progressive potential of mild cervical atypia: prospective cytological, and virological study. *Lancet* 2:237, 1986.

63. **Gusberg SB, Marshall D:** Intraepithelial carcinoma of the cervix; a clinical reappraisal. *Obstet Gynecol* 19:713, 1962.

64. **Anderson FF:** Treatment and follow up of noninvasive cancer of the uterine cervix—report on 205 cases (1948–57). *J Obstet Gynecol Br Comm* 72:172, 1965.

65. **Kolstad P:** Carcinoma of the cervix. Stage Ia. Diagnosis and treatment. *Am J Obstet Gynecol* 104:1015, 1969.

66. **Boyes DA, Worth AJ, Fidler HK:** The results of treatment of 4389 cases of preclinical cervical squamous carcinoma. *J Obstet Gynecol Br Comm* 77:769, 1970.

67. **Creasman WT, Rutledge F:** Carcinoma in situ of the cervix: an analysis of 861 patients. *Obstet Gynecol* 39:373, 1972.

68. **Brundenell M, Cox BS, Taylor CW:** The management of dysplasia, carcinoma in situ and microcarcinoma of the cervix. *J Obstet Gynecol Br Comm* 80:673, 1973.

69. **Burghardt E:** *Colposcopy Cervical Pathology,* ed 2. New York, G Thieme Verlag, 1991.

70. **Foote FW, Stewart FW:** The anatomical distribution of the intraepithelial epidermoid carcinomas of the cervix. *Cancer* 1:431, 1948.

71. **Kolstad P, Stafl A:** *Atlas of Colposcopy,* ed 2. Baltimore, University Park Press, 1982.

72. **Richart RM:** Cervical intraepithelial neoplasia. *Pathol Annu* 8:301, 1973.

73. **Stafl A, Mattingly RF:** Colposcopic diagnosis of cervical neoplasia. *Obstet Gynecol* 41:168, 1973.

74. **Townsend DE, Ostergard DR:** Cryocauterization for preinvasive cervical neoplasia. *J Reprod Med* 6:171, 1971.

75. **Chanen W, Hollyock VE:** Colposcopy and electrocoagulation diathermy for cervical dysplasia and carcinoma in situ. *Obstet Gynecol* 37:623, 1971.

76. **Stafl A, Wilkinson EJ, Mattingly RF:** Laser treatment of cervical and vaginal neoplasia. *Am J Obstet Gynecol* 120:666, 1974.

77. **Richart RM, Townsend D, Crisp W:** An analysis of long term follow-up results in patients with cervical intraepithelial neoplasia treated by cryosurgery. *Am J Obstet Gynecol* 137:823, 1980.

78. **Coppleson M:** Management of preclinical carcinoma of the cervix. In Jordan JA and Singer A (eds): *The Cervix Uteri.* London, WB Saunders, 1976, p 453.

79. **Webb MJ:** Invasive cancer following conservative therapy for previous cervical intraepithelial neoplasia. *Colpo Gynecol Laser Surg* 1:245, 1984.

80. **Anderson MC, Hartley RB:** Cervical crypt involvement by intraepithelial neoplasia. *Obstet Gynecol* 55:546, 1980.

81. **Burke L:** The use of the carbon dioxide laser in cervical intraepithelial neoplasia. *Am J Obstet Gynecol* 144:337, 1982.

82. **Dorsey JH:** Recurrent cervical intraepithelial neoplasia (CIN) and the endocervical button. *Colpo Gynecol Laser Surg* 1:221, 1984.

83. **McIndoe WA, McLean MA, Jones RW, et al:** The invasive potential of carcinoma in situ of the cervis. *Obstet Gynecol* 64:451, 1984.

84. **Murdoch JB, Grimshaw RN, Monaghan JM:** Loop diathermy excision of the abnormal cervical transformation zone. *Int J Gynecol Cancer* 1:105, 1991.

85. **Fu YS, Reagan JW, Richart RM:** Definition of precursors. *Gynecol Oncol* 12:220, 1981.

86. **Meisels A, Fortin R:** Condylomatous lesions of the cervix and vagina. I. Cytologic patterns. *Acta Cytol* 64:451, 1984.

87. **Willett G, Kurman R, Reid R, et al:** Correlation of cervical condylomas and intraepithelial neoplasia with human papillomavirus types. *Int J Gynecol Pathol* 7:350, 1988.

88. **Mitchell H, Drake M, Medley G:** Prospective evaluation of risk of cervical cancer after cytological evidence of human papillomaviral infection. *Lancet* 1:573, 1986.

89. **Nasiell K, Nasiell M, Valcavinkova V:** Behavior of moderate cervical dysplasia during long term follow-up. *Obstet Gynecol* 61:609, 1983.

90. **Becker TM, Wheeler CM, Gouch NM, et al:** Cervical papillomavirus infection and cervical dysplasia in Hispanic, Native American and Non-Hispanic white women in New Mexico. *Am J Public Health* 81:582, 1992.

91. **Reid R, Greenberg MD, Lorincz A, et al:** Should cervical cytologic testing be augmented by cervicography or human papillomavirus deoxyribonucleic acid detection? *Am J Obstet Gynecol* 16:1461, 1991.

92. **Morrison EA, Ho GF, Vermund SH, et al:** Human papillomavirus infection and other risk factors for cervical neoplasia: a case control study. *Int J Cancer* 49:6, 1991.

93. **Koutsky L, Holmes K, Critchlow C, et al:** A cohort study of the risk of cervical intraepithelial neoplasia grade 2 or 3 in relation to papillomavirus infection. *N Eng J Med* 327:1272, 1992.

94. **Reid R:** Biology and colposcopic features of human papillomavirus-associated cervical disease. *Obstet Gynecol Clin Am* 20:123, 1993.

95. **Lorincz A:** Diagnosis of human papillomavirus infection by the new generation of molecular DNA assays. *Clin Immunol Newsletter* 12:123, 1992.

96. **Luesley D, McCrum A, Terry PB, Wade-Evans T:** Complications of cone biopsy related to the dimensions of the cone and the influence of prior colposcopic assessment. *Br J Obstet Gynecol* 92:158, 1985.

97. **Larson G, Gullberg B, Grundsell H:** A comparison of laser and cold knife conization. *Obstet Gynecol* 62:213, 1983.

98. **Jordan JA:** Symposium on cervical neoplasia. I. Excisional methods. *Colpo Gynecol Laser Surg* 1:271, 1984.

99. **Dorsey JH, Diggs ES:** Microsurgical conization of the cervix by carbon dioxide laser. *Obstet Gynecol* 54:565, 1979.

100. **Wright C, Davies E, Riopelle MA:** Laser surgery for cervical intraepithelial neoplasia: principles and results. *Am J Obstet Gynecol* 145:181, 1983.

101. **Indman PD:** Conization of the cervix with CO_2 laser as an office procedure. *J Reprod Med* 30:388, 1985.

102. **Chanen W, Rome RM:** Electrocoagulation diathermy for cervical dysplasia and carcinoma in situ: a 15 year survey. *Obstet Gynecol* 61:673, 1983.

103. **Creasman WT, Hinshaw WM, Clarke-Pearson DL:** Cryosurgery in the management of cervical intraepithelial neoplasia. *Obstet Gynecol* 63:145, 1984.

104. **Ostergard DR:** Cryosurgical treatment of cervical intraepithelial neoplasia. *Obstet Gynecol* 56:233, 1980.

105. **Kaufman RH, Irwin JF:** The cryosurgical therapy of cervical intraepithelial neoplasia. III. Continuing follow-up. *Am J Obstet Gynecol* 131:831, 1978.

106. **Popkin DR, Scali V, Ahmed MN:** Cryosurgery for the treatment of cervical intraepithelial neoplasia. *Am J Obstet Gynecol* 130:551, 1978.

107. **Benedet JL, Nickerson KG, White GW:** Laser therapy for cervical intraepithelial neoplasia. *Obstet Gynecol* 58:188, 1981.

108. **Hatch KD, Shingleton HM, Austin M, et al:** Cryosurgery of cervical intraepithelial neoplasia. *Obstet Gynecol* 57:692, 1981.

109. **Hollyock VE, Chanen W, Wein R:** Cervical function following treatment of intraepithelial neoplasia by electrocoagulation diathermy. *Obstet Gynecol* 61:79, 1982.

110. **Stanhope CR, Phibbs GD, Stewart GC, Reid R:** Carbon dioxide laser surgery. *Obstet Gynecol* 61:624, 1983.

111. **Polanyi TG:** Laser physics: medical applications. *Otolaryngol Clin North Am* 16:753, 1983.

112. **Lipow M:** Laser physics made simple. *Curr Probl Obstet Gynecol Fertil* 9:445, 1986.

113. **Reid R:** Symposium on cervical neoplasia. V. Carbon dioxide laser ablation. *Colpo Gynecol Laser Surg* 1:291, 1984.

114. **Fuller TA:** The physics of surgical lasers. *Lasers Surg Med* 11:5, 1980.

115. **Fuller TA:** Fundamentals of lasers in surgery and medicine. In Dixon JA: *Surgical Applications of Lasers*. Chicago, Yearbook Medical Publishers, 1983, pp 11–28.

116. **Reid R:** Physical and surgical principles governing expertise with the carbon dioxide laser. *Obstet Gynecol North Am* 14:513, 1987.

117. **Fuller TA:** Laser tissue interaction: the influence of power density. In Baggish M (ed): *Basic and Advanced Laser Surgery and Gynecology*. New York, Appleton-Century-Crofts, 1985, pp 51–60.

118. **Reid R:** Physical and surgical principles of laser surgery in the lower genital tract. *Obstet Gynecol Clin North Am* 18:429, 1991.

119. **Reid R, Elson L, Absten G:** A practical guide to laser safety. *Colpo Gynecol Laser Surg* 2:121, 1986.

120. **Burger MPM, Hollema H:** The reliability of the histologic diagnosis in colposcopically directed biopsies. A plea for LETZ. *Int J Gynecol Cancer* 3:385, 1993.

121. **Prendiville W, Cullimore J:** Excision of the transformation zone using the low voltage diathermy (LVD) loop: a superior method of treatment. *Colposc Gynaecol Laser Surg* 3:225, 1987.

122. **Gunasekera PC, Phipps JM, Lewis BV:** Large loop excision of the transformation zone (LLETZ) compared to carbon dioxide laser in the treatment of CIN: a superior mode of treatment. *Br J Obstet Gynaecol* 97:995, 1990.

123. **Prendiville W, Cullimore J, Norman S:** Large loop excision of the transformation zone (LLETZ): a new method of management for women with cervical intraepithelial neoplasia. *Br J Obstet Gynaecol* 96:1054, 1989.

124. **Bigrigg MA, Codling BW, Pearson P, et al:** Colposcopic diagnosis and treatment of cervical dysplasia at a single clinic visit. *Lancet* 2:336:229, 1990.

125. **Luesley DM, Cullimore J, Redman CWE, et al:** Loop diathermy excision of the cervical transformation zone in patients with abnormal cervical smears. *Br Med J* 300:1690, 1990.

239

126. **Whiteley PF, Oláh KS:** Treatment of cervical intraepithelial neoplasia: experience with low voltage diathermy loop. *Am J Obstet Gynecol* 162:1272, 1990.

127. **Murdoch JB, Grimshaw RN, Morgan PR, Monaghan JM:** The impact of loop diathermy on management of early invasive cervical cancer. *Int J Gynecol Cancer* 2:129, 1992.

128. **Mor-Yosef S, Lopes A, Pearson S, Monaghan JM:** Loop diathermy cone biopsy. *Obstet Gynecol* 75:884, 1990.

129. **Wright TC, Richart RM, Ferenczy A, Koulos J:** Comparison of specimens removed by CO_2 laser conization and the loop electrosurgical excision procedure. *Obstet Gynaecol* 79:147, 1992.

130. **Wright T, Richart R, Ferenczy A:** *Electrosurgery for HPV-Related Diseases of the Lower Genital Tract.* New York, Arthur Vision & Anjou, Quebec, Biovision Publishers, 1992, p 127.

131. **Campion MJ:** Natural history and clinical manifestations of HPV infection. *Obstet Gynecol* 14:363, 1988.

132. **Hummer WK, Mussey F, Decker DG, Docherty MB:** Carcinoma in situ of the vagina. *Am J Obstet Gynecol* 108:1109, 1970.

133. **Campion MJ, Clarkson P, McCance DJ:** Squamous neoplasia of the cervix in relation to other genital tract neoplasia. In Singer A (ed): *Clinical Obstetrics and Gynecology.* London, WB Saunders, 1985, pp 265–280.

134. **Pfister H:** Relationship of papillomavirus to anogenital cancer. *Obstet Gynecol Clin North Am* 14:349, 1987.

135. **McCance DJ, Clarkson PK, Dyson JL, et al:** Human papillomavirus types 6 and 16 in multifocal intraepithelial neoplasia of the female lower genital tract. *Br J Obstet Gynaecol* 82:1101, 1985.

136. **Reid R:** Human papillomaviral infection: the key to rational triage of cervical neoplasia. *Obstet Gynecol Clin North Am* 14:407, 1987.

137. **Oriel JD:** Natural history of genital warts. *Br J Vener Dis* 47:1, 1971.

138. **Reid R:** Superficial laser vulvectomy. I. The efficacy of extended superficial ablation for refractory and very extensive condylomas. *Am J Obstet Gynecol* 151:1047, 1985.

139. **Rosenberg SK, Greenberg MD, Reid R:** Sexually transmitted papillomaviral infection in men. *Obstet Gynecol Clin North Am* 14:495, 1987.

140. **Duus BR, Philipsen T, Christensen JD, et al:** Refractory condyloma acuminata: a controlled clinical trial of carbon dioxide laser versus conventional surgical treatment. *Genitourin Med* 61:59, 1985.

141. **Reid R, Elfont EA, Zirkin RM, Fuller TA:** Superficial laser vulvectomy. II. The anatomic and biophysical principles permitting accurate control over the depth of dermal destruction with the carbon dioxide laser. *Am J Obstet Gynecol* 152:261, 1985.

142. **Reid R, Greenberg MD, Lorincz A, et al:** Superficial laser vulvectomy. IV. Extended laser vaporization and adjunctive 5-fluorouracil therapy of human papillomavirus-associated vulvar disease. *Obstet Gynecol* 76:439, 1990.

143. **Sillman FH, Sedlis A, Boyce JG:** A review of lower genital intraepithelial neoplasia and the use of topical 5-fluorouracil. *Obstet Gynecol Surv* 40:190, 1985.

144. **Krebs HB:** Prophylactic topical 5-fluorouracil following treatment of human papillomavirus-associated lesions of the vulva and vagina. *Obstet Gynecol* 68:837, 1986.

145. **Krebs HB:** The use of topical 5-fluorouracil in the treatment of genital condylomata. *Clin Obstet Gynecol* 14:559, 1987.

146. **Friedman-Kien AE, Eron LJ, Conant M, et al:** Natural interferon alpha for treatment of condylomata acuminata. *JAMA* 259:533, 1988.

147. **Gall SA, Hughes CE, Troffatter K:** Interferon for the therapy of condyloma acuminatum. *Am J Obstet Gynecol* 153:157, 1985.

148. **Gall SA, Hughes CE, Mounts P, et al:** Efficacy of human lymphoblastoid interferon in the therapy of resistant condylomas acuminata. *Obstet Gynecol* 67:643, 1986.

149. **Reid R, Greenberg MD, Pizzuti, et al:** Superficial laser vulvectomy. V. Surgical debulking is enhanced by adjuvant systemic interferon. *Am J Obstet Gynecol* 166:815, 1992.

150. **Dorsey JH, Baggish MS:** Multifocal vaginal intraepithelial neoplasia with uterus in situ. In Sharp F, Jordan JA (eds): *Gynaecological Laser Surgery*. Proceedings of the 15th Study Group of the Royal College of Obstetricians and Gynaecologists. Ithaca, New York, Perinatology Press, 1985, p 173.

151. **Rutledge F:** Cancer of the vagina. *Am J Obstet Gynecol* 97:635, 1967.

152. **Woodman C, Jordan JA, Wade-Evans T:** The management of vaginal intraepithelial neoplasia after hysterectomy. *Br J Obstet Gynaecol* 138:321, 1980.

153. **Schmauz R, Owor R:** Epidemiology of malignant degeneration of condylomata acuminata in Uganda. *Pathol Res Pract* 170:91, 1980.

154. **Jordan JA, Sharp F:** CO_2 laser treatment of vaginal intraepithelial neoplasia. In Sharp F, Jordan JA (eds): *Gynaecology Laser Surgery*. Proceedings of the 15th Study Group of the Royal College of Obstetricians and Gynaecologists, Ithaca, New York, Perinatology Press, 1985, p 181.

155. **Buscema J, Woodruff JD, Parmley T, Genadry R:** Carcinoma in situ of the vulva. *Obstet Gynecol* 55:225, 1980.

156. **Friedrich EG, Wilkinson EJ, Fu YS:** Carcinoma in situ of the vulva: a continuing challenge. *Am J Obstet Gynecol* 136:880, 1980.

157. **zur Hausen H:** Human papillomaviruses and their possible role in squamous cell carcinomas. *Curr Top Microbiol Immunol* 78:1, 1977.

158. **Park JS, Kurman R, Schiffman M, et al:** Basaloid and warty carcinoma of the vulva: distinctive types of squamous carcinoma with human papillomavirus. *Lab Invest* 1:62, 1991.

159. **Rutledge F, Sinclair M:** Treatment of intraepithelial carcinoma of the vulva by skin excision and graft. *Am J Obstet Gynecol* 102:806, 1968.

160. **Chafee W, Ferguson K, Wilkinson EJ:** Vulvar intraepithelial neoplasia (VIN); principles of surgical therapy. *Colpo Gynecol Surg* 4:125, 1988.

161. **Friedrich EG Jr, Wilkinson EJ, Fu YW:** Carcinoma in situ of the vulva; a continuing challenge. *Am J Obstet Gynecol* 136:830, 1980.

162. **DiSaia PJ:** Management of superficially invasive vulvar carcinoma. *Clin Obstet Gynecol* 28:196, 1985.

163. **Reid R:** Physical and surgical principles governing expertise with the carbon dioxide laser. *Obstet Gynecol Clin North Am* 14:407, 1987.

164. **McConnell EM:** Squamous carcinoma of the anus: a review of 96 cases. *Br J Surg* 57:89, 1973.

165. **Daling JR, Weiss NS, Klopfenstein LL, et al:** Correlates of homosexual behavior and the incidence of anal cancer. *JAMA* 247:1988, 1982.

166. **Frazer IH, Medley G, Crapper RM, et al:** Association between anorectal dysplasia, human papillomavirus and human immunodeficiency virus infection in homosexual men. *Lancet* 2:657, 1986.

167. **Ferenczy A, Mitao M, Nagai N, et al:** Latent papillomavirus and recurring genital warts. *N Engl J Med* 313:784, 1985.

168. **Reid R:** Superficial laser vulvectomy. III. A new surgical technique for appendage-conserving ablation of refractory condylomas and vulvar intraepithelial neoplasia. *Am J Obstet Gynecol* 152:504, 1985.

Cervical Cancer

Kenneth D. Hatch

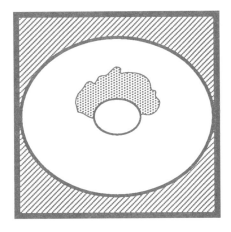

Invasive cancer of the cervix has been considered a preventable cancer because it has a long preinvasive state, cervical cytology screening programs are available, and the treatment for preinvasive lesions is effective. However, 15,000 new cases of invasive cervical cancer and approximately 4600 deaths were anticipated in the United States in 1994 (1). Although cervical cancer has not been eliminated, the incidence of invasive disease is decreasing, and it is being diagnosed earlier, leading to better survival rates (1, 2). The mean age for cervical cancer is 52.2 years, and the distribution of cases is bimodal, with peaks at 35–39 years and 60–64 years (1).

Diagnosis

Vaginal bleeding is the most common symptom occurring in patients with cancer of the cervix. Most often this is postcoital bleeding, but it may occur as irregular or postmenopausal bleeding. Patients with advanced disease may have a malodorous vaginal discharge, weight loss, or obstructive uropathy.

On general physical examination, the supraclavicular and groin lymph nodes should be palpated to exclude metastatic disease. On pelvic examination, a speculum is placed and the cervix is inspected for suspicious areas. The vagina is inspected for extension of disease. With invasive cancer, the cervix is usually firm and expanded, and these features should be evaluated on digital examination. Rectal examination is important to help establish cervical consistency and size, particularly in patients with endocervical carcinomas. It is the only way to determine cervical size if the vaginal fornices have been obliterated by menopausal changes or by the extension of disease. Parametrial extension of disease is best determined by the finding of nodularity beyond the cervix on rectal examination.

When obvious tumor growth is present, an outpatient cervical biopsy is usually sufficient for diagnosis. The colposcope may be helpful in directing the examiner

243

toward the most invasive area for biopsy. If the diagnosis cannot be made conclusively with outpatient biopsy, diagnostic conization may be necessary.

Colposcopy of the Invasive Lesion

For patients with suspected early invasive cancer on Pap smear and a grossly normal-appearing cervix, colposcopic examination is mandatory. **Colposcopically directed biopsies may permit the diagnosis of frank invasion and thus avoid a diagnostic cone biopsy, allowing the physician to proceed directly to treatment.**

Colposcopic findings that suggest invasion are:

1. Abnormal blood vessels

2. Irregular surface contour with loss of surface epithelium

3. Color tone change

Abnormal Blood Vessels The vessels may be looped, branching, or reticular. *Abnormal looped vessels* are the most common and arise from the *punctation* and *mosaic* vessels present in cervical intraepithelial neoplasia (CIN). As the neoplastic growth process proceeds, the need for nutrition leads to proliferation of the blood vessels, and the punctate vessels at the surface produce double and triple loops.

These surface tufting vessels then proliferate and push out over the surface of the epithelium in an erratic fashion. Some are straight, although most have a loop, a corkscrew, of a J-shaped pattern (Fig. 7.1).

Figure 7.1. Abnormal looped vessels in invasive cervical cancer.

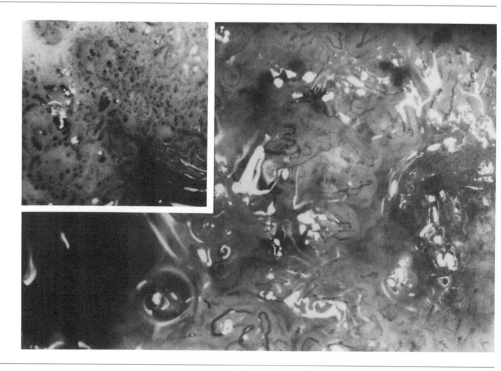

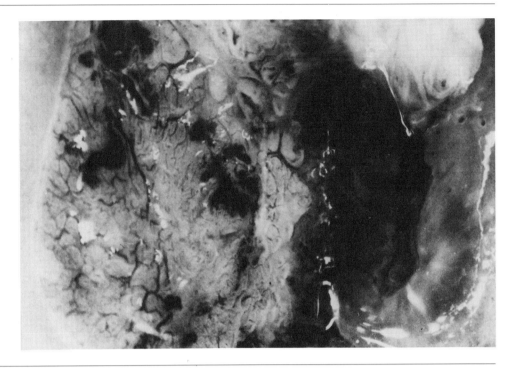

Figure 7.2. Abnormal branching vessels in invasive cervical cancer.

Abnormal branching vessels arise from the cervical stroma and are pushed to the surface as the underlying cancer invades and pushes upward. The normally branching cervical stromal vessels are best observed over nabothian cysts. Here the branches are generally at acute angles, with the caliber of vessels becoming smaller after branching, much like the arborization of a tree. The abnormal branching blood vessels seen with cancer tend to form obtuse or right angles, with the caliber sometimes enlarging after branching (Fig. 7.2). Sharp turns, dilatations, and narrowings also mark the behavior of these vessels. The surface epithelium may be lost in these areas, leading to irregular surface contour and friability.

Abnormal reticular vessels represent the terminal capillaries of the cervical epithelium. Normal capillaries are best seen in a postmenopausal woman with atrophic epithelium. When cancer involves this epithelium, the surface is again eroded, and the capillary network is exposed. These vessels are very fine, short, and composed of small commas without an organized pattern (Fig. 7.3). They are not specific for invasive cancer, as atrophic cervicitis may also have this appearance.

Irregular Surface Contour Abnormal surface patterns are observed as the tumor growth proceeds. The surface epithelium ulcerates as the cells lose intercellular cohesiveness secondary to the loss of desmosomes. Irregular contour also may occur because of a papillary characteristic of the lesion (Fig. 7.4). **This sometimes can be confused with a human papillomavirus papillary growth on the cervix, and for that reason biopsies should be performed on all papillary cervical growths.**

Color Tone Change Color tone may change as a result of the increasing vascularity, surface epithelial necrosis, and in some cases production of keratin. The

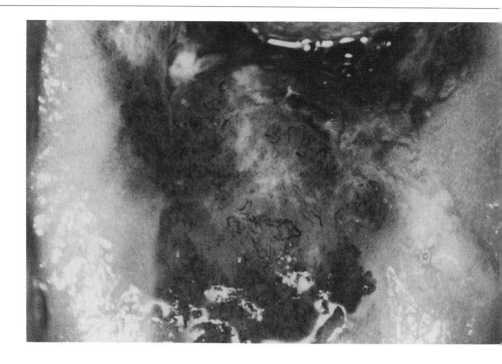

Figure 7.3. Abnormal reticular vessels in invasive cervical cancer.

color tone is a yellow-orange rather than the expected pink of intact squamous epithelium or the red of the endocervical epithelium.

Adenocarcinoma Adenocarcinoma of the cervix does not have a specific colposcopic appearance. All of the blood vessels described above may be seen in these lesions as well. **Because adenocarcinomas tend to develop within the endocervix, an endocervical curettage is required as part of the colposcopic examination.**

Staging

Clinical Staging

The current staging system of the International Federation of Gynecology and Obstetrics (FIGO) is presented in Table 7.1. The staging procedures allowed by FIGO are listed in Table 7.2.

When there is doubt concerning the stage to which a cancer should be allocated, the earlier stage is mandatory. Once a clinical stage is assigned and treatment has been initiated, the stage must not be changed because of subsequent findings by either extended clinical staging or surgical staging. The "upstaging" of patients during treatment will erroneously produce an apparent improvement in the results of treatment of low-stage disease. The distribution of patients by clinical stage is 38% Stage I, 32% Stage II, 26% Stage III, and 4% Stage IV (2).

Extended Clinical Staging Lymphangiography, computerized axial tomography (CT), sonography, and magnetic resonance imaging (MRI) have been used by various investigators in an attempt to improve clinical staging (3–8). Because these tests are not generally available throughout the world and because the

246

interpretation of results is variable, the findings of these studies are not used for assigning the FIGO stage. However, they may be used in planning therapy.

Evaluation of the para-aortic lymph nodes with lymphangiography is associated with a false-positive rate of 20–40% and a false-negative rate of 10–20% (3–5). The accuracy of CT scans is 80–85%, with a false-negative rate of 10–15% and a false-positive rate of 20–25% (6–8). Early MRI data are comparable (9). When abnormalities are noted by these procedures, a fine needle aspiration (FNA) showing metastatic disease will allow the radiation treatment field to be extended and obviate the need for an exploratory laparotomy to determine the status of the lymph nodes.

Surgical Staging   The accuracy of clinical staging is somewhat limited, and surgical evaluation, which is not practical or feasible in many patients, is more accurate. The specifics of surgical staging are discussed later in this chapter.

Patterns of Spread

Cancer of the cervix spreads by:

1. Direct invasion into the cervical stroma, corpus, vagina, and parametrium

2. Lymphatic metastasis

3. Blood-borne metastasis

4. Intraperitoneal implantation

The incidence of pelvic and para-aortic nodal metastasis is shown in Table 7.3.

Figure 7.4.   Irregular surface growth in invasive cervical cancer.

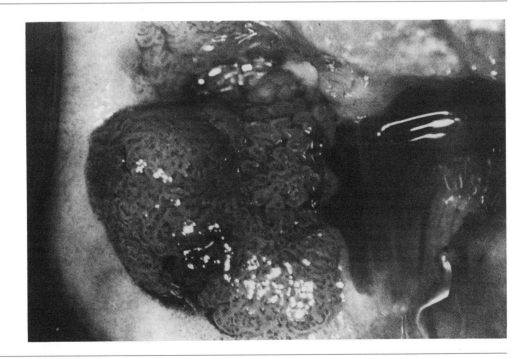

Table 7.1   FIGO Staging of Carcinoma of the Cervix Uteri

Preinvasive Carcinoma

Stage 0   Carcinoma *in situ,* intraepithelial carcinoma (cases of Stage 0 should not be included in any therapeutic statistics).

Invasive Carcinoma

Stage I*   Carcinoma strictly confined to the cervix (extension to the corpus should be disregarded).

Stage Ia   Preclinical carcinomas of the cervix, that is, those diagnosed only by microscopy.

Stage Ia1   Minimal microscopically evident stromal invasion.

Stage Ia2   Lesions detected microscopically that can be measured. The upper limit of the measurement should not show a depth of invasion of more than 5 mm taken from the base of the epithelium, either surface or glandular, from which it originates, and a second dimension, the horizontal spread, must not exceed 7 mm. Larger lesions should be staged as Ib.

Stage Ib   Lesions of greater dimensions than Stage Ia2 whether seen clinically or not. Preformed space involvement should not alter the staging but should be specifically recorded so as to determine whether it should affect treatment decisions in the future.

Stage II†   The carcinoma extends beyond the cervix but has not extended on to the wall. The carcinoma involves the vagina, but not the lower third.

Stage IIa   No obvious parametrial involvement.

Stage IIb   Obvious parametrial involvement.

Stage III‡   The carcinoma has extended on to the pelvic wall. On rectal examination, there is no cancer-free space between the tumor and the pelvic wall. The tumor involves the lower third of the vagina. All cases with hydronephrosis or nonfunctioning kidney.

Stage IIIa   No extension to the pelvic wall.

Stage IIIb   Extension on to the pelvic wall and/or hydronephrosis or nonfunctioning kidney.

Stage IV‡   The carcinoma has extended beyond the true pelvis or has clinically involved the mucosa of the bladder or rectum. A bullous edema as such does not permit a case to be allotted to Stage IV.

Stage IVa   Spread of the growth to adjacent organs.

Stage IVb   Spread to distant organs.

---

*Stage Ia carcinoma should include minimal microscopically evident stromal invasion as well as small cancerous tumors of measurable size. Stage Ia should be subdivided into those lesions with minute foci of invasion visible only microscopically as Stage Ia1 and the macroscopically measurable microcarcinomas as Stage Ia2 to gain further knowledge of the clinical behavior of these lesions. The term Ib occult should be omitted.

The diagnosis of both Stage Ia1 and Ia2 should be based on microscopic examination of removed tissue, preferably a cone, which must include the entire lesion. As noted above, the lower limit of Stage Ia2 should be that it can be measured macroscopically (even if dots need to be placed on the slide before measurement) and the upper limit of Ia2 is given by measurement of the two largest dimensions in any given section. The depth of invasion should not be more than 5 mm taken from the base of the epithelium, either surface or glandular, from which it originates. The second dimension, the horizontal spread, must not exceed 7 mm. Vascular space involvement, either venous or lymphatic, should not alter the staging but should be specifically recorded as it may affect treatment decisions in the future. Lesions of greater size should be staged as Ib. As a rule, it is impossible to estimate clinically whether a cancer of the cervix has extended to the corpus. Extension to the corpus should therefore be disregarded.

†A patient with a growth fixed to the pelvic wall by a short and indurated, but not nodular, parametrium should be allotted to Stage IIb. At clinical examination, it is impossible to decide whether a smooth, indurated parametrium is truly cancerous or only inflammatory. Therefore, the case should be assigned to Stage III only if the parametrium is nodular to the pelvic wall or the growth itself extends to the pelvic wall. The presence of hydronephrosis or nonfunctioning kidney due to stenosis of the ureter by cancer permits a case to be allotted to Stage III even if, according to other findings, it should be allotted to Stage I or II.

‡The presence of the bullous edema as such should not permit a case to be allotted to Stage IV. Ridges and furrows into the bladder wall should be interpreted as signs of submucous involvement of the bladder if they remain fixed to the growth at palpation (i.e., examination from the vagina or the rectum during cystoscopy). A cytologic finding of malignant cells in washings from the urinary bladder requires further examination and a biopsy specimen from the wall of the bladder.

Table 7.2   Staging Procedures

Physical examination*	Palpate lymph nodes Examine vagina Bimanual rectovaginal examination (under anesthesia recommended)
Radiologic studies*	Intravenous pyelogram Barium enema Chest x-ray Skeletal x-ray
Procedures*	Biopsy Conization Hysteroscopy Colposcopy Endocervical curettage Cystoscopy Proctoscopy
Optional studies†	Computerized axial tomography Lymphangiography Ultrasonography Magnetic resonance imaging Radionucleotide scanning Laparoscopy

*Allowed by FIGO.
†Information that is not allowed by FIGO to change the clinical stage.

Table 7.3   Incidence of Pelvic and Para-aortic Nodal Metastasis by Stage

Stage	n	% Positive Pelvic Nodes	% Positive Paraaortic Nodes
Ia1	23*	0	0
Ia2 (1–3 mm)	156†	0.6%	0
(3–5 mm)	84†	4.8%	<1%
Ib	1926††	15.9%	2.2%
IIa	110§	24.5%	11%
IIb	324§	31.4%	19%
III	125§	44.8%	30%
IVa	23§	55%	40%

*References 15, 42.
†References 14, 15, 41, 42.
††References 4, 23, 28, 29, 31, 33, 35, 50.
§References 3, 4, 23, 33, 47, 50.

Treatment

The principles of treatment for cancer of the cervix are those of any other malignancy; i.e., both the primary lesion and the potential sites of spread should be treated.

The two modalities for primary treatment are surgery and radiotherapy. Whereas radiation therapy can be used in all stages of disease, surgery alone is limited to patients with Stage I and IIa disease. The 5-year survival rate for Stage I cancer of the cervix is approximately 85% with either radiation therapy or radical hysterectomy.

249

There are advantages to using surgical therapy instead of radiotherapy, particularly in the younger age group for whom conservation of the ovaries is important. Chronic bladder and bowel problems that require medical or surgical intervention occur in up to 8% of patients undergoing radiation therapy (10). Such problems are difficult to treat because they result from fibrosis and decreased vascularity. This is in contrast to the surgical injuries, which in general are easily repairable and without long-term complications. Sexual dysfunction after radiation therapy is more likely to occur because of vaginal shortening, fibrosis, and atrophy of the epithelium. The surgical approach shortens the vagina, but gradual lengthening is brought about by sexual activity. The epithelium does not become atrophic because it responds either to the patient's endogenous estrogen or to exogenous estrogens if the patient is postmenopausal.

In general, radical hysterectomy is reserved for women who are in good physical condition. Chronologic age should not be a deterrent. With better anesthesia, elderly patients withstand radical surgery almost as well as their younger counterparts (11).

Generally, it is prudent not to operate primarily on lesions that are >4 cm in diameter. When selected in this manner, the urinary fistula rate is <2% (12) and the operative mortality rate is <1% (13). An advantage of radiotherapy is its applicability to all stages and to most patients regardless of their age, size, and medical condition.

Surgical Therapy

Stage Ia—Microinvasive Carcinoma

Until 1985 there was no FIGO recommendation concerning the size of lesion or the depth of invasion that should be considered microinvasive (Stage Ia). This led to considerable confusion and controversy in the literature. Over the years, as many as 18 different definitions have been used to describe "microinvasion." In 1974 the Society of Gynecologic Oncologists (SGO) recommended a definition that is in common use today:

"A microinvasive lesion is one in which neoplastic epithelium invades the stroma to a depth ≤3 mm beneath the basement membrane and in which lymphatic or blood vascular involvement is not demonstrated." The purpose of defining microinvasion is to identify a group of patients who are not at risk of lymph node metastases or recurrence and who therefore may be treated with less than radical therapy. Diagnosis must be based on a cone biopsy of the cervix. Because the treatment decision rests with the gynecologist, treatment must be based on a review of the conization specimen with the pathologist. It is important to have the pathologic condition described in terms of:

1. Depth of invasion

2. Width and breadth of the invasive area

3. Presence or absence of lymphatic vascular space invasion

These variables are used to determine how extensive the operation should be and whether the regional lymph nodes should be treated.

Stage Ia1—Early Stromal Invasion

A group of patients with invasion ≤1 mm in depth with isolated projections arising at the base of carcinoma in situ (CIS) has been defined by Lohe et al. (14). Lymph vascular space invasion is rare in these patients, and lymph node metastases are extremely rare. The width of the invasive prongs is generally less than their depth.

In the absence of lymph vascular space invasion, patients may be treated with cone biopsy or simple hysterectomy. If a therapeutic conization is performed, the surgical margins must be free of disease.

Stage Ia2—≤5 mm Invasion

When the depth of invasion exceeds 1 mm, the incidence of lymph vascular space invasion increases and the risk of pelvic node metastasis increases.

1–3 mm Invasion **Lesions with invasion between 1 and 3 mm in depth have a less than 1% incidence of pelvic node metastases.** Although this is still controversial, it appears that the patients most at risk of nodal metastases or central pelvic recurrence are those with definitive evidence of tumor emboli in lymph vascular spaces (15, 16).

Therefore patients with invasion between 1 and 3 mm and no lymph vascular space invasion may be treated with extrafascial hysterectomy without node dissection. Therapeutic conization appears to be adequate therapy for this group if childbearing capability is desired. Surgical margins must be free of disease. If there is lymph vascular space invasion, an alternative would be a pelvic node dissection together with a type I or II hysterectomy.

3–5 mm Invasion **Lesions with invasion between 3 and 5 mm have a 3.8% incidence of pelvic node metastases** (16, 17); thus pelvic node dissection is necessary in this group. The primary tumor may be treated with a modified radical hysterectomy (type II).

Stage Ib/IIa Invasive Cancer	**Surgical therapy of Stage Ib and IIa carcinoma of the cervix involves radical hysterectomy, pelvic lymphadenectomy, and para-aortic lymph node evaluation.**

Types of Hysterectomy

Modified Radical Hysterectomy (Type II) The hysterectomy described by Wertheim is less extensive than a radical hysterectomy and removes the medial half of the cardinal ligaments and the uterosacral ligaments (18). This is commonly referred to as the modified radical or type II hysterectomy. Wertheim's original

251

Table 7.4 Surgical Management of Early Invasive Cancer of the Cervix

Stage Ia1	*Early stromal invasion (<1 mm)*	Conization Type I hysterectomy
Stage Ia2	*1–3 mm invasion* No lymph-vascular space invasion With lymph-vascular space invasion	Conization Type I hysterectomy Type I or II hysterectomy with (?) pelvic lymph node dissection
	3–5 mm invasion	Type II hysterectomy with pelvic lymphadenectomy
Stage Ib	*>5 mm invasion*	Type III hysterectomy with pelvic lymphadenectomy

operation did not include a pelvic lymph node dissection but, rather, selective removal of enlarged lymph nodes.

Radical Hysterectomy (Type III) The radical hysterectomy performed most often in this country is that described by Meigs (19) in 1944. The operation includes a pelvic lymph node dissection along with removal of most of the uterosacral and cardinal ligaments and the upper third of the vagina. Piver and Rutledge (18) have referred to this operation as the type III radical hysterectomy.

A summary of the surgical management of early cervical cancer is presented in Table 7.4.

Further classification of radical hysterectomies is as follows:

Extended Radical Hysterectomy (Type IV) In the type IV operation, the periureteral tissue, superior vesicle artery, and up to three-fourths of the vagina are removed (18).

Partial Exenteration (Type V) In the type V operation, portions of the distal ureter and bladder are resected. These procedures are rarely performed because radiotherapy should be used if such extensive disease is encountered (18).

Radical Hysterectomy and Pelvic Node Dissection

Incision The abdomen is opened through either a midline incision or a low transverse incision after the methods of Maylard or Cherney. The low transverse incision, which is described in Chapter 15, requires division of the rectus muscles and provides excellent exposure of the lateral pelvis. It allows adequate pelvic node dissection and wide resection of the primary tumor.

Exploration After the abdomen is entered, the peritoneal cavity is explored to exclude metastatic disease. The stomach is palpated to make certain that it has been decompressed to facilitate packing of the intestines. The liver is palpated, and the omentum is inspected for metastases. Both kidneys are palpated to ensure their proper placement and lack of congenital and other abnormalities. The para-aortic nodes are palpated transperitoneally.

During exploration of the pelvis, the fallopian tubes and ovaries are inspected for any abnormalities. In the patient who is less than 40 years of age, the ovaries

252

are generally conserved. The peritoneum of the vesicouterine fold and the rectouterine pouch should be inspected for signs of tumor extension or implantation. The cervix is then palpated between the thumb anteriorly and the fingers posteriorly to determine its extent, and the cardinal ligaments are palpated for evidence of lateral tumor extension or nodularity.

Para-aortic Lymph Node Evaluation   If the patient has no evidence of disease extending beyond the cervix or vaginal fornix, i.e., "surgical Stage Ib or IIa," the operation proceeds. The bowel is packed so as to expose the peritoneum overlying the bifurcation of the aorta. The peritoneum is incised medial to the ureter and over the right common iliac artery. A retractor is placed retroperitoneally to expose the aorta and the vena cava.

Any enlarged para-aortic lymph nodes are dissected, hemoclips are applied for hemostasis, and specimens are sent for frozen section. If the lymph nodes are positive for metastatic cancer, an option is to discontinue the operation and use radiation therapy (19). If the lymph nodes are negative for disease, the left side of the aorta is palpated through the peritoneal incision with a finger passed under the inferior mesenteric artery. The lymph nodes on this side of the aorta are more lateral and nearly behind the aorta and the common iliac artery (Fig. 7.5). If the left para-aortic lymph nodes are not clinically suspicious and the cervical tumor is small with no suspicious pelvic lymph nodes, these additional lymph nodes are not submitted for frozen section. If they are removed, they may be dissected through the incision made for the right para-aortic nodes, or they may be dissected after reflection of the sigmoid colon medially.

Pelvic Lymphadenectomy   The pelvic lymphadenectomy can proceed at this time, or it can be deferred until the hysterectomy has been completed. This is a matter of preference for the operating surgeon. The surgeon begins the pelvic lymph node dissection by opening the round ligaments at the pelvic sidewall and developing the paravesical and pararectal spaces. The ureter is elevated on the medial flap by a Deaver retractor to expose the common iliac artery. The common iliac and external iliac nodes are dissected, with care taken not to injure the genitofemoral nerve, which lies laterally on the psoas muscle. At the bifurcation of the common iliac artery, the external iliac node chain is divided into a lateral and a medial portion.

The lateral chain is stripped free from the artery to the circumflex iliac vein distally. A hemoclip is placed across the distal portion of the lymph node chain to reduce the incidence of lymphocyst formation. The medial chain is then dissected. The obturator lymph nodes are dissected next; for this the lymph nodes are grasped just under the external iliac vein and traction is applied medially. Although the majority of patients have both the obturator artery and vein dorsal to the obturator nerve, 10% will have an aberrant vein arising from the external iliac vein. The node chain is separated from the nerve and vessels and clipped caudally. They are dissected cephalad to the hypogastric artery. The cephalad portion of the obturator space should be entered lateral to the external iliac artery and medial to the psoas muscle, where the remainder of the obturator node tissue can be dissected as far cephalad as the common iliac artery.

Development of Pelvic Spaces   The pelvic spaces are developed by sharp and blunt dissection (Fig. 7.6).

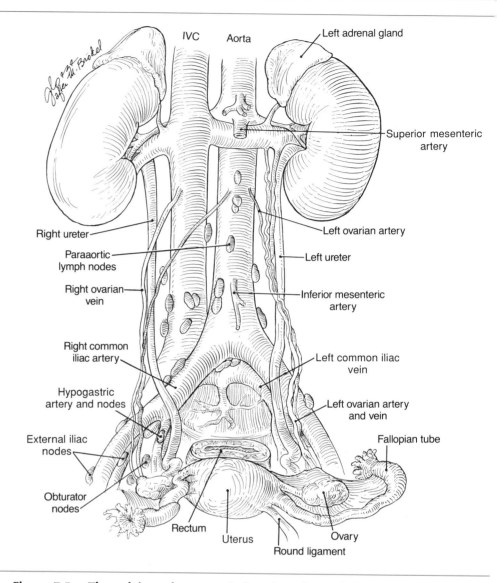

Figure 7.5.   The pelvic and paraaortic lymph nodes and their relationship to the major retroperitoneal vessels. (Reproduced, with permission, from Hacker NF, Moore JG (eds): *Essentials of Obstetrics and Gynecology.* Philadelphia, WB Saunders, 1986, p 8.)

The paravesical space is bordered by:

1. The obliterated umbilical artery running along the bladder medially

2. The obturator internus muscle along the pelvic sidewall laterally

3. The cardinal ligament posteriorly

4. The pubic symphysis anteriorly

The attachments of the vagina to the tendinous arch form the floor of the paravesicle space.

The pararectal space is bordered by:

254

1. The rectum medially

2. The cardinal ligament anteriorly

3. The hypogastric artery laterally

4. The sacrum posteriorly

The coccygeus (levator ani) muscle forms the floor of the pararectal space.

Takedown of the Bladder   A critical step is the dissection of the bladder from the anterior part of the cervix and vagina. Occasionally, tumor extension into the base of the bladder (which cannot be detected with cystoscopy) precludes adequate mobilization of the bladder flap, leading to the abandonment of the operation. Therefore, this portion of the operation should be undertaken early in the procedure.

Dissection of the Uterine Artery   The superior vesicle artery is dissected away from the cardinal ligament at a point near the uterine artery. The uterine artery, which usually arises from the superior vesicle artery, is thus isolated and divided while the vesicle arteries are preserved. The uterine vessels are then brought over the ureter by application of gentle traction. Occasionally, the uterine vein will pass under the ureter.

Dissection of the Ureter   The ureter is dissected free from its medial peritoneal flap at the level of the uterosacral ligament. As the ureter passes near the uterine

Figure 7.6.   The pelvic ligaments and spaces.

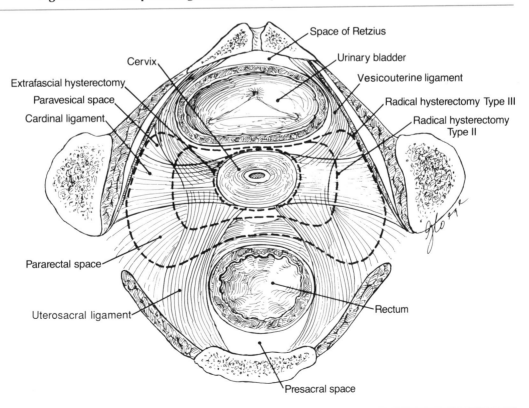

255

artery, there is a consistent branch from the uterine artery to the ureter. This is sacrificed in the standard radical (type III) hysterectomy but preserved in the modified radical (type II) hysterectomy.

Dissection of the ureter from the vesicouterine ligament (ureteral tunnel) now may be accomplished. If the patient has a deep pelvis, ligation of the uterosacral and cardinal ligaments may be undertaken first in order to bring the ureteral tunnel dissection closer to the operator. The roof of the ureteral tunnel is the anterior vesicouterine ligament. It should be ligated and divided to expose the posterior ligament. This ligament is also divided in the radical (type III) hysterectomy but conserved in the modified radical (type II) hysterectomy (Fig. 7.7).

Posterior Dissection The peritoneum across the cul-de-sac is incised, exposing the uterosacral ligaments. The rectum is rolled free from the uterosacral ligaments, and these ligaments are divided midway to the sacrum in a radical (type III) hysterectomy and near the rectum in the modified radical (type II) operation. This allows the operator to develop the cardinal ligament separate from the rectum. A surgical clamp is placed on the cardinal ligament at the lateral pelvic sidewall in a radical hysterectomy and at the level of the ureteral bed in the modified radical procedure. A clamp is placed on the specimen side to maintain traction and is left on to ensure that the full cardinal ligament is excised with the specimen. A right-angled clamp then is placed caudad to this clamp across the paravaginal tissues. A second paravaginal clamp is usually needed to reach the vagina.

Vagina The vagina is entered anteriorly, and the upper third of the vagina is removed with the specimen. More vaginal epithelium can be excised if necessary,

Figure 7.7. Radical hysterectomy. Uterine artery is ligated, ureter is dissected, and sites for division of the vesicouterine and uterosacral ligaments are shown.

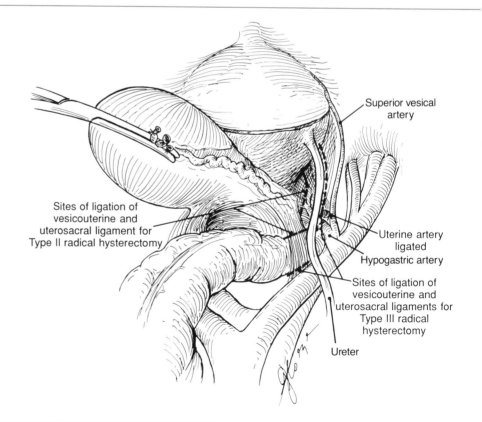

Superior vesical artery

Sites of ligation of vesicouterine and uterosacral ligament for Type II radical hysterectomy

Uterine artery ligated
Hypogastric artery

Sites of ligation of vesicouterine and uterosacral ligaments for Type III radical hysterectomy

Ureter

depending on the previous colposcopic findings. The vaginal edge may be sutured in a hemostatic fashion and left open with a drain from the pelvic space or closed with a suction drain placed percutaneously. The ureteral fistula and pelvic lymphocyst rates from these two techniques are similar.

Modified Radical Hysterectomy

The modified radical hysterectomy differs from the radical hysterectomy in the following ways:

1. The uterine artery is transected at the level of the ureter, thus preserving the ureteral branch to the ureter.

2. The cardinal ligament is not divided near the sidewall but instead is divided at approximately its midportion near the ureteral dissection.

3. The anterior vesicouterine ligament is divided, but the posterior vesicouterine ligament is conserved.

4. A smaller margin of vagina is removed.

Complications of Radical Hysterectomy

Acute Complications   The acute complications (15) include:

1. Blood loss (average 0.8 liter)

2. Ureterovaginal fistula (1–2%)

3. Vesicovaginal fistula (<1%)

4. Pulmonary embolus (1–2%)

5. Small-bowel obstruction (1%)

6. Febrile morbidity (25–50%)

The febrile morbidity is most often pulmonary (10%), with pelvic cellulitis (7%) and urinary tract infection (6%) seen frequently. Wound infection, pelvic abscess, and phlebitis all occur in fewer than 5% of patients (20).

Subacute Complications   The subacute effects of radical hysterectomy are postoperative bladder dysfunction and lymphocyst formation. For the first few days after radical hysterectomy, the patient's bladder volume is decreased and the filling pressure is increased. The sensitivity to filling is diminished and the patient is unable to initiate voiding. The cause of this dysfunction is unclear.

It is important to maintain adequate bladder drainage during this time to prevent overdistention. Bladder drainage is best accomplished with a suprapubic catheter. It is more comfortable for the patient and allows the physician to perform a cystometrogram and determine residual urine without the need for frequent catheterization. In addition, the patient is able to accomplish trial voiding at home by clamping the catheter, voiding, and releasing to check the residual. A cystometrogram may be performed 3 to 4 weeks postoperatively. The patient must be able to sense the fullness of the bladder, initiate voiding, and void with a residual urine of <75 ml for use of the catheter to be discontinued. If she cannot, voiding trials at home should ensue until this can be accomplished.

Lymphocyst formation occurs in fewer than 5% of patients (21), and the cause is uncertain. Adequate drainage of the pelvis after radical hysterectomy may be an important step in prevention. Ureteral obstruction and partial venous obstruction and thrombosis may occur from lymphocyst formation. Simple aspiration of the lymphocyst is generally not curative, but percutaneous catheters with chronic drainage may allow healing. If this is unsuccessful, operative intervention with excision of a portion of the lymphocyst wall and placement of either large bowel or omentum into the lymphocyst should be performed.

Chronic Complications The most common chronic effect of radical hysterectomy is *bladder hypotonia* or, in extreme instances, *atony*. This occurs in approximately 3% of patients, regardless of the method of bladder drainage (22, 23). It may be a result of bladder denervation and not simply a problem associated with bladder overdistention (24). Voiding every 4 to 6 hours by the clock, increasing intraabdominal pressure with the Credé's maneuver, and intermittent self-catheterization may be used to manage the hypotonic bladder.

Ureteral strictures are uncommon in the absence of postoperative radiation therapy, recurrent cancer, or lymphocyst formation (12). If the stricture is associated with lymphocyst formation, treatment of the lymphocyst will usually alleviate the problem. Strictures after radiation therapy should be managed with ureteral stenting. If a ureteral stricture is noted in the absence of radiotherapy or lymphocyst formation, recurrent carcinoma is the most common cause. A CT scan of the area of obstruction should be obtained and FNA cytology should be performed to exclude carcinoma if there is a target lesion. If these tests are negative, a ureteral stent may be placed to relieve the stricture. Close observation for recurrent carcinoma is necessary, and diagnosis of recurrence may ultimately require laparotomy.

Results of Surgical Therapy

The survival of patients after radical hysterectomy and pelvic lymphadenectomy is dependent on (15, 25–39):

1. The status of the lymph nodes

2. The size of tumor

3. Involvement of paracervical tissues

4. The depth of invasion

5. The presence or absence of lymph vascular space invasion

Lymph Nodes The most dependent variable associated with survival is the status of the lymph nodes. **Patients with negative nodes will have an 85–90% 5-year survival rate** (38, 40), **whereas the survival rate for those with positive nodes ranges from 20% to 74%, depending on the number of nodes involved, the location, and the size of the metastases** (34–36, 40–43).

Other data on lymph node status can be summarized as follows:

1. When the common iliac lymph nodes are positive, the 5-year survival is about 25% versus about 65% when the pelvic lymph nodes only are involved (44–46).

2. Bilateral positive pelvic lymph nodes portend a worse prognosis (22–40% survival rate) than unilateral positive pelvic nodes (59–70%) (44, 45).

3. More than three positive pelvic lymph nodes is accompanied by a 68% recurrence rate, versus 30–50% when three or fewer lymph nodes are positive (34, 41).

4. Patients in whom tumor emboli are the only findings in the positive pelvic lymph node have an 82.5% 5-year survival rate, whereas the survival rate with microscopic invasion of the lymph nodes is 62.1% and that with macroscopic disease is 54% (25).

The influence of the addition of postoperative radiotherapy on survival is discussed below.

Lesion Size   Lesion size is an independent predictor of survival. Patients with lesions <2 cm have approximately a 90% survival rate, and those with lesions >2 cm have a 60% survival rate (28). When the primary tumor is >4 cm, the survival rate drops to 40% (26, 37). An analysis of a Gynecologic Oncology Group (GOG) prospective study of 645 patients shows a 94.6% 3-year disease-free survival rate for patients with occult lesions, 85.5% for those with tumors <3 cm, and 68.4% for patients with tumors >3 cm (38).

Depth of Invasion   Patients in whom the depth of invasion is <1 cm have a 5-year survival rate around 90%, but the survival rate falls to 63–78% if the depth of invasion is >1 cm (15, 38, 42).

Parametrial Spread   Patients with spread to the parametrium have a 5-year survival rate of 69% versus 95% when the parametrium is negative. When the parametrium is involved and pelvic lymph nodes are also positive, the 5-year survival rate falls to 39–42% (29, 39).

Lymph Vascular Space Involvement   The significance of the finding of lymph vascular space involvement is somewhat controversial. Several reports have shown a 50–70% 5-year survival rate when lymph vascular space invasion is present and a 90% 5-year survival rate in its absence (15, 28, 32, 46–50). Others have found no significant difference in survival if the study is controlled for other risk factors (37, 38, 51–53). Lymph vascular space involvement may be a predictor of lymph node metastasis and not an independent predictor of survival.

Postoperative Radiotherapy

In an effort to improve survival, postoperative radiotherapy has been recommended for patients with high-risk factors, such as metastasis to pelvic lymph nodes (15, 26, 40, 46), invasion of paracervical tissue (29, 30), deep cervical invasion (54), or positive surgical margins (41, 55). Although most authors agree that postoperative radiotherapy is necessary for positive surgical margins, the use of radiation in patients with other high-risk factors is controversial. Particularly controversial but best studied is the use of radiation in the presence of positive pelvic lymph nodes. The rationale for treatment is the knowledge that radiotherapy can sterilize cancer in pelvic lymph nodes and that pelvic node dissection does not remove all of the nodal and lymphatic tissue. The hesitancy to recommend postoperative radiotherapy relates to the significant rate of postradiotherapy bowel and urinary tract complications (56). A prospective randomized study has not been performed, and all the data currently available are retrospective.

From these retrospective studies, it appears that postoperative radiation therapy for positive pelvic nodes can decrease pelvic recurrence but does not improve 5-year actuarial survival. Morrow (41) reported a multi-institutional study that showed no difference in survival in patients with three or fewer pelvic nodes (59% versus 60%). However, there seemed to be a benefit when radiotherapy was given to those with more than three positive nodes.

Kinney et al. (57) matched 60 pairs of irradiated and nonirradiated women for age, lesion size, and number and location of positive nodes after radical hysterectomy. They found no significant difference in projected 5-year survival rate (72% surgery alone, 64% surgery plus radiation). The proportion of recurrences in the pelvis only was 67% in the surgery-only group and 27% in the postoperative radiation group ($P < 0.03$).

Soisson et al. (34) performed a Cox regression analysis on 320 women who underwent radical hysterectomy, 72 of whom received postoperative radiation. They reported a significant decrease in pelvic recurrence but no survival benefit.

Alvarez et al. (36) performed a multi-institutional retrospective study in 185 women with positive pelvic nodes after radical hysterectomy, 103 of whom received postoperative radiotherapy. With multivariate analysis, radiotherapy was not found to be an independent predictor of survival, whereas age, lesion diameter, and number of positive nodes were.

These authors all conclude that additional treatment is needed to improve survival. Because the survival is limited by distant site recurrence, the addition of chemotherapy to postoperative radiotherapy has been proposed. Lai et al. (58) reported a 75% disease-free survival rate at 3 years in 40 high-risk patients given cisplatin, vinblastine, and bleomycin after radical hysterectomy and a 46% disease-free survival in 79 comparable patients who refused treatment. Only 4 of 34 (11.8%) with positive pelvic nodes had recurrences, whereas disease recurred in 8 of 24 (33%) untreated patients with positive nodes. Wertheim et al. (59) reported an 82% rate of disease-free survival at 2 years among 32 patients who were treated with postoperative radiation therapy plus cisplatin and bleomycin. These results have led to the prospective randomized trial of postoperative radiotherapy alone versus radiotherapy plus 5-FU and cisplatin currently being performed by the GOG and the Southwest Oncology Group (SWOG).

The location of lymph node metastases is apparently relevant to postradiation recurrence rates. When common iliac lymph nodes are involved, the survival rate drops to 20% (46). As the number of positive pelvic nodes increases, the percentage of positive common iliac and low para-aortic nodes increases (46), i.e., 0.6% when pelvic lymph nodes are negative, 6.3% with one positive pelvic node, 21.4% with two or three positive nodes, and 73.3% with four or more positive nodes. Inoue et al. (46) have used this information to recommend "extended-field" radiotherapy to patients with positive pelvic lymph nodes in an attempt to treat undetected extrapelvic nodal disease. They reported a 3-year disease-free survival rate of 85% in patients with positive pelvic nodes and 51% in patients with positive common iliac nodes, which is better than the survival rates of 50% and 23%, respectively, for historical control groups receiving radiotherapy to the pelvis alone.

Postoperative radiotherapy for patients with the other high-risk factors has not been shown to be effective, with the possible exception of patients with parametrial extension, where a 77.8% survival rate with radiotherapy versus a 72.7% survival rate without radiotherapy has been shown (25). The GOG has identified risk groups by proportional hazards modeling for patients with Stage I disease and no pelvic node metastasis (38). The relative risk of recurrence was calculated for the three most important risk factors:

1. Depth of stromal invasion

2. Clinical size of the primary tumor

3. Capillary-lymphatic space involvement

Patients with a high risk of recurrence are being randomized to no further treatment versus pelvic radiotherapy in a current GOG protocol.

Neoadjuvant Chemotherapy

The use of chemotherapy to shrink the tumor before radical hysterectomy or radiotherapy is termed neoadjuvant chemotherapy. No randomized studies have been reported. However, the information available from current studies suggests that, compared with historical controls, neoadjuvant therapy can achieve a 22–44% complete response rate, decrease the number of positive pelvic lymph nodes, and improve the 2- and 3-year disease-free survival rates, particularly in patients with Stage I and II disease.

Kim et al. (60) used cisplatin, vinblastine, and bleomycin before radical hysterectomy in 54 patients with Stage I and IIa tumors >4 cm in size. They reported a complete response rate of 44% and a partial response rate of 50% based on evaluation of the radical hysterectomy specimen. Tumors recurred in only three patients, giving a 94% disease-free survival with a minimum of 2 years follow-up. Of the 11 patients with positive nodes, three had recurrences and all had three or more positive nodes. A comparison with historical controls for a tumor of this size revealed a 40% disease-free survival rate.

In treating 75 patients with Stage I, II, and III disease whose tumors were >4 cm, Panici et al. (61) administered cisplatin, bleomycin, and methotrexate before surgery or radiation therapy. A 3-year disease-free survival rate of 100%, 81%, and 66% was achieved for Stages I, II and III, respectively. Initial large tumor size and parametrial infiltration were significantly correlated with a lower response to neoadjuvant therapy. Recurrence was significantly correlated with FIGO stage, parametrial infiltration, and residual cervical tumor. Eleven of the 12 recurrences involved the pelvis, indicating that additional local treatment is needed for this high-risk group.

In treating 151 patients who had Stage IIb and III tumors, Sardi et al. (62) administered cisplatin, vinblastine, and bleomycin before surgery plus radiation (62.5%) or radiation alone (37.7%). They reported a 2-year disease-free survival rate in Stages II and III of 79% and 50%, respectively, compared with survival rates of 47% and 26% in historical controls treated with radiation alone. For the 25 patients (22%) who experienced a complete response to the chemotherapy, there was a 96% disease-free survival rate and a 0% incidence of lymph node metastasis.

To determine the efficacy of neoadjuvant chemotherapy, randomized trials have been initiated in the GOG and in other centers.

Radiation Therapy

Radiotherapy can be used to treat all stages of cervical squamous cell cancer, with cure rates of approximately 70% for Stage I, 60% for Stage II, 45% for Stage III, and 18% for Stage IV (2). The treatment plan generally consists of a combination of *external teletherapy* to treat the regional nodes and to shrink the primary tumor and *intracavitary brachytherapy* to boost the central tumor. Intracavitary therapy alone may be used in patients with early disease when the incidence of lymph node metastasis is negligible.

The treatment sequence depends on tumor volume. Stage Ib lesions <2 cm may be treated first with an intracavitary source to treat the primary lesion, followed by external therapy to treat the pelvic nodes. Larger lesions will require external radiotherapy first to shrink the tumor and to reduce the anatomic distortion caused by the cancer. This enables the therapist to achieve better intracavitary dosimetry.

The usual dosages delivered will be 7000–8000 cGy to point A and 6000 cGy to point B, limiting the bladder and rectal dosage to less than 6000 cGy. To achieve this, it is necessary to have adequate packing of the bladder and bowel away from the intracavitary sources. Localization films and careful calculation of dosimetry are mandatory to optimize the dose of radiotherapy and to reduce the incidence of bowel and bladder complications. Local control depends on adequate dosage to the tumor from the intracavitary source.

Extended-Field Radiotherapy

Clinical staging fails to predict the extension of disease to the para-aortic nodes in 7% of patients with Stage Ib disease, 18% with Stage IIb, and 28% with Stage III (63). Such patients will have "geographic" treatment failures if standard pelvic radiotherapy ports are used.

Surgical Staging

Surgical staging procedures designed to discover the presence of positive nodes have been devised. Transperitoneal exploration was first used, but it was associated with a 16–33% mortality rate from radiotherapy-induced bowel complications and a 5-year survival rate of only 9–12% (64, 65). The radiotherapy dose to the para-aortic chain was 5500–6000 cGy, which is now known to be excessive. Postsurgical adhesions entrap the intestine in the radiotherapy field, and therefore the bowel receives the full dose of radiotherapy. In the absence of postsurgical adhesions, the small bowel would move in and out of the radiotherapy field and receive a lesser dose. To avoid these postsurgical adhesions, extraperitoneal dissection of the para-aortic nodes is now recommended, and the radiotherapy dosage should be reduced to 5000 cGy or less (66, 67).

When such an approach is used, postradiotherapy bowel complications occur in fewer than 5% of the patients (68, 69), and the 5-year survival rate is 15–26% in patients with positive para-aortic nodes (8, 69). Survival appears to be related to the amount of disease in the para-aortic nodes and to the size of the primary tumor. In patients whose metastases to the para-aortic lymph nodes are microscopic and whose central tumor is not extending to the pelvic sidewall, the 5-year survival rate improves to 20–50% (70, 71).

Supraclavicular Lymph Node Biopsy Although not standard practice, the performance of a supraclavicular lymph node biopsy has been advocated in patients with positive para-aortic lymph nodes before the initiation of extended-field irradiation and also in patients with a central recurrence before exploration for possible exenteration. The incidence of metastatic disease in the supraclavicular lymph nodes in patients with positive para-aortic lymph nodes is 5–30% (72). Fine needle aspiration cytology should be performed if there are any enlarged nodes, as this can obviate the performance of an excisional biopsy.

Technique for Supraclavicular Lymph Node Biopsy   An incision is made in a transverse direction about 1–2 cm above and parallel to the clavicle. The subcutaneous tissue is incised, and the scalene fat pad and lymph nodes are isolated and resected. The lymph nodes are situated in the supraclavicular triangle, which is bounded medially by the sternocleidomastoid muscle, inferiorly by the clavicle, and laterally and posteriorly by the omohyoid muscle. The floor of the triangle consists of the scalenus anterior and medius muscles. The phrenic nerve courses through this triangle on the surface of the scalenus muscles, and the internal jugular vein lies just deep and posterior to the scalenus medius. Deep to the scalenus muscle lies the internal carotid artery. Biopsy procedures in this area must avoid these vital structures.

Radiation Plus Chemotherapy	Primary pelvic radiotherapy fails to control the disease in 30–82% of patients with cervical carcinoma (2). Approximately two-thirds of these failures occur in the pelvis (73). A variety of agents have been used in an attempt to increase the effectiveness of radiation therapy in patients with large primary tumors. Hydroxyurea has produced some improvement in response rate and survival when compared with radiation therapy alone in a controlled series of patients (74, 75). 5-FU and mitomycin-C have also been reported to improve response rates for advanced cervical cancer (76). Cisplatin has been shown to have cytotoxic activity against cervical carcinoma (77) and recently has been demonstrated to be a radiation sensitizer (78). It has produced some improvement in response and survival when used with radiation therapy for cervical cancer as compared with radiation therapy alone (78, 79). Currently, randomized trials are being conducted to determine the best chemotherapy to combine with radiation therapy (80) (see Chapter 2).
Complications of Radiotherapy	*Perforation* of the uterus may occur at the time of insertion of the uterine tandem. This is a problem particularly in the elderly patient or in the patient who has had a previous diagnostic conization. When perforation is recognized, the tandem should be removed and the patient should be observed for bleeding or signs of peritonitis. Survival may be decreased in patients who have had uterine perforation (81), possibly because these patients have more extensive uterine disease, which predisposes them to perforation. *Fever* may occur after insertion of the uterine tandem and ovoids. This most often results from infection of the necrotic tumor and occurs 2–6 hours after insertion of the intracavitary system. Provided that uterine perforation has been excluded by ultrasonography, intravenous broad-spectrum antibiotic coverage, usually with a cephalosporin, should be started. If the fever does not decrease promptly, or if the fever is >38.5°C, an aminoglycoside and a bacteroides-specific antibiotic should be added. If the fever persists or if the patient shows signs of septic shock or peritonitis, the intracavitary system must be removed. Antibiotics are continued

263

until the patient has recovered and the intracavitary application is delayed for 1–2 weeks.

Acute Morbidity

The acute effects of radiotherapy occur after 2000–3000 cGy and are due to ionizing radiation on the epithelium of the intestine and bladder. Symptoms include diarrhea, abdominal cramps, nausea, frequent urination, and occasionally bleeding from the bladder or bowel mucosa. The bowel symptoms can be treated with a low-gluten, low-lactose, and low-protein diet. Antidiarrheal and antispasmodic agents may also help. The bladder may be treated with antispasmodics. Severe symptoms may require a week of rest from radiotherapy.

Chronic Morbidity

The chronic effects of radiotherapy result from the induction of vasculitis and fibrosis, and they are more serious. These complications occur several months to several years after the radiotherapy has been completed. The bowel and bladder fistula rate after pelvic radiation therapy for cervical cancer is 1.4–5.3% (10, 12). Other serious toxicity (e.g., bowel bleeding, stricture, stenosis, or obstruction) occurs in 6.4–8.1% of patients (10, 12).

Proctosigmoiditis Bleeding from proctosigmoiditis should be treated with a low-residue diet, antidiarrheal medications, and steroid enemas. In extreme cases, a colostomy may be required to rest the bowel completely, and occasionally resection of the rectosigmoid must be performed.

Rectovaginal Fistula Rectovaginal fistulas or rectal strictures occur in ≤2% of patients. The successful closure of fistulas with bulbocavernosus flaps has been reported (82). Bricker and Johnston (83) have reported a technique of sigmoid colon transposition to repair rectosigmoid fistulas or rectal strictures. Occasionally, resection with anastomosis is feasible.

Small-Bowel Complications Patients with previous abdominal surgery are more likely to have pelvic adhesions and thus sustain more radiotherapy complications in the small bowel. The terminal ileum may sustain chronic damage because of its relatively fixed position at the cecum. The patient typically has a long history of crampy abdominal pain, intestinal rushes, and distention characteristic of partial small-bowel obstruction. Often low-grade fever and anemia accompany the symptoms. Patients who have no evidence of disease should be treated aggressively with total parenteral nutrition, nasogastric suction, and early operation after the anemia has resolved and good nutritional status has been attained. The operation performed depends on individual circumstances (84).

A side-to-side ileocolonic bypass is the quickest and easiest procedure to perform in the patient who is a poor operative risk. However, it leaves behind a mass of bowel with fibrosis, low-grade inflammation, and multiple obstructions. This mass of bowel can lead to continued discomfort, perforation, or enterocutaneous fistula. Resection of this bowel should be performed if necrosis is present or if the patient is able to undergo a more extensive operation. Approximately 100 cm of small bowel beyond the ligament of Treitz is needed for adequate oral nutrition; supplementation with vitamin K, vitamin B_{12}, and bile salts is necessary if the terminal ileum has been resected.

Small bowel fistulas after radiotherapy will rarely close spontaneously while the patient is on total parenteral nutrition. Recurrent cancer should be excluded; then aggressive fluid replacement, nasogastric suction, and wound care should be employed. A fistulogram and a barium enema should be performed to exclude a combined large and small bowel fistula. The fistula-containing loop of bowel may be either resected or isolated and left *in situ*. In the latter case, the fistula will act as its own mucous fistula.

Urinary Tract   Chronic urinary tract complications occur in 1–5% of patients and depend on the dose to the base of the bladder. *Vesicovaginal fistulas* are the most common complication and usually require supravesicular urinary diversion. Occasionally, a small fistula can be repaired with either a bulbocavernosus flap or an omental pedicle. *Ureteral strictures* are usually a sign of recurrent cancer, and FNA cytology under CT scan control should be obtained at the site of the obstruction. If this is negative, the patient should be explored to determine disease status. If radiation fibrosis is the cause, then ureterolysis may be possible or indwelling ureteral stents may be passed through the open urinary bladder.

A comparison of surgery and radiation for the treatment of low-stage cervical cancer is presented in Table 7.5.

Post-treatment Surveillance

The patient who receives radiotherapy should be closely monitored for response. Regression of tumor may be expected to continue for up to 3 months after radiotherapy. If disease obviously progresses during this interval, however, surgical treatment should be considered.

The pelvic examination should note progressive shrinkage of the cervix and possible stenosis of the cervical os and surrounding upper vagina. The *rectovaginal examination,* with careful palpation of the uterosacral and cardinal ligaments for nodularity, is most important. FNA cytology of suspicious areas should be used to make an early diagnosis of persistent disease. In addition to the pelvic

Table 7.5   Comparison of Surgery Versus Radiation for Stage Ib/IIa Cancer of the Cervix

	Surgery	*Radiation*
Survival	85%	85%
Serious complications	Urologic fistulas 1–2%	Intestinal and urinary strictures and fistulas 1.4–5.3%
Vagina	Initially shortened, but may lengthen with regular intercourse	Fibrosis and possible stenosis, particularly in postmenopausal patients
Ovaries	Can be conserved	Destroyed
Chronic effects	Bladder atony in 3%	Radiation fibrosis of bowel and bladder in 6–8%
Applicability	Best candidates are <65, <200 lb., and in good health	All patients are potential candidates
Surgical mortality	1%	<1% (from pulmonary embolism during intracavitary therapy)

examination, the supraclavicular and inguinal lymph nodes should be carefully examined, and cervical or vaginal cytology should be performed every 3 months for 2 years and then every 6 months for the next 3 years. An endocervical curettage may be added for those patients with large central tumors.

An x-ray film of the chest may be obtained yearly in patients who have advanced disease. Metastasis to the lung has been reported in 1.5% of cases, with solitary nodules present in one-fourth. Resection of a solitary nodule in the absence of any other persistent disease may yield some long-term survivors (85). Although an intravenous pyelogram (IVP) is not a part of the routine postradiotherapy surveillance, it should be obtained if a pelvic mass is detected or if urinary symptoms warrant it. The finding of ureteral obstruction after radiotherapy in the absence of a palpable mass may indicate unresectable pelvic sidewall disease, but this should be confirmed, usually by FNA cytology (86).

Patients who have had radical hysterectomy and who are at high risk of recurrence may benefit from early recognition of recurrence, because they might be saved with radiation therapy. In these patients, a routine IVP at 6–12 months may be beneficial. After radical hysterectomy, about 80% of recurrences are detected within 2 years (87). The larger the primary lesion, the shorter the median time to recurrence (88).

Special Problems

Adenocarcinoma

The incidence of adenocarcinoma of the cervix appears to be increasing relative to that of squamous cancers. Older reports indicated that 5% of all cervical cancers were adenocarcinomas (89), whereas newer reports show an incidence as high as 18.5–27% (90, 91). The FIGO annual report indicates a poorer prognosis for adenocarcinoma than for squamous cell carcinoma in every stage. This has been supported by Hopkins and Morley (91), who performed a Cox proportional hazard analysis of 203 women with adenocarcinoma and 756 women with squamous carcinoma. They reported 5-year survival rates of 90% versus 60%, 62% versus 47% and 36% versus 8% for Stages I, II, and III, respectively. Although some have attributed this to a relative resistance to radiation, it is more likely a reflection of the tendency of adenocarcinomas to grow endophytically and to be undetected until a larger volume of tumor is present.

The clinicopathologic features of Stage I adenocarcinomas have been well studied (90, 92–94). These studies have identified size of tumor, depth of invasion, grade of tumor, and age of the patient as significant correlates of lymph node metastasis and survival. When matched with squamous carcinomas for lesion size, age, and depth of invasion, the incidence of lymph node metastases and the survival rate appear to be the same (92, 93). Patients with Stage I adenocarcinomas can be selected for treatment according to the same criteria as for those with squamous cancers (93).

The proper treatment for bulky Stage I tumors and Stage II tumors is controversial. Radiation alone has been advocated by some (95), but others support radiation plus extrafascial hysterectomy (96, 97). In 1975 Rutledge et al. (96) reported an 85.2% 5-year survival rate for all patients with Stage I disease treated with radiation alone and an 83.8% survival for those who had radiation plus surgery.

The central persistent disease rate was 8.3% versus 4%. In Stage II disease, the 5-year survival rate was 41.9% for radiation alone and 53.7% for radiation plus surgery. A recent report from the M.D. Anderson Hospital again revealed no significant difference in survival among patients treated with either radiation alone or radiation plus extrafacial hysterectomy (98).

Patients with adenosquamous carcinoma of the cervix have been reported to have a poorer prognosis than those with pure adenocarcinoma or squamous carcinoma (99). Whether or not this is true when corrected for size of lesion is controversial (92, 93).

The association of adenocarcinoma with squamous intraepithelial neoplasia is well documented (100). A squamous intraepithelial lesion may be observed colposcopically and treated with outpatient therapy, and the coexistent adenocarcinoma in the canal may be overlooked. Performance of an endocervical curettage at colposcopy will help prevent such an occurrence.

Cervical Cancer in Pregnancy

After a review of the literature, Hacker et al. (101) reported that the incidence of invasive cervical cancer associated with pregnancy was one in 2200. All pregnant patients should have a Pap smear at the initial antenatal visit, and any grossly suspicious lesion should be subjected to biopsy. Diagnosis is often delayed during pregnancy because bleeding is attributed to pregnancy-related complications. If the Pap smear is positive for malignant cells and the diagnosis of invasive cancer cannot be made with colposcopy and biopsy, a diagnostic conization may be necessary. Because conization subjects the mother and fetus to complications, it should be performed only in the second trimester, and only in patients with an inadequate colposcopy and strong cytologic evidence of invasive cancer. Conization in the first trimester of pregnancy is associated with an abortion rate of up to 33% (101, 102).

Microinvasive Carcinoma   After conization, there appears to be no harm in delaying definitive treatment until fetal maturity is achieved in patients with Stage Ia cervical cancer (101, 103, 104). Patients with <3 mm of invasion and no lymph vascular space involvement may be followed to term and delivered vaginally. A 6-week postpartum vaginal hysterectomy may be performed if further childbearing is not desired.

Patients with 3–5 mm of invasion and those with lymph vascular space invasion may also be followed to term (101, 104). They may be delivered by cesarean section, followed immediately by modified radical hysterectomy and pelvic lymph node dissection.

Stage Ib Carcinoma   Patients with >5 mm invasion should be treated as having frankly invasive carcinoma of the cervix. Treatment will depend on the stage of gestation and the wishes of the patient. Modern neonatal care affords a 75% survival rate for infants delivered at 28 weeks of gestational age and 90% for those delivered at 32 weeks. Fetal pulmonary maturity can be determined by amniocentesis, and prompt treatment can be instituted when pulmonary maturity is documented. Although controversial, it is probably unwise to delay therapy for longer than 4 weeks (103, 104). The recommended treatment is classic cesarean section followed by radical hysterectomy with pelvic lymph node dissection. There should be a thorough discussion of the risks and options with both parents before any treatment is undertaken.

Advanced-Stage Carcinoma Those patients with cervical cancer in Stages II–IV should be treated with radiotherapy. If the fetus is viable, it is delivered by classic cesarean section and therapy is begun postoperatively. If the pregnancy is in the first trimester, external radiation therapy can be started with the expectation that spontaneous abortion will occur before the delivery of 4000 cGy. In the second trimester, a delay of therapy may be entertained to improve the chances of fetal survival. If the patient wishes to delay therapy, it is important to ensure fetal pulmonary maturity before delivery is undertaken.

Prognosis The clinical stage is the most important prognostic factor. Overall survival is slightly better for patients with cervical cancer in pregnancy, because an increased proportion of these patients have Stage I disease. For patients with advanced disease, there is evidence that pregnancy impairs the prognosis (101, 104). The diagnosis of cancer in the postpartum period is associated with a more advanced clinical stage and a corresponding decrease in survival.

Cancer of the Cervical Stump

Cancer of the cervical stump is less common today than it was several decades ago when supracervical hysterectomy was popular. Early-stage disease is treated surgically, with very little change in technique from that used when the uterus is intact (105). Advanced-stage disease may present a therapeutic problem for the radiotherapist if the length of the cervical canal is <2 cm. This length is necessary to allow satisfactory placement of the uterine tandem. If the uterine tandem cannot be placed, radiation therapy can be completed with vaginal ovoids or with an external treatment plan in which lateral ports are used to augment the standard anterior and posterior ports. Such a technique will reduce the dosage to the bowel and bladder and thus reduce the incidence of complications.

Coexistent Pelvic Mass

The origin of a pelvic mass must be clarified before treatment. An IVP will exclude a pelvic kidney, and a barium enema will help identify diverticular disease or carcinoma of the colon. The abdominal x-ray film may show typical calcifications associated with benign ovarian teratomas or uterine leiomyomas. A pelvic ultrasonogram will differentiate between solid and cystic masses and indicate uterine or adnexal origin. Solid masses of uterine origin are most often leiomyomas and generally do not need further investigation.

Coexistent Ovarian Cancer Undiagnosed adnexal masses must be explored to exclude coexistent cancer of the ovary. If such disease is encountered, treatment is determined by the stage of both tumors, as follows:

1. If the cervical cancer is Stage I, radical hysterectomy, bilateral salpingo-oophorectomy, pelvic lymphadenectomy, and appropriate staging or debulking of the ovarian cancer are indicated. This surgical treatment of the cervical cancer will obviate the need for both radiotherapy and chemotherapy, which may lead to significant morbidity and to substandard treatment of both cancers.

2. If the cervical cancer cannot be treated surgically, the ovarian disease should be debulked without removal of the uterus, allowing for sub-

sequent radiation. Further therapy for the ovarian cancer will depend on the stage of disease.

Pyometra/Hematometra   An enlarged fluid-filled uterine cavity may be a *pyometra* or a *hematometra*. The *hematometra* can be drained by dilatation of the cervical canal and will not interefere with treatment. The *pyometra* also should be drained and the patient placed on antibiotics to cover *Bacteroides,* anaerobic *Staphylococcus* and *Streptococcus,* and aerobic coliform bacteria. Placement of a large mushroom catheter through the cervix has been advocated, but the catheter itself may become obstructed and lead to further occlusion of the drainage. Repeated dilation of the cervix with aspiration of pus every 2–3 days is more effective.

If the disease is Stage I, a radical hysterectomy and pelvic node dissection may be performed. However, a pyometra is usually found in patients with advanced disease, and thus radiotherapy is required. External beam therapy can begin when the pyometra has cleared. Patients often have a significant amount of pus in the uterus or a tubo-ovarian abscess without signs of infection; therefore a normal temperature and a normal white blood cell count do not necessarily exclude infection. Repeat physical examination or pelvic ultrasonography will be necessary to ensure adequate drainage.

Invasive Cancer Found at Simple Hysterectomy

When invasive cervical cancer is found after simple hysterectomy, it may be treated with radiotherapy or reoperation involving a pelvic node dissection and radical excision of parametrial tissue, cardinal ligaments, and the vaginal stump (106).

Reoperation   Reoperation is particularly indicated for a young patient who has a small lesion and in whom preservation of ovarian function is desirable. It is not indicated for patients who have positive margins or obvious residual disease (106). Survival after radical reoperation is similar to that after radical hysterectomy for Stage I disease.

Radiation Therapy   Survival after radiotherapy depends on the volume of disease, the status of the surgical margins, and the length of delay from surgery to radiotherapy. Patients with microscopic disease have a 95–100% 5-year survival rate; those with macroscopic disease and free margins, 82–84%; those with microscopically positive margins, 38–87%; and those with obvious residual cancer, 20–47% (107–109). More than 6 months' delay in treatment is associated with a 20% survival (109).

Stage IVa Cervical Cancer

Although primary exenteration may be considered for patients with direct extension to the rectum or bladder, it is rarely performed. For patients with extension to the bladder, the survival rate with radiation therapy is as high as 30%, with a urinary fistula rate of only 3.8% (110).

The presence of tumor in the bladder may prohibit cure with radiation therapy alone, so consideration must be given to removal of the bladder on completion of external beam radiation. This is particularly true if the disease persists at that time and the geometry is not conducive to implant therapy. Rectal extension is less commonly observed but may require diversion of the fecal stream before therapy to avoid septic episodes from fecal contamination.

Pelvic Inflammatory Disease

Acute pelvic inflammatory disease (PID) is not common in patients with cancer of the cervix. Fever and pelvic tenderness most often result from local infection of the necrotic tumor. Broad-spectrum antibiotic treatment should be undertaken until the patient is afebrile. More common is chronic PID with an accompanying hydrosalpinx, chronic abscess, or pelvic adhesions. Patients with chronic abscesses should undergo drainage, preferably from an extraperitoneal approach.

The proper management of a hydrosalpinx is not as well defined. Resection of such masses may lead to more bowel adhesions and a higher rate of bowel complications; leaving the tubo-ovarian disease intact may allow for reactivation of a smoldering infection when the intracavitary system is placed. Adhesions of small bowel to the uterus, cul-de-sac, or adnexae after PID result in a higher dose of radiotherapy to these loops of bowel and subsequently a higher rate of complications. Some oncologists advocate dissection of such adhesions and interposition of the omentum or the more radioresistant sigmoid colon between the uterus and the small bowel.

Cervical Hemorrhage

Occasionally a patient will be seen with a large lesion that produces life-threatening hemorrhage. A biopsy of the lesion should be performed to verify neoplasia, and a vaginal pack soaked in Monsel's solution (ferric subsulfate) should be packed tightly against the cervix. After proper staging, external radiation therapy can be started with the expectation that control of bleeding may require 8–10 daily treatments at 180–200 cGy/day. Broad-spectrum antibiotics should be used to reduce the incidence of infection. If the patient becomes febrile, the pack should be removed. Rapid replacement of the pack may be necessary, and a fresh pack should be immediately available.

This management of hemorrhage in the previously untreated patient is preferable to exploration and vascular ligation. Occasionally, vascular embolization under fluoroscopic control is required in severe cases, and this procedure may obviate a laparotomy. However, vascular occlusion may lead ultimately to decreased blood flow and oxygenation of the tumor, and, because the effect of radiotherapy is dependent on tissue oxygen content, the efficacy of the radiotherapy may be compromised.

Ureteral Obstruction

Untreated patients with bilateral ureteral obstruction and uremia deserve individualization of treatment. Transvesicle or percutaneous ureteral catheters should be placed in those patients with no evidence of distant disease, and radiotherapy with curative intent should be instituted. Those with metastatic disease beyond curative treatment fields should have the options presented to them concerning ureteral stenting, palliative radiotherapy, and chemotherapy for the metastatic disease. A median survival of 17 months for these patients may be achieved with aggressive management (111).

Barrel-Shaped Cervix

The expansion of the upper endocervix and lower uterine segment by tumor has been referred to as a barrel-shaped cervix. Patients with tumors >6 cm in diameter have a 17.5% central failure rate when treated with radiotherapy alone, because the tumor at the periphery of the lower uterine segment is too far from the standard intracavitary source to receive a tumoricidal dose (112). Attempts have been made to overcome this problem radiotherapeutically by means of interstitial implants into the tumor with a perineal template, but high central failure rates have also been reported with this technique (113).

Most oncologists prefer a combination of radiotherapy and surgery for these patients. The usual approach is to perform an extrafascial hysterectomy 6 weeks after the completion of radiation therapy in an effort to resect a small, centrally persistent tumor. The dose of external radiotherapy is reduced to 4000 cGy and a single intracavitary treatment is given, followed by an extrafascial hysterectomy (114, 115). This approach appears to result in a lower rate of central failure (2%), although it is not clear that overall survival is improved. There is disagreement concerning the need for extrafascial hysterectomy, and the GOG is currently undertaking a randomized study to compare adjuvant hysterectomy with radiotherapy alone in patients who have no evidence of occult metastases in the para-aortic nodes.

Poor Vaginal Geometry

The narrow upper vagina of the older patient may preclude the use of an intracavitary source. Such patients will have to receive their entire course from external sources, leading to a higher central failure rate and more significant bowel and bladder morbidity. If Stage I disease is present in such a patient, a radical hysterectomy with pelvic node dissection is preferable if the patient's medical condition allows.

Small Cell Carcinoma

Van Nagell et al. (116) have described the aggressive nature of small cell (neuroendocrine-type) carcinoma of the cervix and have noted its similarity to that arising from the bronchus. At the time of diagnosis, it is commonly disseminated, with bone, brain, liver, and bone marrow being the most common sites of metastases. Pathologically, the diagnosis is aided by the finding of neuroendocrine granules on electron microscopy, as well as by immunoperoxidase studies that are positive for a variety of neuroendocrine proteins such as calcitonin, insulin, glucagon, somatostatin, gastrin, and ACTH. In addition to the traditional staging for cancer of the cervix, these patients should have bone, liver, and brain scans, as well as bone marrow aspiration and biopsy.

Local therapy alone gives almost no chance of cure. Regimens of combination chemotherapy have improved the median survival in small cell bronchogenic carcinoma, and these regimens are now being used for treatment of small cell (neuroendocrine-type) carcinoma of the cervix. Combination chemotherapy may consist of either VAC (vincristine, Adriamycin, and cytoxan), or EP (VP-16 [etoposide] and cisplatin) (117). Patients must be followed carefully because they are at high risk of developing recurrent metastatic disease (118).

Recurrent Cervical Cancer

Treatment for recurrent cervical cancer depends on the mode of primary therapy and the site of recurrence. **Patients who have been treated initially with surgery should be considered for radiation therapy, and those who have had radiation therapy should be considered for surgical treatment.** Chemotherapy is palliative only, reserved for patients who are not considered curable by the other two modalities.

Radiotherapy for recurrence after surgery consists primarily of external treatment. In patients with isolated vaginal cuff recurrences, vaginal ovoids also may be placed. Patients with a regional recurrence may require interstitial implantation with a Syed type of template in addition to the external therapy. A 25% survival rate can be expected in patients treated with radiation for a postsurgical recurrence (87).

Radiation Re-treatment

Re-treatment of recurrent pelvic disease by means of radiotherapy with curative intent is confined to those patients who had suboptimal or incomplete primary therapy. This may allow the radiotherapist to deliver curative doses to the tumor. The proximity of the bladder and rectum to the cancer and their relative sensitivity to radiation injury are the major deterrents to reirradiation.

The use of multiple interstitial radiation sources into the locally recurrent cancer through a perineal template may help to overcome these dosimetric considerations (106, 119). However, the fistula rates are high and the consequences must be seriously considered before one embarks on interstitial therapy. In general, patients considered curable with interstitial implant therapy would be better served by a pelvic exenteration.

Localized metastatic lesions may be palliated successfully with radiotherapy. Painful bony metastases, central nervous system lesions, and severe urologic or vena caval obstructions are specific indications.

Surgical Therapy

Surgical therapy for postradiation recurrence is limited to patients with central pelvic disease. A few carefully selected patients with small-volume disease limited to the cervix may be treated with an extrafascial or radical hysterectomy. However, the difficulty of assessing tumor volume and the 30–50% rate of serious urinary complications in these previously irradiated patients lead most gynecologic oncologists to recommend pelvic exenteration because this is the patient's last chance for cure (120, 121).

Exenteration

The operation can be an *anterior exenteration* (removal of the bladder, vagina, cervix, and uterus), a *posterior exenteration* (removal of the rectum, vagina, cervix, and uterus), or a *total exenteration* (removal of both bladder and rectum with the vagina, cervix, and uterus). A total exenteration that includes a large perineal phase includes the entire rectum and leaves the patient with a permanent colostomy as well as a urinary conduit. In selected patients, a total exenteration may take place above the levator muscle *(supralevator)*, leaving a rectal stump that may be anastomosed to the sigmoid, thus avoiding a permanent colostomy.

Preoperative Evaluation and Patient Selection   The search for metastatic disease is imperative. Physical examination includes careful palpation of the peripheral lymph nodes with FNA cytology of any suspicious nodes. A random biopsy of nonsuspicious supraclavicular lymph nodes has been advocated (72, 122) but is not routinely practiced. A CT scan of the lung will detect disease missed on routine x-ray examination of the chest. An abdominal and pelvic CT scan is helpful in the detection of liver metastases and enlarged para-aortic nodes. CT-directed FNA cytologic study of any abnormality should be undertaken. If a positive cytologic diagnosis is obtained, it will obviate the need for exploratory laparotomy.

Extension of the tumor to the pelvic sidewall is a contraindication to exenteration; however, this may be difficult for even the most experienced ex

aminer to determine because of radiation fibrosis. If any question of resectability arises, the patient should be given the benefit of exploratory laparotomy and parametrial biopsies, because this is the patient's last hope for cure (123–126). **The clinical triad of unilateral leg edema, sciatic pain, and ureteral obstruction is nearly always pathognomonic of unresectable disease on the pelvic sidewall.**

Preoperatively, the patient should be prepared for a major operation. Total parenteral nutrition may be necessary to place the patient in an anabolic state for optimal healing. A bowel preparation, preoperative antibiotics, and prophylaxis for deep venous thrombosis with low-dose heparin or pneumatic calf compression should be used (127).

The surgical mortality increases with age, and the operation should rarely be considered in the patient who is more than 70 years old. Other medical illnesses should be taken into account; when life expectancy is limited, exenterative surgery is unwise.

Anterior Exenteration   Candidates for anterior exenteration are those in whom the disease is limited to the cervix and anterior part of the upper vagina. Proctoscopic examination should be performed, because a positive finding would mandate a total exenteration. However, a negative proctoscopic examination finding does not exclude disease in the rectal muscularis, and findings at laparotomy still must be considered. Generally, the presence of disease in the posterior vaginal mucosa directly over the rectum mandates removal of the underlying rectum.

Posterior Exenteration   A posterior exenteration is rarely performed for recurrent cervical cancer but is indicated for the patient with an isolated posterior vaginal recurrence where dissection of the ureters through the cardinal ligaments will not be necessary.

Total Exenteration   Total exenteration with a large perineal phase is indicated when the disease extends down to the lower part of the vagina. Because distal vaginal lymphatics may empty into the inguinal node region, these nodes should be carefully evaluated preoperatively. A surgically removed specimen is presented in Figure 7.8.

A supralevator total exenteration with low rectal anastomosis is indicated in the patient whose disease is confined to the upper vagina and cervix. Frozen-section margins of the rectal edge should be obtained, because occult metastases to the muscularis may occur.

Technique   The patient is placed in the low lithotomy or "ski" position. This will enable the operators to perform the abdominal and perineal phases of the operation simultaneously. The abdominal incision is made in the lower midline. The liver and omentum should be palpated carefully. The rest of the abdomen is explored, and the para-aortic nodes are palpated. Both the right and left para-aortic nodes are sent for frozen section. If they are negative, the pelvic spaces are opened by division of the round ligament at the pelvic sidewall. The prevesicle, paravesicle, pararectal, and presacral spaces are all developed, and the ligaments are evaluated for resectability. Enlarged or suspicious pelvic lymph nodes should be removed and sent for frozen section. Positive lymph nodes, peritoneal breakthrough of the tumor, or tumor implants in the abdomen or pelvis should lead to abandonment of the operation.

273

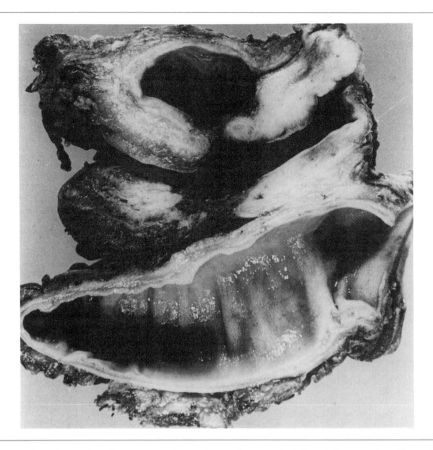

Figure 7.8. A surgically removed specimen from a total pelvic exenteration. Note the bladder above with a fistulous tract to the vagina and the rectum below.

When the patient is judged to be a candidate for resection, the procedure begins with ligation of the portion of the anterior hypogastric artery that includes the uterine artery, the vesicle arteries, and the obliterated umbilical artery. This exposes the cardinal ligament, which is likewise ligated. The broad attachments of the rectum to the sacrum are divided. Then the vaginal attachments to the tendinous arch are divided, and the vaginal arteries and vein are located at the lateral margin of this pedicle. The specimen is completely mobilized, and the penetration of the rectum and vagina through the pubococcygeous muscle can be identified. The various sites for ligation of the pubococcygeous muscle for total exenteration versus anterior exenteration are identified, and the perineal phase of the operation is initiated (Fig. 7.9).

Even if the patient is to have an anterior exenteration, the pubourethral ligaments are isolated by first passing a long, sharp clamp directly in the midline under the pubic symphysis. The abdominal hand guides the instrument into the correct space cephalad. A second clamp is placed under the pubic arch to ligate the pubococcygeal muscles that surround the vagina. The posterior vaginal wall is then dissected free from the rectal muscularis, and the attachment of the pubococcygeal muscle to the lower third of the rectum is divided and ligated.

If the patient is to have a total exenteration with a large perineal phase, the pubourethral and pubococcygeal muscles are identified and divided at their attachments to the pubic arch as before. In addition, the pubococcygeal attachment to the perineal body are divided, as is the anococcygeal ligament, which is attached to the anus.

When low colonic resection is performed in a posterior or total exenteration, an effort should be made to reanastomose the colon. The technique for this procedure is discussed in Chapter 15. The end-to-end anastomosis (EEA) stapler is employed to facilitate the low reanastomosis (128). The omentum is mobilized, leaving the left gastroepiploic artery as the vascular pedicle, and used to wrap the anastomosis and fill the pelvic defect posterior to the anastomosis. If there is no tension on the anastomotic line and there are two complete "doughnuts" in the stapler with no leak of the anastomosis when air is introduced through the rectum, a colostomy does not have to be performed (129). Total parenteral nutrition is used for 2–3 weeks to decrease colonic content while the anastomosis heals. Stricture and incontinence rates are decreased when the anastomosis is handled in this manner.

The recent development of techniques to establish continent urinary diversion has further improved the woman's physical appearance after exenteration (130–132) (see Chapter 15). When both a rectal anastomosis and a continent diversion are performed, the patient has no permanent external appliance and the psychological trauma associated with this is avoided.

Every effort should be made to create a neovagina simultaneous with the exenteration (133). The surgical techniques are outlined in Chapter 15. This procedure also helps in the reconstruction of the pelvic floor after extirpation of the pelvic viscera. Whether or not a neovagina is constructed, it is desirable to mobilize the omentum on the left gastroepiploic artery and use it to create a new pelvic floor.

Figure 7.9.   Cross-section diagram of pelvis showing lines of excision through the pubococcygeus muscle for anterior and total exenterations.

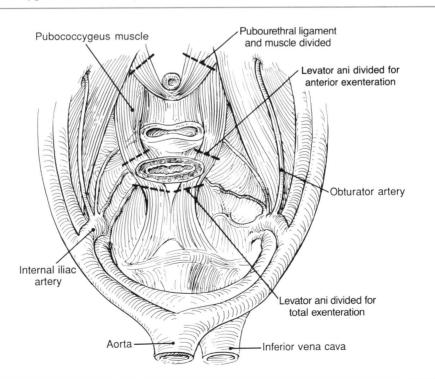

Results Surgical mortality has steadily decreased to an acceptable level of less than 10%. The most common causes of postoperative death are sepsis, pulmonary thromboembolism, and hemorrhage. Fistulas of the gastrointestinal and genitourinary tract are serious surgical complications, with a 30–40% mortality rate despite attempts at surgical repair. The risk of such fistulas has been decreased by the use of unirradiated segments of bowel for formation of the urinary conduit (127).

The 5-year survival rate is 33–60% for patients undergoing anterior exenteration and 20–46% for those undergoing total exenteration (121, 123–133). Survival is poorer for those patients with recurrent disease >3 cm, invasion into the bladder, positive pelvic lymph nodes, and recurrence diagnosed within 1 year after radiotherapy (126). The 5-year survival rate of patients with positive pelvic lymph nodes is less than 5%. Thus the performance of an extensive lymphadenectomy in the irradiated field is not warranted, but discontinuation of the procedure is advisable if any nodes are positive for metastatic cancer. Survival of patients who have any disease in the peritoneal cavity is nil.

Chemotherapy

Recurrent cervical cancer is not considered curable with chemotherapy. A number of clinical trials with various drugs have shown response rates of up to 45% (134). Complete responses are unusual and are generally limited to patients with chest metastases, where the dose of drug delivered to the disease is better than that delivered to the fibrotic postirradiation pelvis (135).

Vermorken (136) has recently reviewed the literature on the role of chemotherapy in cervical cancer. He concludes that present data do not support the claim that toxic combination chemotherapy regimens are superior to cisplatin alone in terms of survival benefit, although further studies are required to determine whether combination chemotherapy may offer a benefit for certain subgroups of patients. The response rates for simple agents and combination chemotherapy in squamous cell cervical cancer are shown in Tables 7.6 and 7.7 (136).

Table 7.6   Combination Chemotherapy in Cervical Carcinoma*

Regimens	*Patients (Response/Treated)*	*% Response*
Non-cisplatin-based combinations		
DOX/MTX	66/169	39
DOX/BLM	5/52	10
DOX/CTX (±5FU)	17/94	18
DOX (other)	48/186	26
BLM/MTX (±VCR)	26/45	58
BLM/MMC	83/200	41
VRC/BLM/MMC	80/180	43
Cisplatin-based combinations		
2-drug	142/368	38
3-drug	174/416	41
4-drug	131/313	42

*Cumulative data, DOX = doxorubicin, MTX = methotrexate, CTX = cyclophosphamide, 5FU = 5-fluorouracil, BLM = bleomycin, VCR = vincristine, MMC = mitomycin C.
Reproduced, with permission, from Vermorken JB: The role of chemotherapy in squamous cell carcinoma of the uterine cervix: a review. *Int J Gynecol Cancer* 3:129, 1993.

Table 7.7   Single Conventional Agent Chemotherapy in Cervical Carcinoma

Drugs	Patients (Response/Treated)	% Response
Alkylating agents		
Cyclophosphamide	36/271	13
Chlorambucil	11/44	25
Melphalan	4/20	20
CCNU	3/63	5
Methyl-CCNU	7/94	7
Antimetabolites		
5-Fluorouracil	36/270	13
Methotrexate	12/73	16
6-Mercaptopurine	1/18	5
Hydroxyurea	0/27	0
Antibiotics		
Doxorubicin	32/172	19
Bleomycin	19/176	11
Mitomycin-C	5/23	22
Porfiromycin	17/78	22
Plant alkaloids		
Vincristine	10/58	17
Vinblastine	2/20	10
Miscellaneous		
Cisplatin	238/968	25
Carboplatin	50/250	19
Ifosfamide	34/93	37
Hexamethylmelamine	11/50	22
DTIC (Dacarbazine)	3/12	25

Modified, with permission, from Vermorken JB: The role of chemotherapy in squamous cell carcinoma of the uterine cervix: a review. *Int J Gynecol Cancer* 3:129, 1993.

References

1. **Boring CC, Squires TS, Tong T:** Cancer statistics, 1994. *CA-Cancer J Clin* 44:7, 1994.

2. **Pettersson F** (ed): Annual report on the results of treatment in gynecological cancer. *Int J Gynecol Obstet* 36:1, 1991.

3. **Lagasse LD, Ballon SC, Berman ML, Watring WG:** Pretreatment lymphangiography and operative evaluation in carcinoma of the cervix. *Am J Obstet Gynecol* 134:219, 1979.

4. **Averette HE, Ford JH Jr, Dudan RC, et al:** Staging of cervical cancer. *Clin Obstet Gynecol* 18:215, 1975.

5. **Koehler PR:** Current status of lymphangiography in patients with cancer. *Cancer* 37:503, 1976.

6. **King LA, Talledo OE, Gallup DG, EL Gammal TAM:** Computed tomography in evaluation of gynecologic malignancies: a retrospective analysis. *Am J Obstet Gynecol* 155:960, 1986.

7. **Bandy LC, Clarke-Pearson DL, Silverman PM, Creasman WT:** Computed tomography in evaluation of extrapelvic lymphadenopathy in carcinoma of the cervix. *Obstet Gynecol* 65:73, 1986.

8. **Hacker NF, Berek JS:** Surgical staging. In Surwit E, Alberts D (eds): *Cervix Cancer.* Boston, Martinus Nijhoff, 1987, pp 43–57.

9. **Worthington JL, Balfe DM, Lee JKT, et al:** Uterine neoplasms: MR imaging. *Radiology* 159:725, 1986.

10. **Van Nagell JR Jr, Parker JC Jr, Maruyama Y, et al:** Bladder or rectal injury following radiation therapy for cervical cancer. *Am J Obstet Gynecol* 119:727, 1974.

11. **Lawton FG, Hacker NF:** Surgery for invasive gynecologic cancer in the elderly female population. *Obstet Gynecol* 76:287, 1990.

12. **Hatch KD, Parham G, Shingleton HM, et al:** Ureteral strictures and fistulae following radical hysterectomy. *Gynecol Oncol* 19:17, 1984.

13. **Webb M, Symmonds R:** Wertheim hysterectomy: a reppraisal. *Obstet Gynecol* 54:140, 1979.

14. **Lohe KJ:** Early squamous cell carcinoma of the uterine cervix. I. Definition and histology. *Gynecol Oncol* 6:10, 1978.

15. **Boyce J, Fruchter R, Nicastri A:** Prognostic factors in stage I carcinoma of the cervix. *Gynecol Oncol* 12:154, 1981.

16. **Simon NL, Gore H, Shingleton HM, et al:** Study of superficially invasive carcinoma of the cervix. *Obstet Gynecol* 68:19, 1986.

17. **Delgado G, Bundy BN, Fowler WC, et al:** A prospective surgical pathological study of stage I squamous carcinoma of the cervix: a Gynecologic Oncology Group study. *Gynecol Oncol* 35:314, 1989.

18. **Piver M, Rutledge F, Smith J:** Five classes of extended hysterectomy for women with cervical cancer. *Obstet Gynecol* 44:265, 1974.

19. **Meigs J:** Radical hysterectomy with bilateral pelvic node dissections: a report of 100 patients operated five or more years ago. *Am J Obstet Gynecol* 63:854, 1951.

20. **Orr JW Jr, Shingleton HM, Hatch KD:** Correlation of perioperative morbidity in conization to radical hysterectomy interval. *Obstet Gynecol* 59:726, 1982.

21. **Potter ME, Alvarez RD, Shingleton HM, et al:** Early invasive cervical cancer with pelvic lymph node involvement: to complete or not to complete radical hysterectomy? *Gynecol Oncol* 37:78, 1990.

22. **Mann WJ Jr, Orr JW Jr, Shingleton HM, et al:** Perioperative influences on infectious morbidity in radical hysterectomy. *Gynecol Oncol* 11:207, 1981.

23. **Green T:** Ureteral suspension for prevention of ureteral complications following radical Wertheim hysterectomy. *Obstet Gynecol* 28:1, 1966.

24. **Lowe J, Mauger G, Carmichael J:** The effect of Wertheim hysterectomy upon bladder and urethral function. *Am J Obstet Gynecol* 139:826, 1981.

25. **Baltzer J, Lohe K, Kopke W, Zander J:** Histologic criteria for the prognosis of patients with operated squamous cell carcinoma of the cervix. *Gynecol Oncol* 13:184, 1982.

26. **Chung C, Nahhas W, Stryker J, Curry S:** Analysis of factors contributing to treatment failures in stage IB and IIa carcinoma of the cervix. *Am J Obstet Gynecol* 138:550, 1980.

27. **Creasman W, Soper J, Clarke-Pearson D:** Radical hysterectomy as therapy for early carcinoma of the cervix. *Am J Obstet Gynecol* 155:964, 1986.

28. **Van Nagell J, Donaldson E, Parker J:** The prognostic significance of cell type and lesion size in patients with cervical cancer treated by radical surgery. *Gynecol Oncol* 5:142, 1977.

29. **Inoue T, Okumura M:** Prognostic significance of parametrial extension in patients with cervical carcinoma stage Ib, IIa, and IIIb. *Cancer* 54:1714, 1984.

30. **Bleker O, Ketting B, Wayjean-eecen B, Kloosterman G:** The significance of microscopic involvement of the parametrium and/or pelvic lymph nodes in cervical cancer stages Ib and IIa. *Gynecol Oncol* 16:56, 1983.

31. **Gauthier P, Gore I, Shingleton HM:** Identification of histopathologic risk groups in stage Ib squamous cell carcinoma of the cervix. *Obstet Gynecol* 66:569, 1985.

32. **Van Nagell J, Donaldson E, Wood E, Parker J:** The significance of vascular invasion and lymphocytic infiltration in invasive cervical cancer. *Cancer* 41:228, 1978.

33. **Nahhas W, Sharkey F, Whitney C:** The prognostic significance of vascular channel involvement in deep stromal penetration in early cervical carcinoma. *Am J Clin Oncol* 6:259, 1983.

34. **Soison AP, Soper JT, Clarke-Pearson DL, et al:** Adjuvant radiotherapy following radical hysterectomy for patients with stage Ib and IIA cervical cancer. *Gynecol Oncol* 37:390, 1990.

35. **Tinga DJ, Timmer PR, Bouma J, Aalder JG:** Prognostic significance of single versus multiple lymph node metastases in cervical carcinoma stage IB. *Gynecol Oncol* 39:175, 1990.

36. **Alvarez RD, Soong S-J, Kinney WK, et al:** Identification of prognostic factors and risk groups in patients found to have nodal metastasis at the time of radical hysterectomy for early stage squamous carcinoma of the cervix. *Gynecol Oncol* 35:130, 1990.

37. **Fuller AF, Elliott N, Kosloff C, et al:** Determinants of increased risk for recurrence in patients undergoing radical hysterectomy for stage IB and IIA carcinoma of the cervix. *Gynecol Oncol* 33:34, 1989.

38. **Delgado G, Bundy B, Zaino R, et al:** Prospective surgical-pathological study of disease free interval in patients with stage IB squamous cell carcinoma of the cervix: a Gynecologic Oncology Group study. *Gynecol Oncol* 38:352, 1990.

39. **Gonzalez DG, Ketting BW, Van Bunningen B, Van Duk, JDP:** Carcinoma of the uterine cervix stage IB and IIA: results of postoperative irradiation in patients with microscopic infiltration in the parametrium and/or lymph node metastasis. *Int J Radiat Oncol Biol Phys* 16:389, 1989.

40. **Martinbeau P, Kjorstad K, Iversen T:** Stage Ib carcinoma of the cervix: the Norwegian Radium Hospital. II. Results when pelvic nodes are involved. *Obstet Gynecol* 60:215, 1982.

41. **Morrow P:** Panel report: Is pelvic irradiation beneficial in the postoperative management of stage Ib squamous cell carcinoma of the cervix with pelvic node metastases treated by radical hysterectomy and pelvic lymphadenectomy? *Gynecol Oncol* 10:105, 1980.

42. **Inoue T:** Prognostic significance of the depth of invasion relating to nodal metastases, parametrial extension, and cell types. *Cancer* 54:3035, 1984.

43. **Piver M, Chung W:** Prognostic significance of cervical lesion size and pelvic node metastases in cervical carcinoma. *Obstet Gynecol* 46:507, 1975.

44. **Hsu CT, Cheng YS, Su SC:** Prognosis of uterine cervical cancer with extensive lymph node metastasis. *Am J Obstet Gynecol* 114:954, 1972.

45. **Pilleron J, Durand J, Hamelin J:** Prognostic value of node metastasis in cancer of the uterine cervix. *Am J Obstet Gynecol* 119:458, 1974.

46. **Inoue T, Chihara T, Morita K:** Postoperative extended field irradiation in patients with pelvic and/or common iliac node metastasis from cervical carcinoma stages Ib to IIb. *Gynecol Oncol* 25:234, 1986.

47. **Larsson G, Alm P, Gullberg B, Grundsell H:** Prognostic factors in early invasive carcinoma of the uterine cervix. *Am J Obstet Gynecol* 146:145, 1983.

48. **Lohe KJ, Burghardt E, Hillemanns HG, et al:** Early squamous cell carcinoma of the uterine cervix. II. Clinical results of a cooperative study in the management of 419 patients with early stromal invasion and microcarcinoma. *Gynecol Oncol* 6:31, 1978.

49. **Burghardt E, Holzer E:** Diagnosis and treatment of microinvasive carcinoma of the cervix uteri. *Obstet Gynecol* 49:641, 1977.

50. **Van Nagell J Jr, Greenwell N, Powell D, Donaldson E:** Microinvasive carcinoma of the cervix. *Am J Obstet Gynecol* 145:981, 1983.

51. **Leman M, Benson W, Kurman R, Park R:** Microinvasive carcinoma of the cervix. *Obstet Gynecol* 48:571, 1976.

52. **Seski JC, Abell MR, Morley GW:** Microinvasive squamous cell carcinoma of the cervix: definition, histologic analysis, late results of treatment. *Obstet Gynecol* 50:410, 1977.

53. **Roche WO, Norris HC:** Microinvasive carcinoma of the cervix. *Cancer* 36:180, 1975.

54. **Nahhas WA, Sharkey FE, Whitney CW, et al:** The prognostic significance of vascular channel involvement and deep stromal invasion in early cervical cancer. *Am J Clin Oncol* 6:259, 1983.

55. **Shingleton HM, Orr JW Jr:** Primary surgical and combined treatment. In Singer A, Jordan J (eds): *Cancer of the Cervix.* New York, Churchill Livingstone, 1983, p 79.

56. **Barter JF, Soong S-J, Shingleton HM, et al:** Complications of combined radical hysterectomy: postoperative radiation therapy in women with early stage cervical cancer. *Gynecol Oncol* 32:292, 1989.

57. **Kinney WK, Alvarez RD, Reid GC, et al:** Value of adjuvant whole-pelvic irradiation after Wertheim hysterectomy for early-stage squamous carcinoma of the cervix with pelvic nodal metastasis: a matched-control study. *Gynecol Oncol* 34:258, 1989.

58. **Lai C-H, Lin T-S, Soong Y-K, et al:** Adjuvant chemotherapy after radical hysterectomy for cervical carcinoma. *Gynecol Oncol* 35:193, 1989.

59. **Wertheim MS, Hakes TB, Daghestani AN, et al:** A pilot study of adjuvant therapy in patients with cervical cancer at high risk of recurrence after radical hysterectomy and pelvic lymphadenectomy. *J Clin Oncol* 3:912, 1985.

60. **Kim DS, Moon H, Kim KT, et al:** Two-year survival: preoperative adjuvant chemotherapy in the treatment of cervical cancer stages Ib and II with bulky tumor. *Gynecol Oncol* 33:225, 1989.

61. **Panici PB, Scambia G, Baiocchi G, et al:** Neoadjuvant chemotherapy and radical surgery in locally advanced cervical cancer: Prognostic factors for response and survival. *Cancer* 67:372, 1991.

62. **Sardi J, Sananes C, Giaroli A, et al:** Neoadjuvant chemotherapy in locally advanced carcinoma of the cervix uteri. *Gynecol Oncol* 38:486, 1990.

63. **Berman M, Keys N, Creasman W, DiSaia P:** Survival and patterns of recurrence in cervical cancer metastatic to paraaortic lymph nodes. *Gynecol Oncol* 19:8, 1984.

64. **Piver MS, Barlow JJ, Krishnamsetty R:** Five-year survival (with no evidence of disease) in patients with biopsy-confirmed aortic node metastasis from cervical carcinoma. *Am J Obstet Gynecol* 193:575, 1981.

65. **Wharton JT, Jones HW III, Day TG, et al:** Preirradiation celiotomy and extended field irradiation for invasive carcinoma of the cervix. *Obstet Gynecol* 49:333, 1977.

66. **Ballon SC, Berman ML, Lagasse LD, et al:** Survival after extraperitoneal pelvic and paraaortic lymphadenectomy and radiation therapy in cervical carcinoma. *Obstet Gynecol* 57:90, 1981.

67. **Twiggs LB, Potish RA, George RJ, Adcock LL:** Pretreatment extraperitoneal surgical staging in primary carcinoma of the cervix uteri. *Surg Gynecol Obstet* 158:243, 1984.

68. **Weiser EB, Bundy BN, Hoskins WJ, et al:** Extraperitoneal versus transperitoneal selective paraaortic lymphadenectomy in the pretreatment surgical staging of advanced cervical carcinoma (a Gynecologic Oncology Group study). *Gynecol Oncol* 33:283, 1989.

69. **Stehman FB, Bundy BN, DiSaia PJ, et al:** Carcinoma of the cervix treated with radiation therapy. I. A multi-variate analysis of prognostic variables in the Gynecologic Oncology Group. *Cancer* 67:2776, 1991.

70. **Lovecchio JL, Averette HE, Donato D, Bell J:** 5-year survival of patients with periarotic nodal metastases in clinical stage IB and IIA cervical carcinoma. *Gynecol Oncol* 38:446, 1990.

71. **Rubin SC, Brookland R, Mikuta JJ, et al:** Paraaortic nodal metastases in early cervical carcinoma: long-term survival following extended-field radiotherapy. *Gynecol Oncol* 18:213, 1984.

72. **Buchsbaum JH, Lifshitz S:** The role of scalene lymph node biopsy in advanced carcinoma of the cervix uteri. *Surg Gynecol Obstet* 143:246, 1976.

73. **Jampolis S, Andras J, Fletcher GH:** Analysis of sites and causes of failure of irradiation in invasive squamous cell carcinoma of the intact uterine cervix. *Radiology* 115:681, 1975.

74. **Hreshchyshyn MM, Aron BS, Boronow RC, et al:** Hydroxyurea or placebo combined with radiation to treat stage IIIb and IV cervical cancer confined to the pelvis. *Int J Radiat Oncol Biol Phys* 5:317, 1979.

75. **Piver MS, Barlow JJ, Vongtama V, Blumenson L:** Hydroxyurea: a radiation potentiator in carcinoma of the uterine cervix. *Am J Obstet Gynecol* 147:803, 1983.

76. **Thomas G, Dembo A, Beale F:** Concurrent radiation, mitomycin-C and 5-fluorouracil in poor prognosis carcinoma of the cervix: preliminary results of a Phase I-II study. *Int J Radiat Oncol Biol Phys* 10:1785, 1984.

77. **Bonomi P, Blessing JA, Stehman FB:** A randomized trial of three Cisplatinum dose schedules in squamous cell carcinoma of the uterine cervix. *J Clin Oncol* 3:1079, 1985.

78. **Choo YC, Choy TK, Wong LC, Ma HK:** Potentiation of radiotherapy by cis-dichlorodiammine platinum (II) in advanced cervical carcinoma. *Gynecol Oncol* 23:94, 1986.

79. **Twiggs LB, Potish RA, McIntyre S, et al:** Concurrent weekly cis-platinum and radiotherapy in advanced cervical cancer: a preliminary dose escalating toxicity study. *Gynecol Oncol* 24:143, 1986.

80. **Thomas G, Dembo A, Fyles A, et al:** Concurrent chemoradiation in advanced cervical cancer. *Gynecol Oncol* 38:446, 1990.

81. **Kim RY, Levy DS, Brascho DJ, Hatch KD:** Uterine perforation during intracavitary application: prognostic significance in carcinoma of the cervix. *Radiology* 147:249, 1983.

82. **White AJ, Buchsbaum HJ, Blythe JG, Lifshitz S:** Use of the bulbocavernosus muscle (Martius procedure) for repair of radiation-induced rectovaginal fistulas. *Obstet Gynecol* 60:114, 1982.

83. **Bricker EM, Johnston WD:** Repair of postirradiation rectovaginal fistula and stricture. *Surg Gynecol Obstet* 148:499, 1979.

84. **Smith ST, Seski JC, Copeland LJ, et al:** Surgical management of irradiation-induced small bowel damage. *Obstet Gynecol* 65:563, 1985.

85. **Gallousis S:** Isolated lung metastases from pelvic malignancies. *Gynecol Oncol* 7:206, 1979.

86. **Nordqvist SRB, Sevin BU, Nadji M, et al:** Fine-needle aspiration cytology in gynecologic oncology. I. Diagnostic accuracy. *Obstet Gynecol* 54:719, 1979.

87. **Krebs HB, Helmkamp BF, Sevin B-U, et al:** Recurrent cancer of the cervix following radical hysterectomy and pelvic node dissection. *Obstet Gynecol* 59:422, 1982.

88. **Shingleton HM, Orr JW Jr:** Posttreatment surveillance. In Singer A, Jordan J (eds): *Cancer of the Cervix*. New York, Churchill Livingstone, 1983, p 136.

89. **Kjorstad KE:** Adenocarcinoma of the uterine cervix. *Gynecol Oncol* 5:219, 1977.

90. **Berek JS, Hacker NF, Fu YS, et al:** Adenocarcinoma of the uterine cervix: histologic variables associated with lymph node metastasis and survival. *Obstet Gynecol* 65:46, 1985.

91. **Hopkins MP, Morley GW:** A comparison of adenocarcinoma and squamous cell carcinoma of the cervix. *Obstet Gynecol* 77:912, 1991.

92. **Shingleton HM, Gore H, Bradley DH, Soong SJ:** Adenocarcinoma of the cervix. I. Clinical evaluation and pathologic features. *Am J Obstet Gynecol* 139:799, 1981.

93. **Kilgore LC, Soong S-J, Gore H, et al:** Analysis of prognostic features in adenocarcinoma of the cervix. *Gynecol Oncol* 31:137, 1988.

94. **Berek JS, Castaldo TW, Hacker NF, et al:** Adenocarcinoma of the uterine cervix. *Cancer* 48:2734, 1981.

95. **Mayer EG, Galindo J, Davis J, et al:** Adenocarcinoma of the uterine cervix: incidence and the role of radiation therapy. *Radiology* 121:725, 1976.

96. **Rutledge FN, Galakatos AE, Wharton JT, Smith JP:** Adenocarcinoma of the uterine cervix. *Am J Obstet Gynecol* 122:236, 1975.

97. **Gallup DG, Abell MR:** Invasive adenocarcinoma of the uterine cervix. *Obstet Gynecol* 49:596, 1977.

98. **Eifel PJ, Morris M, Oswald MJ, et al:** Adenocarcinoma of the uterine cervix: prognosis and patterns of failure in 367 cases. *Cancer* 65:2507, 1990.

99. **Gallup DG, Harper RH, Stock RJ:** Poor prognosis in patients with adenosquamous cell carcinoma of the cervix. *Obstet Gynecol* 65:416, 1985.

100. **Maier RC, Norris HJ:** Coexistence of cervical intraepithelial neoplasia with primary adenocarcinoma of the endocervix. *Obstet Gynecol* 56:361, 1980.

101. **Hacker NF, Berek JS, Lagasse LD, et al:** Cervical cancer in pregnancy. *Obstet Gynecol* 59:735, 1982.

102. **Averette HE, Nasser N, Yankow SL, Little WA:** Cervical conization in pregnancy. *Am J Obstet Gynecol* 106:543, 1970.

103. **Lee RB, Neglia W, Park RC:** Cervical carcinoma in pregnancy. *Obstet Gynecol* 58:584, 1981.

104. **Shingleton HM, Orr JW Jr:** Cancer complicating pregnancy. In Singer A, Jordan J (eds): *Cancer of the Cervix.* New York, Churchill Livingstone, 1983, p 203.

105. **Green TH, Morse WJ Jr:** Management of invasive cervical cancer following inadvertent simple hysterectomy. *Obstet Gynecol* 33:763, 1969.

106. **Orr JW Jr, Ball GC, Soong SJ, et al:** Surgical treatment of women found to have invasive cervix cancer at the time of total hysterectomy. *Obstet Gynecol* 68:353, 1986.

107. **Durrance FY:** Radiotherapy following simple hysterectomy in patients with stage I and II carcinoma of the cervix. *Am J Roentgenol Radium Ther Nucl Med* 102:165, 1968.

108. **Andras EJ, Fletcher GH, Rutledge F:** Radiotherapy of carcinoma of the cervix following simple hysterectomy. *Am J Obstet Gynecol* 115:647, 1973.

109. **Heller PB, Barnhill DR, Mayer AR, et al:** Cervical carcinoma found incidentally in a uterus removed for benign indications. *Obstet Gynecol* 67:187, 1986.

110. **Million RR, Rutledge F, Fletcher GH:** Stage IV carcinoma of the cervix with bladder invasion. *Am J Obstet Gynecol* 113:239, 1972.

111. **Taylor PT, Andersen WA:** Untreated cervical cancer complicated by obstructive uropathy and renal failure. *Gynecol Oncol* 11:162, 1981.

112. **Fletcher GH, Wharton JT:** Principles of irradiation therapy for gynecologic malignancy. *Curr Probl Obstet Gynecol* 2:2, 1978.

113. **Gaddis O Jr, Morrow CP, Klement V, et al:** Treatment of cervical carcinoma employing a template for transperineal interstitial Iridium brachytherapy. *Int J Radiol Oncol Biol Phys* 9:819, 1983.

114. **O'Quinn AG, Fletcher GH, Wharton JT:** Guidelines for conservative hysterectomy after irradiation. *Gynecol Oncol* 9:68, 1980.

115. **Homesley HD, Raben M, Blake DD, et al:** Relationship of lesion size to survival in patients with stage IB squamous cell carcinoma of the cervix uteri treated by radiation therapy. *Surg Gynecol Obstet* 150:529, 1980.

116. **Van Nagell JR Jr, Donaldson ES, Wood EC, et al:** Small cell carcinoma of the cervix. *Cancer* 40:2243, 1979.

117. **Oldham RK, Greco FA:** Small cell lung cancer, a curable disease. *Cancer Chem Pharmacol* 4:173, 1980.

118. **Sheets EE, Berman ML, Hrountas CK, et al:** Surgically treated early-stage neuroendocrine small-cell cervical carcinoma. *Obstet Gynecol* 71:(1)10, 1988.

119. **Feder BH, Syed AMN, Neblett D:** Treatment of extensive carcinoma of the cervix with the "transperineal parametrial butterfly"—a preliminary report on the revival of Waterman's approach. *Int J Radiat Oncol Biol Phys* 4:735, 1978.

120. **Mikuta JJ, Giuntoli RL, Rubin EL, Mangan CE:** The radical hysterectomy. *Am J Obstet Gynecol* 128:119, 1977.

121. **Symmonds RE, Pratt JH, Welch JS:** Extended Wertheim operation for primary, recurrent, or suspected recurrent carcinoma of the cervix. *Obstet Gynecol* 24:15, 1964.

122. **Ketcham AS, Chretien PB, Hoye RC, et al:** Occult metastases to the scalene lymph nodes in patients with clinically operable carcinoma of the cervix. *Cancer* 31:180, 1973.

123. **Morley GW, Lindenauer SM:** Pelvic exenteration therapy for gynecologic malignancy: an analysis of 70 cases. *Cancer* 38:581, 1976.

124. **Rutledge FN, Smith JP, Wharton JT, O'Quinn AG:** Pelvic exenteration: an analysis of 296 patients. *Am J Obstet Gynecol* 129:881, 1977.

125. **Averette HE, Lichtinger M, Sevin BU, Girtanner RE:** Pelvic exenteration: a 150-year experience in a general hospital. *Am J Obstet Gynecol* 150:179, 1984.

126. **Hatch KD, Shingleton H, Soong S, et al:** Anterior pelvic exenteration. *Gynecol Oncol* 31:135, 1988.

127. **Orr JW Jr, Shingleton HM, Hatch KD, et al:** Gastrointestinal complications associated with pelvic exenteration. *Am J Obstet Gynecol* 145:325, 1983.

128. **Berek JS, Hacker NF, Lagasse LD:** Rectosigmoid colectomy and reanastamosis to facilitate resection of primary and recurrent gynecologic cancer. *Obstet Gynecol* 64:715, 1984.

129. **Hatch KD, Shingleton HM, Potter ME, et al:** Low rectal resection and anastomosis at the time of pelvic exenteration. *Gynecol Oncol* 32:262, 1988.

130. **Kock ND, Nilson AE, Nilsson LO, et al:** Urinary diversion via a continent ileal reservoir: clinical results in 12 patients. *J Urol* 128:469, 1982.

131. **Penalver MA, Bejany DE, Averette HE, et al:** Continent urinary diversion in gynecologic oncology. *Gynecol Oncol* 34:274, 1989.

132. **Mannel RS, Braly PS, Buller RE:** Indiana pouch continent urinary reservoir in patients with previous pelvic irradiation. *Obstet Gynecol* 75(6):891, 1990.

133. **Berek JS, Hacker NF, Lagasse LD:** Vaginal reconstruction performed simultaneously with pelvic exenteration. *Obstet Gynecol* 63:318, 1984.

134. **Thigpen JT:** Single agent chemotherapy in carcinoma of the cervix. In Surwit EA, Alberts DS (eds): *Cervix Cancer.* Boston, Martinus Nijhoff, 1987, pp 119–136.

135. **Barter JF, Soong SJ, Hatch KD, et al:** Diagnosis and treatment of pulmonary metastases from cervical carcinoma. *Gynecol Oncol* 38:347, 1990.

136. **Vermorken JB:** The role of chemotherapy in squamous cell carcinoma of the uterine cervix: a review. *Int J Gynecol Cancer* 3:129, 1993.

8

Uterine Cancer

Neville F. Hacker

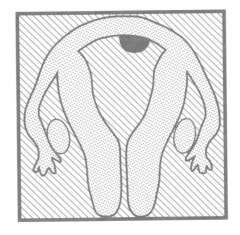

Endometrial carcinoma is the most common malignancy of the female genital tract in the United States. For 1994, 31,000 new cases and 5900 deaths were anticipated (1). This is predominantly a disease of affluent, obese, postmenopausal women of low parity, although an increasing proportion of younger patients with endometrial cancer has been reported (2). Over the last few decades, age-standardized incidence rates have risen in most countries and in urban populations. Developing countries (and Japan) have incidence rates 4–5 times lower than Western industrialized nations, the lowest rates being in India and South Asia (3). Significant advances in our knowledge of endometrial cancer have occurred in the past two decades. A better definition of the histologic subtypes has evolved, clearly defining different prognostic groups. The etiologic significance of estrogen has been clearly elucidated. Careful surgical staging has more accurately defined patterns of spread, and the move away from preoperative radiation has allowed more individualization of treatment.

Any factor that increases exposure to unopposed estrogen (e.g., hormone replacement therapy, obesity, anovulatory cycles, estrogen-secreting tumors) increases the risk of endometrial cancer, whereas factors that decrease exposure to estrogens or increase progesterone levels (e.g., oral contraceptives or smoking) tend to be protective (3). The impact of these factors differs in various populations, however, and in Northern Italy established risk factors account for only about 50% of the cases (4).

Because it generally presents as early-stage disease and can be treated without radical surgery, endometrial carcinoma has frequently been regarded as a relatively benign type of cancer. However, a more critical evaluation of survival data indicates that this concept is erroneous (5).

Screening of Asymptomatic Women

The ideal method for outpatient sampling of the endometrium has not yet been devised, and no blood test of sufficient sensitivity and specificity has been de-

285

Table 8.1   Patients for Whom Screening for Endometrial Cancer Is Justified

1. Postmenopausal women on exogenous estrogens

2. Obese postmenopausal women, particularly if there is a family history of endometrial, breast, bowel, or ovarian cancer

3. Women whose menopause occurred after 52 years of age

4. Premenopausal women with anovulatory cycles, such as those with polycystic ovarian disease

veloped. Therefore mass screening of the population is not practical. However screening for endometrial carcinoma or its precursors is justified for certain high-risk persons, including those shown in Table 8.1.

Only about 50% of women with endometrial cancer will have malignant cells on a Papanicolaou (Pap) smear (6, 7). However, compared with patients who have normal cervical cytology, patients with suspicious or malignant cells are more likely to have deeper myometrial invasion, higher tumor grade, positive peritoneal cytology, and a more advanced stage of disease (8).

The appearance of normal- as well as abnormal-appearing endometrial cells in cervical smears taken in the second half of the menstrual cycle or in postmenopausal women should alert the clinician to the possibility of endometrial disease. About 6% of postmenopausal patients with *normal* endometrial cells in cervical smears will have endometrial carcinoma, and about 13% will have endometrial hyperplasia (9). If morphologically abnormal endometrial cells are present, about 25% of women will have endometrial carcinoma (10). The likelihood of endometrial carcinoma being present increases with the patient's age (11).

The unsatisfactory results obtained with conventional Pap smears are due to the indirect sampling of the endometrium and several commercially available devices have been developed to allow direct sampling (e.g., Pipelle, Vabra aspirator). A satisfactory endometrial biopsy specimen also may be obtained in the office with the Karman cannula or a small curette, such as a Novak or Kevorkian (Fig. 8.1).

Figure 8.1.   Devices used for sampling endometrium. From top to bottom: Serrated Novak, Novak, Kevorkian, Explora® (Mylex), and Pipelle® (Unimar).

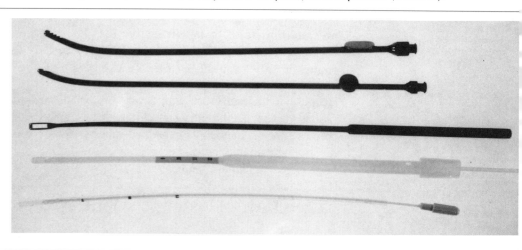

With these devices, an endometrial smear may be made for cytologic evaluation and a cell block may be prepared for histologic examination. Even in experienced hands, endometrial smears are difficult to interpret, and optimal information is obtained by the combined use of endometrial smears and cell blocks (12). All of these office techniques for endometrial sampling cause the patient some discomfort, and in about 8% of patients it is not possible to obtain a specimen because of a stenotic os. This failure rate increases to about 18% for women over 70 years of age (12). Although the accuracy of endometrial sampling has not been definitively determined, it is probably on the order of 90% (13). The clinician should be comfortable with one of these techniques.

More recently, transvaginal ultrasonography with or without color flow imaging has been investigated as a screening technique (14). Preliminary data suggest a strong association between the thickness of the endometrial strip and endometrial disease, normal endometrium being usually < 5 mm thick. One indication for this screening technique would be postmenopausal women who are receiving unopposed estrogen, but Bourne et al. (15) recently reported an 11% false-positive rate for this group.

Clinical Features

Symptoms

Endometrial carcinoma should be excluded in all patients shown in Table 8.2. Ninety percent of patients with endometrial carcinoma will have abnormal vaginal bleeding, most commonly postmenopausal bleeding. The usual causes of postmenopausal bleeding are shown in Table 8.3. **Intermenstrual bleeding or heavy prolonged bleeding in perimenopausal or anovulatory premenopausal women should arouse suspicion. The diagnosis may be delayed unnecessarily in these women because the bleeding is usually ascribed to "hormonal imbalance."** A high index of suspicion also is needed to make an early diagnosis in women under 40 years of age.

Occasionally, vaginal bleeding does not occur because of cervical stenosis, particularly in thin, elderly estrogen-deficient patients. Smith and McCartney (16) have called this group "estrogen independent," and they suggest that an *estrogen provocation test* may allow earlier diagnosis: daily vaginal or oral estrogen for 4 weeks will soften the cervix and will be followed by vaginal bleeding if endometrial carcinoma is present. Some patients with cervical stenosis develop a hematometra, and a small percentage have a purulent vaginal discharge resulting from a pyometra.

Signs

Physical examination commonly reveals an obese, hypertensive, postmenopausal woman, although about 35% of patients are not obese and show no signs of

---

Table 8.2   Patients in Whom a Diagnosis of Endometrial Cancer Should Be Excluded

1. All patients with postmenopausal bleeding

2. Postmenopausal women with a pyometra

3. Asymptomatic postmenopausal women with endometrial cells on a Papanicolaou smear

4. Perimenopausal patients with intermenstrual bleeding or increasingly heavy periods

5. Premenopausal patients with abnormal uterine bleeding, particularly if there is a history of anovulation

Table 8.3 Etiology of Postmenopausal Bleeding

Factor	Approximate Percentage
Exogenous estrogens	30
Atrophic endometritis/vaginitis	30
Endometrial cancer	15
Endometrial or cervical polyps	10
Endometrial hyperplasia	5
Miscellaneous (e.g., cervical cancer, uterine sarcoma, urethral caruncle, trauma)	10

Reproduced, with permission, from Hacker NF, Moore JG (eds): *Essentials of Obstetrics and Gynecology* Philadelphia, WB Saunders, 1986, p 467.

hyperestrogenism (17). Abdominal examination is usually unremarkable except in advanced cases when ascites may be present, and hepatic or omental metastases may be palpable. Occasionally, a hematometra will appear as a large, smooth midline mass arising from the pelvis. On pelvic examination, it is important to inspect and palpate the vulva, vagina, and cervix carefully to exclude metastatic spread or other causes of abnormal vaginal bleeding. The uterus may be bulky, but often it is not significantly enlarged. Rectovaginal examination should be performed to evaluate the fallopian tubes, ovaries, and cul-de-sac. Endometrial carcinoma may metastasize to these sites or, alternatively, coexistent ovarian tumors such as a granulosa cell tumor, thecoma, or epithelial ovarian carcinoma may be noted.

Diagnosis

All patients suspected of having endometrial carcinoma should have an endocervical curettage and an office endometrial biopsy. Any of the techniques previously described may be used, and hysteroscopy may prove to be a useful adjunct to biopsy (18). A histologically positive endometrial biopsy allows the planning of definitive treatment.

Because there is a false-negative rate of about 10%, a negative endometrial biopsy in a symptomatic patient must be followed by a fractional curettage under anesthesia. A diagnosis of endometrial hyperplasia on endometrial biopsy does not obviate the need for further investigation.

Fractional Curettage

While the patient is under anesthesia, careful bimanual rectovaginal examination is performed, a weighted speculum is placed in the vagina, and the cervix is grasped with a tenaculum. The endocervical canal is curetted prior to cervical dilatation, and the tissue is placed in a specially labeled container. The uterus then is sounded, the cervix is dilated, and the endometrium is systematically curetted. The tissue is placed in a separate container so that the histopathology of the endocervix and endometrium can be determined separately.

Preoperative Investigations

Routine preoperative investigations for early-stage endometrial carcinoma are shown in Table 8.4. If a fractional curettage has not been performed, an *endocervical curettage* should be performed to evaluate the endocervix.

Nonroutine tests are sometimes indicated, particularly for more advanced cases. *Cystoscopy* and *sigmoidoscopy* are necessary only if bladder or rectal involvement is suspected clinically (19). A *barium enema* should be performed if there is occult blood in the stool or a recent change in bowel habits, as concomitant colon cancer occasionally occurs (20). A *pelvic and abdominal computed tomography (CT) scan* may be helpful to determine the extent of metastatic disease in the following circumstances:

1. Abnormal liver function tests

2. Clinical hepatomegaly

3. Palpable upper abdominal mass

4. Palpable extrauterine pelvic disease

5. Clinical ascites

Magnetic resonance scanning was evaluated as a tool for preoperative staging in a recent National Cancer Institute cooperative study (21). Eighty-eight patients from five participating hospitals were entered in the study. For evaluating the depth of myometrial invasion, the overall accuracy was 66%, and the imaging was considered adequate for the evaluation of para-aortic lymph nodes in only 8% of the cases. Until image quality and techniques improve significantly, magnetic resonance imaging (MRI) is not a cost-effective method for the preoperative evaluation of patients with endometrial cancer.

Staging

The 1971 staging system for endometrial carcinoma devised by the International Federation of Gynecologists and Obstetricians (FIGO) is shown in Table 8.5. It was a *clinical staging*, based on examination under anesthesia, sounding of the uterus, and a limited number of investigations such as endocervical curettage, hysteroscopy, cystoscopy, proctoscopy, and x-ray examinations of the lungs and skeleton. This staging system is still used if a patient is considered unsuitable for surgery.

Several studies in the literature demonstrated significant understaging when patients were subjected to adequate surgical evaluation (22–27). Therefore, in 1988, the Cancer Committee of FIGO introduced a *surgical staging* system (Table 8.6).

Although more accurate information should be obtained if thorough surgical staging is carried out on all patients, this is unlikely to happen; therefore staging

Table 8.4   Routine Preoperative Investigations for Early-Stage Endometrial Carcinoma

Full blood count
Serum creatinine and electrolytes
Liver function tests
Blood sugar
Urinalysis
Electrocardiogram
Chest x-ray

Table 8.5   1971 FIGO Clinical Staging for Endometrial Carcinoma

Stage 0	Carcinoma *in situ*.
Stage I	The carcinoma is confined to the corpus.
Stage Ia	The length of the uterine cavity is 8 cm or less.
Stage Ib	The length of the uterine cavity is more than 8 cm.

Stage I cases should be subgrouped with regard to the histologic grade of the adenocarcinoma as follows:

Grade 1	Highly differentiated adenomatous carcinoma.
Grade 2	Moderately differentiated adenomatous carcinoma with partly solid areas.
Grade 3	Predominantly solid or entirely undifferentiated carcinoma.
Stage II	The carcinoma has involved the corpus and the cervix but has not extended outside the uterus.
Stage III	The carcinoma has extended outside the uterus but not outside the true pelvis.
Stage IV	The carcinoma has extended outside the true pelvis or has obviously involved the mucosa of the bladder or rectum. A bullous edema as such does not permit a case to be allocated to Stage IV.
Stage IVa	Spread of the growth to adjacent organs.
Stage IVb	Spread to distant organs.

Table 8.6   1988 FIGO Surgical Staging for Endometrial Carcinoma

Stage Ia	**G123**	Tumor limited to endometrium
Stage Ib	**G123**	Invasion to less than one-half the myometrium
Stage Ic	**G123**	Invasion to more than one-half the myometrium
Stage IIa	**G123**	Endocervical glandular involvement only
Stage IIb	**G123**	Cervical stromal invasion
Stage IIIa	**G123**	Tumor invades serosa and/or adnexa, and/or positive peritoneal cytology
Stage IIIb	**G123**	Vaginal metastases
Stage IIIc	**G123**	Metastases to pelvic and/or para-aortic lymph nodes
Stage IVa	**G123**	Tumor invasion of bladder and/or bowel mucosa
Stage IVb		Distant metastases including intra-abdominal and/or inguinal lymph nodes

Histopathology—degree of differentiation:
Cases of carcinoma of the corpus should be classified (or graded) according to the degree of histologic differentiation, as follows:
   G1 = 5% or less of a nonsquamous or nonmorular solid growth pattern
   G2 = 6–50% of a nonsquamous or nonmorular solid growth pattern
   G3 = more than 50% of a nonsquamous or nonmorular solid growth pattern

Notes on pathological grading:
1. Notable nuclear atypia, inappropriate for the architectural grade, raises the grade of a grade 1 or grade 2 tumor by 1.
2. In serous adenocarcinomas, clear-cell adenocarcinomas, and squamous cell carcinomas, nuclear grading takes precedence.
3. Adenocarcinomas with squamous differentiation are graded according to the nuclear grade of the glandular component.

Rules related to staging:
1. Because corpus cancer is now staged surgically, procedures previously used for determination of stages are no longer applicable, such as the findings from fractional D&C to differentiate between stage I and stage II.
2. It is appreciated that there may be a small number of patients with corpus cancer who will be treated primarily with radiation therapy. If that is the case, the clinical staging adopted by FIGO in 1971 would still apply, but designation of that staging system would be noted.
3. Ideally, width of the myometrium should be measured along with the width of tumor invasion.

Reproduced, with permission, from International Federation of Gynecology and Obstetrics. Annual report on the results of treatment in gynecologic cancer. *Int J Gynecol Obstet* 28:189–190, 1989.

reports will lack uniformity. Routine lymphadenectomy is unlikely to be performed for a number of reasons:

1. Many patients with endometrial carcinoma are treated in the community, where the necessary surgical skills may not be available to perform lymphadenectomy.

2. Many patients are obese and are not suitable for extensive nodal resections.

3. Patients with early tumors do not justify routine lymphadenectomy.

In addition, the extent of the lymphadenectomy has not been defined (i.e., random sampling of pelvic and para-aortic nodes, complete pelvic and/or para-aortic lymphadenectomy, or resection of any enlarged nodes).

The distribution of endometrial carcinoma by surgical stage at initial presentation is shown in Table 8.7.

Spread Patterns

Endometrial carcinoma spreads by the following routes:

1. Direct extension to adjacent structures

2. Transtubal passage of exfoliated cells

3. Lymphatic dissemination

4. Hematogenous dissemination

Direct Extension   Direct extension is the most common route of spread, and it results in penetration of the myometrium and eventually the serosa of the uterus. The cervix and fallopian tubes and ultimately the vagina and parametrium may be invaded. Tumors arising in the upper corpus may involve the tube or serosa before involving the cervix, whereas tumors arising from the lower segment of the uterus will involve the cervix early. The exact anatomic route by which endometrial cancer involves the cervix has not been clearly defined, but it probably involves a combination of contiguous surface spread, invasion of deep tissue planes, and lymhphatic dissemination (29, 30).

Transtubal Dissemination   The presence of malignant cells in peritoneal washings and the development of widespread intra-abdominal metastases in some

Table 8.7   Carcinoma of the Endometrium: Distribution by Surgical Stage

Stage	Number	Percent
I	5730	74.8
II	871	11.4
III	818	10.7
IV	227	2.9
No stage	17	0.2
Total	**7663**	**100.0**

Reproduced from the Annual Report on the Results of Treatment in Gynaecological Cancer, *Int J Gynecol Obstet* 36:140, 1991.

patients with early-stage endometrial cancer strongly suggest that cells may be exfoliated from the primary tumor and transported to the peritoneal cavity by retrograde flow along the fallopian tubes. Although this is probably the most common mechanism of spread, other mechanisms also must have some role, as positive peritoneal washings have been reported in patients who have had a prior tubal ligation (31).

Lymphatic Dissemination   Lymphatic dissemination is clearly responsible for spread to pelvic and para-aortic lymph nodes. **Although lymphatic channels pass directly from the fundus to the para-aortic nodes via the infundibulopelvic ligament, it is rare to find positive para-aortic nodes in the absence of positive pelvic nodes.** However, it is quite common to find microscopic metastases in both pelvic and para-aortic nodes, suggesting simultaneous spread to pelvic and para-aortic nodes in some patients. This is in contrast to cervical cancer, where para-aortic nodal metastases are always secondary to pelvic nodal metastases.

It seems likely that vaginal metastases also result from lymph-vascular spread. They commonly occur in the absence of cervical involvement (32), excluding direct spread as the mechanism, and may occur despite preoperative sterilization of the uterus with intracavitary radiation, excluding implantation of cells at the time of surgery as the mechanism (33).

Hematogenous Spread   Hematogenous spread most commonly results in lung metastases, but liver, brain, bone, and other sites are involved less commonly.

Prognostic Variables

Although stage of disease is the most significant prognostic variable, a number of factors have been shown to correlate with outcome in patients with the same stage of disease. These prognostic variables are summarized in Table 8.8. Knowledge of them is essential if appropriate treatment programs are to be devised.

Age

In general, younger women have a better prognosis than older women. Malkasian et al. (34) reported grade 3 lesions in only 3.5% of premenopausal women (4 of 114), compared with 12.5% of postmenopausal women (58 of 463). Aalders et al. (35) noted a recurrence rate of 8.5% among 294 patients under 60 years of age with stage I disease, compared with 17.5% among 246 women aged 60 years or older. The incidence of poorly differentiated lesions was similar in the two groups, but in the older group there were more patients with deep myometrial invasion (46.3% vs 24.1%). **Thus the improved prognosis for younger women seems to be related to the presence of better-differentiated, less invasive tumors** (36). It is important to carefully review the histologic characteristics of these well-differentiated lesions in young women, as Crissman et al. (37) have reported overdiagnosis of atypical endometrial hyperplasias in 41% of 54 cases.

Histologic Type

A retrospective review of 388 patients treated at the Mayo Clinic recorded an uncommon histologic subtype in 52 patients (13%). There were 20 adenosquamous, 14 serous papillary, 11 clear cell, and 7 undifferentiated carcinomas (38). In contrast to the 92% survival rate among patients with endometrioid carci-

Table 8.8 Prognostic Variables in Endometrial Cancer Other Than FIGO Stage

Age

Histologic type

Histologic grade

Nuclear grade

Myometrial invasion

Vascular space invasion

Tumor size

Peritoneal cytology

Hormone receptor status

DNA ploidy

Type of therapy (surgery vs radiation)

noma, the overall survival rate for these patients was only 33%. At the time of surgical staging, 62% of the patients with an unfavorable histologic subtype had extrauterine spread of disease.

The prognostic significance of squamous elements in endometrial carcinoma has been debated for decades (39). Recently, Zaino et al. (40) investigated the prognostic significance of squamous differentiation in 456 patients with typical adenocarcinomas and in 175 women with areas of squamous differentiation who had been entered into a Gynecologic Oncology Group (GOG) clinicopathologic study of Stage I and II disease. They reported that the biologic behavior of these tumors reflected the histologic grade and depth of invasion of the glandular component. Although prognostically valuable information was provided by dividing these tumors into adenoacanthomas and adenosquamous carcinomas, more information was gained when they were stratified by the histologic grade of the glandular component. Zaino et al. recommended that the terms "adenoacanthoma" and "adenosquamous carcinoma" be replaced by the simple term *adenocarcinoma with squamous differentiation*.

Papillary serous carcinomas have only recently been described in the endometrium (41, 42). They tend to invade the myometrium and lymph-vascular spaces, but even in the absence of deep myometrial invasion, they may disseminate widely (41, 43, 44), with a particular predilection for recurrence in the upper abdomen (42, 45).

Sherman et al. (44) studied 13 pure uterine papillary serous carcinomas (UPSC), 19 tumors consisting of UPSC admixed with other types of endometrial carcinomas, and 9 UPSCs confined to or associated with an endometrial polyp. Only cases in which ≥ 25% of the tumor consisted of UPSC were included. Survival was similar for the three groups, with more than 80% of the patients either dead of disease or alive with residual or recurrent tumor.

The mechanisms that have been proposed to explain the characteristic intra-abdominal dissemination of these tumors include transtubal spread, vascular-lymphatic invasion, and multifocal disease. Sherman et al. (44) made the interesting observation that "intraepithelial serous carcinoma" was present in the endocervix in 22% of their cases, in the fallopian tube in 5%, on the surface of the ovary in 10%, and on peritoneal surfaces or omentum in 25%.

Clear cell carcinomas represent fewer than 5% of endometrial carcinomas, although clear cell elements are commonly present in papillary serous tumors (44). Vascular space invasion is more common in these lesions (46), and depth of myometrial infiltration and vessel invasion are important prognosticators. Only patients with intramucosal tumors have a prognosis comparable to those with endometrioid adenocarcinomas (47).

Squamous cell carcinomas of the endometrium are rare. In a review of the literature Abeler et al. (48) estimated that the survival rate for patients with clinical Stage I disease was 36%.

Histologic Grade and Myometrial Invasion

There is a strong correlation between histologic grade, myometrial invasion, and prognosis. **Increasing tumor grade and myometrial penetration are associated with an increasing risk of pelvic and para-aortic lymph node metastases, adnexal metastases, positive peritoneal cytology, local vault recurrence, and hematogenous spread** (42).

The GOG reported the surgical pathologic features of 621 patients with Stage I endometrial carcinoma (27). The frequency of positive pelvic and para-aortic nodal metastases in relation to histologic grade and depth of myometrial invasion is shown in Tables 8.9 and 8.10. When grade 1 carcinomas are confined to the inner third of the myometrium, the incidence of positive pelvic nodes is < 3%, whereas when grade 3 lesions involve the outer third, the incidence of positive pelvic nodes is 34%. For aortic nodes, the corresponding figures are < 1% and 23%.

It is difficult to correlate accurately the risk of local recurrence with histologic grade and depth of myometrial invasion because of the prophylactic value of adjuvant radiation. The risk of distant metastases in relation to histologic grade and myometrial invasion is shown in Table 8.11 (49).

Vascular Space Invasion

Vascular space invasion appears to be an independent risk factor for recurrence and for death from endometrial carcinoma of all histologic types (37,

---

Table 8.9   Grade, Depth of Invasion, and Pelvic Node Metastasis of Endometrial Carcinoma

Depth of Myometrial Invasion	Histologic Grade		
	G1 (N = 180)	*G2* (N = 288)	*G3* (N = 153)
Endometrium only (N = 86)	0 (0%)	1 (3%)	0 (0%)
Inner third (N = 281)	3 (3%)	7 (5%)	5 (9%)
Middle third (N = 115)	0 (0%)	6 (9%)	1 (4%)
Outer third (N = 139)	2 (11%)	11 (19%)	22 (34%)

Reproduced, with permission, from Creasman WT, Morrow CP, Bundy BN, et al: Surgical pathologic spread patterns of endometrial cancer: a Gynecologic Oncology Group study. *Cancer* 60:2035, 1987.

Table 8.10   Grade, Depth of Invasion, and Aortic Node Metastasis of Endometrial Carcinoma

Depth of Myometrial Invasion	Histologic Grade		
	G1 (N = 180)	G2 (N = 288)	G3 (N = 153)
Endometrium only (N = 86)	0 (0%)	1 (3%)	0 (0%)
Inner third (N = 281)	1 (1%)	5 (4%)	2 (4%)
Middle third (N = 115)	1 (5%)	0 (0%)	0 (0%)
Outer third (N = 139)	1 (6%)	8 (14%)	15 (23%)

Reproduced, with permission, from Creasman WT, Morrow CP, Bundy BN, et al: Surgical pathologic spread patterns of endometrial cancer: a Gynecologic Oncology Group study. *Cancer* 60:2035, 1987.

Table 8.11   Clinical Stage I Endometrial Carcinoma: Distant Metastases Versus Histologic Grade and Myometrial Invasion

Variable	Number	Metastases	Percent
Histologic grade			
Grade 1	93	2	2.2
Grade 2	88	9	10.2
Grade 3	41	16	39.0
Myometrial invasion			
None	92	4	4.3
Inner third	80	8	10.0
Middle third	17	2	11.8
Outer third	33	13	39.4

Gynecologic Oncology Group data: Reproduced, with permission, from DiSaia PJ, Creasman WT, Boronow RC, Blessing JA: Risk factors and recurrent patterns in stage I endometrial cancer. *Am J Obstet Gynecol* 151:1009, 1985.

50, 51). Aalders et al. (35) reported recurrences and deaths in 26.7% of patients with Stage I disease who had vascular space invasion compared with 9.1% of those without vessel invasion ($P < 0.01$). Abeler et al. (51) reviewed 1974 cases of endometrial carcinoma from the Norwegian Radium Hospital and reported an 83.5% 5-year survival rate for patients without demonstrable vascular invasion compared with 64.5% for those in whom invasion was present (51).

The overall incidence of lymph-vascular invasion in Stage I endometrial carcinoma is about 15%, although it increases with increasing myometrial invasion and decreasing tumor differentiation. Hanson et al. (50) reported vascular space invasion in 5% of patients with invasion limited to the inner one-third of the myometrium compared with 70% of those with invasion to the outer one-third. Similarly, it was present in 2% of grade 1 carcinomas and 42% of grade 3 lesions. Ambros and Kurman (52), using multivariate analysis, reported that only depth of myometrial invasion, DNA ploidy, and vascular invasion–associated changes (VIAC) correlated significantly with survival for patients with Stage I endometrioid adenocarcinomas. VIAC was defined as vascular invasion by tumor, and/or the presence of myometrial perivascular lymphocytic infiltrates.

Peritoneal Cytology

The significance of positive peritoneal cytology is controversial (53). The incidence of positive cytology in Stage I disease is shown in Table 8.12. Positive washings are most commonly present in patients with grade 3 histology, metastases

Table 8.12   Incidence of Positive Peritoneal Cytology in Clinical Stage I Endometrial Carcinoma

Author	Cases	Positive Cytology	Percent
Creasman et al., 1981 (54)	167	26	15.5
Szpak et al., 1981 (55)	54	12	22.2
Yazigi et al., 1983 (56)	93	10	10.8
Creasman et al., 1987 (27)	621	76	12.2
Harouny et al., 1988 (57)	276	47	17.1
Hirai et al., 1989 (58)	173	25	14.5
Lurain et al., 1989 (59)	157	30	19.1
Total	**1,541**	**226**	**14.7**

to the adnexae, deep myometrial invasion, and/or positive pelvic or para-aortic nodes (27, 53–60).

Creasman et al. (54) reported that 6 of 13 patients (46%) with positive cytology but no extrauterine disease died of disseminated intraperitoneal carcinomatosis, although a recent study by Kadar et al. (60) of 269 patients with clinical Stage I and Stage II endometrial cancer reported that if the disease was confined to the uterus, positive peritoneal cytology did not influence survival. Interestingly, if the disease had spread to the adnexa, lymph nodes, or peritoneum, positive peritoneal cytology decreased survival from 73% to 13% at 5 years, but all recurrences were at distant sites.

The recent GOG study reported by Morrow et al. (61) analyzed 697 patients with information on peritoneal cytology and adequate follow-up. Disease recurred in 25 of 86 patients (29%) with positive washings, whereas 64 of 611 patients (10.5%) with negative washings had recurrence of disease. Morrow et al. noted, however, that 17 of the 25 recurrences were outside the peritoneal cavity.

In a recent review of the literature concerning patients with clinical Stage I endometrial cancer, Milosevic et al. (62) reported positive peritoneal cytology in 8.3%, 12.1%, and 15.9% of patients with grades 1, 2, and 3 histology, respectively. Superficial and deep myometrial invasion was associated with positive washings in 7.6% and 17.2% of the cases, respectively. They concluded that the poor prognosis associated with malignant washings was largely a reflection of other adverse prognostic factors. They suggested that a high technical false-positive rate made it difficult to determine the clinical usefulness of the test in patients with low-grade, superficially invasive tumors.

Hormone Receptor Status   In general, mean estrogen receptor (ER) and progesterone receptor (PR) levels are inversely proportional to histologic grade (63–66). However, ER and PR content have been shown to be independent prognostic indicators for endometrial cancer; i.e., patients whose tumors are positive for one or both receptors have longer survival than patients whose carcinoma lacks the corresponding receptors (63–65, 67, 68) (Table 8.8). Liao et al. (64) reported that, even for patients with lymph node metastases, the prognosis was significantly improved if the tumor was receptor positive. PR appears to be a stronger predictor of survival than ER and, at least for the ER, the absolute level of the receptors may be important: the higher the level, the better the prognosis (69).

Nuclear Grade

Nuclear grading has been reported by only a few investigators, but it is a significant prognostic indicator (69). Christopherson et al. (70) found nuclear grading to be a more accurate prognosticator than histologic grade.

The new FIGO grading system takes into account the nuclear grade of the tumor, and "nuclear atypia" inappropriate for the architectural grade raises the grade by 1. However, there is great variability in the literature regarding the criteria for nuclear grading, and intraobserver and interobserver reproducibility of nuclear grading are poor (71).

Tumor Size

In an analysis of 142 patients with clinical Stage I endometrial carcinoma, Schink et al. (72) recently reported tumor size as an independent prognostic factor. Lymph node metastases occurred in 4% of the patients with tumors $\leq$ 2 cm diameter, 15% with tumors > 2 cm diameter, and 35% with tumors involving the entire uterine cavity. The incidence of nodal metastases in relation to tumor size and depth of invasion is shown in Table 8.13.

DNA Ploidy

Recent studies have indicated that approximately one-fourth of the patients with endometrial carcinomas have aneuploid tumors, which is a low incidence in comparison with many other solid tumors, including ovarian and cervical carcinomas. However, patients with aneuploid tumors are at significantly increased risk of early recurrence and death from disease (52, 73, 74).

Method of Treatment

In contrast to cervical cancer, patients with endometrial cancer treated with hysterectomy alone or hysterectomy and radiation do significantly better than those treated with radiation alone (75–77). This appears to be related to the inability of radiation therapy to effectively eliminate disease in the myometrium (78, 79). Grigsby et al. (76) reported on 116 patients with Stage II endometrial carcinoma. Ninety were treated with combined radiation and surgery, whereas 26 received radiation alone. The results of treatment are shown in Table 8.14.

Table 8.13   Incidence of Lymph Node Metastasis in Endometrial Cancer by Tumor Size and Depth of Myometrial Invasion

Depth of Invasion	Tumor Size		
	$\leq$ 2 cm Diameter (%)	> 2 cm Diameter (%)	Entire Surface (%)
None	0/17 (0)	0/8 (0)	0/0 (0)
< ½	0/27 (0)	5/41 (12)	2/9 (22)
$\geq$ ½	2/9 (22)	6/23 (26)	4/8 (50)

Reproduced, with permission, from Schink JC, Lurain JR, Wallemark CB, Chmiel JS: Tumor size in endometrial cancer: a prognostic factor for lymph node metastasis. *Obstet Gynecol* 70:216, 1987.

Table 8.14 Clinical Stage II Carcinoma of the Endometrium: Comparison of Treatment Methods

	No. of Patients	Distant Metastases	Pelvic Recurrence	Five-Year Survival
Radiation and surgery	90	13.3%	8.9%	78%
Radiation alone	26	11.5%	34.6%	48%

Reproduced, with permission, from Grigsby PW, Perez CA, Camel HM, Galakatos AE: Stage II carcinoma of the endometrium: results of therapy and prognostic factors. *Int J Radiat Oncol Biol Phys* 11:1915, 1985.

Endometrial Hyperplasia

Classical teaching has been that endometrial hyperplasias represent a continuum of morphologic severity; the most severe form, termed atypical adenomatous hyperplasia or carcinoma *in situ*, was considered the immediate precursor of endometrial carcinoma (80–82).

In recent years this continuum concept has been challenged. Independent studies by Kurman et al. (83) and Ferenczy et al. (84) have suggested that:

1. Endometrial hyperplasia and endometrial neoplasia are two biologically different diseases.

2. The only important distinguishing feature is the presence or absence of cytologic atypia.

Ferenczy et al. (84) suggested that the term *endometrial hyperplasia* be used for any degree of glandular proliferation devoid of cytologic atypia and the term *endometrial intraepithelial neoplasia* for lesions with cytologic atypia. Using similar criteria in a long-term follow-up study of 170 patients with endometrial hyperplasia, Kurman et al. (83) reported a 1.6% risk of progression to carcinoma in patients devoid of cytologic atypia, compared with a 23% risk in patients with cytologic atypia.

Subsequently, Ferenczy and Gelfand (85) reported 85 menopausal women with endometrial hyperplasia. Sixty-five patients had no cytologic atypia, and 84% of this group responded to medroxyprogesterone acetate (MPA). Four (6%) had recurrent hyperplasia after discontinuing the MPA, and none developed carcinoma, with a mean follow-up of 7 years. By contrast, 20 patients had cytologic atypia, and only 50% of them responded to MPA. Five (25%) developed recurrent hyperplasia, and 5 (25%) developed adenocarcinoma.

These data suggest that most women with endometrial hyperplasia will respond to progestin therapy and are not at increased risk of developing cancer. Patients who do not respond are at a significantly increased risk of progressing to invasive cancer and should be advised to have a hysterectomy. Patients who are unlikely to respond can be identified on the basis of cytologic atypia. A suggested scheme of management is outlined in Figure 8.2.

Treatment of Endometrial Cancer

The cornerstone of treatment for endometrial cancer is total abdominal hysterectomy and bilateral salpingo-oophorectomy, and this operation should

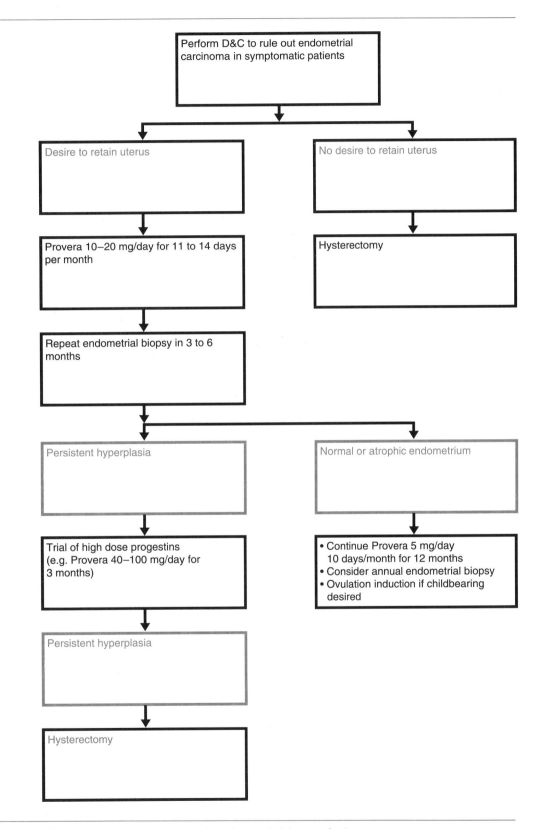

Figure 8.2.   Management of endometrial hyperplasia.

be performed in all cases whenever feasible. In addition, many patients will require some type of adjuvant radiation therapy to help prevent vaginal vault recurrence and to sterilize occult disease in lymph nodes.

Very few controlled studies have been undertaken to assess properly the role of radiation in the management of endometrial cancer, and the studies that have been conducted are not controlled adequately for prognostic variables. Therefore it is difficult to document that radiation actually improves survival (35, 86). With the recent information available on surgicopathologic staging, pathways for early metastases have been elucidated and prognostic variables better defined, allowing a more individualized approach to adjuvant radiation.

Individualization of treatment is best accomplished when all significant pathologic information is available. Therefore, there has been a significant move toward postoperative rather than preoperative radiation. Some workers, including those at the Radiumhemmet, continue to advocate preoperative brachytherapy for patients with grade 3 histology (75).

Stage I and Stage II Occult

Microscopic cervical involvement (positive endocervical curettage) is often designated (unofficially) Stage II occult disease. For practical purposes, such patients can be managed the same as patients with Stage I disease.

When the carcinomatous tissue obtained at endocervical curettage is completely separate from the endocervical tissue, it presumably represents contamination from the corpus, as the prognosis in such circumstances is similar to that of Stage I disease (28, 29). **False-positive rates of 40–50% have been reported for endocervical curettage** (28, 75, 87, 88). Extension of endometrial carcinoma into the cervical stroma in the absence of involvement of the surface epithelium may be missed on endocervical curettage (89). If the cervix is firm and expanded and the endocervical curettage is negative, a wedge biopsy to include the underlying stroma may be necessary to determine cervical involvement.

A recommended treatment plan is shown in Figure 8.3.

The initial approach for all medically fit patients should be total abdominal hysterectomy and bilateral salpingo-oophorectomy. Removal of a vaginal cuff is not necessary. The adnexae should be removed because they may be the site of microscopic metastases. In addition, patients with endometrial carcinoma are at increased risk of ovarian cancer. Such tumors sometimes occur concurrently (90). Surgical staging, including lymphadenectomy, should be performed in those patients shown in Table 8.15.

Operative Technique

The laparotomy is best performed through a lower midline abdominal incision, although a Pfannenstiel incision is commonly used. The probability that this type of low transverse incision will be inadequate is substantial in the presence of a poorly differentiated carcinoma, an enlarged uterus, cervical extension, or an adnexal mass because in these situations, omentectomy and removal of enlarged aortic nodes or abdominal metastases may be necessary (91). An alternative to this approach is to use a transverse, muscle-dividing incision (e.g., the Maylard or Cherney), as discussed in Chapter 15. In the presence of obesity and a large abdominal panniculus, which is not uncommon in patients with endometrial carcinoma, a lower midline incision may offer better exposure (92).

300

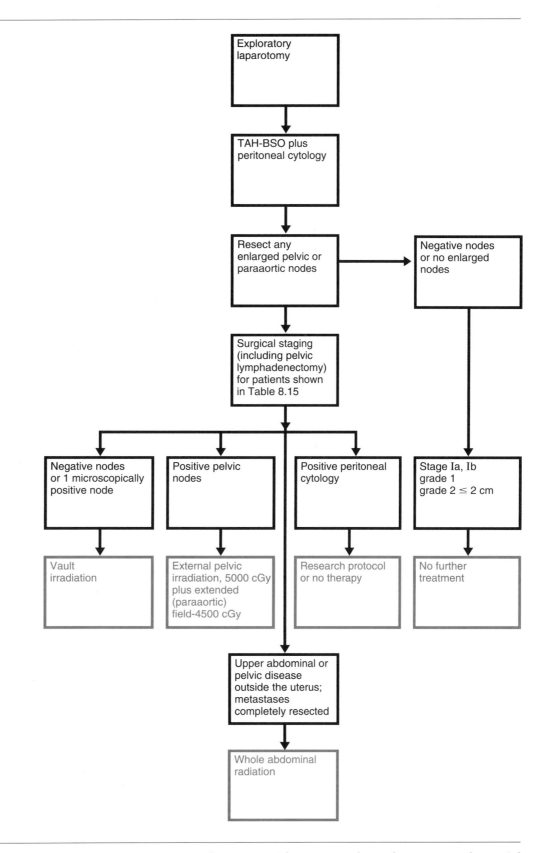

Figure 8.3.   Management of patients with Stage I and occult Stage II endometrial carcinoma.

Table 8.15 Endometrial Carcinoma Stages I and Occult II: Patients Requiring Surgical Staging

1. Patients with grade 3 lesions
2. Patients with grade 2 tumors >2 cm in diameter
3. Patients with adenosquamous, clear cell, or papillary serous carcinomas
4. Patients with greater than 50% of myometrial invasion
5. Patients with cervical extension

After the abdomen is opened, peritoneal washings are taken from the pelvis, paracolic gutters, and subdiaphragmatic area with 50 ml normal saline solution. The fluid is withdrawn immediately and sent to the cytology laboratory. Thorough exploration of the abdomen and pelvis is performed, with particular attention to the liver, diaphragm, omentum, and para-aortic nodes. Any suspicious lesions are excised or subjected to biopsy.

The uterus is grasped with clamps that encompass the round and ovarian ligaments and the fallopian tube. After the round ligaments are divided, the incision is carried anteriorly around the vesicouterine fold of peritoneum and posteriorly parallel and lateral to the infundibulopelvic ligaments. With a narrow Deaver retractor in the retroperitoneum providing gentle traction cephalad in the direction of the common iliac vessels, the iliac vessels and ureter are displayed. The pelvic lymph nodes can be visualized and palpated, and any enlarged nodes can be removed.

With each ureter under direct vision, the infundibulopelvic ligaments are divided and tied. The bladder is dissected off the front of the cervix, and then the uterine vessels are skeletonized and divided at the level of the isthmus. Straight Kocher clamps are used to secure the cardinal and uterosacral ligaments; angled clamps then are used to secure the vaginal angles. The uterus, tubes, and ovaries are removed and the vaginal vault is closed. No vaginal cuff need be taken.

The specimen is opened on the operating table to determine the need for surgical staging in patients with grade 1 or 2 tumors. All patients with grade 3 tumors require surgical staging. For grade 1 tumors, gross examination accurately predicts depth of myometrial invasion. In an analysis of 113 patients with surgical Stage I endometrial carcinoma, Goff and Rice (93) reported that macroscopic examination of the fresh specimen correctly predicted depth of invasion in 55 of 63 grade 1 lesions (87.3%), 24 of 37 grade 2 lesions (64.9%), and 4 of 13 grade 3 lesions (30.8%). They recommended that frozen section should be done for patients with grade 2 or 3 tumors. An alternative approach, used by the author, is to measure tumor diameter for grade 2 lesions to determine the need for surgical staging. Schink et al. (72) reported a 22% incidence of lymph node metastases for grade 2 tumors > 2 cm in diameter (7 of 32). None of 19 grade 2 tumors < 2 cm in diameter had nodal metastases.

Surgical staging requirements have not been detailed by the Cancer Committee of FIGO. If accurate surgical staging is to be obtained, full pelvic lymphadenectomy should be performed on all patients who meet the criteria in Table 8.15, and this is the author's current approach. The dissection includes removal of common iliac nodes and of the fat pad overlying the distal inferior vena cava. Any enlarged para-aortic nodes are also removed. If full pelvic lymphadenectomy is considered inadvisable because of the patient's general medical condition, which is uncommon, resection of any enlarged pelvic or para-aortic nodes should be performed. An omental biopsy specimen is also taken.

It is not the author's current approach to perform full para-aortic lymphadenectomy on patients with endometrial carcinoma. The GOG data (61) would suggest that patients with positive para-aortic nodes are likely to have:

1. Grossly positive pelvic nodes

2. Grossly positive adnexae, or

3. Grade 2 or 3 lesions with outer-third myometrial invasion

The pelvic peritoneum is not closed, and it usually is not necessary to place drains in the pelvis. The sigmoid colon is placed in the pelvis to help exclude loops of small bowel. The abdominal wound is best closed with a continuous Smead-Jones type of internal retention suture, particularly if high-risk factors for postoperative wound dehiscence, such as obesity, are present.

Vaginal Hysterectomy **In selected patients with marked obesity and medical problems that place them at high risk for abdominal operations, vaginal hysterectomy should be considered.** Peters et al. (94) reported a 94% survival rate among 56 patients with Stage I endometrial carcinoma who underwent vaginal hysterectomy. Seventy-five percent had grade 1 lesions, and 32 patients received adjuvant radiation, mainly brachytherapy. Others have reported a similar experience (34, 95), and this approach is clearly preferable to treatment of these patients with radiation alone. Vaginal hysterectomy is particularly applicable to patients with grade 1 lesions. The diminished ability to remove the ovaries is an obvious shortcoming with the vaginal approach, although adnexectomy may be facilitated by laparoscopy.

Adjuvant Radiation

Adjuvant radiation has not been shown to improve survival for patients with endometrial cancer (86). However, most patients with Stage I disease have a good prognosis, provided the uterus, tubes, and ovaries are removed; therefore, very large numbers of patients would be needed to show any benefit for adjuvant radiation. **Logical reasoning would suggest that appropriate irradiation should improve survival for selected high-risk patients, because it has been shown to decrease significantly the incidence of both pelvic and vaginal recurrences.** Vault recurrences may be decreased by either external irradiation or intracavitary radium (25, 96); pelvic recurrences may be decreased by external irradiation (97–99). As about 5000 cGy is probably necessary to sterilize micrometastases in lymph nodes, it seems unlikely that grossly enlarged nodes will be sterilized with the usual dose of adjuvant pelvic irradiation unless they are surgically resected initially.

Before the move toward surgicopathologic staging of endometrial carcinoma, preoperative intracavitary or external irradiation was usually given. The rationale was that the radiation would sterilize the malignant cells, impairing their implantability and thereby decreasing the likelihood of vaginal implantation or systemic dissemination at the time of uterine manipulation.

Truskett and Constable (33) reported a vaginal recurrence rate of 6.2% for patients with no residual disease in the operative specimen after preoperative radiation.

Therapy was given with intrauterine Heyman capsules but without vault radium sources. This observation eliminates the risk of implantation as a rationale for preoperative irradiation and suggests that vaginal recurrences are due to lymphatic spread, which takes place before any surgical manipulation.

The remaining argument in favor of preoperative irradiation is the possibility of decreasing systemic dissemination. It seems unlikely that the manipulation associated with intracavitary therapy would be less likely to cause tumor dissemination than would surgical manipulation. Bean et al. (100) reported distant metastases in 4 of 130 patients treated with preoperative radiation, compared with 1 of 150 patients treated with primary surgery. Although this was not a properly randomized, prospective study, these data do suggest that primary surgery is associated with minimal risk of tumor dissemination.

With primary surgery, a significant number of patients will be found to have such good-prognosis tumors that adjuvant radiation can be safely eliminated. For those patients who require postoperative radiation, the therapy can be better tailored to the needs of the individual patient. The proper role of adjuvant radiation for endometrial cancer will not be known until large randomized studies with a control (no treatment) arm have been performed, but with our present state of knowledge, the options for postoperative management are as follows:

1. Observation

2. Vault irradiation

3. External pelvic irradiation

4. Extended-field irradiation

5. Whole abdominal irradiation

6. Intraperitoneal ^{32}P

Observation

Patients with grade 1 or 2 lesions confined to the inner third of the myometrium have an excellent prognosis, and no adjuvant radiation is necessary for this group. Danish workers have reported a 96% 5-year survival for patients with Stage I, grade 1 lesions treated with surgery alone (101). Fanning and colleagues (102) compared surgery and adjuvant radiation with surgery alone for patients with Stage I, grade 2 adenocarcinomas of favorable histologic subtype and less than one-third myometrial invasion. The 5-year survival rate for surgery and radiation was 94% (128 of 136), and the recurrence rate was 2.2% (3 of 136). The 5-year survival rate for the surgery-alone group was 98% (51 of 52), and the recurrence rate was 1.9% (1 of 52). Gal et al. (103) reported a 100% survival for 64 patients with surgical Stage Ia or Ib disease. Half of these patients received no adjuvant radiation.

Vaginal Radiation

Vault recurrence carries a poor prognosis, and intracavitary vaginal radiation significantly reduces the incidence of vault recurrence. Lotocki et al. (25

304

reported that preoperative or postoperative vault radium decreased the incidence of vault recurrence from 14% to 1.7%. Morbidity is low, although vaginal stenosis and dyspareunia may be a problem for postmenopausal patients if there is no regular vaginal dilatation. Colpostats alone usually are used to deliver a surface dose of 5500–6000 cGy. The author currently uses vault cesium alone for patients with negative lymph nodes after full surgical staging. Although pelvic lymphadenectomy is not likely to improve survival or pelvic control compared with removal of palpably suspicious nodes and external beam therapy (104), it does obviate the need for external beam therapy in the majority of cases.

External Pelvic Irradiation

With an increasing number of patients in cancer centers having pelvic lymphadenectomy as part of their primary surgery, the indications for external pelvic irradiation are decreasing. However, external pelvic irradiation will significantly decrease the risk of pelvic recurrence (97) and is recommended for high-risk patients who have not undergone surgical staging. Such patients include all those with grade 3 tumors and all those with invasion into the outer half of the myometrium or cervical extension. Patients who have multiple positive pelvic nodes after surgical staging are at significant risk of aortic nodal metastases; therefore such patients should receive extended-field (pelvic and para-aortic) radiation, unless the para-aortic nodes have been dissected and proven negative.

External irradiation should be as effective as vaginal irradiation for sterilizing micrometastases at the vaginal vault; thus there seems to be no reason to give both external and vault irradiation postoperatively, as morbidity will be significantly increased. Stokes et al. (105) reported a serious complication rate of 8.8% (7 of 79) when external irradiation and intracavitary radium were combined. Similarly, among 1011 cases treated at the Radiumhemmet, there was a 1.8% incidence of late complications in the group receiving postoperative external irradiation compared with 15.9% in the group treated with preoperative intrauterine radium plus postoperative whole-pelvic irradiation (106).

Extended-Field Radiation

Risk factors for pelvic lymph node metastases portend a lower but significant risk of para-aortic metastases, and failure rates of 15–20% in the para-aortic area have been reported for patients receiving pelvic radiation only (97, 99). Fairly extensive experience with extended-field radiation in patients with cervical cancer indicates about a 25% 5-year survival rate for patients with positive para-aortic nodes (107). Limited information is available on extended-field radiation for patients with endometrial cancer, but workers at the University of Minnesota reported a 5-year survival of about 40% for 20 patients with surgically confirmed para-aortic spread (108) (Fig. 8.4). This experience was recently confirmed by the Gynecologic Oncology Group (61). **According to the GOG data, those patients who should be given extended field radiation are those with:**

1. Biopsy-proven para-aortic nodal metastasis

2. Grossly positive pelvic nodes, or multiple positive pelvic nodes

3. Grossly positive adnexal metastases

4. Outer-third myometrial invasion and grade 2 or 3 tumors.

305

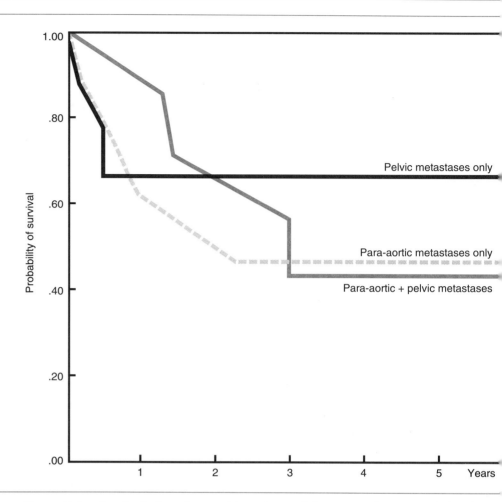

Figure 8.4. Survival of patients with endometrial cancer after extended-field irradiation for surgically confirmed para-aortic lymph node metastasis. (Reproduced, with permission, from Potish RA, Twiggs LB, Adcock LL, et al: Para-aortic lymph node radiotherapy in cancer of the uterine corpus. *Obstet Gynecol* 65:251, 1985.)

Tolerance to para-aortic radiation is limited to 4500–5000 cGy by the small bowel and spinal cord. Potish et al. (108) reported only one case of severe enteric morbidity in 48 patients, for a complication rate of 2%.

Whole Abdominal Radiation

Management of patients with positive peritoneal washings or adnexal or peritoneal metastases is controversial. Potish et al. (109) treated 27 patients with open-field external beam abdominal irradiation. Nine patients had positive peritoneal cytology only. Patients with spread to the adnexae, peritoneal fluid, or both had a 5-year relapse-free rate of 90%, whereas the disease recurred in all patients with macroscopic disease beyond the adnexae. Similar results have been reported with the moving-strip technique (110). For patients with peritoneal or omental metastases that have been completely excised, it seems reasonable to use whole-abdominal radiation. In the presence of gross residual disease, systemic therapy should be offered.

Intraperitoneal ^{32}P

Investigators at Duke University have reported favorable results with intraperitoneal ^{32}P for patients with malignant peritoneal cytology (111). However, most patients with malignant washings are also at risk of vaginal vault and pelvic sidewall recurrences and thus require external pelvic irradiation. When the latter was combined with intraperitoneal ^{32}P, 5 of 17 patients (29%) developed chronic intestinal morbidity necessitating surgical intervention (111). Other problems associated with ^{32}P include the uneven distribution of fluid commonly present and the potential for bowel injury from "hot spots."

At the present time, the significance of positive peritoneal washings in patients with endometrial cancer remains controversial. After reviewing the literature, Milosevic et al. (62) believed that routine adjuvant therapy for patients with malignant cytology was not justified. Usually there are other adverse prognostic factors, which necessitate adjuvant therapy in their own right.

Adjuvant Progestins	**Although the role of progestins in the management of patients with advanced and recurrent endometrial cancer has been established, they have not been shown to be of value in an adjuvant setting** (112–114). In a randomized study of 1148 patients with clinical Stage I or II endometrial cancer at the Norwegian Radium Hospital, death due to intercurrent disease, particularly cardiovascular disease, was actually more common in the progesterone-treated group ($p = 0.04$) (115). In 461 high-risk patients, a tendency toward fewer cancer-related deaths and a better disease-free survival in the treatment group was observed, but crude survival was unchanged. It was concluded that further studies were needed in high-risk patients but that the evidence suggested that prophylactic progestin therapy was not likely to be a cost-effective approach for patients with endometrial cancer unless there was a high-risk, receptor-positive tumor.
Stage II	**When both the cervix and the endometrium are clinically involved with adenocarcinoma, it may be difficult to distinguish between a Stage Ib adenocarcinoma of the cervix and a Stage II endometrial carcinoma.** Histopathologic evaluation is not helpful in the differentiation of these two conditions, and the diagnosis must be based on clinical and epidemiologic features. The obese, elderly woman with a bulky uterus is most likely to have endometrial cancer, whereas the younger woman with a bulky cervix and a normal corpus is most likely to have cervical cancer.

The small number of cases in all reported series and the lack of randomized, prospective studies preclude dogmatic statements about the optimal mode of therapy. Patients with Stage II endometrial cancer have about a 35% incidence of positive pelvic nodes (116); therefore any treatment protocol should include treatment of these nodes (Table 8.14). For optimal prognosis, the uterus also should be removed in all patients (75, 76, 117).

Two main approaches have been used for patients with Stage II disease:

1. Radical hysterectomy, bilateral salpingo-oophorectomy, and bilateral pelvic lymphadenectomy

2. Combined radiation and surgery (i.e., preoperative external pelvic irradiation and intracavitary radium or cesium), followed in 6 weeks by total abdominal hysterectomy and bilateral salpingo-oophorectomy.

Radical Surgery	Radical surgery allows accurate surgicopathologic information to be obtained, but many of these patients are obese, elderly, hypertensive, and diabetic and thus

307

are unsuitable candidates for this approach. In addition, results are no better than with the combined approach. Rutledge (118) stated that radical hysterectomy should be limited to patients with anatomic problems or other conditions that conflict with the use of radiation.

Combined Radiation and Surgery	The most common approach is to use external and intracavitary radiation followed by extrafascial hysterectomy (79, 117, 119–121). The hysterectomy usually is performed about 6 weeks after irradiation to allow the inflammatory edema to settle, although Boronow (122) reported no significant difference in survival when the hysterectomy was performed at 0 to 10 weeks. Preoperative external radiation optimizes the geometry of the intracavitary insertion, and there is less risk of fixed bowel in the pelvis.

Bruckman et al. (120) treated 25 patients with 4000 cGy whole-pelvis irradiation and 4000 mg-hours of intracavitary radium at a single insertion. There were no vaginal recurrences, and all relapses in the pelvis were accompanied by distant metastases. Nahhas et al. (78) reported no improvement in survival when radical hysterectomy was performed after the external radiation in lieu of intracavitary radium plus extrafascial hysterectomy.

Most papers on combined therapy report significant bowel morbidity. Workers at the Joint Center for Radiation Therapy in Boston reported significant morbidity in 5 of 55 patients (9%) (121). Rectovaginal fistulas developed in two patients, and three patients had small- or large-bowel obstructions requiring surgical intervention. Four required diverting colostomies.

A recent study from the M.D. Anderson Hospital of 83 patients with Stage II endometrial cancer treated with a combined radiosurgical approach reported severe gastrointestinal or urologic complications in 10 patients (12%). Complications included proctitis with rectal stricture (2), radiation enteritis (1), small bowel obstruction (3), rectovaginal fistula (1), recurrent hemorrhagic cystitis (3), bilateral ureteral obstruction (1), and enterovesicle fistula (2). Six patients required surgery, and three patients (4%) died of the complications (117).

Radiation Therapy Alone	Radiation therapy alone is reserved for patients with medical contraindications to surgery but may provide good pelvic control in patients with minimal myometrial invasion. These are usually patients with well-differentiated lesions (123), particularly if the primary lesion is arising in the lower segment of the uterus.

Proposed Management	Current management protocols for Stage II endometrial cancer fail to address the problem of extrapelvic spread. **Although the incidence of metastases to the para-aortic lymph nodes, adnexal structures, and upper abdomen would be expected to be higher than for Stage I lesions, there is currently no staging information available on patients with clinically overt Stage II disease; thus the role of extended-field or whole-abdominal radiation for these patients has not been explored.**

Our current approach to Stage II endometrial carcinoma is to perform primary surgery and surgical staging, provided the patient is medically fit. The surgery, which should be performed only if the parametrial tissues are free of disease, is as follows:

1. Modified (type II) radical hysterectomy

2. Bilateral salpingo-oophorectomy

3. Pelvic and abdominal peritoneal washings for cytologic study

4. Pelvic lymphadenectomy to the aortic bifurcation

5. Resection of grossly enlarged para-aortic nodes

6. Omental biopsy

7. Biopsy of any suspicious peritoneal nodules

Postoperatively, adjuvant radiation is individualized. If lymph nodes are negative, vault cesium, without external beam therapy, is given. Patients with multiple positive pelvic nodes or grossly positive pelvic nodes are given extended-field external beam therapy, without vault cesium. Patients with completely resected upper abdominal disease receive whole-abdomen radiation. As at all centers, our experience with Stage II endometrial cancer is limited and firm data to support this approach are not currently available.

Clinical Stage III	Patients with FIGO clinical Stage III carcinoma of the endometrium usually have involvement of the parametrium, pelvic sidewall, or adnexal structures. Involvement of the vagina or cul-de-sac is less common (32). Because it usually is not possible to be certain of the nature of an adnexal mass without laparotomy, some cases will have a lower surgicopathologic stage when benign adnexal disease is found. On the other hand, subclinical involvement of the adnexae occurs in about 5–10% of patients with Stage I and II endometrial carcinoma, and these patients often are included in papers reviewing Stage III endometrial cancer. Aalders et al. (124) reported a 5-year survival rate of 40% for patients with surgicopathologic Stage III disease, compared with 16% for patients with clinical Stage III. Bruckman et al. (125) reported a 5-year survival rate of 80% when only the ovary and/or the fallopian tube were involved, compared with 15% when other extra-uterine pelvic structures were involved.

Treatment for Stage III endometrial carcinoma must be individualized but should aim to include total abdominal hysterectomy and bilateral salpingo-oophorectomy. In the presence of an adnexal mass, surgery usually should be performed initially to determine the nature of the mass and to remove the bulk of the diseased tissue. In the presence of parametrial extension, it will usually be more appropriate to commence with external irradiation and intracavitary radium.

Surgical eradication of all macroscopic tumor is of major prognostic importance for all patients with clinical Stage III disease (124). The surgery should include removal of any enlarged pelvic or para-aortic lymph nodes. If all gross disease can be removed from the pelvis, thorough surgical staging is warranted. This should include peritoneal washings from the paracolic gutters and subdiaphragmatic areas, para-aortic lymph node sampling, and biopsy of the omentum and parietal peritoneum.

Genest et al. (126) reported that the site of first recurrence was limited to the abdominal cavity in 79% of their patients in whom treatment failed (23 of 29), suggesting a role for whole-abdomen radiation in Stage III endometrial cancer, particularly in patients with positive peritoneal washings or demonstrable micrometastases to the upper abdomen. However, Mackillop and Pringle (32) noted that although abdominal failure was common, it was rarely the only site of failure. Morbid obesity or other general medical conditions may limit the use of whole-abdominal irradiation in these patients.

Systemic metastases are a major problem, but the value of adjuvant systemic therapy is unproven. These patients generally have tumors that are less well-differentiated, so their hormone receptor content is usually low, making response to progestins unlikely. No chemotherapeutic agents have any apparent prophylactic value in endometrial cancer.

Stage IV

Stage IV endometrial carcinoma is uncommon, and results of therapy are generally poor. However, an occasional patient will be seen with a well-differentiated adenocarcinoma that has metastasized because of prolonged patient delay or prolonged physician delay or because cervical stenosis has prevented the appearance of abnormal bleeding. Such tumors usually contain estrogen and progesterone receptors, and prolonged survival may occur with progestin therapy, followed later by total abdominal hysterectomy, bilateral salpingo-oophorectomy, and possibly radiation therapy.

In a series of 83 patients reported by Aalders et al. (127) from the Norwegian Radium Hospital, the lung was the main site of extrapelvic spread, with 36% of patients having lung metastases. Ballon et al. (128) reported 33 patients (2.3%) with pulmonary metastases among 1434 patients who had endometrial cancer. Only 10 of the 33 patients had the lung metastases at initial presentation, and the lungs were the sole site of metastatic disease in only 8 of the 33 patients.

Treatment of Stage IV disease must be individualized but will usually involve a combination of surgery, radiation therapy, and progestins. The objective of the surgery is to try to achieve local disease control in the pelvis in order to help palliate bleeding, discharge, and complications involving the bowel and/or the bladder. Aalders et al. (127) reported that control of the pelvic disease could be achieved in 20 of 72 patients (28%) with radiation alone or in combination with surgery and/or progestins. If tumor is removed, it should be sent for ER and PR determination to help guide subsequent systemic therapy.

Pelvic exenteration may be considered in the occasional patient in whom disease extension is limited to the bladder and/or rectum.

Special Clinical Circumstances

Endometrial Cancer Diagnosed After Hysterectomy This situation is best avoided by routine opening of the excised uterus in the operating room so that the adnexa can be removed and appropriate staging performed if unsuspected endometrial cancer is discovered. When the diagnosis is made during the postoperative period, the following approach is recommended:

1. Grade 1 or 2 lesions with less than one-third myometrial invasion: no further treatment, although prophylactic oophorectomy is advisable because of the risk of subsequent ovarian cancer. This is particularly important if there is any family history of breast, ovarian, or colon cancer (Lynch II syndrome).

2. All other lesions: further laparotomy with removal of adnexae, surgical staging, and appropriate postoperative radiation

Synchronous Primary Tumors in the Endometrium and Ovary This is an uncommon but well-recognized occurrence. In about half of the cases, both endometrial and ovarian tumors will be of the endometrioid type. These patients are often premenopausal and have a favorable prognosis. Treatment should be determined on the premise that each represents a primary lesion, and many will require surgery only without adjuvant radiation (90, 129). When more aggressive histologic subtypes are involved, or if the uterine and ovarian tumors are histologically dissimilar, the prognosis is much poorer, and adjuvant radiotherapy should be used.

Well-differentiated Carcinomas in Very Young Women Adenocarcinomas of the endometrium occasionally occur in very young women (under 30 years), usually in association with the polycystic ovarian (PCO) syndrome. About 90% of the lesions are well differentiated and limited to the endometrium (130). For the well-differentiated lesions, a 2-month trial of progestins (e.g., Megace orally, 160–320 mg per day) may be undertaken if childbearing capability is desired. If a repeat curettage shows no evidence of carcinoma, conservative treatment may continue. If the lesion persists, or if childbearing capability is not desired, hysterectomy is the treatment of choice (131, 132). Castration should be avoided unless it is necessary for cure (131). Lesions other than well-differentiated adenocarcinomas should be treated in the standard manner.

Recurrent Disease

According to figures reported in the *Annual Report on the Results of Treatment in Gynecological Cancer* (volume 21), about 33% of patients treated for endometrial cancer will die within 5 years (Table 8.16). Risk increases with stage of disease. Serum CA-125 titers are usually elevated in patients with recurrent disease, although Pastner et al. (133) reported that none of six patients with an isolated vaginal recurrence had elevated levels. They also reported that CA-125 titers may be falsely elevated in the presence of severe radiation injury of the bowel (133).

Recurrent endometrial carcinoma has received relatively little attention in the past, but the large series of 379 patients with recurrent disease reported by Aalders

Table 8.16   Carcinoma of the Corpus Uteri, 1982–1986: 3- and 5-Year Actuarial Survival Rate by Clinical Stage

Stage	Patients Treated		Survival			
			3-Year		5-Year	
	No.	%	No.	%	No.	%
I	7,092	70.2	5,540	83.2	2,824	76.3
II	1,803	17.8	1,153	69.0	531	59.2
III	818	8.1	270	37.1	120	29.4
IV	364	3.6	44	14.2	23	10.3
No stage	32	0.3	16	60.1	8	51.8
Total	**10,109**	**100.0**	**7,023**	**74.8**	**3,506**	**66.9**

Reproduced from the Annual Report on the Results of Treatment of Gynecological Cancer, TABLE BIVa, 21:140, 1992.

et al. (134) from the Norwegian Radium Hospital provides some important information. Local recurrence was found in 50% of the patients, distant metastases in 29%, and simultaneous local and distant metastases in 21%. The median time from primary treatment to detection of recurrence was 14 months for patients with local recurrence and 19 months for those with distant metastases. Thirty-four percent of all recurrences were detected within 1 year and 76% within 3 years of primary treatment. In 10% of the patients, recurrence was diagnosed more than 5 years after primary treatment. At the time of diagnosis, 32% of all patients were free of symptoms and the diagnosis was made on routine physical or radiologic examination. For patients with local recurrence, 36% were free of symptoms, 37% had vaginal bleeding, and 16% had pelvic pain.

Treatment of recurrent endometrial cancer must be individualized but will generally commence with hormone therapy. If there is progressive disease, cytotoxic chemotherapy may be offered. However, the results of treatment with cytotoxic agents are poor (135).

Isolated vaginal metastases are the most amenable to therapy with curative intent. Phillips et al. (136) reported on 81 patients with vaginal recurrences and noted that 68% had an isolated vaginal recurrence, 23% had both vaginal and pelvic recurrences, and 9% had vaginal and extrapelvic recurrences. Among the 54 patients with isolated vaginal recurrences, 39 lesions (71%) recurred in the proximal half of the vagina, nine (17%) recurred in the distal half, three (6%) recurred in the proximal and distal parts of the vagina, and in three patients (6%) the location of the vaginal recurrence was not recorded.

Patients with a vaginal recurrence require thorough investigation to detect any associated metastatic foci, and this should commence with a radiograph of the chest and pelvic and abdominal CT scans. Fine needle aspiration cytology may be used to make a definitive diagnosis of a suspicious nodule.

If no other foci are detected, patients who have had prior pelvic radiation may undergo exploratory laparotomy with a view to some type of pelvic exenteration, provided the disease is found to be central and there are no lymph node metastases. In patients who have received no prior pelvic irradiation, external irradiation plus some type of brachytherapy may be appropriate. Phillips et al. (136) reported apparent cure in 11 of 39 patients (28%) with a proximal vaginal recurrence and in 4 of 9 patients (44%) with a distal vaginal recurrence. Survival was directly proportional to the interval between the primary therapy and development of the recurrence. Surgical resection of the metastatic nodule before radiation may improve local control, particularly for lesions > 2 cm in diameter. Laparotomy has the advantage of allowing a thorough search of the pelvis and abdomen for other metastatic foci.

Hormone Therapy

In 1961, Kelley and Baker (137) reported on the use of moderate doses of progesterone for 21 patients with recurrent endometrial cancer. Six objective responses were seen, ranging from 9 months to 4.5 years. Thigpen et al. (138) reported the GOG experience with 331 women with measurable disease treated with 150 mg of medroxyprogesterone acetate (MPA) daily. Only 32 complete responses (10%) and 26 partial responses (8%) were observed. The median progression-free interval was brief (138). Podratz et al. (139) reported similar findings from the Mayo Clinic—only 10% of patients had an objective response to therapy, and fewer than 50% were alive at 1 year.

The route of administration does not appear to influence response rate or survival (140), and the type of progestin seems to be of no significance (141). High-dose therapy (1000 mg MPA daily) also seems to offer no advantage (142). Side effects are usually minor and include weight gain, edema, thrombophlebitis, headache, and occasionally hypertension.

Because of their low toxicity, progestins should be used initially in all patients with recurrent endometrial cancer, particularly those with positive hormone receptors. If an objective response is obtained, the progesterone should be continued indefinitely. Some responses may be sustained for several years. If no response is obtained within 2 months but progesterone receptors are known to be present, a higher dose may be worth trying before therapy is changed.

The nonsteroidal antiestrogen, tamoxifen, has also been used to treat patients with recurrent endometrial cancer. It inhibits the binding of estradiol to uterine ER, presumably blocking the proliferative stimulus of circulating estrogens. Responses are usually seen in patients who have previously responded to progestins, but an occasional response may occur in a patient who is unresponsive to progestins (143, 144). Tamoxifen may be administered orally in a dose of 10–20 mg twice daily and continued for as long as the disease is responding. In a review of the literature, Moore et al. (142) reported a pooled response rate of 22% for single-agent tamoxifen.

The potential for combined tamoxifen-progestin therapy has been explored, as these two agents have been shown to have a synergism that may relate to the induction of increased levels of PR by the weak estrogenic action of tamoxifen (143). Results to date have been disappointing (142).

Cytotoxic Chemotherapy

Cytotoxic chemotherapy for endometrial cancer is of only palliative value, and the results are generally disappointing. Adriamycin is the most active agent. The GOG reported an overall response rate of 38%, with 26% of the patients achieving a complete clinical response. Median survival for the complete responders was 14 months (145). Other single agents that show activity against endometrial cancer include cisplatin, carboplatin, hexamethylmelamine, Cytoxan, and 5-fluorouracil (5-FU). The GOG conducted a trial to compare melphalan, 5-FU, and Megace with Adriamycin, 5-FU, Cytoxan, and Megace. The response rate in both arms of the trial was 36% (146), which is no better than that achieved with Adriamycin alone. Although superior results have been reported for cisplatin, Cytoxan, Adriamycin, and Megace (147), only small numbers of patients were treated, and direct comparative trials will be necessary to demonstrate any benefit over single-agent Adriamycin. Uterine papillary serous carcinomas are histologically the same as ovarian serous tumors, but the reported response rate to cisplatin-containing combination chemotherapy is only about 20% (148).

The availability of recombinant hemopoietic colony-stimulating factors (e.g., granulocyte-CSF, granulocyte-macrophage-CSF, interleukin-3) has stimulated interest in dose-intensity trials, and the emergence of carboplatin as an active drug provides a basis for development of high-dose regimens (142).

Hormone Replacement Therapy

Particularly for younger women, hormone replacement therapy is an important issue after treatment for endometrial cancer. **Patients with Stage I disease have a good prognosis, and protection against osteoporosis and the cardiovascular**

effects of estrogen deficiency is important. Although it has been frequently stated that estrogen replacement therapy is contraindicated in patients who have had endometrial cancer, Creasman et al. (149) have challenged this concept. In a nonrandomized study, they reported no deleterious effect from estrogen given to 47 patients with Stage I endometrial cancer when compared with 174 patients with similar risk factors who did not receive estrogen. In fact, the estrogen group experienced a significantly longer disease-free survival.

Our current practice is to offer all patients a combination of Premarin 0.625 mg and Provera 2.5 mg, both taken daily without interruption.

Prognosis

Although individual institutions may report superior results, the most comprehensive survival data are provided in the *Annual Report on the Results of Treatment in Gynecological Cancer*. Results for the years 1982 through 1986 are shown in Tables 8.16 and 8.17. These data highlight the significance of histologic grade: patients with Stage II, grade 1 tumors have a better prognosis than patients with Stage Ic, grade 3 lesions.

Survival in relation to grade and depth of myometrial invasion for Stage I disease is shown in Table 8.18. These data are from a series reported from McMaster University in Canada, and many of the patients received preoperative radiation therapy.

Survival in relation to the various histologic types is shown in Table 8.19. The poor prognosis associated with adenosquamous, papillary serous, and clear cell carcinoma is apparent.

Uterine Sarcomas

Uterine sarcomas are rare mesodermal tumors that account for about 3% of uterine cancers (150). They are a heterogeneous group of tumors, and thus individual experience with each lesion is limited. Hence treatment protocols are not standardized, and there are few controlled studies evaluating different therapeutic approaches.

There are no known predisposing epidemiologic factors, except possibly pelvic irradiation (151), and criteria for histopathologic classification are not standardized, particularly for the more borderline lesions. As a group, their behavior is

Table 8.17 Surgical Stage I and II Endometrial Cancer: Actuarial 5-Year Survival by Histologic Grade and Stage

	Stage I						Stage II			
	Ia		Ib		Ic		IIa		IIb	
Grade	No.	%	No.	%	No.	%	No.	%	No.	%
1	1049	92.3	1011	94.1	386	83.2	77	86.1	73	72.7
2	529	89.7	755	84.9	368	79.8	84	71.8	105	71.1
3	184	81.5	250	76.3	183	68.3	41	65.9	63	49.0
Not Graded	71	85.9	88	84.8	30	68.8	12	80.0	13	59.6

Adapted from the *Annual Report on the Results of Treatment of Gynecological Cancer*. Table BVb, 21:145, 1992.

Table 8.18   Stage I Endometrial Carcinoma: 5-Year Actuarial Survival Related to Grade and Depth of Myometrial Invasion in 718 "Operable" Patients

	Actuarial Survival		
Depth of Invasion	Grade 1 (%)	Grade 2 (%)	Grade 3 (%)
No residual	97.6	98	79.9
Endometrial	97.1	97.5	79.8
Myometrial (< ⅓)	92.6	87	61.1
Myometrial (> 50%)	90.9	71	26.3

Reproduced, with permission, from Lotocki RJ, Copeland LJ, DePetrillo AD, Muirhead W: Stage I endometrial adenocarcinoma: treatment results in 835 patients. *Am J Obstet Gynecol* 146:141, 1983.

Table 8.19   Stage I Endometrial Cancer: 5-Year Survival in Relation to Histologic Subtypes (N = 595)

Subtype	Alive (%)	DOD (%)
Adenoacanthoma	87.5	6.3
Adenocarcinoma	79.8	6.2
Papillary serous	69.7	21.2
Adenosquamous	53.1	32.7
Clear cell	44.2	51.2

Reproduced, with permission, from Christopherson WM, Connelly PJ, Alberhasky RC: Carcinoma of the endometrium. V. An analysis of prognosticators in patients with favorable subtypes and stage I disease. *Cancer* 51:1705, 1983.
DOD = dead of disease.

characterized by rapid clinical progression, and they carry a poor overall prognosis. **The number of mitoses per 10 high-power fields seems to be the most reliable predictor of biologic behavior, but criteria for diagnosis of uterine sarcomas have varied between observers and over time.**

Classification

Mesodermal derivatives from which sarcomas may arise include uterine smooth muscle, endometrial stroma, and blood and lymphatic vessel walls. Uterine sarcomas can be divided basically into two types:

1. *Pure*, in which only malignant mesodermal elements are present (e.g., leiomyosarcoma).

2. *Mixed*, in which malignant mesodermal and malignant epithelial elements are present (e.g., carcinosarcoma).

They also may be subdivided into *homologous* and *heterologous* tumors, depending on whether the malignant mesodermal elements are normally present in the uterus. Malignant smooth muscle and stroma represent homologous elements, whereas malignant striated muscle and cartilage represent heterologous elements.

A working classification, modified from the more extensive classifications of Ober (152) and Kempson and Bari (153), is shown in Table 8.20. For practical purposes, the three common malignant uterine sarcomas are leiomyosarcomas, endometrial stromal sarcomas, and mixed mesodermal sarcomas.

315

Table 8.20   Classification of Uterine Sarcomas

Type	Homologous	Heterologous
Pure	Leiomyosarcoma Stromal sarcoma (i) endolymphatic stromal myosis (ii) Endometrial stromal sarcoma	Rhabdomyosarcoma Chondrosarcoma Osteosarcoma Liposarcoma
Mixed	Carcinosarcoma	Mixed mesodermal sarcoma

Reproduced, with permission, from Hacker NF, Moore, JG (eds): *Essentials of Obstetrics and Gynecology,* Philadelphia, WB Saunders, 1986, p 472.

Staging

There is no official staging system for uterine sarcomas, but it is usual to use the FIGO system for corpus carcinoma (Table 8.6). More accurate prognostic information is obtained by surgical staging.

Spread Patterns

Like endometrial carcinomas, these tumors infiltrate the myometrium and extend locally. However, they have a propensity for early hematogenous spread, and lymphatic dissemination occurs in about 35% of the patients whose disease is clinically confined to the uterus and cervix (154).

Smooth Muscle Tumors

Leiomyosarcomas, which must be distinguished from the cellular leiomyomas and atypical leiomyomas (see Chapter 4), occur most commonly in the 45- to 55-year age group and account for 30% of uterine sarcomas. They usually arise *de novo* from uterine smooth muscle, although rarely they may arise in a preexisting leiomyoma. A review of 1432 patients undergoing hysterectomy for presumed fibroids at the University of Southern California revealed leiomyosarcoma in the hysterectomy specimen in 10 patients (0.7%). The incidence increased steadily from the fourth to the seventh decades of life (0.2%, 0.9%, 1.4%, and 1.7%, respectively) (155). Rapid enlargement of a fibroid is a possible sign of malignancy.

Most leiomyosarcomas are accompanied by pain, a sensation of pressure, abnormal uterine bleeding, or a lower abdominal mass. A few patients may have signs of metastatic disease, such as a persistent cough, back pain, or ascites. On physical examination, it is impossible to distinguish leiomyosarcomas from large leiomyomas or from other uterine sarcomas. Papanicolaou smears are unrewarding, and uterine curettings are diagnostic for only the 10–20% of tumors that are submucosal (153, 156). Diagnosis usually is not made preoperatively.

Intravenous leiomyomatosis is a rare, relatively benign uterine smooth muscle tumor in which much of the tumor is present in (and may arise from) veins (157). It may extend as rubbery cords beyond the uterus into the parametrium or occasionally into the vena cava. Some patients may survive for prolonged periods in spite of incomplete resection of diseased tissue. High levels of ER and PR are present in some tumors, and regression may occur after menopause.

Leiomyomatosis peritonealis disseminata is a condition in which numerous nodules of histologically benign smooth muscle are present on peritoneal surfaces

(158). It is frequently associated with a term pregnancy or with the use of oral contraceptives, and regression may occur after termination of pregnancy.

Endometrial Stromal Tumors

Endometrial stromal tumors include the benign stromal nodule, the low-grade stromal sarcoma, and the frankly malignant endometrial stromal sarcoma (Table 8.21). Endometrial stromal sarcomas constitute 15–25% of uterine sarcomas (150). Most patients are in the age range of 42–53 years. More than half the patients are premenopausal, and young women and girls may be affected (150). Abnormal vaginal bleeding is the most common presenting symptom and abdominal pain and uterine enlargement may occur (159). Although they may be intramural, most endometrial stromal sarcomas involve the endometrium and usually uterine curettage leads to diagnosis.

Low-grade stromal sarcomas, which usually have fewer than 5 mitoses per 10 high-power fields, also have been termed *endometrial stromatosis* and *endolymphatic stromal myosis*. They have infiltrating margins and demonstrate venous and lymphatic invasion. Although their behavior is relatively indolent, recurrences and distant metastases have been documented, indicating that they are a form of malignant neoplasm (160). Prolonged survival and even cure are not uncommon after surgical resection of recurrent or metastatic lesions.

Mixed Mesodermal Tumors

Mixed mesodermal tumors usually occur in an older age group, most patients being postmenopausal (161). The frankly malignant variants grow rapidly, and usually they are accompanied by postmenopausal bleeding, pelvic pain, a palpable lower abdominal mass, or symptoms of metastatic disease. Most patients have an enlarged or irregular uterus, and the tumor protrudes through the cervical os like a polyp in about half the patients (150). Uterine curettage will usually detect malignant tissue in the uterus, although determination of the exact nature of the tumor may require histologic examination of the entire specimen.

Treatment

Surgery

The only treatment of any proven curative value for the frankly malignant uterine sarcomas is surgical excision. This will typically involve total abdominal hysterectomy and bilateral salpingo-oophorectomy, although in young patients it may be reasonable to preserve the ovaries in a patient with a leiomyosarcoma, particularly if the tumor has arisen in a fibroid (162).

Table 8.21   AFIP Classification of Endometrial Stromal Tumors

Tumor	Malignant Potential	Cytologic Atypia	Mitoses/ 10 HPF
Stromal nodule	None	Mild–Moderate (pushing margins)	Less than 10; usually 0–3
Low-grade stromal sarcoma	Low to intermediate	Mild–Moderate (infiltrating margins)	Less than 10; usually 1–3
Stromal sarcoma	High	Moderate–Marked	10 or more

Reproduced, with permission, from Zaloudek CJ, Norris HG: Mesenchymal tumors of the uterus. In Fengolio C, Wolff M (eds): *Progress in Surgical Pathology*, vol 3, New York, Mason Publishing, 1981, pp 1–35.
AFIP = Armed Forces Institute of Pathology.

Surgical staging offers prognostic information, but there is no evidence that the information can be used to improve survival.

Radiation Therapy

Although the value of adjuvant radiation is controversial (163), it seems likely that it improves tumor control in the pelvis without influencing final outcome (164–166). This would be expected because of the high incidence of distant failure, particularly in the lungs and upper abdomen. It is not known whether extended-field or whole-abdominal radiation after surgical staging can influence prognosis, although whole-abdominal radiation has been reported to prevent abdominal relapse (165).

Chemotherapy

A number of chemotherapeutic agents are active against uterine sarcomas, the most important being Adriamycin, cisplatin, and ifosfamide. Unfortunately, most responses are partial and of short duration. For cisplatin (50 mg/M^2 every 3 weeks), the GOG reported a complete-response rate of 8% and a partial-response rate of 11% among 63 patients with advanced or recurrent mixed mesodermal tumors who had received no prior chemotherapy (167). Among 33 patients with leiomyosarcomas, there was only one partial response (3%). By contrast, leiomyosarcomas appear to be more responsive to Adriamycin. In the GOG trials, the response rate for leiomyosarcomas was 25% (7 of 28), compared with 10% (4 of 41) for mixed mesodermal sarcomas (168). Ifosfamide also has good activity against mixed mesodermal sarcomas, the GOG demonstrating 9 responses among 28 patients (31.2%) (169). For leiomyosarcomas, the response rate for ifosfamide was 17.2% (6 of 35), and all responses were partial (170).

Peters et al. (171) treated 11 patients with advanced or recurrent uterine stromal sarcomas or mixed mesodermal tumors with cisplatin 100 mg/M^2 and Adriamycin 40–60 mg/M^2 every 3–4 weeks for six cycles and reported a response in eight patients (73%) (171). Three patients had a negative second-look procedure and two were alive and free of disease > 24 months.

Because of the propensity for early hematogenous spread, adjuvant chemotherapy after hysterectomy to eliminate micrometastases is an attractive concept. However, in a randomized GOG study of Adriamycin after total abdominal hysterectomy and bilateral salpingo-oophorectomy for Stage I or II uterine sarcoma, neither survival nor progression-free interval was prolonged by the adjuvant chemotherapy (172). In a nonrandomized study, Peters et al. (171) reported 17 patients with high-risk clinical Stage I uterine stromal sarcomas or mixed mesodermal tumors who were treated with six cycles of cisplatin and Adriamycin as described above. Fourteen of the patients had invasion to the outer third of the myometrium, seven had documented lymph node metastases, and five had positive peritoneal washings. With a median follow-up of 34 months, there were only four recurrences, giving a projected 5-year survival rate of 75%. This combination certainly justifies further study in a phase III trial of adjuvant chemotherapy.

Prognosis

The frankly malignant uterine sarcomas generally have a poor prognosis. Surgical stage is the most important prognostic variable. If the tumor is confined to the uterus at laparotomy (surgical Stage I), the 5-year survival rate is about 50%. If there is spread beyond the uterus, the 5-year survival rate is about 20%. **When corrected by stage, there is no significant difference in failure rates, spread**

patterns, or survival among the three main histologic variants (164, 166). For mixed mesodermal tumors, there is also no difference in patterns of recurrence or survival between homologous, heterologous, or undifferentiated sarcomatous elements. Leiomyosarcomas in premenopausal patients carry a better overall prognosis, but this relates to their earlier stage at diagnosis (156). If the leiomyosarcoma arises in a benign fibroid, the prognosis is improved (156,173). Similarly, mixed mesodermal sarcomas and endometrial stromal sarcomas carry a worse overall prognosis, but this relates to the generally later stage at diagnosis (163, 164).

References

1. **Boring CC, Squires TS, Tony S:** Cancer statistics, 1994. *CA-Cancer J Clin* 44:7, 1994.

2. **Gallup DG, Stock RJ:** Adenocarcinoma of the endometrium in women 40 years of age or younger. *Obstet Gynecol* 64:417, 1984.

3. **Parazzini F, LaVecchia C, Bocciolone L, Franceschi S:** The epidemiology of endometrial cancer. *Gynecol Oncol* 41:1, 1991.

4. **Parazzini F, Negri E, LaVecchia C, et al:** Population attributable risk for endometrial cancer in Northern Italy. *Eur J Cancer Clin Oncol* 25:1451, 1989.

5. **Boronow RC:** Endometrial cancer: not a benign disease. *Obstet Gynecol* 47:630, 1976.

6. **Gusberg SB, Milano C:** Detection of endometrial carcinoma and its precursors. *Cancer* 47:1173, 1981.

7. **Bibbo M, Rice AM, Wied GL, Zuspan FP:** Comparative specificity and sensitivity of routine cytologic examination and the Gravlee jet wash technique for diagnosis of endometrial changes. *Obstet Gynecol* 43:253, 1974.

8. **DuBeshter B, Warshal DP, Angel C, et al:** Endometrial carcinoma: the relevance of cervical cytology. *Obstet Gynecol* 77:458, 1991.

9. **Ng ABP, Reagan JW, Hawliczek CT, Wentz BW:** Significance of endometrial cells in the detection of endometrial carcinoma and its precursors. *Acta Cytol* 18:356, 1974.

10. **Zucker PK, Kasdon EJ, Feldstein ML:** The validity of Pap smear parameters as predictors of endometrial pathology in menopausal women. *Cancer* 56:2256, 1985.

11. **Cherkis RC, Patten SF, Andrews TJ, et al:** Significance of normal endometrial cells detected by cervical cytology. *Obstet Gynecol* 71:242, 1988.

12. **Koss LG, Schreiber K, Oberlander SG, et al:** Screening of asymptomatic women for endometrial cancer. *Obstet Gynecol* 57:681, 1981.

13. **Hofmeister FJ:** Endometrial biopsy: another look. *Am J Obstet Gynecol* 118:773, 1974.

14. **Goldstein SR, Nachtigall M, Snyder JR, Nachtigall L:** Endometrial assessment by vaginal ultrasonography before endometrial sampling in patients with postmenopausal bleeding. *Am J Obstet Gynecol* 163:119, 1990.

15. **Bourne TH, Campbell S, Steer CV, et al:** Detection of endometrial cancer by transvaginal ultrasonography with color flow imaging and blood flow analysis: a preliminary report. *Gynecol Oncol* 40:253, 1991.

16. **Smith M, McCartney AJ:** Occult, high-risk endometrial carcinoma. *Gynecol Oncol* 22:154, 1985.

17. **Bokhman JV:** Two pathogenetic types of endometrial carcinoma. *Gynecol Oncol* 15:10, 1983.

18. **Stelmachow J:** The role of hysteroscopy in gynecologic oncology. *Gynecol Oncol* 14:392, 1982.

19. **Abayomi O, Dritschilo A, Emami B, et al:** The value of "routine tests" in the staging evaluation of gynecologic malignancies: a cost effectiveness analysis. *Int J Radiat Oncol Biol Phys* 8:241, 1982.

20. **Malkasian GD, McDonald TW, Pratt JH:** Carcinoma of the endometrium—Mayo Clinic experience. *Mayo Clin Proc* 52:175, 1977.

21. **Hricak H, Rubinstein LV, Gherman GM, Karstaedt N:** MR imaging evaluation of endometrial carcinoma: results of an NCI cooperative study. *Radiology* 179:829, 1991.

22. **Musumeci R, De Palo G, Conti U, et al:** Are retroperitoneal lymph node metastases a major problem in endometrial adenocarcinoma? *Cancer* 46:1887, 1980.

23. **Tiitinen A, Forss M, Aho I, et al:** Endometrial adenocarcinoma: clinical outcome in 881 patients and analysis of 146 patients whose deaths were due to endometrial cancer. *Gynecol Oncol* 25:11, 1986.

24. **Cowles TA, Magrina JF, Masterson BJ, Capen CV:** Comparison of clinical and surgical staging in patients with endometrial carcinoma. *Obstet Gynecol* 66:413, 1985.

25. **Lotocki RJ, Copeland LJ, DePetrillo AD, Muirhead W:** Stage I endometrial adenocarcinoma: treatment results in 835 patients. *Am J Obstet Gynecol* 146:141, 1983.

26. **Boronow RC, Morrow CP, Creasman WT, et al:** Surgical staging in endometrial cancer: clinicopathologic findings of a prospective study. *Obstet Gynecol* 63:825, 1984.

27. **Creasman WT, Morrow CP, Bundy BN, et al:** Surgical pathologic spread patterns of endometrial cancer. *Cancer* 60:2035, 1987.

28. **Onsrud M, Aalders J, Abeler V, Taylor P:** Endometrial carcinoma with cervical involvement (stage II): prognostic factors and value of combined radiological-surgical treatment. *Gynecol Oncol* 13:76, 1982.

29. **Kadar NRD, Kohorn EI, Li Volsi VA, Kapp DS:** Histologic variants of cervical involvement by endometrial carcinoma. *Obstet Gynecol* 59:85, 1982.

30. **Bigelow B, Vekshtein V, Demopoulos RI:** Endometrial carcinoma, stage II: route and extent of spread to the cervix. *Obstet Gynecol* 62:363, 1983.

31. **Creasman WT, Lukeman J:** Role of the fallopian tube in dissemination of malignant cells in corpus cancer. *Cancer* 29:456, 1972.

32. **Mackillop WJ, Pringle JF:** Stage III endometrial carcinoma: a review of 90 cases. *Cancer* 56:2519, 1985.

33. **Truskett ID, Constable WC:** Management of carcinoma of the corpus uteri. *Am J Obstet Gynecol* 101:689, 1968.

34. **Malkasian GD, Annegers JF, Fountain KS:** Carcinoma of the endometrium: stage I. *Am J Obstet Gynecol* 136:872, 1980.

35. **Aalders J, Abeler V, Kolstad P, Onsrud M:** Postoperative external irradiation and prognostic parameters in stage I endometrial carcinoma. *Obstet Gynecol* 56:419, 1980.

36. **Quinn MA, Kneale BJ, Fortune DW:** Endometrial carcinoma in premenopausal women: a clinicopathological study. *Gynecol Oncol* 20:298, 1985.

37. **Crissman JD, Azoury RS, Barnes AE, Schellhas HF:** Endometrial carcinoma in women 40 years of age or younger. *Obstet Gynecol* 57:669, 1981.

38. **Wilson TD, Podratz KC, Gaffey TA, et al:** Evaluation of unfavourable histologic subtypes in endometrial adenocarcinoma. *Am J Obstet Gynecol* 162:418, 1990.

39. **Silverberg SG, Bolin MG, De Giorgi LS:** Adenoacanthoma and mixed adenosquamous carcinoma of the endometrium: a clinicopathologic study. *Cancer* 30:1307, 1972.

40. **Zaino RJ, Kurman R, Herbold D, et al:** The significance of squamous differentiation in endometrial carcinoma. *Cancer* 68:2293, 1991.

41. **Lauchlan SC:** Tubal (serous) carcinoma of the endometrium. *Arch Pathol Lab Med* 15:615, 1981.

42. **Hendrickson M, Ross J, Eifel PJ, et al:** Adenocarcinoma of the endometrium: analysis of 256 cases with carcinoma limited to the uterine corpus. *Gynecol Oncol* 13:373, 1982.

43. **Chambers JT, Merino M, Kohorn EI, et al:** Uterine papillary serous carcinoma. *Obstet Gynecol* 69:109, 1987.

44. **Sherman ME, Bitterman P, Rosenshein NB, et al:** Uterine serous carcinoma. *Am J Surg Pathol* 16:600, 1992.

45. **Jeffrey JF, Krepart GV, Lotocki RJ:** Papillary serous adenocarcinoma of the endometrium. *Obstet Gynecol* 67:670, 1986.

46. **Christopherson WM, Alberhasky RG, Connelly PJ:** Carcinoma of the endometrium. I. A clinicopathologic study of clear cell carcinoma and secretory carcinoma. *Cancer* 49:1511, 1982.

47. **Abeler VM, Kjorstad KE:** Clear cell carcinoma of the endometrium: a histopathological and clinical study of 97 cases. *Gynecol Oncol* 40:207, 1991.

48. **Abeler VM, Kjorstad KE:** Endometrial squamous cell carcinoma: report of three cases and review of the literature. *Gynecol Oncol* 36:321, 1990.

49. **DiSaia PJ, Creasman WT, Boronow RC, Blessing JA:** Risk factors and recurrent patterns in stage I endometrial cancer. *Am J Obstet Gynecol* 151:1009, 1985.

50. **Hanson MB, Van Nagell JR, Powell DE, et al:** The prognostic significance of lymph-vascular space invasion in stage I endometrial cancer. *Cancer* 55:1753, 1985.

51. **Abeler VM, Kjorstad KE, Berle E:** Carcinoma of the endometrium in Norway: a histopathological and prognostic survey of a total population. *Int J Gynecol Cancer* 2:9, 1992.

52. **Ambros RA, Kurman RJ:** Identification of patients with stage I uterine endometrioid adenocarcinoma at high risk of recurrence by DNA ploidy, myometrial invasion, and vascular invasion. *Gynecol Oncol* 45:235, 1992.

53. **Lurain JR:** The significance of positive peritoneal cytology in endometrial cancer. *Gynecol Oncol* 46:143, 1992.

54. **Creasman WT, DiSaia PJ, Blessing J, et al:** Prognostic significance of peritoneal cytology in patients with endometrial cancer and preliminary data concerning therapy with intraperitoneal radiopharmaceuticals. *Am J Obstet Gynecol* 141:921, 1981.

55. **Szpak CA, Creasman WT, Vollmer RT, Johnston WW:** Prognostic value of cytologic examination of peritoneal washings in patients with endometrial carcinoma. *Acta Cytol* 25:640, 1981.

56. **Yazigi R, Piver S, Blumenson L:** Malignant peritoneal cytology as a prognostic index in stage I endometrial cancer. *Obstet Gynecol* 62:359, 1983.

57. **Harouny VR, Sutton GP, Clark SA, et al:** The importance of peritoneal cytology in endometrial carcinoma. *Obstet Gynecol* 72:394, 1988.

58. **Hirai Y, Fujimoto I, Yamauchi K, et al:** Peritoneal fluid cytology and prognosis in patients with endometrial carcinoma. *Obstet Gynecol* 73:335, 1989.

59. **Lurain JR, Rumsey NK, Schink JC, et al:** Prognostic significance of positive peritoneal cytology in clinical stage I adenocarcinoma of the endometrium. *Obstet Gynecol* 74:175, 1989.

60. **Kadar N, Homesley HD, Malfetano JH:** Positive peritoneal cytology is an adverse factor in endometrial carcinoma only if there is other evidence of extrauterine disease. *Gynecol Oncol* 46:145, 1992.

61. **Morrow CP, Bundy BN, Kurman RJ, et al:** Relationship between surgical-pathologic risk factors and outcome in clinical stage I and II carcinoma of the endometrium: a Gynecologic Oncology Group study. *Gynecol Oncol* 40:55, 1991.

62. **Milosevic MF, Dembo AJ, Thomas GM:** The clinical significance of malignant peritoneal cytology in stage I endometrial carcinoma. *Int J Gynecol Cancer* 2:225, 1992.

63. **Ehrlich CE, Young PCM, Stehman FB:** Steroid receptors and clinical outcome in patients with adenocarcinoma of the endometrium. *Am J Obstet Gynecol* 158:796, 1988.

64. **Liao BS, Twiggs LB, Leung BS, et al:** Cytoplasmic estrogen and progesterone receptors as prognostic parameters in primary endometrial carcinoma. *Obstet Gynecol* 67:463, 1986.

65. **Creasman WT, Soper JT, McCarty KS, et al:** Influence of cytoplasmic steroid receptor content on prognosis of early stage endometrial carcinoma. *Am J Obstet Gynecol* 151:922,1985.

66. **Zaino RJ, Satyaswaroop PG, Mortel R:** The relationship of histologic and histochemical parameters to progesterone receptor status in endometrial adenocarcinomas. *Gynecol Oncol* 16:196, 1983.

67. **Martin JD, Hahnel R, McCartney AJ, Woodings TL:** The effect of estrogen receptor status on survival in patients with endometrial cancer. *Am J Obstet Gynecol* 147:322, 1983.

68. **Palmer DC, Muir IM, Alexander AI, et al:** The prognostic importance of steroid receptors in endometrial carcinoma. *Obstet Gynecol* 72:388, 1988.

69. **Geisinger KR, Homesley HD, Morgan TM, et al:** Endometrial adenocarcinoma: a multiparameter clinicopathologic analysis including DNA profile and the sex steroid hormone receptors. *Cancer* 58:1518, 1986.

70. **Christopherson WM, Connelly PJ, Alberhasky RC:** Carcinoma of the endometrium. V. An analysis of prognosticators in patients with favorable subtypes and stage I disease. *Cancer* 51:1705, 1983.

71. **Nielson AL, Thomsen HK, Nyholm HCJ:** Evaluation of the reproducibility of the revised 1988 International Federation of Gynecology and Obstetrics grading system of endometrial cancers with special emphasis on nuclear grading. *Cancer* 68:2303, 1991.

72. **Schink JC, Lurain JR, Wallemark CB, Chmiel JS:** Tumor size in endometrial cancer: a prognostic factor for lymph node metastasis. *Obstet Gynecol* 70:216, 1987.

73. **Iversen OE:** Flow cytometric doxyribonucleic acid index: a prognostic factor in endometrial carcinoma. *Am J Obstet Gynecol* 155:770, 1986.

74. **Stendahl U, Wagenius G, Strang P, Tribukait B:** Flow cytometry in invasive endometrial carcinoma. *In Vivo* 2:123, 1988.

75. **Surwit EA, Joelsson I, Einhorn N:** Adjuvant radiation therapy in the management of stage I cancer of the endometrium. *Obstet Gynecol* 58:590, 1981.

76. **Grigsby PW, Perez CA, Camel HM, Galakatos AE:** Stage II carcinoma of the endometrium: results of therapy and prognostic factors. *Int J Radiat Oncol Biol Phys* 11:1915, 1985.

77. **Bickenbach W, Lochmuller H, Dirlich G, et al:** Factor analysis of endometrial carcinoma in relation to treatment. *Obstet Gynecol* 29:632, 1967.

78. **Nahhas WA, Whitney CW, Stryker JA, et al:** Stage II endometrial carcinoma. *Gynecol Oncol* 10:303, 1980.

79. **Hernandez W, Nolan JF, Morrow CP, Jernstrom PH:** Stage II endometrial carcinoma: two modalities of treatment. *Am J Obstet Gynecol* 131:171, 1978.

80. **Hertig AT, Sommers SC, Bengloff H:** Genesis of endometrial carcinoma. III. Carcinoma in situ. *Cancer* 2:964, 1949.

81. **Gusberg SB, Kaplan AL:** Precursors of corpus cancer. IV. Adenomatous hyperplasia as stage O carcinoma of the endometrium. *Am J Obstet Gynecol* 87:662, 1963.

82. **Vellios F:** Endometrial hyperplasias, precursors of endometrial carcinoma. *Pathol Annu* 7:201, 1972.

83. **Kurman RJ, Kaminski PF, Norris HJ:** The behavior of endometrial hyperplasia: a long-term study of "untreated" hyperplasia in 170 patients. *Cancer* 56:403, 1985.

84. **Ferenczy A, Gelfand MM, Tzipris F:** The cytodynamics of endometrial hyperplasia and carcinoma: a review. *Ann Pathol* 3:189, 1983.

85. **Ferenczy A, Gelfand M:** The biologic significance of cytologic atypia in progesten-treated endometrial hyperplasia. *Am J Obstet Gynecol* 160:126, 1989.

86. **Piver MS, Yazigi R, Blumenson L, Tsukada Y:** A prospective trial comparing hysterectomy, hysterectomy plus vaginal radium, and uterine radium plus hysterectomy in stage I endometrial carcinoma. *Obstet Gynecol* 54:85, 1979.

87. **Wallin TE, Malkasian GD, Gaffey TA, et al:** Stage II cancer of the endometrium: a pathologic and clinical study. *Gynecol Oncol* 18:1, 1984.

88. **Berman ML, Afridi MA, Kambour AI, Ball HG:** Risk factors and prognosis in stage II endometrial cancer. *Gynecol Oncol* 14:49, 1982.

89. **Kurman RJ, Norris HJ:** Endometrial neoplasia: Hyperplasia and carcinoma. In Blaustein A (ed): *Pathology of the Female Genital Tract,* ed 2. New York, Springer-Verlag, 1982, p 344.

90. **Eiffel P, Hendrickson M, Ross J, et al:** Simultaneous presentation of carcinoma involving the ovary and the uterine corpus. *Cancer* 50:163, 1982.

91. **Morrow CP, Schlaerth JB:** Surgical management of endometrial carcinoma. *Clin Obstet Gynecol* 25:81, 1982.

92. **Morrow CP, Hernandez WL, Townsend DE, DiSaia PJ:** Pelvic celiotomy in the obese patient. *Am J Obstet Gynecol* 127:335, 1977.

93. **Goff BA, Rice LW:** Assessment of depth of myometrial invasion in endometrial adenocarcinoma. *Gynecol Oncol* 38:46, 1990.

94. **Peters WA III, Andersen WA, Thornton N Jr, Morley GW:** The selective use of vaginal hysterectomy in the management of adenocarcinoma of the endometrium. *Am J Obstet Gynecol* 146:285, 1983.

95. **Bloss JD, Berman ML, Bloss LP, Buller RE:** Use of vaginal hysterectomy for the management of stage I endometrial cancer in the medically compromised patient. *Gynecol Oncol* 40:74, 1991.

96. **Ritcher N, Lucas WE, Yon JL, Sanford FG:** Preoperative whole pelvic external irradiation in stage I endometrial cancer. *Cancer* 48:58, 1981.

97. **Salazar OM, Feldstein ML, DePapp EW, et al:** Endometrial carcinoma: analysis of failures with special emphasis on the use of initial preoperative external pelvic radiation. *Int J Radiat Oncol Biol Phys* 2:1101, 1977.

98. **Onsrud M, Kolstad P, Normann T:** Postoperative external pelvic irradiation in carcinoma of the corpus stage I: a controlled clinical trial. *Gynecol Oncol* 4:222, 1976.

99. **Komaki R, Cox JD, Hartz A, et al:** Influence of preoperative irradiation on failures of endometrial carcinoma with high risk of lymph node metastases. *Am J Clin Oncol* 7:661, 1984.

100. **Bean HA, Bryant AS, Carmichael JA, Mallik A:** Carcinoma of the endometrium in Saskatchewan: 1966 to 1971. *Gynecol Oncol* 6:503, 1978.

101. **Hording U, Hanses U:** Stage I endometrial carcinoma: a review of 140 patients primarily treated with surgery only. *Gynecol Oncol* 22:51, 1985.

102. **Fanning J, Evans MC, Peters AJ, et al:** Adjuvant radiotherapy for stage I, grade 2 endometrial adenocarcinoma and adenoacanthoma with limited myometrial invasion. *Obstet Gynecol* 70:920, 1987.

103. **Gal D, Recio FO, Zamurovic D:** The new International Federation of Gynecology and Obstetrics surgical staging and survival rates in early endometrial carcinoma. *Cancer* 69:200, 1992.

104. **Belinson JL, Lee KR, Badger GJ, et al:** Clinical stage I adenocarcinoma of the endometrium—analysis of recurrences and the potential benefit of staging lymphadenectomy. *Gynecol Oncol* 44:17, 1992.

105. **Stokes S, Bedwinek J, Breaux S, et al:** Treatment of stage I adenocarcinoma of the endometrium by hysterectomy and irradiation: analysis of complications. *Obstet Gynecol* 65:86, 1985.

106. **Joelsson I, Sandri A, Kottmeier HL:** Carcinoma of the uterine corpus: a retrospective survey of individualized therapy. *Acta Radiol* [Suppl] 334:3, 1973.

107. **Hacker NF, Berek JS:** Surgical staging of cervical cancer. In Alberts D, Surwit EA (eds): *Cervix Cancer.* Boston, Martinus Nijhoff, 1987, pp 43–58.

108. **Potish RA, Twiggs LB, Adcock LL, et al:** Paraaortic lymph node radiotherapy in cancer of the uterine corpus. *Obstet Gynecol* 65:251, 1985.

109. **Potish RA, Twiggs LB, Adcock LL, Prem KA:** Role of whole abdominal radiation therapy in the management of endometrial cancer; prognostic importance of factors indicating peritoneal metastases. *Gynecol Oncol* 21:80, 1985.

110. **Greer BE, Hamberger AD:** Treatment of intraperitoneal metastatic adenocarcinoma of the endometrium by the whole-abdomen moving-strip technique and pelvic boost irradiation. *Gynecol Oncol* 16:365, 1983.

111. **Soper JT, Creasman WT, Clarke-Pearson DL, et al:** Intraperitoneal chronic phosphate ^{32}P suspension therapy of malignant peritoneal cytology in endometrial carcinoma. *Am J Obstet Gynecol* 153:191,1985.

112. **DePalo G, Mersom M, Del Vecchio M, et al:** A controlled clinical study of adjuvant medroxyprogesterone acetate (MPA) therapy in pathological Stage I endometrial cancer with myometrial invasion. *Proc Am Soc Clin Oncol* 4:121, 1985.

113. **Lewis GC, Slack NH, Mortel R, Bross IJ:** Adjuvant progestogen therapy in the primary definitive treatment of endometrial cancer. *Gynecol Oncol* 2:368, 1974.

114. **MacDonald RR, Thorogood J, Mason MK:** A randomized trial of progestogens in the primary treatment of endometrial carcinoma. *Br J Obstet Gynaecol* 95:166, 1988.

115. **Vergote I, Kjorstad K, Abeler V, Kolstad P:** A randomized trial of adjuvant protestogen in early endometrial cancer. *Cancer* 64:1011, 1989.

116. **Morrow CP, DiSaia PJ, Townsend DE:** Current management of endometrial carcinoma. *Obstet Gynecol* 42:399, 1973.

117. **Larson DM, Copeland LJ, Gallager HS, et al:** Stage II endometrial carcinoma: results and complications of a combined radiotherapeutic-surgical approach. *Cancer* 61:1528, 1988.

118. **Rutledge F:** The role of radical hysterectomy in adenocarcinoma of the endometrium. *Gynecol Oncol* 2:331, 1974.

119. **Tak WK:** Carcinoma of the endometrium with cervical involvement (stage II). *Cancer* 43:2504, 1979.

120. **Bruckman JE, Goodman RL, Murthy A, Marck A:** Combined irradiation and surgery in the treatment of stage II carcinoma of the endometrium. *Cancer* 42:1146, 1978.

121. **Kinsella TJ, Bloomer WD, Lavin PT, Knapp RC:** Stage II endometrial carcinoma: 10 year follow-up of combined radiation and surgical treatment. *Gynecol Oncol* 10:290, 1980.

122. **Boronow RC:** Carcinoma of the corpus: treatment at M.D. Anderson Hospital. In: *Cancer of the Uterus and Ovary (Anderson Hospital)*. Chicago, Year Book, 1969, pp 35–61.

123. **Goplerud DR, Belgrad R:** The importance of histologic grade in stage II endometrial carcinoma. *Surg Gynecol Obstet* 148:406, 1979.

124. **Aalders J, Abeler V, Kolstad P:** Clinical (Stage III) as compared to subclinical intrapelvic extrauterine tumor spread in endometrial carcinoma: a clinical and histopathological study of 175 patients. *Gynecol Oncol* 17:64, 1984.

125. **Bruckman JE, Bloomer WD, Marck A, et al:** Stage III adenocarcinoma of the endometrium: two prognostic groups. *Gynecol Oncol* 9:12, 1980.

126. **Genest P, Drouin P, Girard A, Gerig L:** Stage III carcinoma of the endometrium: a review of 41 cases. *Gynecol Oncol* 26:77, 1987.

127. **Aalders J, Abeler V, Kolstad P:** Stage IV endometrial carcinoma: a clinical and histopathological study of 83 patients. *Gynecol Oncol* 17:75, 1984.

128. **Ballon SG, Berman ML, Donaldson RC, et al:** Pulmonary metastases of endometrial carcinoma. *Gynecol Oncol* 7:56, 1979.

129. **Farias-Eisner R, Nieberg RK, Berek JS:** Synchronous primary neoplasms of the female reproductive tract. *Gynecol Oncol* 33:335, 1989.

130. **Farhi DC, Nosanchuk J, Silberberg SG:** Endometrial adenocarcinoma in women under 25 years of age. *Obstet Gynecol* 68:741, 1986.

131. **Kempson RL, Pokorny GE:** Adenocarcinoma of the endometrium in women aged forty and younger. *Cancer* 21:650, 1968.

132. **Fechner RE, Kaufman RH:** Endometrial adenocarcinoma in Stein-Levanthol syndrome. *Cancer* 34:444, 1974.

133. **Pastner B, Orr JW, Mann WJ:** Use of serum Ca 125 measurement in posttreatment surveillance of early-stage endometrial carcinoma. *Am J Obstet Gynecol* 162:427, 1990.

134. **Aalders J, Abeler V, Kolstad P:** Recurrent adenocarcinoma of the endometrium: a clinical and histopathological study of 379 patients. *Gynecol Oncol* 17:85, 1984.

135. **Burke TW, Heller PB, Woodward JE, et al:** Treatment failure in endometrial carcinoma. *Obstet Gynecol* 75:96, 1990.

136. **Phillips GL, Prem KA, Adcock LL, Twiggs LB:** Vaginal recurrence of adenocarcinoma of the endometrium. *Gynecol Oncol* 13:323, 1982.

137. **Kelley RM, Baker WH:** Progestational agents in the treatment of carcinoma of the endometrium. *N Engl J Med* 264:216, 1961.

138. **Thigpen T, Blessing J, DiSaia P, et al:** Oral medroxyprogesterone acetate in advanced or recurrent endometrial carcinoma. In Baulieu EE, Iacobelli S, McGuire WL (eds): *Endocrinology and malignancy.* Parthenon, 1986, pp 446–454.

139. **Podratz KC, O'Brien PC, Malkasian GD, et al:** Effects of progestational agents in treatment of endometrial cacinoma. *Obstet Gynecol* 66:106, 1985.

140. **Kauppila A:** Progestin therapy of endometrial, breast and ovarian carcinoma. *Acta Obstet Gynecol Scand* 63:441, 1984.

141. **Piver MS, Barlow JJ, Lurain JR, et al:** Medroxyprogesterone acetate (Depo-Provera) vs hydroxyprogesterone caproate (Delalutin) in women with metastatic endometrial adenocarcinoma. *Cancer* 45:268, 1980.

142. **Moore TD, Phillips PH, Nerenstone SR, Cheson BD:** Systemic treatment of advanced and recurrent endometrial carcinoma: current status and future directions. *J Clin Oncol* 9:1071, 1991.

143. **Swenerton KD:** Treatment of advanced endometrial adenocarcinoma with tamoxifen. *Cancer Treat Rep* 64:805, 1980.

144. **Bonte J, Ide P, Billiet G, Wynants P:** Tamoxifen as a possible chemotherapeutic agent in endometrial adenocarcinoma. *Gynecol Oncol* 11:140, 1981.

145. **Thigpen JT, Buchsbaum HJ, Mangan C, Blessing JA:** Phase II trial of adriamycin in the treatment of advanced or recurrent endometrial carcinoma: a Gynecologic Oncology Group study. *Cancer Treat Rep* 63:21, 1979.

146. **Cohen CJ, Bruckner HW, Deppe G, et al:** Multidrug treatment of advanced and recurrent endometrial carcinoma: a Gynecologic Oncology Group study. *Obstet Gynecol* 63:719, 1984.

147. **Lovecchio JL, Averette HE, Lichtinger M, et al:** Treatment of advanced or recurrent endometrial adenocarcinoma with cyclophosphamide, doxorubicin, cis-platinum and megestrol acetate. *Obstet Gynecol* 63:557, 1984.

148. **Levenback C, Burke TW, Silva E, et al:** Uterine papillary serous carcinoma (UPSC) treated with cisplatin, doxorubicin, and cyclophosphamide (PAC). *Gynecol Oncol* 46:317, 1992.

149. **Creasman WT, Henderson D, Hinshaw W, Clarke-Pearson DL:** Estrogen replacement therapy in the patient treated for endometrial cancer. *Obstet Gynecol* 67:326, 1986.

150. **Zaloudek CJ, Norris HJ:** Mesenchymal tumors of the uterus. In Fengolio C, Wolff M (eds): *Progress in Surgical Pathology,* vol 3. New York, Masson Publishing, 1981, pp 1–35.

151. **Norris HJ, Taylor HB:** Postirradiation sarcomas of the uterus. *Obstet Gynecol* 26:689, 1965.

152. **Ober WB:** Uterine sarcomas: histogenesis and taxonomy. *Ann NY Acad Sci* 75:568, 1959.

153. **Kempson RL, Bari W:** Uterine sarcomas: classification, diagnosis, and prognosis. *Hum Pathol* 1:331, 1970.

154. **DiSaia PJ, Morrow CP, Boronow R, et al:** Endometrial sarcoma: lymphatic spread pattern. *Am J Obstet Gynecol* 130:104, 1978.

155. **Leibsohn S, d'Ablaing G, Mishell DR, Schlaerth JB:** Leiomyosarcoma in a series of hysterectomies performed for presumed uterine leiomyomas. *Am J Obstet Gynecol* 162:968, 1990.

156. **Dinh TV, Woodruff JD:** Leiomyosarcoma of the uterus. *Am J Obstet Gynecol* 144:817, 1982.

157. **Norris HJ, Parmley T:** Mesenchymal tumors of the uterus. V. Intravenous leiomyomatosis: a clinical and pathologic study of 14 cases. *Cancer* 36:2164, 1975.

158. **Goldberg MF, Hurt WG, Frable WJ:** Leiomyomatosis peritonealis disseminata: report of a case and review of the literature. *Obstet Gynecol* 49:465, 1977.

159. **DeFusco PA, Gaffey TA, Malkasian GD, et al:** Endometrial stromal sarcoma: review of Mayo Clinic experience, 1945–1980. *Gynecol Oncol* 35:8, 1989.

160. **Hart WR, Yoonessi M:** Endometrial stromatosis of the uterus. *Obstet Gynecol* 49:393,1977.

161. **Spanos WJ, Wharton JT, Gomez L, et al:** Malignant mixed mullerian tumors of the uterus. *Cancer* 53:311, 1984.

162. **Silverberg SG:** Leiomyosarcoma of the uterus: a clinicopathological study. *Obstet Gynecol* 38:613, 1971.

163. **Kahanpaa KV, Wahlstom T, Grohn P, et al:** Sarcoma of the uterus: a clinicopathologic study of 119 patients. *Obstet Gynecol* 67:417, 1986.

164. **Salazar OM, Bonfiglio TA, Patten SF, et al:** Uterine sarcomas: analysis of failures with special emphasis on the use of adjuvant radiotherapy. *Cancer* 42:1161, 1978.

165. **Spanos WJ, Peters LJ, Oswald MJ:** Patterns of recurrence in malignant mixed mullerian tumor of the uterus. *Cancer* 57:155, 1986.

166. **Echt G, Jepson J, Steel J, et al:** Treatment of uterine sarcomas. *Cancer* 66:35, 1990.

167. **Thigpen JT, Blessing JA, Beecham J, et al:** Phase II trial of cisplatin as first-line chemotherapy in patients with advanced or recurrent uterine sarcomas: a Gynecologic Oncology Group study. *J Clin Oncol* 9:1962, 1991.

168. **Omura GA, Major FJ, Blessing JA, et al:** A randomized study of Adriamycin with and without dimethyl triazenoimidazole carboxamide in advanced uterine sarcomas. *Cancer* 52:626, 1983.

169. **Sutton G, Blessing JA, Rosenshein N, et al:** Phase II trial of ifosfamide and mesna in mixed mesodermal tumors of the uterus (a Gynecologic Oncology Group study). *Am J Obstet Gynecol* 161:309, 1989.

170. **Sutton GP, Blessing JA, Barrett RJ, McGehee R:** Phase II trial of ifosfamide and mesna in leiomyosarcoma of the uterus: a Gynecologic Oncology Group study. *Am J Obstet Gynecol* 166:556, 1992.

171. **Peters WA III, Rivkin SE, Smith MR, Tesh DE:** Cisplatin and adriamycin combination chemotherapy for uterine stromal sarcomas and mixed mesodermal tumors. *Gynecol Oncol* 34:323, 1989.

172. **Omura GA, Blessing JA, Major E, Silverberg S:** A randomized trial of Adriamycin versus no adjuvant chemotherapy in stage I and II uterine sarcomas. *J Clin Oncol* 9:1240, 1985.

173. **Gallup DG, Cordray DR:** Leiomyosarcoma of the uterus: case reports and a review. *Obstet Gynecol Surv* 34:300, 1979.

Epithelial Ovarian Cancer

Jonathan S. Berek

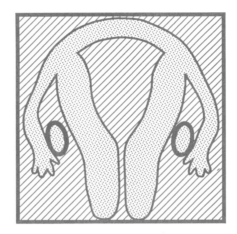

Of all the gynecologic cancers, ovarian malignancies represent the greatest clinical challenge. Epithelial cancers are the most common ovarian malignancies, and, because they are usually asymptomatic until they have metastasized, patients present with advanced disease in more than two-thirds of the cases. Ovarian cancer represents a major surgical challenge, requires intensive and often complex therapies, and is extremely demanding of the patient's psychological and physical energy. It has the highest fatality to case ratio of all the gynecologic malignancies. There are more than 24,000 new cases annually in the United States, and 13,600 women can be expected to succumb to their illness (1).

Classification

Approximately 90% of ovarian cancers are derived from tissues that come from the coelomic epithelium or "mesothelium" (2). The cells are a product of the primitive mesoderm, which can undergo metaplasia. Neoplastic transformation can occur when the cells are genetically predisposed to oncogenesis and/or exposed to an oncogenic agent (3).

Pathology

Invasive Cancer

Seventy-five percent of epithelial cancers are of the serous histologic type. Less common types are mucinous (20%), endometrioid (2%), clear cell, Brenner, and undifferentiated carcinomas, each of the latter three representing < 1% of epithelial lesions (2). Each tumor type has a histologic pattern that reproduces the mucosal features of a section of the lower genital tract (3). For example, the serous or papillary pattern has an appearance similar to that of the glandular epithelium lining the fallopian tube. Mucinous tumors contain cells that resemble the endocervical glands, and the endometrioid tumors resemble the endometrium. More specific details of the histology are discussed in Chapter 4.

Borderline Tumors

An important group of tumors to distinguish is the *tumor of low malignant potential*, also called the *borderline* tumor. Borderline tumors are lesions that tend to remain confined to the ovary for long periods of time, occur predominantly in premenopausal women, and are associated with a very good prognosis (2–6). They are encountered most frequently between the ages of 30 and 50 years, whereas invasive carcinomas are found more commonly between the ages of 50 and 70 years (2).

Although uncommon, metastatic implants may occur with borderline tumors. Such implants have been divided into noninvasive and invasive forms. The latter group have a higher likelihood of developing progressive, proliferative disease in the peritoneal cavity, which can lead to intestinal obstruction and death (2, 6).

Peritoneal Carcinoma

The primary malignant transformation of the peritoneum has been called *primary peritoneal carcinoma* or *primary peritoneal papillary serous carcinoma*. This disease simulates ovarian cancer clinically. This phenomenon can produce a condition in which "ovarian cancer" can arise in a patient whose ovaries were surgically removed many years earlier (7). In such cases, there may be microscopic or small macroscopic cancer on the surface of the ovary and extensive disease in the upper abdomen, particularly in the omentum.

Clinical Features

More than 80% of epithelial ovarian cancers are found in postmenopausal women. The peak incidence of this disease occurs at 62 years. Before the age of 45, these cancers are relatively uncommon. Fewer than 1% of epithelial ovarian cancers occur before the age of 21 years, two-thirds of ovarian malignancies in such patients being germ cell tumors (2, 8, 9). About 30% of ovarian neoplasms in postmenopausal women are malignant, whereas only about 7% of ovarian epithelial tumors in premenopausal patients are frankly malignant (2).

Screening

The value of tumor markers and ultrasonography to screen for epithelial ovarian cancer has not been clearly established by prospective studies. Screening with transabdominal ultrasonography has been encouraging (10), but specificity has been limited. However, recent advances in transvaginal ultrasonography have been shown to have a very high (> 95%) sensitivity for the detection of early-stage ovarian cancer, although this test alone might require as many as 10–15 laparotomies per ovarian cancer detected (11, 12). Routine annual pelvic examinations are disappointing for the early detection of ovarian cancer (13). Transvaginal color flow Doppler to assess the vascularity of the ovarian vessels has been shown to be a useful adjunct to ultrasonography (13, 14), but its role in screening remains to be defined.

CA 125 has been shown to contribute to the early diagnosis of epithelial ovarian cancer (16–21). Regarding the sensitivity of the test, CA 125 can detect 50% of patients with Stage I disease, and 60% if patients with Stage II disease are included (17). Data suggest that the specificity of CA 125 is improved when the test is combined with transvaginal ultrasonography (18) or when the CA 125 levels are followed over time (19, 20). These data have encouraged the development of prospective screening studies in Sweden and the United Kingdom (21, 22). In these studies, patients with elevated CA 125 levels (> 30 U/ml) have undergone abdominal ultrasonography and 14 ovarian cancers have been discovered among 27,000 women screened. About four laparotomies have been performed per cancer detected.

Given the false-positive results for both CA 125 and transvaginal ultrasonography, particularly in premenopausal women, these tests are not cost-effective and should not be used routinely to screen for ovarian cancer. In the future, new markers or technologies may improve the specificity of ovarian cancer screening, but proof of this will require a large prospective study. Screening in women who have a familial risk may have a better yield, but additional study is necessary (24).

Genetic Risk for Epithelial Ovarian Cancer

The lifetime risk of ovarian carcinoma for women in the United States is about 1.4% (23). The risk of ovarian cancer is higher in women with certain family histories (24–30). Most epithelial ovarian cancer is sporadic, with familial or hereditary patterns accounting for fewer than 5% of all malignancies (30). A patient can have a genetic risk of a *site-specific familial ovarian cancer*, a hereditary *breast/ovarian familial cancer syndrome*, or the *Lynch II syndrome*.

Site-Specific Familial Ovarian Cancer   Although the risk of developing epithelial ovarian cancer is higher, the precise risk is difficult to determine but depends on the number of first- and/or second-degree relatives with a history of epithelial ovarian carcinoma.

1. In families with two first-degree relatives (i.e., mother, sister, or daughter) with documented epithelial ovarian cancer, the risk that a female first-degree relative will have an affected gene could be as high as 50% (27). The pedigree type is consistent with an autosomal dominant mode of inheritance (27, 28).

2. In families with a single first-degree relative and a single second-degree relative (i.e., grandmother, aunt, first cousin, or granddaughter) with epithelial ovarian cancer, the risk that a woman will have an affected gene also may be increased, but the degree of risk may be difficult to determine precisely unless one performs a full pedigree analysis. The relative risk may be three- to tenfold higher (24) than in those without a familial history of the disease.

3. In families with a single first-degree relative with epithelial ovarian carcinoma, a woman has a slightly increased risk of having an affected gene, the relative increase being two- to fourfold (24).

Hereditary ovarian cancers generally occur in women about 10 years younger than those with nonhereditary tumors (28). As the median age of epithelial ovarian cancer is about 61 years, a woman with a first- or second-degree relative who had ovarian cancer before the age of 50 will have a higher probability of carrying an affected gene.

Breast/Ovarian Familial Cancer Syndrome Breast/ovarian familial cancer syndrome may exist in a family in which there is a combination of epithelial ovarian and breast cancers, affecting a mixture of first- and second-degree relatives. (25, 29). Women with this syndrome tend to have these tumors at a young age, and the breast cancers may be bilateral. If two first-degree relatives are affected, this pedigree is consistent with an autosomal dominant mode of inheritance (25, 27). The relative risk of developing ovarian cancer may be two- to fourfold greater than the general population (24). Women with a primary history of breast cancer have twice the expected incidence of subsequent ovarian cancer (27). Recently, a gene locus on the 17q chromosome, the BRCA1 gene, has been associated with this syndrome (31).

Lynch II Syndrome The Lynch II syndrome, which includes multiple adenocarcinomas, involves a combination of familial colon cancer (known as the Lynch I syndrome), a high rate of ovarian, endometrial, and breast cancers, and other malignancies of the gastrointestinal and genitourinary systems (27). The risk that a woman who is a member of one of these families will develop epithelial ovarian cancer depends on the frequency of this disease in first- and second-degree relatives, although these women appear to have at least three times the relative risk of the general population (27). A full pedigree analysis of such families should be performed by a geneticist to more accurately determine the risk.

In all of these syndromes, women at risk benefit from a thorough pedigree analysis. A geneticist should evaluate the family pedigree for at least three generations. Decisions about management are best made after careful study and, whenever possible, verification of the histologic diagnosis of the family members' ovarian cancer.

The management of a woman with a strong family history of epithelial ovarian cancer depends on her age, her reproductive plans, and the extent of risk. The plan must be individualized because the value of screening with transvaginal ultrasonography, CA 125 levels, or other procedures has not been clearly established in women at high risk. Bourne et al. (24) have shown that this approach can detect tumors about ten times more often than in the general population, and thus they recommend screening in high-risk women. The current recommendations of the Committee on Gynecologic Practice of the American College of Obstetricians and Gynecologists are summarized below (23):

1. Women who wish to preserve their reproductive capacity should undergo periodic screening by transvaginal ultrasonography every 6 months and should consider prophylactic oophorectomy when the family has been completed. Oral contraceptives may be given to young women before a planned family, although the protective effect in high-risk women has not been evaluated.

2. Women with familial ovarian or hereditary breast/ovarian cancer syndrome who do not wish to maintain their fertility should be offered prophylactic bilateral salpingo-oophorectomy. The risk should be clearly documented, preferably established by pedigree analysis, before oophorectomy. These women should be counseled that this operation does not offer absolute protection because peritoneal carcinomas occasionally can occur after bilateral oophorectomy (7).

3. Women with a documented Lynch II syndrome should be treated as above, but, in addition, they should undergo periodic screening mammography, colonoscopy, and endometrial biopsy.

Symptoms	The majority of women with epithelial ovarian cancer have no symptoms for long periods of time. When symptoms do develop, they are often vague and nonspecific (8, 32). In early-stage disease, the patient may complain of irregular menses if she is premenopausal. If a pelvic mass is compressing the bladder or rectum, she may report urinary frequency or constipation. Occasionally, she may perceive lower abdominal distention, pressure, or pain, such as dyspareunia. Acute symptoms, such as pain secondary to rupture or torsion, are unusual.

In advanced-stage disease, patients most often have symptoms related to the presence of ascites, omental metastases, or bowel metastases. The symptoms include abdominal distention, bloating, constipation, nausea, anorexia, or early satiety. Premenopausal women may complain of irregular or heavy menses, whereas vaginal bleeding may occur in postmenopausal women.

Signs	The most important sign is the presence of a pelvic mass on physical examination. A solid, irregular, fixed pelvic mass is highly suggestive of an ovarian malignancy. If, in addition, an upper abdominal mass or ascites is present, the diagnosis of ovarian cancer is almost certain. Because the patient usually complains of abdominal symptoms, she may not be subjected to a pelvic examination, and the presence of a tumor may be missed.

In patients who are at least 1 year past menopause, the ovaries should have become atrophic and not palpable. Thus any palpable pelvic mass in these patients should be considered suspicious. This situation has been referred to as the *postmenopausal palpable ovary syndrome* (33). This concept has been challenged, as subsequent authors have reported that only about 3% of palpable masses measuring < 5 cm are malignant in postmenopausal women (13).

Diagnosis	The diagnosis of an ovarian cancer requires an exploratory laparotomy. The preoperative evaluation of the patient with an adnexal mass is outlined in Figure 9.1.

In the premenopausal patient, a period of observation is reasonable, provided the adnexal mass is not clinically suspicious (i.e., it is mobile, mostly cystic, unilateral, and of regular contour). Generally, an interval of no more than 2 months is allowed, a period during which hormonal suppression with the oral contraceptive may be used. If the lesion is not neoplastic, it should regress, as measured by pelvic examination and pelvic ultrasonography. If the mass does not regress or if it increases in size, it must be presumed to be neoplastic and must be removed surgically.

The size of the lesion is of importance. If a cystic mass is > 8 cm in diameter, the probability is high that the lesion is neoplastic, unless the patient has been taking clomiphene citrate or other agents to induce ovulation (10–13). Patients

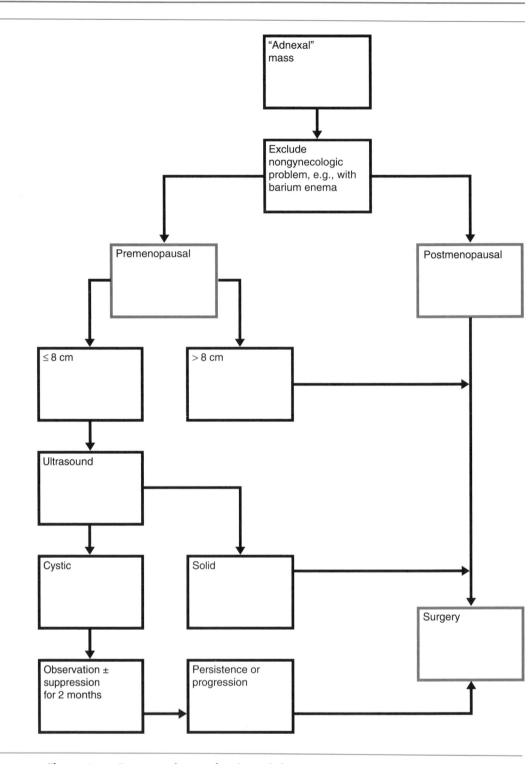

Figure 9.1 Preoperative evaluation of the patient with an adnexal mass.

whose lesions are clinically suspicious (i.e., predominantly solid, relatively fixed, or irregularly shaped) should undergo laparotomy, as should postmenopausal patients with adnexal masses.

Before the planned exploration, the patient should undergo routine hematologic and biochemical assessments. A preoperative evaluation in a patient undergoing laparotomy should include a radiograph of the chest and an assessment of the urinary tract with an intravenous pyelogram. An abdominal and pelvic computed tomography (CT) or magnetic resonance imaging (MRI) scan is of no value in patients with a definite pelvic mass. Patients with ascites and no pelvic mass should have a CT or MRI scan to look particularly for liver or pancreatic tumors. The findings only rarely preclude laparotomy (34). If the hepatic enzymes are normal, the likelihood of liver disease is low. Liver-spleen scans, bone scans, and brain scans are unnecessary unless symptoms or signs suggest metastases to these sites.

The preoperative evaluation should exclude other primary cancers metastatic to the ovary. A barium enema or colonoscopy is indicated in some patients over the age of 45 years to exclude a primary colonic lesion with ovarian metastasis. Any patient who has evidence of occult blood in the stool or evidence of intestinal obstruction should undergo this study. An upper gastrointestinal series or gastroscopy is indicated if there are symptoms indicating gastric involvement (34, 35). Bilateral mammography is indicated if there is any breast mass, because occasionally breast cancer metastatic to the ovaries can simulate primary ovarian cancer.

Cervical cytologic study should be performed, although its value for the detection of ovarian cancer is very limited. Patients who have irregular menses or postmenopausal vaginal bleeding should have an endometrial biopsy and an endocervical curettage to exclude the presence of uterine or endocervical cancer metastatic to the ovary.

Differential Diagnosis   Ovarian epithelial cancers must be differentiated from benign neoplasms and functional cysts of the ovaries. A variety of benign conditions of the reproductive tract, such as pelvic inflammatory disease, endometriosis, and pedunculated uterine leiomyomas, can simulate ovarian cancer. Nongynecologic causes of a pelvic tumor, such as an inflammatory or neoplastic colonic mass, must be excluded (34). A pelvic kidney can simulate ovarian cancer.

Serum CA 125 levels have been shown to be useful in distinguishing malignant from benign pelvic masses (36). In postmenopausal patients with an adnexal mass and a very high serum CA 125 level (> 95 μ/ml), there is a 96% positive predictive value for malignancy. In premenopausal patients, however, the specificity of the test is low because the CA 125 level tends to be elevated in common benign conditions.

Patterns of Spread

Ovarian epithelial cancers spread primarily by exfoliation of cells into the peritoneal cavity, by lymphatic dissemination, and by hematogenous spread.

Transcoelomic   The most common and earliest mode of dissemination is by exfoliation of cells that implant along the surfaces of the peritoneal cavity. The cells tend to follow the circulatory path of the peritoneal fluid. The fluid tends to move with the forces of respiration from the pelvis, up the paracolic gutters, especially on the right, along the intestinal mesenteries, to the right hemidiaphragm. Therefore, metastases are typically seen on the posterior cul-de-sac, paracolic gutters, right hemidiaphragm, liver capsule, the peritoneal surfaces of the intestines and their mesenteries, and the omentum. The disease seldom invades the intestinal lumen but progressively agglutinates loops of bowel, leading to a functional intestinal obstruction. This condition is known as *carcinomatous ileus*.

Lymphatic Lymphatic dissemination to the pelvic and para-aortic lymph nodes is common, particularly in advanced-stage disease (37–39). Spread through the lymphatic channels of the diaphragm and through the retroperitoneal lymph nodes can lead to dissemination above the diaphragm, especially to the supraclavicular lymph nodes (32). Burghardt et al. (38) reported that 78% of patients with Stage III disease have metastases to the pelvic lymph nodes. In another series (39), the rate of positive para-aortic lymph nodes was 18% in Stage I, 20% in Stage II, 42% in Stage III, and 67% in Stage IV.

Hematogenous Hematogenous dissemination at the time of diagnosis is uncommon, with spread to vital organ parenchyma, such as the lungs and liver, in only about 2–3% of patients. Most patients with disease above the diaphragm at the time of presentation have a right pleural effusion (3, 5). Systemic metastases are seen more frequently in patients who have survived for some years. Dauplat et al. (40) reported that distant metastasis consistent with Stage IV disease ultimately occurred in 38% of the patients whose disease was originally intraperitoneal. Malignant pleural effusion developed in one-fourth of the patients, with a subsequent median survival of 6 months. Other sites and their median survivals were as follows: parenchymal lung metastasis in 7.1%, median survival 9 months; subcutaneous nodules in 3.5%, 12 months; malignant pericardial effusion 2.4%, 2.3 months; central nervous system 2%, 1.3 months; and bone metastases in 1.6%, 4 months. Significant risk factors for distant metastases were malignant ascites, peritoneal carcinomatosis, large metastatic disease within the abdomen, and retroperitoneal lymph node involvement at the time of initial surgery.

Prognostic Factors

The outcome of patients after treatment can be evaluated in the context of prognostic factors, which can be grouped into pathologic, biologic, and clinical factors (41). The survivals of groups of patients based on prognostic factors is presented at the end of the chapter.

Pathologic Factors The morphology and histologic pattern, including the architecture and grade of the lesion, are important prognostic variables (3).

Histologic type has not generally been thought to be of prognostic significance, but recently several papers have suggested that clear cell carcinomas are associated with a worse prognosis than the other histologic types (41, 42).

Histologic grade, as determined either by the pattern of differentiation or by the extent of cellular anaplasia and the proportion of undifferentiated cells, seems to be of prognostic significance (43–46). However, studies of the reproducibility of grading ovarian cancers have shown a high degree of intraobserver and interobserver variation (47, 48). Because there is significant heterogeneity of tumors and observational bias, the value of histologic grade as an independent prognostic factor has not been clearly established. Baak et al. (49) have presented a standard grading system based on morphometric analysis, and the system appears to correlate with prognosis, especially in its ability to distinguish low-grade or borderline patterns from other tumors.

Biologic Factors Several biologic factors have been correlated with prognosis in epithelial ovarian cancer. Using *flow cytometry*, Friedlander et al. (50) showed that ovarian cancers were commonly aneuploid. Furthermore, they and others showed that there was a high correlation between FIGO stage and ploidy; i.e., low-stage cancers tend to be diploid and high-stage tumors tend to be aneuploid (51–57). Patients with diploid tumors have a significantly longer median survival than those with aneuploid tumors: 5 years versus 1 year, respectively (51). Multivariate analyses have demonstrated that ploidy is an independent prognostic variable and one of the most significant predictors of survival (51). *Flow cytometric analysis* also provides data on the cell cycle, and the proliferation fraction (S phase) determined by this technique has correlated with prognosis in some studies (58–61).

More than 60 *proto-oncogenes* have been identified, and studies have focused on the amplification or expression of these genetic loci and their relationship to the development and progression of ovarian cancer. For example, Slamon et al. (62) reported that 30% of epithelial ovarian tumors expressed HER-2/*neu* oncogene and that this group had a poorer prognosis, especially those patients with > 5 copies of the gene (62). Berchuck et al. (63) reported a similar incidence (32%) of HER-2/*neu* expression. In their series, patients whose tumors expressed the gene had a poorer median survival (15.7 months versus 32.8 months). Others have not substantiated this finding (64), and a review of the literature by Leary et al. (65) revealed an overall incidence of HER-2/*neu* expression of only 11%. Thus the prognostic value of HER-2/*neu* expression in ovarian cancer is unclear, and further study is required.

The *in vitro clonogenic assay* has been studied in ovarian cancer. A significant inverse correlation has been reported between clonogenic growth *in vitro* and survival (66, 67). Multivariate analysis has found that clonogenic growth in a semisolid culture medium is a significant independent variable (66). Further study will be needed to evaluate the clinical usefulness of this assay.

Clinical Factors   In addition to stage, the extent of residual disease after primary surgery, the volume of ascites, patient age, and performance status are all independent prognostic variables (68–71). Among patients with Stage I disease, Dembo et al. (72) showed, in a multivariate analysis, that tumor grade and "dense adherence" to the pelvic peritoneum had a significant adverse impact on prognosis, whereas intraoperative tumor spillage or rupture did not.

Staging

Ovarian epithelial malignancies are staged according to the International Federation of Gynecology and Obstetrics (FIGO) system, and the staging system of 1987 is listed in Table 9.1. The FIGO staging is based on findings at surgical exploration. A preoperative evaluation should exclude the presence of extraperitoneal metastases.

The importance of thorough surgical staging cannot be overemphasized, because subsequent treatment will be determined by the stage of disease. In patients in whom exploratory laparotomy does not reveal any macroscopic evidence of disease on inspection and palpation of the entire intra-abdominal space, a careful search for microscopic spread must be undertaken.

In earlier series in which patients did not undergo careful surgical staging, the overall 5-year survival for patients with apparent Stage I epithelial ovarian cancer was only about 60% (8). Since then, survival rates of 90–100% have been reported for patients who were properly staged and found to have Stage Ia or Ib disease (73, 74).

Table 9.1   FIGO Staging for Primary Carcinoma of the Ovary

Stage I		Growth limited to the ovaries.
	Stage Ia	Growth limited to one ovary; no ascites containing malignant cells. No tumor on the external surface; capsule intact.
	Stage Ib	Growth limited to both ovaries; no ascites containing malignant cells. No tumor on the external surfaces; capsules intact.
	Stage Ic*	Tumor either Stage Ia or Ib but with tumor on the surface of one or both ovaries; or with capsule ruptured; or with ascites present containing malignant cells or with positive peritoneal washings.
Stage II		Growth involving one or both ovaries with pelvic extension.
	Stage IIa	Extension and/or metastases to the uterus and/or tubes.
	Stage IIb	Extension to other pelvic tissues.
	Stage IIc*	Tumor either Stage IIa or IIb but with tumor on the surface of one or both ovaries; or with capsule(s) ruptured; or with ascites present containing malignant cells or with positive peritoneal washings.
Stage III		Tumor involving one or both ovaries with peritoneal implants outside the pelvis and/or positive retroperitoneal or inguinal nodes. Superficial liver metastasis equals Stage III. Tumor is limited to the true pelvis, but with histologically proven malignant extension to small bowel or omentum.
	Stage IIIa	Tumor grossly limited to the true pelvis with negative nodes but with histologically confirmed microscopic seeding of abdominal peritoneal surfaces.
	Stage IIIb	Tumor of one or both ovaries with histologically confirmed implants of abdominal peritoneal surfaces, none exceeding 2 cm in diameter. Nodes negative.
	Stage IIIc	Abdominal implants > 2 cm in diameter and/or positive retroperitoneal or inguinal nodes.
Stage IV		Growth involving one or both ovaries with distant metastasis. If pleural effusion is present, there must be positive cytologic test results to allot a case to Stage IV. Parenchymal liver metastasis equals Stage IV.

These categories are based on findings at clinical examination and/or surgical exploration. The histologic characteristics are to be considered in the staging, as are results of cytologic testing as far as effusions are concerned. It is desirable that a biopsy be performed on suspicious areas outside the pelvis.
*In order to evaluate the impact on prognosis of the different criteria for allotting cases to stage Ic or IIc, it would be of value to know if rupture of the capsule was (1) spontaneous or (2) caused by the surgeon and if the source of malignant cells detected was (1) peritoneal washings or (2) ascites.

Technique for Surgical Staging

In patients whose preoperative evaluation suggests a probable malignancy, a midline or paramedian abdominal incision is recommended to allow adequate access to the upper abdomen. When a malignancy is unexpectedly discovered in a patient who has a lower transverse incision, the rectus muscles can be either divided or detached from the symphysis pubis to allow better access to the upper abdomen (see Chapter 15). If this is not sufficient, the incision can be extended on one side to create a "J" incision.

The ovarian tumor should be removed intact, if possible, and a frozen histologic section obtained. If ovarian malignancy is present and the tumor is apparently confined to the ovaries or the pelvis, thorough surgical staging should be carried out. This involves the following steps:

1. *Any free fluid, especially in the pelvic cul-de-sac, should be submitted for cytologic evaluation.*

336

2. *If no free fluid is present, peritoneal "washings" should be performed* by instilling and recovering 50–100 ml of saline from the pelvic cul-de-sac, each paracolic gutter, and from beneath each hemidiaphragm. Obtaining the specimens from under the diaphragms can be facilitated with the use of a red rubber catheter attached to the end of a bulb syringe.

3. *A systematic exploration of all the intra-abdominal surfaces and viscera is performed,* proceeding in a clockwise fashion from the cecum cephalad along the paracolic gutter and the ascending colon to the right kidney, the liver and gallbladder, the right hemidiaphragm, the entrance to the lesser sac at the para-aortic area, across the transverse colon to the left hemidiaphragm, down the left gutter and the descending colon to the rectosigmoid colon. The small intestine and its mesentery from the ligament of Trietz to the cecum should be inspected.

4. *Any suspicious areas or adhesions on the peritoneal surfaces should be biopsied. If there is no evidence of disease, multiple intraperitoneal biopsies should be performed.* The peritoneum of the pelvic cul-de-sac, both paracolic gutters, the peritoneum over the bladder, and the intestinal mesenteries should be biopsied.

5. *The diaphragm should be sampled either by biopsy or by scraping with a tongue depressor and making a cytologic smear.* Biopsies of any irregularities on the surface of the diaphragm can be facilitated by use of the laparoscope and the associated biopsy instrument.

6. *The omentum should be resected from the transverse colon, a procedure called an infracolic omentectomy.* The procedure is initiated on the underside of the greater omentum, where the peritoneum is incised just a few millimeters away from the transverse colon. The branches of the gastroepiploic vessels are clamped, ligated, and divided, along with all the small branching vessels that feed the infracolic omentum. If the gastrocolic ligament is palpably normal, it does not need to be resected.

7. *The retroperitoneal spaces should be explored to evaluate the pelvic and para-aortic lymph nodes.* The retroperitoneal dissection is performed by incision of the peritoneum over the psoas muscles. This may be done on the ipsilateral side only for unilateral tumors. Any enlarged lymph nodes should be resected and submitted for frozen section. If no metastases are present, a formal pelvic lymphadenectomy should be performed.

Results

Metastases in apparent Stage I and II epithelial ovarian cancer are summarized in Table 9.2. As many as three in 10 patients whose tumor appears confined to the pelvis have occult metastatic disease in the upper abdomen or the retroperitoneal lymph nodes (39, 74–83).

The importance of careful initial surgical staging is emphasized by the findings of a cooperative national study (74) in which 100 patients with apparent Stage I and II disease who were referred for subsequent therapy underwent additional surgical staging. In this series, 28% of the patients initially thought to have Stage

337

Table 9.2   Site of Metastases in Patients with Apparent Stage I and II Ovarian Cancer

Ref.	Diaphragm		Aortic Lymph Nodes		Pelvic Nodes		Omentum		Positive Cytology	
18			4/21	(19.1%)	2/21	(9.6%)				
21	2/58	(3.4%)	6/52	(11.5%)	1/11	(9.1%)	6/57	(10.5%)		
22	3/72	(4.2%)					7/79	(8.9%)		
23									7/36	(19.4%)
24	1/31	(3.2%)	0/5	(0%)			0/5	(0%)	8/31	(25.8%)
25			2/10	(20.0%)	0/10	(0%)				
26	7/16	(43.7%)								
27			5/26	(19.2%)	0/9	(0%)	1/21	(4.7%)		
28									16/44	(36.0%)
29									1/10	(10.0%)
Total	**13/177**	**(7.3%)**	**17/114 (18.1%)**		**3/51 (5.9%)**		**14/162**	**(8.6%)**	**32/121 (26.4%)**	

Modified, with permission, from Berek JS, Hacker NF: Staging and second-look operations in ovarian cancer. In Piver MS (ed): *Ovarian Malignancies*. Edinburgh, Churchill Livingstone, 1987, p 112.

I disease were "upstaged" and 43% of those thought to have Stage II disease had more advanced lesions. A total of 31% of the patients were upstaged as a result of additional surgery, and 77% were reclassified as having Stage III disease. Histologic grade was a significant predictor of occult metastasis; i.e., 16% of the patients with grade 1 lesions were upstaged, compared with 34% with grade 2 disease and 46% with grade 3 disease.

Treatment

Stage I

The primary treatment for Stage I epithelial ovarian cancer is surgical, i.e., a total abdominal hysterectomy, bilateral salpingo-oophorectomy, and surgical staging (73, 74). In certain circumstances, a unilateral oophorectomy may be permitted, as discussed below.

Borderline Tumors

The principal treatment of borderline ovarian tumors is surgical resection of the primary tumor. There is no evidence that either subsequent chemotherapy or radiation therapy improves survival. After a frozen section has determined that the histology is borderline, premenopausal patients who desire preservation of ovarian function may be managed with a "conservative" operation, i.e., a unilateral oophorectomy (84). In a study of patients who underwent unilateral ovarian cystectomy only for apparent Stage I borderline serous tumors, Lim-Tan et al. (85) found that this conservative operation was also safe; only 8% of the patients had recurrences 2–18 years later, all with curable disease confined to the ovaries. Recurrence was associated with "positive margins" of the removed ovarian cyst (85). Thus, hormonal function and fertility can be maintained (5, 84, 85). In patients in whom an oophorectomy or cystectomy has been performed and a borderline tumor is later documented in the permanent pathology, no additional immediate surgery is necessary.

Stages Ia and Ib, Grade 1

In patients who have undergone a thorough staging laparotomy and in whom there is no evidence of spread beyond the ovary, an abdominal hysterectomy and bilateral salpingo-oophorectomy is appropriate therapy. **The uterus and the contralateral ovary can be preserved in women with Stage Ia, grade 1 disease who desire to preserve fertility.** These women should be followed carefully with routine periodic pelvic examinations and determinations of serum CA 125 level. Generally, the other ovary and the uterus are removed at the completion of childbearing.

Guthrie et al. (83) studied the outcome of 656 patients with early-stage epithelial ovarian cancer. No untreated patients who had Stage Ia, grade 1 cancer died of their disease; thus adjuvant radiation and chemotherapy are unnecessary. Furthermore, the Gynecologic Oncology Group (GOG) carried out a prospective, randomized trial of observation versus melphalan for patients with Stage Ia and Ib, grade 1 disease. Five-year survival for each group was 94% and 96%, respectively, confirming that no further treatment is needed for such patients.

Stages Ia and Ib (Grades 2 and 3) and Stage Ic

In patients whose disease is more poorly differentiated or in whom there are malignant cells either in ascitic fluid or in peritoneal washings, additional therapy is indicated. Although the optimal therapy in these patients is not known, treatment options include chemotherapy or radiation therapy, the latter with intraperitoneal radiocolloids or whole-abdominal radiation. Some comparisons of these modalities have been made, although most are retrospective and therefore inconclusive.

Chemotherapy

Chemotherapy for patients with Stages Ia and Ib, grade 2 or 3, and Stage Ic epithelial ovarian cancer can be either single agent or multiagent. The most frequently used single-agent chemotherapy has been melphalan given orally on a "pulse" basis for 5 consecutive days every 28 days. In the past, this treatment has been given for up to 24 months. The advantage of this approach is the relative ease of administration. The principal disadvantage is that about 10% of the patients who receive more than 12 cycles of alkylating agent therapy will develop an acute nonlymphocytic leukemia over the next 5–10 years (87). This is an important issue in patients with Stage I disease, and melphalan should not be given for more than six cycles in such patients.

Because cisplatin, carboplatin, and Taxol are active single agents against epithelial ovarian cancer, they may be preferable to melphalan in patients with low-stage disease. There are some series in which cisplatin and cyclophosphamide, with or without Adriamycin (PC or PAC), have been used to treat patients with Stage I disease (42, 83–88), but there are no data comparing the use of cisplatin combination chemotherapy with either single-agent chemotherapy or radiation therapy (88). There is an ongoing GOG trial of PC versus intraperitoneal ^{32}P in patients with Stage Ib and Ic disease. There are no data yet available on the use of Taxol in low-stage ovarian cancer. A summary of randomized phase III trials for the treatment of patients with low-stage disease is presented in Table 9.3 (42, 86, 89, 90).

Radiation Therapy

There are two general approaches to the treatment of these low-stage epithelial cancers with radiation: intraperitoneal radiocolloids or whole-abdominal radiation

339

Table 9.3   Randomized Trials in Stage I Epithelial Ovarian Cancer

Author	Number Entered/ Analyzed	Stages	Treatment	Outcome	P-Value
Dembo (89)	63/54	Ia	Observation vs. Pelvic XRT	4/27* 5/27	NS
Hreshchyshyn (86)	168/86	All Stage I	Pelvic XRT vs. Observation vs. Melphalan	7/23* 5/29 2/34	NS NS
Young (42)	92/81	Stage I, grades 1 and 2: no ascites, rupture, or penetration	Observation vs. Melphalan	88%† 93%	NS
Young (42)	143/141	All other Stage I, optimal Stage II	Melphalan vs. IP ^{32}P	65%‡ 69%	NS
Bolis (90)	57/47	Stage I, grades 1 and 2: ascites, rupture, or penetration	Observation vs. Cisplatin × 6	70%§ 71%	NS
Bolis (90)	124/104	All other Stage I	IP ^{32}P vs. Cisplatin × 6	69%§ 79%	NS

Reproduced, with permission, from Dembo AJ: Epithelial ovarian cancer: the role of radiotherapy. *Int J Rad Oncol Biol Phys* 22:835, 1992.
*Relapses; †10-year relapse-free survival; ‡10-year survival; §4-year relapse-free survival.

therapy. In one retrospective trial of ^{32}P, the 5-year survival for patients thus treated was 85% (91). In a series of patients with Stage I disease treated with whole abdominal radiation (92), the 5-year relapse-free survival was only 78%, but many of these patients had high-risk variables (e.g., poor histologic grade).

A prospective trial was conducted by the GOG in patients with Stage Ib, grade 3, Stage Ic, or Stage II with no residual disease. Twelve cycles of melphalan were compared with intraperitoneal ^{32}P; there was no difference in survival (Figure 9.2) (42). In a multicenter Italian trial (90), a randomized comparison of six cycles of cisplatin as a single agent versus ^{32}P showed an 84% disease-free survival with cisplatin and 61% with ^{32}P ($p < 0.1$). Therefore it appears that the use of ^{32}P produces results similar to single-agent melphalan chemotherapy, although cisplatin as a single agent may be preferable (Table 9.3). If further relapses are to be prevented, the use of combination chemotherapy may be indicated, but the data are as yet unavailable. Pelvic radiation alone is not as effective as melphalan in these patients and should not be used in ovarian cancer (86).

Current recommendations for treatment of patients with Stage Ia and Ib (high-grade) and Stage Ic epithelial ovarian cancer depend on the patient's overall health and status. Treatment with cisplatin or PC combination chemotherapy for 3–4 cycles seems desirable in young patients, whereas a short course of melphalan (4–6 cycles) may be preferable for older women. Intraperitoneal ^{32}P is an acceptable alternative, provided there are no significant adhesions. The role of Taxol in these patients warrants investigation.

Stages II, III, and IV

The treatment of all patients with advanced-stage disease is approached in a similar manner, with modifications made for the overall status and general health of the patient, as well as the extent of residual disease present at the time treatment is initiated. A treatment scheme is outlined in Figure 9.3

The patient should undergo an initial exploratory procedure with removal of as much disease as possible. The operation to remove the primary tumor as well as the associated metastatic disease is referred to as "debulking," or *cytoreductive* surgery. Most patients subsequently receive combination chemotherapy for an empiric number of cycles. In some patients with completely resected disease, whole-abdominal radiation therapy may be used. In patients with no clinical evidence of disease and negative tumor markers at the completion of chemotherapy, a reassessment laparotomy, or *"second-look,"* may be performed. In patients with persistent disease at second-look laparotomy, second-line or "salvage" therapy may be recommended. There are many possible salvage therapies available, but all are of limited effectiveness.

Cytoreductive Surgery   Patients with advanced-stage epithelial ovarian cancer documented at initial exploratory laparotomy should undergo cytoreductive surgery to remove as much of the tumor and its metastases as possible (93–100). The operation typically includes the performance of a total abdominal hysterectomy and bilateral salpingo-

Figure 9.2   Overall survival of patients with Stage I or II epithelial ovarian cancer treated on two GOG trials. (Reproduced, with permission, from Young RC, Walton LA, Ellenberg SS, et al: Adjuvant therapy in stage I and stage II epithelial ovarian cancer: results of two prospective randomized trials. *N Engl J Med* 322:1021, 1990.)

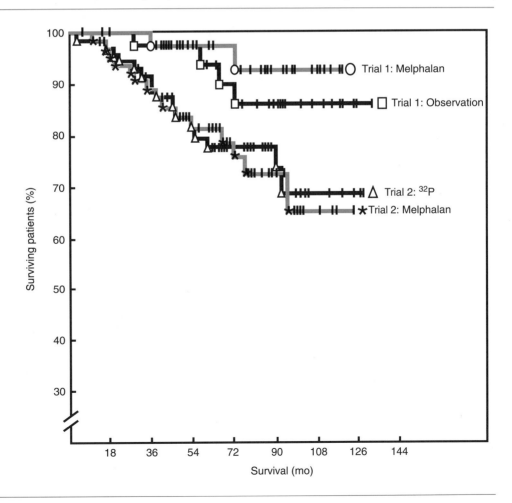

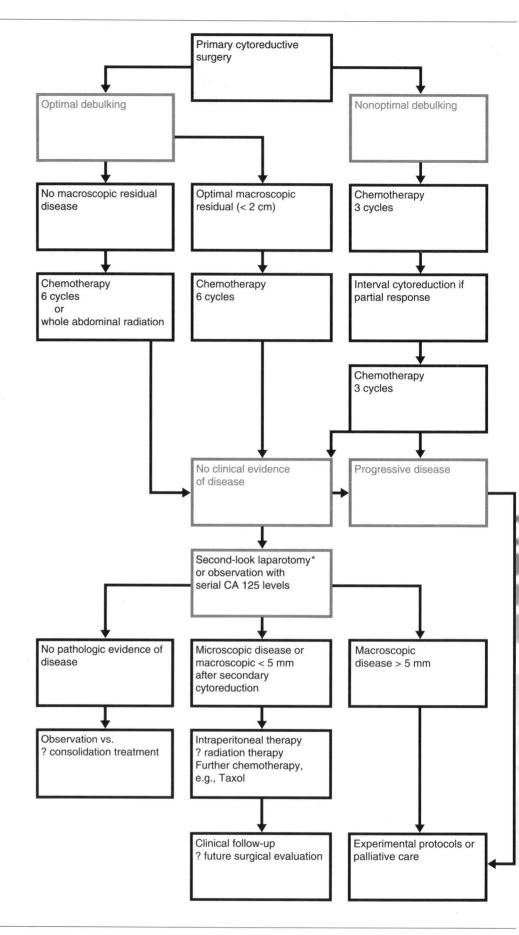

Figure 9.3 Treatment scheme for patients with advanced-stage ovarian cancer.

oophorectomy, along with a complete omentectomy and resection of any metastatic lesions from the peritoneal surfaces or from the intestines. The pelvic tumor often directly involves the rectosigmoid colon, the terminal ileum, and the cecum (Figure 9.4). In a minority of patients, most or all of the disease is confined to the pelvic viscera and the omentum, so that removal of these organs will result in extirpation of all gross tumor, a situation that is associated with a reasonable chance of prolonged progression-free survival.

Theoretic Rationale

The rationale for cytoreductive surgery relates to three general theoretic considerations (93, 94, 100–101):

1. The physiologic benefits of tumor mass excision.

2. The improved tumor perfusion and increased growth fraction, both of which increase the likelihood of response to chemotherapy or radiation therapy.

3. The enhanced immunologic competence of the patient.

Physiologic Benefits   The removal of bulky tumor masses may reduce the volume of ascites present. Often, ascites will completely disappear after removal of

Figure 9.4   Extensive ovarian carcinoma involving the bladder, rectosigmoid, and ileocecal area. (Reproduced, with permission, from Heintz APM, Berek JS: Cytoreductive surgery for ovarian carcinoma. In Piver MS (ed): *Ovarian Malignancies*. Edinburgh, Churchill Livingstone, 1987, p 134.)

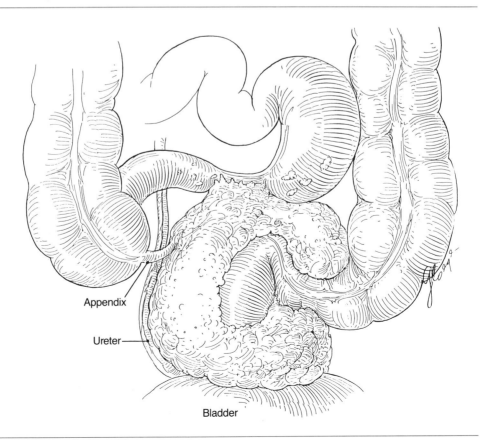

Appendix

Ureter

Bladder

the primary tumor and a large omental "cake." Also, removal of the omental cake often alleviates the nausea and early satiety that many patients experience. Removal of intestinal metastases may restore adequate intestinal function and lead to an improvement in the overall nutritional status of the patient, thereby facilitating the patient's ability to tolerate subsequent chemotherapy.

Tumor Perfusion and Cell Kinetics A large, bulky tumor may contain areas that are poorly vascularized, and such areas will be exposed to suboptimal concentrations of chemotherapeutic agents. Similarly, these areas are poorly oxygenated, so radiation therapy, which requires adequate oxygenation to achieve maximal cell kill, will be less effective. Thus surgical removal of these bulky tumors may eliminate areas that are most likely to be relatively resistant to treatment.

In addition, larger tumor masses tend to be composed of a higher proportion of cells that are either nondividing or in the "resting" phase (i.e., G_o cells, which are essentially resistant to the therapy). A low *growth fraction* is characteristic of bulky tumor masses, and cytoreductive surgery can result in smaller residual masses with a relatively higher growth fraction.

The *fractional cell kill hypothesis* of Skipper (100) postulates that a constant proportion of the tumor cells are destroyed with each treatment. This theory suggests that a given dose of a drug will kill a constant fraction of cells as long as the growth fraction and phenotype are the same. Therefore a treatment that reduces a population of tumor cells from 10^9 to 10^4 cells also would reduce a population of 10^5 cells to a single cell. If the absolute number of tumor cells is lower at the initiation of treatment, fewer cycles of therapy should be necessary to eradicate the cancer, provided that the cells are not inherently resistant to the therapy.

The larger the initial tumor burden, the longer the necessary exposure to the drug and, therefore, the greater the chance of developing *acquired* drug resistance. However, because the spontaneous mutation rate of tumors is an inherent property of the malignancy, the likelihood of developing *phenotypic* drug resistance also increases as the size of the tumor increases. The chance of developing a clone of cells resistant to a specific agent is related to both the tumor size and its mutation frequency (101). This is one of the inherent problems with cytoreductive surgery for large tumor masses: phenotypic drug resistance may have already developed before any surgical intervention.

Immunologic Factors Larger tumor masses appear to be more immunosuppressive than smaller tumors. In addition to the nonspecific immunocompromise that occurs with large tumors, bulky tumors may be much less amenable to control by the host defense mechanisms. The normal mechanisms of recognition of abnormal antigens may be overwhelmed and abrogated by the relatively large number of cancer cells. Excess tumor antigen can block the function of cytotoxic lymphocytes. Indeed, large tumors may result in the inherent production of immunologically suppressive substances, as well as the induction of suppressor lymphocyte activity (102).

Some have questioned the ability of cytoreductive surgery to improve the overall outcome of patients with ovarian cancer (103). Concern has been expressed that these operations are excessively morbid and that modern chemotherapies are sufficient. While no randomized prospective study has ever been performed to define the value of primary cytoreductive surgery, a recent prospective trial of "interval" cytoreductive surgery (performed after three cycles of platinum-combination chemotherapy) demonstrated a survival benefit for those patients who had an optimal resection of their disease at that time compared with those who did not (104). All retrospective studies indicate that the diameter of the largest residual tumor nodule before the initiation of chemotherapy is significantly related to progression-free survival in patients with advanced ovarian cancer. In addition, quality of life is likely to be significantly enhanced by removal of bulky tumor masses from the pelvis and upper abdomen.

Goals of Cytoreductive Surgery

The principal goal of cytoreductive surgery is removal of all of the primary cancer and, if possible, all metastatic disease. If resection of all metastases is not feasible, the goal is to reduce the tumor burden by resection of all individual tumors to an "optimal" status. Griffiths (93) initially proposed that all metastatic nodules should be reduced to ≤ 1.5cm in maximum diameter and showed that survival was significantly longer in such patients.

Subsequently, Hacker and Berek (94) showed that patients whose largest residual lesions were $\leq$ 5mm had a superior survival, and this was substantiated by Van Lindert et al. (95). The median survival of patients in this category was 40 months, compared with 18 months for patients whose lesions were < 1.5 cm and 6 months for patients with nodules > 1.5 cm (Fig. 9.5).

The resectability of the metastatic tumor is usually determined by the location of the disease. Optimal cytoreduction is difficult to achieve in the presence of extensive disease on the diaphragm, in the parenchyma of the liver, along the base of the small-bowel mesentery, in the lesser omentum, or in the porta hepatis.

The ability of cytoreductive surgery to influence survival is limited by the extent of metastases prior to cytoreduction, presumably because of the presence of phenotypically resistant clones of cells in large metastatic masses. Patients whose metastatic tumor is very large (i.e., > 10 cm before cytoreductive surgery) have a shorter survival than those with smaller areas of disease (96) (Fig. 9.6). Extensive carcinomatosis, the presence of ascites, and poor tumor grade, even with lesions that measure < 5 mm, may also worsen the survival (99, 101).

Exploration

The supine position on the operating table may be sufficient for most patients. However, for those with extensive pelvic disease for whom a low resection of the colon may be necessary, the low lithotomy position should be used. Debulking operations should be performed through a vertical incision in order to gain adequate access to the upper abdomen as well as to the pelvis.

After the peritoneal cavity is opened, ascitic fluid, if present, should be evacuated. In some centers, fluid is submitted routinely for appropriate *in vitro* studies, particularly the clonogenic assay. In cases of massive ascites, careful attention must be given to hemodynamic monitoring, especially in patients with borderline cardiovascular function. In such patients, monitoring of the central venous pressure alone may be inadequate, and a Swan-Ganz catheter may be used, as discussed in Chapter 16.

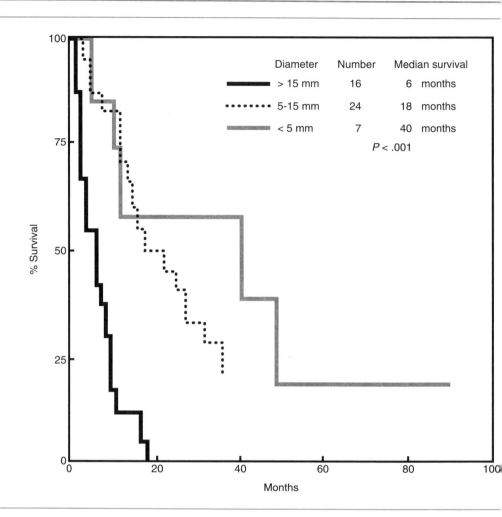

Figure 9.5 Survival versus diameter of largest residual disease. (Reprinted, with permission, from the American College of Obstetrics and Gynecology. Hacker NF, Berek JS, Lagasse LD, et al: *Obstet Gynecol* 61:413, 1983.)

A thorough inspection and palpation of the peritoneal cavity and retroperitoneum are carried out to assess the extent of the primary tumor and the metastatic disease. All abdominal viscera must be palpated to exclude the possibility that the ovarian disease is metastatic, particularly from the stomach, colon, or pancreas. If optimal status is *not* considered achievable, extensive bowel and urologic resections are not indicated except to overcome a bowel obstruction. However, removal of the primary tumor and omental cake is usually both feasible and desirable.

Pelvic Tumor Resection

The essential principle of removal of the pelvic tumor is to use the retroperitoneal approach (105). To accomplish this, the retroperitoneum is entered laterally, along the surface of the psoas muscles, which avoids the iliac vessels and the ureters. The procedure is initiated by division of the round ligaments bilaterally if the uterus is present. The peritoneal incision is extended cephalad, lateral to the ovarian vessels within the "infundibulopelvic ligament," and caudally toward the bladder. With careful dissection, the retroperitoneal space is explored, and the ureter and pelvic vessels are identified. The pararectal and paravesicle spaces are identified and developed as described in Chapter 7.

The peritoneum overlying the bladder is dissected to connect the peritoneal incisions anteriorly. The vesicouterine plane is identified, and, with careful sharp dissection, the bladder is mobilized from the anterior surface of the cervix. The ovarian vessels are isolated, doubly ligated, and divided.

The hysterectomy, which is often not a "simple" operation, is performed. The ureters need to be carefully displayed in order to avoid injury. During this procedure, the uterine vessels can be identified. The hysterectomy and resection of the contiguous tumor are completed by ligation of the uterine vessels and the remainder of the tissues within the cardinal ligaments.

Because epithelial ovarian cancers tend not to invade the lumina of the colon or bladder, it is usually feasible to resect pelvic tumors without having to resect portions of the lower colon or the urinary tract (106, 107). However, if the disease surrounds the rectosigmoid colon and its mesentery, it may be necessary to remove that portion of the colon to clear the pelvic disease (Fig. 9.7) (106). This is justified if the patient will be left with "optimal" disease at the end of the cytoreduction. After the pararectal space is identified in such patients, the proximal site of colonic involvement is identified, the colon and its mesentery are divided,

Figure 9.6 Survival versus diameter of largest metastatic disease before cytoreduction. (Reprinted, with permission, from the American College of Obstetrics and Gynecology. Hacker NF, Berek JS, Lagasse LD, et al.: *Obstet Gynecol* 61:413, 1983.)

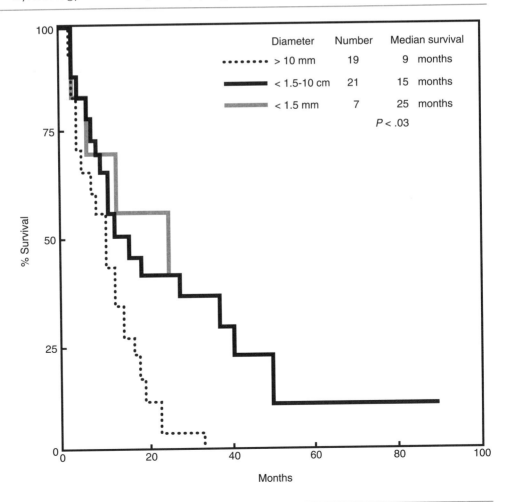

Diameter	Number	Median survival
> 10 mm	19	9 months
< 1.5–10 cm	21	15 months
< 1.5 mm	7	25 months

$P < .03$

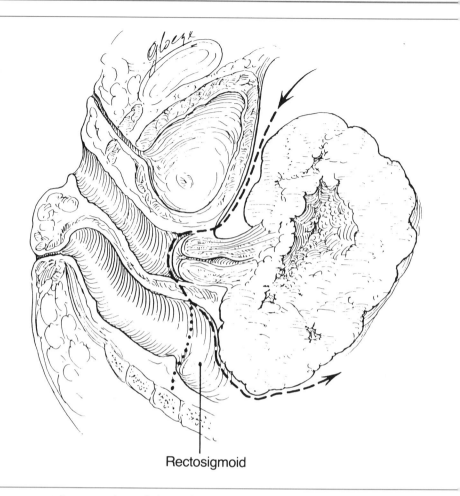

Rectosigmoid

Figure 9.7 **The resection of the pelvic tumor** may include removal of the uterus, tubes, and ovaries, as well as portions of the lower intestinal tract. The arrows represent the plane of resection.

and the rectosigmoid is removed along with the uterus *en bloc*. A reanastomosis of the colon is performed, as described in Chapter 15.

It is rarely necessary to resect portions of the lower urinary tract (107). Occasionally, resection of a small portion of the bladder may be required. If so, a cystotomy should be performed to assist in resection of the disease. Rarely, partial ureteric resection may be necessary, followed by primary reanastomosis (ureteroureterostomy), ureteroneocystostomy, or transureteroureterostomy, as described in Chapter 15.

Omentectomy

Advanced epithelial ovarian cancer often completely replaces the omentum, forming an "omental cake." This disease may be adherent to the parietal peritoneum of the anterior abdominal wall, making entry into the abdominal cavity difficult. After freeing the omentum from any adhesions to parietal peritoneum, adherent loops of small intestine are freed by sharp dissection. The omentum is then lifted and pulled gently in the cranial direction, exposing the attachment of the infracolic omentum to the transverse colon. The peritoneum is incised to open the appropriate plane, which is developed by sharp dissection along the serosa of the transverse colon. Small vessels are ligated with hemoclips. The omentum is then separated from the greater curvature of the stomach by ligation of the right and left gastroepiploic arteries and ligation of the short gastric arteries (Fig. 9.8).

The disease in the gastrocolic ligament can extend to the hilus of the spleen and splenic flexure of the colon on the left and to the capsule of the liver and the hepatic flexure of the colon on the right. Usually, the disease does not invade the parenchyma of the liver or spleen, and a plane can be found between the tumor and these organs. However, it will occasionally be necessary to perform splenectomy to remove all the omental disease (108).

Intestinal Resection

The disease may involve focal areas of the small or large intestine, and resection should be performed if it would permit the removal of all or most of the abdominal metastases. Apart from the rectosigmoid colon, the most frequent sites of intestinal metastasis are the terminal ileum, the cecum, and the transverse colon. Resection of one or more of these segments of bowel may be necessary (106, 108).

Resection of Other Metastases

Other large masses of tumor that are located on the parietal peritoneum should be removed, particularly if they are isolated masses, and their removal will permit

Figure 9.8   Separation of the omentum from stomach and transverse colon. (Reproduced, with permission, from Heintz APM, Berek JS: Cytoreductive surgery for ovarian carcinoma. In Piver MS (ed): *Ovarian Malignancies*. Edinburgh, Churchill Livingstone, 1987, p 134.)

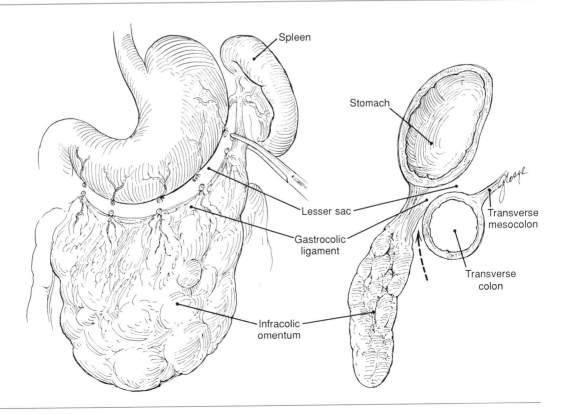

optimal cytoreduction. Resection of extensive disease from the surfaces of the diaphragm is generally neither practical nor feasible, although solitary metastases may be resected, the diaphragm sutured, and a chest tube placed for a few days (109, 110). The use of the CUSA (Cavitron Ultrasonic Surgical Aspirator) and the argon beam laser may help facilitate resection of small tumor nodules, especially those on flat surfaces (111, 112).

Feasibility and Outcome

An analysis of the retrospective data available suggests that these operations are feasible in 70–90% of patients when performed by gynecologic oncologists (108, 113). Major morbidity is in the range of 5% and operative mortality in the range of 1% (108, 114). Intestinal resection in these patients does not appear to increase the overall morbidity of the operation (106, 108). The performance of a pelvic lymphadenectomy in patients with Stage III disease has been reported to prolong survival (38), although verification of this awaits a prospective, randomized study.

Chemotherapy

Systemic chemotherapy is the standard treatment for metastatic epithelial ovarian cancer. For many years, oral single-agent alkylating therapy was used (115), but the introduction of cisplatin in the latter half of the 1970s changed the therapeutic approach for most patients, and cisplatin-based combination chemotherapy has been the most frequently used treatment regimen in the United States for the past decade. Recently, Taxol has become available, and comparative trials of Taxol, cisplatin, and their combination are now ongoing.

Single-Agent Therapy

The standard dose for the single alkylating agent, melphalan, is 0.2 mg/kg/day given for 5 consecutive days every 28 days. In three separate GOG studies of suboptimal Stage III ovarian cancer, 193 patients were treated with this regimen. Sixty-two patients (33%) had a clinical response, with a 16% complete response rate and a 17% partial response rate (116). However, the median duration of response was only 7 months and median survival was 12 months. The results of these prospective studies are comparable to many retrospective studies in the literature.

Other active drugs that have been used as single agents include cisplatin, carboplatin, Taxol, ifosfamide, Adriamycin, hexamethylmelamine, and 5-FU (88, 116–124). Cisplatin, carboplatin and Taxol appear to be more active than alkylating agents, whereas the others are somewhat less active. Cisplatin and/or carboplatin produce sufficiently high response rates to justify their routine use in primary therapy, and the role of Taxol is yet to be determined. The individual activities and their complementary toxicities serve as the rationale for their incorporation into combination regimens.

The use of single-agent chemotherapy for metastatic epithelial ovarian cancer is generally reserved for patients whose overall physical condition precludes the use of more toxic therapy. In elderly or debilitated patients, or in those who refuse intravenous chemotherapy, the use of an oral agent is simple and appealing.

Single-agent drugs, orally administered, are sometimes used for second-line chemotherapy because of their relative ease of administration and low toxicity. Sec-

350

ond-line responses to Taxol (120), hexamethylmelamine (122), carboplatin (123), and cisplatin (124) in those patients who have responded previously to cisplatin have been observed in 10–36% of patients.

Combination Chemotherapy

A variety of combination chemotherapeutic regimens have been tested in the treatment of advanced epithelial ovarian cancer. A summary of the most common regimens is presented in Table 9.4.

Single-Agent Versus Combination Chemotherapy   Combination chemotherapy has been shown to be superior to single-agent therapy in most patients with advanced epithelial ovarian cancer (125). The era of this testing began in the latter half of the 1970s when combinations of agents found to have activity against epithelial tumors were compared with single-agent therapy. The first study to show any benefit for combination therapy compared a regimen called Hexa-CAF (hexamethylmelamine, Cytoxan, methotrexate, 5-FU) with melphalan (126). This randomized prospective study showed that the response rate and the median survival with the combination regimen were better than with the single drug. The Hexa-CAF regimen produced a complete response rate of 33% with a median survival of 29 months, compared with 16% and 17 months, respectively, for melphalan.

Cisplatin-Based Combination Chemotherapy   Very soon after these data were published, cisplatin became available for the treatment of ovarian cancer, and it was soon recognized as a very active single agent against the disease. In a prospective study in England, it was shown that cisplatin was better than an alkylator, cyclophosphamide (Cytoxan) as a single agent (127). Concurrently, cisplatin was tested in a variety of different combinations. One such regimen, CHAP (Cytoxan, hexamethylmelamine, Adriamycin, cisplatin), was shown to be active and generally tolerable (128). A prospective randomized study (129) com-

Table 9.4   Chemotherapeutic Regimens for Advanced Ovarian Cancer

	Regimen	*Interval*
PC	Cisplatin (75–100 mg/M²) Cyclophosphamide (650–1000 mg/M²)	Q 3 weeks
CC	Carboplatin (AUC = 5–7) Cyclophosphamide (600 mg/M²)	Q 4 weeks
PAC	Cisplatin 50 mg/M² Adriamycin 50 mg/M² Cyclophosphamide 500 mg/M²	Q 3–4 weeks

CHAP	Hexamethylmelamine 150 mg/M²
	   orally days 1–14
	 Cyclophosphamide 350 mg/M² IV day
	   1 and day 8
	 Adriamycin 20 mg/M² IV day 1 and
	   day 8
	 Cisplatin 60 mg/M² IV day 1
		Q 3–4 weeks

PT	Cisplatin (75–100 mg/M²) Taxol (135–210 mg/M²)	Q 3 weeks
CT	Carboplatin (starting dose, AUC = 5) Taxol (135–175 mg/M²)	Q 3–4 weeks

AUC = area under the curve.

351

paring CHAP to Hexa-CAF showed a surgically documented complete response rate of 40% for the CHAP regimen, compared with 19% for patients treated with Hexa-CAF. The median survivals were 26 months and 19 months, respectively. Therefore, the cisplatin-based combination regimen appeared superior. Because of the toxicity of hexamethylmelamine, particularly the depression that some patients experience with the drug, many physicians omitted that agent.

In a meta-analysis performed on studies of patients with advanced-stage disease, those given cisplatin-containing combination chemotherapy were compared with those treated with regimens that did not include cisplatin (125). Survival differences between the groups were seen from 2 to 5 years, with the cisplatin group having a slight survival advantage, but this difference disappeared by 8 years (Figure 9.9) (125).

The PAC (cisplatin, Adriamycin, and Cytoxan) regimen has been extensively used for advanced ovarian cancer. Ehrlich et al. (130) reported on 56 patients treated with the PAC regimen every 3 weeks for 12 cycles. The median survival of patients with optimal residual disease was 45 months, compared with 23 months for those with suboptimal disease.

Most studies using the PC (cisplatin and Cytoxan) or PAC regimen report response rates and survivals similar to those produced by the CHAP regimen (118, 131). However, recently updated survival data suggest that the addition of hexamethylmelamine may be of benefit in some subsets of patients with advanced disease (132, 133). In the Mayo Clinic study, the initial analysis of a randomized prospective trial of CHAP versus PC in 181 patients with advanced-stage ovarian cancer showed no survival difference (132). An updated analysis showed a small, statistically significant difference in survival for the CHAP regimen for patients with no gross residual or minimal residual disease (132). Therefore the precise role of hexamethylmelamine in the long-term survival of patients with minimal residual disease epithelial ovarian cancer has not been determined and will require additional randomized trials.

Because of the cardiotoxicity of Adriamycin, it would be desirable to omit the drug if overall response rates were not significantly changed. A large prospective randomized Dutch study of CHAP versus PC showed that the response rates and median survivals were almost identical (131). Because the toxicity of PC was significantly less than that of the four-drug treatment, it was concluded that PC should be considered the treatment of choice.

There have been several trials comparing PAC with PC (134–137). No study showed a significant difference in survival between treatment arms. The GOG's randomized prospective comparison of equitoxic doses of PAC versus PC showed no benefit to the inclusion of Adriamycin in the combination (137). However, a recent meta-analysis of the combined data from these four trials showed a 7% survival advantage at 6 years for those patients treated with the Adriamycin-containing regimen (Figure 9.10) (138). The survival curves appear to converge at 8 years.

The GOG study used a higher dose of Cytoxan in the PC arm to produce the same amount of myelosuppression as the PAC arm, but in the other trials Adriamycin was added to the standard doses of PC (134–137). Therefore the

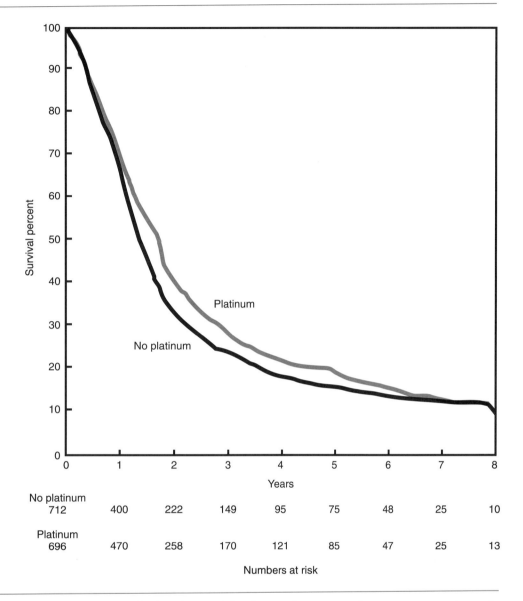

No platinum								
712	400	222	149	95	75	48	25	10

Platinum								
696	470	258	170	121	85	47	25	13

Numbers at risk

Figure 9.9   Survival of patients with advanced-stage ovarian cancer: a meta-analysis of multiple trials comparing cisplatin-containing combination chemotherapy with regimens without cisplatin. (Reproduced, with permission, from Advanced Ovarian Cancer Trialists Group: Chemotherapy in advanced ovarian cancer: an overview of randomized clinical trials. *Br Med J* 303:884, 1991.)

slightly higher survival at 6 years may be due to either the addition of Adriamycin or the increased dose intensity of the three-drug regimen. A randomized trial of a higher dose of cisplatin and/or Cytoxan in the PC arm compared with the PAC would be necessary to resolve this issue.

Dose-Intensification with Cisplatin   With the two-drug regimen PC, higher doses of each drug can be used. This is particularly important for cisplatin, because it has a clinically relevant dose-response curve (i.e., the higher the dose, the greater the theoretical probability of response). The principle of *dose-intensity* is discussed more fully in Chapter 1.

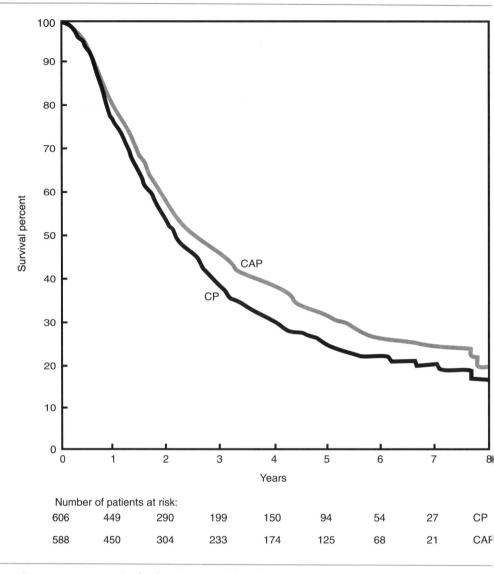

Number of patients at risk:

| 606 | 449 | 290 | 199 | 150 | 94 | 54 | 27 | CP |
| 588 | 450 | 304 | 233 | 174 | 125 | 68 | 21 | CAP |

Figure 9.10   Survival of patients with advanced ovarian cancer: a meta-analysis of trials comparing CP to CAP chemotherapy. (Reproduced, with permission, from Ovarian Cancer Meta-Analysis Project: Cyclophosphamide plus cisplatin versus cyclophosphamide, doxorubicin, and cisplatin chemotherapy of ovarian carcinoma: a meta-analysis. *J Clin Oncol* 9:1668, 1991.)

The issue of dose-intensification of cisplatin was examined in a prospective trial conducted by the GOG (139). In this study, 243 patients with suboptional ovarian cancer were randomized to receive either 50 mg/M^2 or 100 mg/M^2 cisplatin plus 500 mg/M^2 Cytoxan. There was no difference in response rates in those patients with measurable disease, and the overall survival times were identical. There was greater toxicity associated with the high-dose regimen. By contrast, the Scottish group reported that patients who received 100 mg/M^2 cisplatin plus 750 mg/M^2 Cytoxan had a significantly longer median survival compared with those receiving 50 mg/M^2 cisplatin plus the same dose of Cytoxan (140). The overall median survival time was 114 weeks in the high-dose group and 69 weeks in the low-dose group ($p = 0.0008$). The difference was especially striking in patients with optimal residual disease. Therefore the issue remains unsettled.

A randomized, prospective trial of intraperitoneal cisplatin versus intravenous cisplatin (100 mg/M²), each given with 750 mg/M² Cytoxan, has been performed jointly by the Southwest Oncology Group (SWOG) and the GOG in patients with minimal residual disease. The study has been completed, but because median survivals have not yet been reached, an analysis of toxicity and survival is pending. Presumably, the study will help us determine the potential role of primary intraperitoneal cisplatin in these patients with minimal residual disease.

Carboplatin   The second-generation platinum analogue, carboplatin, was introduced and developed to have less toxicity than its parent compound, cisplatin. In toxicity and early efficacy trials, carboplatin was shown to have lower toxicity (141–145). Fewer gastrointestinal side effects, especially nausea and vomiting, were observed than with cisplatin, and there was less nephrotoxicity, neurotoxicity, and ototoxicity.

The initial studies showed that carboplatin and cisplatin have approximately a 4:1 equivalency ratio (142). Thus a standard single-agent dose of about 400 mg/M² has been used in most phase II trials (118). The dose is calculated by using the area under the curve (AUC) and the glomerular filtration rate (GFR) according to the Calvert formula (142), as discussed in Chapter 1. The target AUC is 7 for untreated patients with ovarian cancer. Alternatively, a dose of approximately 350–450 mg/M² carboplatin can be used initially in patients with a normal serum creatinine and adjusted to toxicity. A platelet nadir of approximately 50,000/ml is a suitable target (118).

Prospective randomized trials of carboplatin plus Cytoxan (CC) versus PC have been carried out in patients with Stage III and IV disease. A summary of these trials is presented in Table 9.5 (143, 144). These studies show that the CC regimen has a better therapeutic index in these patients (i.e., equivalent survival with a lower toxicity). **Thus both studies conclude that CC should be the treatment of choice in patients with suboptimal disease.** A comparison of the two regimens has not been made in a sufficient number of patients with optimal disease, so the

Table 9.5 Randomized Trials of Carboplatin + Cyclophosphamide Versus Cisplatin + Cyclophosphamide				
	SWOG Trial		**NCI-C Trial**	
Patients	342		417	
Stage	III (sub) and IV		III (opt + sub) and IV	
Drugs	*Dose*		*Dose*	
Carboplatin	300 mg/M² or		300 mg/M² or	
Cisplatin	100 mg/M²		75 mg/M²	
Cyclophosphamide	600 mg/M²		600 mg/M²	
Response	*Carboplatin*	*Cisplatin*	*Carboplatin*	*Cisplatin*
Total	61%	50%	59%	57%
Complete	33%	30%	27%	36%
Complete pathologic*	10%	7%	12%	16%
Survival	*Carboplatin*	*Cisplatin*	*Carboplatin*	*Cisplatin*
Median	20 mo	17.4 mo	110 wk	100 wk
3-yr	20%	21%	—	—
Time to progression	—	—	58 wk	56 wk

*Negative second-look; opt = optimal; sub = suboptimal.

question of relative efficacy in this group is unresolved. However, Ozols (118) has argued that carboplatin should replace cisplatin in the primary treatment of all of these patients on the basis of available comparative efficacy data. Until the issue has been settled, it is reasonable to use cisplatin in those patients with optimal disease, unless its use is precluded by toxicity or compromised renal or neurologic function. The gastrointestinal toxicities of cisplatin can now be ameliorated reasonably effectively by use of the potent antiemetic, ondancetron. In general, older patients (over 65 years) or those with significant medical conditions (e.g., diabetes mellitus) tolerate cisplatin less well, and carboplatin should be preferred.

Taxol The recent introduction of Taxol as an active agent in ovarian cancer requires the examination of this agent in first-line therapeutic strategies (117–121). Taxol is the most active agent since cisplatin, with overall response rates in phase II trials of 36% in previously treated patients. This is a higher rate than was seen for cisplatin when it was first tested (120). The current randomized trials being carried out by the GOG are:

1. A two-arm comparison of Taxol plus cisplatin (PT) versus PC in optimal Stage III patients (121)

2. A three-arm comparison of Taxol (T) versus cisplatin (P) versus PT in suboptimal Stage III and IV patients

An interim analysis of the first trial shows progression-free survival benefit for the PT arm (17 versus 12 months), and if these data are borne out in future analyses, the preferred regimen in patients with optimally cytoreduced disease may be the Taxol plus platinum combination (121).

Chemotherapeutic Recommendation in Advanced Ovarian Cancer On the basis of the data presented, combination chemotherapy with cisplatin or carboplatin and Taxol is the treatment of choice for patients with advanced disease. It is our preference to use cisplatin (75 mg/M^2) plus Taxol (135–210 mg/M^2) (PT), or for those in whom the toxicity of cisplatin is likely to preclude administration, carboplatin (starting dose AUC = 5) plus Taxol (135–175 mg/M^2) (CT). Dose escalations of Taxol and carboplatin that require G-CSF because of the combined myelosuppressive effects are currently undergoing clinical trials. The roles of Adriamycin and Hexalan (hexamethylmelamine) in combination chemotherapy regimens remain controversial, and their toxicities are significant.

Administration of Chemotherapy and Amelioration of Toxicity

Cisplatin Cisplatin combination chemotherapy is given every 3–4 weeks by intravenous infusion over 1–1.5 hours. Cisplatin requires appropriate hydration, and can be administered on either an inpatient or outpatient basis. Hydration is administered with one-half normal saline given intravenously at a rate of 300–500 ml per hour for 2–4 hours until the urinary output is greater than 100 ml per hour. It is preferable to place a Foley catheter to monitor the output. Immediately before chemotherapy, 12.5 g of mannitol in 50 ml of normal saline solution is infused. When the urinary output is satisfactory, the cisplatin is infused in normal saline; the intravenous fluid rate is decreased to 150–200 ml per hour for 6 hours and then is discontinued if the patient is stable.

The principal toxicities of this regimen are renal, gastrointestinal, hematologic, and neurologic. The renal and neurologic toxicities limit the duration of treatment to no more than 10–12 cycles, although the optimal duration may be shorter (i.e., 6–9 cycles), according to second-look laparotomy data.

The acute gastrointestinal toxicity of cisplatin (i.e., nausea and vomiting) can be minimized with a strong antiemetic, ondancetron, given as a 32 mg intravenous bolus, followed every 4–6 hours with 10 mg intravenously. Alternative regimens include Benadryl, 25 mg orally, and Ativan, 2 mg sublingually, both given 1 hour before the initiation of treatment, followed by Ativan, 2 mg sublingually every 3 hours, Reglan, 100 mg intravenously every 3–4 hours, and one dose of Decadron, 20 mg intravenously.

Carboplatin   The renal and gastrointestinal toxicities of carboplatin are modest compared with cisplatin; thus patients do not require prehydration and outpatient administration is more feasible. Carboplatin does tend to have appreciable bone marrow toxicity, and growth factors such as G-CSF and GM-CSF have facilitated the administration of drug combinations that have neutropenia as a dose-limiting toxicity. The combination of carboplatin with cisplatin, Cytoxan, or Taxol can produce considerable neutropenia, and the concomitant administration of 250 mg/M^2 of G-CSF given subcutaneously on days 1–10 of a treatment cycle may be protective (145, 146). The use of growth factors is discussed more fully in Chapter 1.

Radiation Therapy

An alternative to combination chemotherapy for selected patients with metastatic ovarian cancer is the use of whole-abdominal radiation therapy. Although this approach is not commonly used in the United States, it is standard treatment in some institutions in Canada for patients with no residual macroscopic tumor in the upper abdomen (92). The treatment involves a radiation field that extends from 1–2 cm above the level of the diaphragm to include the entire pelvis. Details of this approach are discussed in Chapter 2.

Whole-abdominal radiation appears useful in patients whose metastatic disease is microscopic or completely resected. The treatment has not been tested against combination chemotherapy. Radiation therapy has been compared with oral chlorambucil and appears to be superior (92). The currently available data suggest that whole-abdominal radiation is inappropriate for patients with macroscopic residual disease.

A trial of three cycles of high-dose cisplatin and Cytoxan "induction" chemotherapy followed by whole-abdominal radiation therapy to "consolidate" the initial response has been reported (147). No apparent benefit could be shown by adding whole-abdominal radiation after chemotherapy in patients with optimal disease.

Immunotherapy

There have been various trials using nonspecific immunostimulants to treat patients with ovarian cancer (102). Most frequently, agents such as *Corynebacterium parvum* and *Bacillus Calmette-Guerin (BCG)* have been used systemically in conjunction with cytotoxic chemotherapy. In trials of *C. parvum* given with melphalan and *BCG* given with PAC chemotherapy, the nonspecific immunostimulant did not provide any additional benefit. Although there is currently a great deal of interest in the use of biologic response modifiers in ovarian cancer, none as yet has demonstrated efficacy as primary treatment. The use of cytokines has been tested in a salvage setting, and the activity of α-interferon, γ-interferon, and interleukin-2 has been demonstrated, as discussed below. Trials of these and other biologics are developing, because they have become increasingly available through recombinant DNA technology. The rationale for the use of these agents in ovarian cancer is discussed in Chapter 3.

Hormonal Therapy

There is no evidence that hormonal therapy alone is appropriate primary therapy for advanced ovarian cancer. The use of progestational agents in the treatment of recurrent well-differentiated endometrioid carcinomas is supported by the current data (148). In a study by Rendina et al. (148), 30 evaluable patients with recurrent epithelial cancers were treated; 17 (57%) had an objective response, with 3 (10%) of these achieving a complete response. All responding patients had well-differentiated, estrogen receptor–positive tumors. A trial of tamoxifen in combination with multiagent chemotherapy is being conducted at Yale University. Hormonal treatments for ovarian cancer are discussed in Chapter 17.

Treatment Assessment

Many patients who undergo optimal cytoreductive surgery and subsequent chemotherapy for epithelial ovarian cancer will have no evidence of disease at the completion of treatment. Tumor markers and radiologic assessments have proved to be too insensitive to exclude the presence of subclinical disease. Therefore a common technique used to evaluate these patients has been the "second-look" operation (73, 149–163). Most often, patients have undergone a formal reassessment laparotomy, although the laparoscope has also been used in this circumstance (161–163). However, there is a 35% false-negative rate if laparoscopy is used for a second-look procedure (73, 162).

Tumor Markers

Tumor markers are not reliable enough to predict accurately which patients with epithelial tumors have had their disease completely eradicated by a particular therapy. Carcinoembryonic antigen (CEA) is often elevated in patients with ovarian cancer, but it is too nonspecific and insensitive to have much use in the management of patients with ovarian cancer (102).

The level of CA 125, a surface glycoprotein associated with müllerian epithelial tissues, is elevated in about 80% of patients with epithelial ovarian cancers, particularly those with nonmucinous tumors. The levels frequently become undetectable after the initial surgical resection and one or two cycles of chemotherapy.

The levels of CA 125 have been correlated with the findings at second-look operations. Positive levels are useful in predicting the presence of disease, but negative levels are an insensitive determinant of the absence of disease. In a prospective study (164), the predictive value of a positive test was shown to be 100%; i.e., if the level of CA 125 was positive (> 35 U/ml), disease was always detectable in patients at the second look. The predictive value of a negative test was only 56%; i.e., if the level was < 35 U/ml, disease was present in 44% of the patients at the time of the second look. **A review of the literature suggests that an elevated CA 125 level predicts persistent disease at second-look in 97% of the cases (17), but the CA 125 level is not sensitive enough to exclude subclinical disease in many patients.**

Serum CA 125 levels can be used during chemotherapy to follow those patients whose level was positive at the initiation of therapy (17, 165). The change in level generally correlates with response. Those patients with persistently elevated titers after three cycles of treatment most likely have resistant clones. Rising levels on treatment almost invariably indicate treatment failure and suggest that continuation of the current regimen is futile.

Radiologic Assessment

In patients with Stage I to III epithelial ovarian cancer, radiologic tests have generally been of limited value in assessing the response to therapy for subclinical disease. Ascites can be readily detected, but even quite large omental metastases can be missed on CT scan (166). If liver enzymes are abnormal, the liver can be evaluated with a CT scan or ultrasonography. A positive CT scan and fine needle aspiration (FNA) cytology indicating tumor persistence could obviate the need for second-look surgery, but the false-negative rate of a CT scan is about 45% (166).

Second-Look Operations

A second-look operation is one performed on a patient who has no clinical evidence of disease after a prescribed course of chemotherapy in order to determine the response to therapy.

Second-Look Laparotomy

The technique of the second-look laparotomy is essentially identical to that for the staging laparotomy (73). The operation should be performed through a vertical abdominal incision. The incision should be initiated below the level of the umbilicus, so that if pelvic disease is detected in the absence of any palpable upper abdominal disease, a smaller incision might suffice. The incision can be extended cranially as needed.

After multiple cytologic specimens have been obtained, biopsies of the peritoneal surfaces should be performed, particularly in any areas of previously documented tumor. These are the most important areas to sample for biopsy because they are most likely to give a positive result. Any adhesions or surface irregularities should be sampled. In addition, biopsy specimens should be taken from the pelvic side walls, the pelvic cul-de-sac, the bladder, the paracolic gutters, the residual omentum, and the diaphragm. A pelvic and para-aortic lymph node dissection should be performed in those patients whose nodal tissues have not been previously removed.

About 30% of patients with no evidence of macroscopic disease will have microscopic metastases (149). Also, in many patients with microscopic disease, it will be detected in only the occasional biopsy or cytologic specimen. Therefore, a large number of specimens (20–30) should be obtained to minimize the "false-negative" rate of the operation. In selected patients in whom gross residual tumor is discovered at second-look surgery, resection of isolated masses may be performed. The removal of all macroscopic areas of disease might facilitate response to salvage therapies (167, 168), and it also permits the collection of tissue for *in vitro* analyses.

359

Results

Second-look laparotomies have not been shown to influence patient survival (158, 160). Therefore they should be performed only in a research setting, where second-line or "salvage" therapies are undergoing clinical trials.

The findings at second-look correlate with subsequent outcome and survival (73, 149–160). Patients who have no histologic evidence of disease have a significantly longer survival than those in whom microscopic or macroscopic disease is documented at laparotomy (155, 156).

The attainment of a negative second-look is not tantamount to a cure (147, 149). Indeed, the reported probability that a patient will have a recurrence after a negative second-look laparotomy ranges from 30–50% at 5 years (73, 149–160). Clearly, it is not possible to sample every potential site of disease. In addition, disease can become clinically apparent in sites that are occult, such as the liver parenchyma (40). The majority of recurrences after a negative second-look laparotomy are in patients with poorly differentiated cancers (160).

Variables associated with the outcome of the second-look laparotomy are:

1. Initial stage

2. Tumor grade

3. The size of the residual tumor and the size of the largest metastatic tumor before treatment

4. The type of chemotherapy

No single variable or combination of variables is sufficiently predictive to obviate a planned second-look laparotomy (73).

Stage Patients whose tumors are initially Stage I and II have negative second-look laparotomy rates of 85–95% and 60–80%, respectively, whereas the rate for patients with Stage III or IV disease is 30–45% (73, 149–157, 160).

Grade The majority of patients with low-stage disease who have evidence of persistent disease at second-look operation have more poorly differentiated tumors (149). The likelihood of a negative second look in patients at all stages is about 60–70% for those with grade 1 tumors, 40–50% for those with grade 2, and only 20% for those with grade 3 (73, 151, 160).

Residual Tumor The maximum size of the residual tumor before therapy is an important predictor of outcome; i.e., the probability of a negative second-look is higher in those patients whose tumor burden before initiation of chemotherapy is smaller. Patients whose disease is microscopic or ≤ 5 mm at the start of therapy have a much higher likelihood of a complete pathologic remission than those patients with more extensive disease (149, 160). Whereas smaller primary tumors seem to be associated with a poorer prognosis, those patients with very extensive metastatic tumors have little likelihood of a negative second-look, regardless of the extent of tumor reduction.

Chemotherapy The likelihood of a negative second-look laparotomy is greater in patients who have been treated with a cisplatin-containing regimen than in

360

those treated without cisplatin (e.g., AC or melphalan alone) (125). In patients with advanced-stage disease treated with the cisplatin-containing regimen, the negative second-look rate is about 35–50%, compared with only about 15–25% in patients treated with regimens that do not include cisplatin.

The second-look laparotomy has helped to define the number of cycles of chemotherapy necessary to achieve a complete response. Six cycles of cisplatin-containing combination chemotherapy produce about the same negative second-look laparotomy rate in patients with advanced-stage disease as do 10–12 cycles (149). These data suggest that epithelial carcinomas that are sensitive to the chemotherapy are likely to respond early in the course of treatment. Additional treatment beyond six cycles does not appear to increase the probability of achieving a complete pathologic remission and will only increase the treatment toxicity.

Second-Look Laparoscopy The advantage of laparoscopy is that it is a less invasive operation; the disadvantage is that visibility may be limited by the frequent presence of intraperitoneal adhesions (151–155). The development of newer techniques for retroperitoneal lymph node dissection has potentially increased the utility of the endoscopic approach to second-look. The morbidity and role of this technique are currently being studied by the GOG.

One technique that has been used for second-look is "open" laparoscopy. This procedure allows placement of the scope after a "cutdown" to the fascia of the rectus abdominus. The peritoneum is entered under direct vision, thus avoiding the blind insertion that can be associated with intestinal injury (162).

The sensitivity of the laparoscopic technique has been determined by an exploratory laparotomy performed immediately after a negative laparoscopy. Thirty-five percent of those who have a negative laparoscopy have evidence of disease at laparotomy (163), but these patients did not undergo a lymphadenectomy at laparoscopy.

The laparoscope has been used immediately before a planned laparotomy. If gross disease is detected and secondary resection of the tumor is not possible, a laparotomy may be omitted (162).

Thus the role of the laparoscope in epithelial ovarian cancer patients is still being defined. It may be used to stage disease in patients who have undergone a prior laparotomy for a tumor that was incompletely staged. Second-look laparoscopy may also be useful for patients on experimental treatment protocols, especially second-line treatments that require some evaluation of response.

Salvage Therapy

Secondary Cytoreduction Patients with persistent or recurrent pelvic and abdominal tumors after primary therapy for ovarian cancer are occasionally candidates for surgical excision of their disease. This operation has been referred to as "secondary" cytoreductive surgery (167). Tumor resection under these circumstances should be restricted to carefully selected patients for whom resection has a reasonable chance of either prolonging life or significantly palliating symptoms, because the majority of patients with persistent or progressive disease after primary therapy do not benefit. The patient in whom secondary cytoreduction might be appropriate should be in good general medical condition. A suitable patient would be one who has no evidence of ascites, has not yet received cisplatin combination chemotherapy, has had at least a partial response to prior alkylating agent therapy, and has had a reasonably long interval since primary diagnosis (longer than 9–12 months). If the patient has previously received cisplatin, secondary cytoreduction is justified if there has been a long disease-free survival (> 24 months) because such patients are likely to respond again to the primary chemotherapy (168–173).

The goal of secondary debulking is to remove all residual gross tumor, if possible, or to reduce the metastatic tumor burden to < 5 mm maximum dimension. Some patients with minimal residual disease will respond to second-line treatment. Those patients in whom the residual disease is completely resected have a significantly longer survival than those who do not (168).

Second-Line Chemotherapy

If disease persists at the time of second-look laparotomy, or if clinically progressive disease develops during primary therapy, patients usually have been switched to an alternative treatment, often a second-line chemotherapy. The response rates for second-line chemotherapies have been less than 10–30% for most drugs tested by the oral or intravenous route (88, 116, 118).

Because response to cisplatin is dose-dependent, secondary response rates as high as 30% have been reported for high-dose cisplatin (100–150 mg/M^2) in patients in whom alkylating agents or low-dose cisplatin (50 mg/M^2) have failed (118, 169, 170). Unfortunately, this approach is associated with considerable toxicity, particularly renal and neural. **The cisplatin analogue, carboplatin, is active as a second-line agent in patients who have responded to prior cisplatin treatment, and response rates in these patients have been 20–30%** (146, 171–173). In cisplatin-refractory patients, response rates to second-line carboplatin are < 10% (171, 173).

Depending on the prior chemotherapy, persistent disease can be treated with cisplatin, carboplatin, Taxol, ifosfamide, or hexamethylmelamine (Hexalan), with or without other agents. Although responses occur, this approach is not curative. **For patients treated initially with platinum therapy, Taxol is an active salvage drug, with responses occurring in 20–36% of patients** (117–120). Hexalan produced second-line complete clinical responses in 15% of the patients (8 of 52) (122) and ifosfamide in 20% of the patients (9 of 26) in a GOG trial (174). In patients with minimal residual (≤ 5 mm) or microscopic disease confined to the peritoneal cavity, consideration can be given to intraperitoneal chemotherapy or immunotherapy (175).

Intraperitoneal Therapy

The failure of second-line intravenous chemotherapy to control residual disease has led to great interest in intraperitoneal therapies. Cytotoxic chemotherapeutic agents, such as cisplatin, 5-fluorouracil (5-FU), cytosine arabinoside (Ara-C), Etoposide (VP-16), and mitoxantrone, have been used in patients with persistent epithelial ovarian cancer (175–183), and complete responses have been seen in patients who start their treatment with minimal residual disease. The surgically documented response rates reported with this approach are about 20–40% for carefully selected patients, and the complete response rate is about 10–20%. Cisplatin appears to be the best drug, although various combinations of agents (e.g., cisplatin plus Etoposide) have been shown to have significant activity (180, 181). Although it has been suggested that this approach produces a significant subsequent improvement in survival (183), there are no prospective phase III data, and the patients so treated tend to be those with a more favorable prognosis regardless of subsequent therapy.

Another approach is the use of intraperitoneal biologic response modifiers (BRMs), such as interferon (184–190). The latter has been found to have some activity in patients with minimal residual disease (184, 185). Because of recombinant DNA technology, other BRMs, particularly the cytokines, are becoming increasingly available for clinical testing. Trials of intraperitoneal α-interferon, γ-interferon, tumor necrosis factor, and interleukin 2 have been performed. The response rate for the intraperitoneal cytokines, α-interferon and γ-interferon, is the same as that for the cytotoxic agents, i.e., about 30–50% (184, 185, 188). The intraperitoneal administration of α-interferon has produced a 32% (9/28) surgically documented complete response rate, and a 50% (14/28) total response rate in patients with minimal residual disease after primary combination chemotherapy with cisplatin (184, 185).

The interferons have been combined with cytotoxic agents in an effort to increase the overall response rates. In two trials, the combination of cisplatin and α-interferon appeared to produce a 50% complete response rate, which was greater than that produced by either single agent (186, 187). However, in a prospective single-arm phase II trial conducted by the GOG, the intraperitoneal administration of cisplatin and α-interferon produced only a 7% response rate (190). In this GOG trial, most patients had cisplatin-refractory tumors with > 5 mm residual disease, generalized carcinomatosis, and ascites. Surgically documented responses to intraperitoneal therapy have been generally limited to patients with minimal residual disease (i.e., < 5 mm maximum tumor dimension) and those whose tumors have been responsive to cisplatin chemotherapy.

Intraperitoneal treatment is not suitable for all patients because it can be cumbersome, requiring catheters that remain functional. Patients with extensive intraperitoneal adhesions are not appropriate candidates, and neither are patients with extraperitoneal disease. On the basis of these issues and the failure to achieve responses in the majority of patients with bulky, platinum-refractory disease, Ozols (191) has argued that this approach has been unsuccessful and should be abandoned. Therefore salvage intraperitoneal chemotherapy and immunotherapy should still be considered experimental.

Whole-Abdominal Radiation

Whole-abdominal radiation therapy given as a "salvage" treatment has been shown to be potentially effective in a small subset of selected patients with microscopic disease, but it is associated with a relatively high morbidity. The principal problem associated with this approach is the development of acute and chronic intestinal morbidity. As many as 30% of patients treated with this approach develop intestinal obstruction, which will necessitate potentially morbid exploratory surgery (192).

Experimental Combination Chemotherapy Regimens

In light of the poor responses to second-line drugs in phase II trials, several new combinations of chemotherapy are now being tested in advanced epithelial ovarian cancer. Some of these approaches are presented in Table 9.6.

363

Table 9.6   New Chemotherapeutic Regimes Undergoing Clinical Trials

Combination				
Taxol (135–210 mg/M²)	+	Cisplatin (75 mg/M²)		
Taxol (135–210 mg/M²)	+	Carboplatin ± G-CSF (starting dose calculated for AUC = 5)		
Carboplatin (600 mg/M²)	+	Cisplatin (50 mg/M² × 2)	+	Cyclophosphamide + Growth factors (250 mg/M²)
Carboplatin (300–350 mg/M²)	+	Cyclophosphamide (600 mg/M²)	+	Hexamethylmelamine (150 mg/M² q d × 14)
Cisplatin (100 mg/M²)	+	Cyclophosphamide (1000 mg/M²)	+	WR2721 (740 mg/M²)

Modified, with permission, from Ozols RF: Chemotherapy for advanced epithelial ovarian cancer. *Hematol Oncol Clin North Am* 6:879, 1992.

The use of Taxol is being studied by the GOG in combination with cisplatin and carboplatin, the latter with G-CSF because both agents produce dose-limiting neutropenia (118). Also, combinations of carboplatin and cisplatin are being tested (175). The rationale for this approach is that the two agents have complementary toxicities, and theoretically the dose intensity of platinum can be enhanced by this combination of two active platinum analogues. Various neuroprotective and myelosuppressive "protectors," such as WR2721, are being tested in high-dose cisplatin regimens.

The use of autologous bone marrow transplantation (ABMT) and peripheral stem cell protection is being tested in patients with advanced ovarian cancer (193–195). In one trial of high-dose carboplatin with autologous bone marrow transplantation, 7 of the 11 patients with extensive refractory disease had an objective response. The maximum tolerated dose of high-dose carboplatin was 2 gm/M² (193). In a retrospective analysis of 35 patients treated with high-dose melphalan and ABMT, 9 of 12 with evaluable residual disease had a measurable response (194). The morbidity of this approach is high, and its role remains to be determined. The use of peripheral stem cell transplantation as an alternative to autologous bone marrow harvest and transplantation is currently being investigated.

Intestinal Obstruction

Patients with epithelial ovarian cancer often develop intestinal obstruction, either at the time of initial diagnosis or, more frequently, in association with recurrent disease (196–203). Obstruction may be related to a mechanical blockage or to carcinomatous ileus.

Correction of the intestinal blockage can be accomplished in most patients whose obstruction appears at the time of initial diagnosis (94). However, the decision to perform an exploratory procedure to palliate intestinal obstruction in patients with recurrent disease is more difficult. In patients whose life expectancy is very short (e.g., less than 2 months), surgical relief of the obstruction is not indicated (196). In those whose projected life span is longer, features that predict a reasonable likelihood of correcting the obstruction include young age, good nutritional status, and the absence of rapidly accumulating ascites (197).

For most patients with recurrent ovarian cancer who present with intestinal obstruction, initial management should include proper radiographic documentation of the obstruction, hydration, correction of any electrolyte disturbances, parenteral alimentation, and intestinal intubation. For the latter, a long gastrointestinal tube (e.g., Cantor tube) should be used, as discussed in Chapter 15. In some patients the obstruction may be alleviated by this conservative approach. A preoperative upper gastrointestinal series and a barium enema will define possible sites of obstruction.

If exploratory surgery is deemed appropriate, the type of operation to be performed will depend on (1) the site and (2) the number of obstructions. Multiple sites of obstruction are not uncommon in patients with recurrent epithelial ovarian cancer. More than one-half of the patients have small-bowel obstruction, one-third have colonic obstruction, and one-sixth have both (198–202). If the obstruction is principally contained in one area of the bowel (e.g., the terminal ileum), this area can either be resected or bypassed, depending on whether a concomitant effort at secondary cytoreduction is indicated. The techniques for these intestinal operations are discussed in Chapter 15. If multiple obstructions are present, resection of several segments of intestine in patients with recurrent disease is usually not indicated, and intestinal bypass and/or colostomy should be performed. A gastrostomy may also be useful in this circumstance (32, 199).

Intestinal bypass is generally less morbid than resection (198, 199), and in patients with recurrent, progressive cancer, the survival time after these two operations is the same (198). Most frequently, an enteroenterostomy or an enterocolostomy is performed (199–202). Colostomy may be necessary when there is a distal large bowel obstruction. Occasionally, the performance of an ileostomy or a jejunostomy is warranted when the large bowel is completely encased in tumor (32). In very advanced cases, a palliative gastrostomy may be used, and this can be placed percutaneously if there is no carcinomatosis around the stomach (203).

Among 268 patients reported to have undergone operations for intestinal obstruction resulting from ovarian cancer, the operative mortality was 14% and major complications were seen in 34% of the patients (196–199). The need for multiple reanastamoses and prior radiation therapy increased the morbidity, which consisted primarily of sepsis and enterocutaneous fistulas.

The median survival time for patients who have undergone intestinal surgery for obstruction secondary to ovarian cancer ranges from 2.5 to 7 months, although Castaldo et al. (196) reported that 17% of such patients survived longer than 12 months.

Survival

As discussed, the prognosis for patients with epithelial ovarian cancer is related to several clinical variables. Survival analyses based on the most commonly used prognostic variables are presented below (68–71):

Age   Including patients at all stages, patients less than 50 years of age have a 5-year survival rate of about 40%, compared with about 15% for patients older than 50 years (2–4, 32, 42, 68–71, 88).

Stage The 5-year survival rate for carefully and properly staged patients with Stage I and II tumors is 80–100%, depending on the tumor grade. Survival for patients with low-stage disease is presented in Figure 9.2. The 5-year survival rate for Stage IIIa is about 30–40%, compared with about 20% for Stage IIIb and only 5% for those with Stages IIIc and IV (68–71, 73, 125, 138).

Grade Including patients of all stages, the overall 5-year survival rate for grade 1 epithelial ovarian cancers is about 40%, compared with about 20% for grade 2 and 5–10% for grade 3 (3, 73, 43–46, 49). The 10- and 20-year survival rate among patients with borderline ovarian tumors is about 95% and 90%, respectively (3, 5, 84, 85).

Residual Disease Patients with microscopic residual disease at the start of treatment have a 5-year survival rate of about 40–75%, compared with about 30–40% for those with optimal disease and only 5% for those with nonoptimal disease (73, 94–97) (Figure 9.4).

Second-Look Status Patients without any evidence of disease at second-look laparotomy have a 5-year survival rate of 50% compared with about 35% for those with microscopic disease and about 5% for those with macroscopic disease (73, 149–157, 160).

Performance Status Patients whose Karnofsky's index (KI) is low (< 70) have a significantly shorter survival than those with a KI > 70 (204).

References

1. **Boring CC, Squires TS, Tong S:** Cancer statistics, 1994. *Ca-Cancer J Clin* 44:7, 1994.

2. **Scully RE:** *Tumors of the Ovary and Maldeveloped Gonads.* Armed Forces Institute of Pathology, Fascicle 16. Washington, D.C., 1979.

3. **Julian CG, Goss J, Blanchard K, Woodruff JD:** Biologic behavior of primary ovarian malignancy. *Gynecol Oncol* 44:873, 1974.

4. **Julian CG, Woodruff JD:** The biologic behavior of low-grade papillary serous carcinoma of the ovary. *Obstet Gynecol* 40:860, 1972.

5. **Genedry R, Poliakoff S, Rotmensch J, et al:** Primary papillary peritoneal neoplasia. *Obstet Gynecol* 58:730, 1981.

6. **Bell DA, Weinstock MA, Scully RE:** Peritoneal implants of ovarian serous borderline tumors: histologic features and prognosis. *Cancer* 62:2212, 1988.

7. **Tobachman JK, Greene MH, Tucker MA, et al:** Intraabdominal carcinomatosis after prophylactic oophorectomy in ovarian cancer-prone families. *Lancet* 2:794, 1982.

8. **Aure JC, Hoeg K, Kolstad P:** Clinical and histologic studies of ovarian carcinoma: Long-term follow-up of 950 cases. *Obstet Gynecol* 37:1, 1971.

9. **Norris HJ, Jensen RD:** Relative frequency of ovarian neoplasms in children and adolescents. *Cancer* 30:713, 1972.

10. **Campbell S, Bhan V, Royston P, et al:** Transabdominal ultrasound screening for early ovarian cancer. *Br Med J* 299:1363, 1989.

11. **van Nagell JR Jr, Donaldson ES, Gallion HH, et al:** Transvaginal sonography as a screening method for ovarian cancer. *Gynecol Oncol* 34:402, 1989.

12. **van Nagell JR Jr, DePriest PD, Puls LE, et al:** Ovarian cancer screening in asymptomatic postmenopausal women by transvaginal sonography. *Cancer* 68:458, 1991.

13. **Rulin MC, Preston AL:** Adnexal masses in postmenopausal women. *Obstet Gynecol* 70:578, 1987.

14. **Kurjak A, Zalud I, Jurkovic D, et al:** Transvaginal color flow Doppler for the assessment of pelvic circulation. *Acta Obstet Gynecol Scand* 68:131, 1989.

15. **Kurjak A, Zalud I, Alfirevic Z:** Evaluation of adnexal masses with transvaginal color ultrasound. *J Ultrasound Med* 10:295, 1991.

16. **Zurawski VR, Broderick SF, Pickens P, et al:** Serum CA 125 levels in a group of nonhospitalized women: relevance for the early detection of ovarian cancer. *Obstet Gynecol* 69:606, 1987.

17. **Jacobs I, Bast RC:** The CA 125 tumour associated antigen: a review of the literature. *Hum Reprod* 4:1, 1989.

18. **Jacobs I, Bridges J, Reynolds C, et al:** Multimodal approach to screening for ovarian cancer. *Lancet* 2:268, 1988.

19. **Zurawski VR Jr, Orjaseter H, Andersen A, Jellum E:** Elevated serum CA-125 prior to diagnosis of ovarian neoplasia: relevance for early detection of ovarian cancer. *Int J Cancer* 42:677, 1988.

20. **Zurawski VR Jr, Sjovall K, Schoenfeld DA, et al:** Prospective evaluation of serum CA-125 levels in a normal population, phase I: the specification of single and serial determinations in testing for ovarian cancer. *Gynecol Oncol* 36:299, 1990.

21. **Einhorn N, Sjovall K, Knapp RC, et al:** A prospective evaluation of serum CA 125 levels for early detection of ovarian cancer. *Obstet Gynecol* 80:14, 1992.

22. **Jacobs I, Prys Davies A, Oram D:** Role of CA 125 in screening for ovarian cancer. In Sharp F, Mason WP, Creasman W (eds): *Ovarian Cancer. 2. Biology, Diagnosis and Management.* London, Chapman and Hall Medical, 1992, p 265.

23. **Genetic risk and screening techniques for epithelial ovarian cancer.** *ACOG Committee Opinion* 117, 1992.

24. **Bourne TH, Whitehead MI, Campbell S, et al:** Ultrasound screening for familial ovarian cancer. *Gynecol Oncol* 43:92, 1991.

25. **Lynch HT, Harris RE, Guirgis HA, et al:** Familial association of breast/ovarian carcinoma. *Cancer* 41:1543, 1978.

26. **Lynch HT, Lynch PM:** Tumor variations in the cancer family syndrome: ovarian cancer. *Am J Surg* 138:439, 1979.

27. **Lynch HT, Conway T, Lynch J:** Hereditary ovarian cancer. In Sharp F, Mason WP, Leake RE (eds): *Ovarian Cancer: Biological and Therapeutic Challenges.* Cambridge, Chapman and Hall Medical, 1990, p 719.

28. **Lynch HT, Watson P, Bewtra TA, et al:** Hereditary ovarian cancer: Heterogeneity in age at diagnosis. *Cancer* 61:1460, 1991.

29. **Schildkraut JM, Thompson WD:** Familial ovarian cancer: a population-based case-control study. *Am J Epidemiol* 128:456, 1988.

30. **Ponder BAJ, Easton DF, Peto J:** Risk of ovarian cancer associated with a family history: preliminary report of the OPCS study. In Sharp F, Mason WP, Leake RE (eds): *Ovarian Cancer: Biological and Therapeutic Challenges.* Cambridge, Chapman and Hall Medical, 1990, p 3.

31. **Hall JM, Lee MK, Newman B, et al:** Linkage of early-onset familial breast cancer to chromosome 17q 21. *Science* 250:1684, 1990.

32. **Berek JS, Hacker NF:** Ovarian and fallopian tubes. In Haskell CM (ed): *Cancer Treatment.* Third ed. Philadelphia, WB Saunders, 1990, pp 295–325.

33. **Barber HK, Grober EA:** The PMPO syndrome (postmenopausal palpable ovary syndrome). *Obstet Gynecol* 38:921, 1971.

34. **Lewis E, Wallace S:** Radiologic diagnosis of ovarian cancer. In Piver MS (ed): *Ovarian Malignancies.* Edinburgh, Churchill Livingstone, 1987, pp 59–80.

35. **Hacker NF, Berek JS, Lagasse LD:** Gastrointestinal operations in gynecologic oncology. In Knapp RE, Berkowitz RS (eds): *Gynecologic Oncology.* Second ed. New York, McGraw-Hill, 1993, pp 361–375.

36. **Malkasian GD, Knapp RC, Lavin PT, et al:** Preoperative evaluation of serum CA 125 levels in premenopausal and postmenopausal patients with pelvic masses: discrimination of benign from malignant disease. *Am J Obstet Gynecol* 159:341, 1988.

37. **Plentl AM, Friedman EA:** *Lymphatic System of the Female Genitalia*. Philadelphia, WB Saunders, 1971.

38. **Burghart E, Hellmuth P, Lahousen M, Stettner H:** Pelvic lymphadenectomy in operative treatment of ovarian cancer. *Am J Obstet Gynecol* 155:315, 1986.

39. **Chen SS, Lee L:** Incidence of paraaortic and pelvic lymph node metastasis in epithelial ovarian cancer. *Gynecol Oncol* 16:95, 1983.

40. **Dauplat J, Hacker NF, Neiberg RK, Berek JS:** Distant metastasis in epithelial ovarian carcinoma. *Cancer* 60:1561, 1987.

41. **Krag KJ, Canellos GP, Griffiths CT, et al:** Predictive factors for long term survival in patients with advanced ovarian cancer. *Gynecol Oncol* 34:88, 1989.

42. **Young RC, Walton LA, Ellenberg SS, et al:** Adjuvant therapy in stage I and stage II epithelial ovarian cancer: results of two prospective randomized trials. *N Engl J Med* 322:1021, 1990.

43. **Bjorkholm E, Pettersson F, Einhorn N, et al:** Long term follow-up and prognostic factors in ovarian carcinoma. The Radiumhemmet series 1958 to 1973. *Acta Radiol Oncol* 21:413, 1982.

44. **Malkasian GD, Decker DG, Webb MJ, et al:** Histology of epithelial tumours of the ovary: clinical usefulness and prognostic significance of histologic classification and grading. *Semin Oncol* 2:191, 1975.

45. **Silverberg SG:** Prognostic significance of pathologic features of ovarian carcinoma. *Curr Top Pathol* 78:85, 1989.

46. **Jacobs AJ, Deligdisch L, Deppe G, Cohen CJ:** Histologic correlations of virulence in ovarian adenocarcinoma. 1. Effects of differentiation. *Am J Obstet Gynecol* 143:574, 1982.

47. **Baak JP, Langley FA, Talerman A, et al:** Interpathologist and intrapathologist disagreement in ovarian tumor grading and typing. *Anal Quant Cytol Histol* 8:354, 1986.

48. **Hernandez E, Bhagavan BS, Parmley TH, et al:** Interobserver variability in the interpretation of epithelial ovarian cancer. *Gynecol Oncol* 17:117, 1984.

49. **Baak JP, Chan KK, Stolk JG, et al:** Prognostic factors in borderline and invasive ovarian tumours of the common epithelial type. *Pathol Res Pract* 182:755, 1987.

50. **Friedlander ML, Hedley DW, Swanson C, et al:** Prediction of long term survivals by flow cytometric analysis of cellular DNA content in patients with advanced ovarian cancer. *J Clin Oncol* 6:282, 1988.

51. **Friedlander ML, Taylor IW, Russell P, et al:** Ploidy as a prognostic factor in ovarian cancer. *Int J Gynaecol Pathol* 1:55, 1983.

52. **Punnonen R, Kallioniemi OP, Mattila J, et al:** Prognostic assessment in stage I ovarian cancer using a discriminant analysis with clinicopathological and DNA flow cytometric data. *Gynecol Obstet Invest* 27:213, 1989.

53. **Murray K, Hopwood L, Volk D, et al:** Cytofluorometric analysis of the DNA content in ovarian cancer and its relation to patient survival. *Cancer* 63:2456, 1989.

54. **Volm M, Bruggemann A, Gunther M, et al:** Prognostic relevance of ploidy, proliferation and resistance predictive tests in ovarian carcinoma. *Cancer Res* 45:5180, 1985.

55. **Friedlander ML, Russell P, Taylor IN, et al:** Flow cytometric analysis of cellular DNA content as an adjunct to the diagnosis of ovarian tumours of borderline malignancy. *Pathology* 16:301, 1984.

56. **Blumenfeld D, Braly PS, Ben-Ezra J, et al:** Tumor DNA content as a prognostic feature in advanced epithelial ovarian carcinoma. *Gynecol Oncol* 27:389, 1987.

57. **Khoo SK, Hurst T, Kearsley J, et al:** Prognostic significance of tumour ploidy in patients with advanced ovarian carcinoma. *Gynecol Oncol* 39:284, 1990.

58. **Kallioniemi OP, Punnonen R, Mattila J, et al:** Prognostic significance of DNA index, multiploidy and S-phase fraction in ovarian cancer. *Cancer* 61:334, 1988.

59. **Wils J, van Guens H, Baak J:** Proposal for therapeutic approach based on prognostic factors including morphometric and flow-cytometric features in stage III-IV ovarian cancer. *Cancer* 61:1920, 1988.

60. **Conte PF, Alama A, Rubagotte A, et al:** Cell kinetics in ovarian cancer: relationship to clinicopathologic features, responsiveness to chemotherapy and survival. *Cancer* 64:1188, 1989.

61. **Kuhn W, Kaufmann M, Feichter GE, et al:** DNA flow cytometry, clinical and morphological parameters as prognostic factors for advanced malignant and borderline tumors. *Gynecol Oncol* 33:360, 1989.

62. **Slamon DJ, Godolphin W, Jones LA, et al:** Studies of the HER-2/neu protooncogene in human breast and ovarian cancer. *Science* 244:707, 1989.

63. **Berchuck A, Kamel A, Whitaker R, et al:** Overexpression of HER-2/*neu* is associated with poor survival in advanced epithelial ovarian cancer. *Cancer Res* 50:4087, 1990.

64. **Rubin SC, Finstad CL, Wong GY, et al:** Prognostic significance of HER-2/*neu* expression in advanced epithelial ovarian cancer: a multivariate analysis. *Am J Obstet Gynecol* 168:162, 1993.

65. **Leary JA, Edwards BG, Houghton CRS:** Amplification of HER-2/*neu* oncogene in human ovarian cancer. *Int J Gynecol Oncol* 2:291, 1993.

66. **Dittrich C, Dittrich E, Sevelda P, et al:** Clonogenic growth in vitro: an independent biologic prognostic factor in ovarian carcinoma. *J Clin Oncol* 9:381, 1991.

67. **Hertoncello I, Bradley TR, Campbell JJ, et al:** Limitations of the clonal agar assay for the assessment of primary human ovarian tumour biopsies. *Br J Cancer* 45:803, 1982.

68. **Voest EE, van Houwelingen JC, Neijt JP:** A meta-analysis of prognostic factors in advanced ovarian cancer with median survival and overall survival measured with log (relative risk) as main objectives. *Eur J Cancer Clin Oncol* 25:711, 1989.

69. **Swenerton KD, Hislop TG, Spinelli J, et al:** Ovarian carcinoma: a multivariate analysis of prognostic factors. *Obstet Gynecol* 65:264, 1985.

70. **van Houwelingen JC, Bokkel Huinink W, van der Burg ATM, Neijt JP:** Predictability of the survival of patients with ovarian cancer. *J Clin Oncol* 7:769, 1989.

71. **Omura GA, Brady MF, Homesley HD, et al:** Long-term follow-up and prognostic factor analysis in advanced ovarian carcinoma: the Gynecologic Oncology Group experience. *J Clin Oncol* 9:1138, 1991.

72. **Dembo AJ, Davy M, Stenwig AE:** Prognostic factors in patients with stage I epithelial ovarian cancer. *Obstet Gynecol* 75:263, 1990.

73. **Berek JS, Hacker NF:** Staging and second-look operations in ovarian cancer. In Alberts DS, Surwit EA (eds): *Ovarian Cancer.* Boston, Martinus Nijhoff, 1985, pp 109–127.

74. **Young RC, Decker DG, Wharton JT, et al:** Staging laparotomy in early ovarian cancer. *JAMA* 250:3072, 1983.

75. **Buchsbaum HJ, Lifshitz S:** Staging and surgical evaluation of ovarian cancer. *Semin Oncol* 11:227, 1984.

76. **Yoshimuna S, Scully RE, Bell DA, Taft PD:** Correlation of ascitic fluid cytology with histologic findings before and after treatment of ovarian cancer. *Am J Obstet Gynecol* 148:716, 1984.

77. **Piver MS, Barlow JJ, Lele SB:** Incidence of subclinical metastasis in stage I and II ovarian carcinoma. *Obstet Gynecol* 52:100, 1978.

78. **Delgado G, Chun B, Caglar H:** Paraaortic lymphadenectomy in gynecologic malignancies confined to the pelvis. *Obstet Gynecol* 50:415, 1977.

79. **Rosenoff SH, Young RC, Anderson T:** Peritoneoscopy: a valuable staging tool in ovarian carcinoma. *Ann Intern Med* 83:37, 1975.

80. **Knapp RC, Friedman EA:** Aortic lymph node metastases in early ovarian cancer. *Am J Obstet Gynecol* 119:1013, 1974.

81. **Keetel WC, Pixley EL, Buchsbaum HJ:** Experience with peritoneal cytology in the management of gynecologic malignancies. *Am J Obstet Gynecol* 120:174, 1974.

82. **Creasman WT, Rutledge F:** The prognostic value of peritoneal cytology in gynecologic malignant disease. *Am J Obstet Gynecol* 110:773, 1971.

83. **Guthrie D, Davy MLJ, Phillips PR:** Study of 656 patients with "early" ovarian cancer. *Gynecol Oncol* 17:363, 1984.

84. **Bostwick DG, Tazelaar HD, Ballon SC, et al:** Ovarian epithelial tumors of borderline malignancy: a clinical and pathologic study of 109 cases. *Cancer* 58:2052, 1986.

85. **Lim-Tan SK, Cajigas HE, Scully RE:** Ovarian cystectomy for serous borderline tumors: a follow-up study of 35 cases. *Obstet Gynecol* 72:775, 1988.

86. **Hreshchyshyn MM, Park RC, Blessing JA, et al:** The role of adjuvant therapy in Stage I ovarian cancer. *Am J Obstet Gynecol* 138:139, 1980.

87. **Greene MH, Boice JD, Greer BE, et al:** Acute nonlymphocytic leukemia after therapy with alkylating agents for ovarian cancer. *N Engl J Med* 307:1416, 1982.

88. **Young RC, Knapp RC, Di Saia PJ, Fuks Z:** Cancer of the ovary. In DeVita VT, Hellman S, Rosenberg SA (eds): *Principles and Practices of Oncology.* Philadelphia, JB Lippincott, 1985, pp 1083–1117.

89. **Dembo AJ, Bush RS, DeBoer G:** Therapy in stage I ovarian cancer. *Am J Obstet Gynecol* 14:231, 1981.

90. **Bolis G, Marsoni S, Chiari N, et al:** Cooperative randomized clinical trial for stage I ovarian carcinoma. In Conte PF, Ragni N, Rosso R, Vermorken JB (eds): *Multimodal Treatment of Ovarian Cancer.* New York, Raven Press, 1989, p 87.

91. **Piver MS, Barlow JJ, Lele SB, et al:** Intraperitoneal chromic phosphate in peritoneoscopically confirmed Stage I ovarian adenocarcinoma. *Am J Obstet Gynecol* 144:836, 1982.

92. **Dembo AJ, Bush RS, Beale FA, et al:** The Princess Margaret Hospital Study of Ovarian Cancer: stages I, II and asymptomatic III presentations. *Cancer Treat Rep* 63:149, 1979.

93. **Griffiths CT:** Surgical resection of tumor bulk in the primary treatment of ovarian carcinoma. *Natl Cancer Inst Monogr* 42:101, 1975.

94. **Hacker NF, Berek JS:** Cytoreductive surgery in ovarian cancer. In Albert PS, Surwit EA (eds): *Ovarian Cancer.* Boston, Martinus Nijhoff, 1986, pp 53–67.

95. **Heintz APM, Berek JS:** Cytoreductive surgery in ovarian cancer. In Piver MS (ed): *Ovarian Cancer.* Edinburgh, Churchill Livingstone, 1987, pp 129–143.

96. **Hacker NF, Berek JS, Lagasse LD, et al:** Primary cytoreductive surgery for epithelial ovarian cancer. *Obstet Gynecol* 61:413, 1983.

97. **Van Lindert AM, Alsbach GJ, Barents JW, et al:** The role of the abdominal radical tumor reduction procedure (ARTR) in the treatment of ovarian cancer. In Heintz APM, Griffiths CT, Trimbos JB (eds): *Surgery in Gynecologic Oncology.* The Hague, Netherlands, Martinus Nijhoff, 1984, pp 275–287.

98. **Hoskins WJ, Bundy BN, Thigpen TJ, Omura GA:** The influence of cytoreductive surgery on recurrence-free interval and survival in small volume stage III epithelial ovarian cancer: a Gynecologic Oncology Group study. *Gynecol Oncol* 47:159, 1992.

99. **Farias-Eisner R, Teng F, Oliveira M, et al:** The influence of tumor grade, distribution and extent of carcinomatosis in minimal residual epithelial ovarian cancer after optimal primary cytoreductive surgery. *Proc Soc Gynecol Oncol* 24:26, 1993.

100. **Skipper HE:** Adjuvant chemotherapy. *Cancer* 41:936, 1978.

101. **Goldie JH, Coldman AJ:** A mathematical model for relating the drug sensitivity of tumors to their spontaneous mutation rate. *Cancer Treat Rep* 63:1727, 1979.

102. **Bookman M, Berek JS:** Biologic and immunologic therapy of ovarian cancer. *Hematol Oncol Clin North Am* 6:941, 1992.

103. **Hunter RW, Alexander NDE, Soutter WP:** Meta-analysis of surgery in advanced ovarian carcinoma: is maximum cytoreductive surgery an independent determinant of prognosis. *Am J Obstet Gynecol* 166:504, 1992.

104. **van der Burg MEL, van Lent M, Kobierska A, et al:** Interval debulking surgery does improve survival in advanced epithelial ovarian cancer: an EROTC Gynecologic Cancer Cooperative Group study. *Proc Am Soc Clin Oncol* 29:818, 1993.

105. **Hudson CN:** Surgical treatment of ovarian cancer. *Gynecol Oncol* 1:370, 1973.

106. **Berek JS, Hacker NF, Lagasse LD:** Rectosigmoid colectomy and reanastamosis to facilitate resection of primary and recurrent gynecologic cancer. *Obstet Gynecol* 64:715, 1984.

107. **Berek JS, Hacker NF, Lagasse LD:** Lower urinary tract resection as part of cytoreductive surgery for ovarian cancer. *Gynecol Oncol* 13:87, 1982.

108. **Heintz AM, Hacker NF, Berek JS, et al:** Cytoreductive surgery in ovarian carcinoma: feasibility and morbidity. *Obstet Gynecol* 67:783, 1986.

109. **Deppe G, Malviya VK, Boike G, Hampton A:** Surgical approach to diaphragmatic metastases from ovarian cancer. *Gynecol Oncol* 24:258, 1986.

110. **Montz FJ, Schlaerth J, Berek JS:** Resection of diaphragmatic peritoneum and muscle: role in cytoreductive surgery for ovarian carcinoma. *Gynecol Oncol* 35:338, 1989.

111. **Brand E, Pearlman N:** Electrosurgical debulking of ovarian cancer: a new technique using the argon beam coagulator. *Gynecol Oncol* 39:115, 1990.

112. **Deppe G, Malviya VK, Boike G, Malone JM, Jr:** Use of Cavitron surgical aspirator for debulking of diaphragmatic metastases in patients with advanced carcinoma of the ovaries. *Surg Gynecol Obstet* 168:455, 1989.

113. **Chen SS, Bochner R:** Assessment of morbidity and mortality in primary cytoreductive surgery for advanced ovarian cancer. *Gynecol Oncol* 20:190, 1985.

114. **Venesmaa P, Ylikorkala O:** Morbidity and mortality associated with primary and repeat operations for ovarian cancer. *Obstet Gynecol* 79:168, 1992.

115. **Smith JP, Day TG:** Review of ovarian cancer at the University of Texas Systems Cancer Center, M.D. Anderson Hospital and Tumor Institute. *Am J Obstet Gynecol* 135:984, 1979.

116. **Thigpen JT:** Single agent chemotherapy in the management of ovarian carcinoma. In Alberts DS, Surwit EA (eds): *Ovarian Cancer.* Boston, Martinus Nijhoff, 1985, pp 115–146.

117. **Rowinsky EK, Czaenave LA, Donehower RC:** Taxol: a novel investigational antimicrotubule agent. *J Natl Cancer Inst* 82:247, 1990.

118. **Ozols RF:** Chemotherapy for advanced epithelial ovarian cancer. *Hematol Oncol Clin North Am* 6:879, 1992.

119. **McGuire WP, Rowinski EK, Rosensheim NE, et al:** Taxol: a unique antineoplastic agent with significant activity in advanced ovarian epithelial neoplasms. *Ann Intern Med* 111:273, 1989.

120. **Thigpen T, Blessing J, Ball H, et al:** Phase II trial of Taxol as a second-line therapy for ovarian carcinoma: a Gynecologic Oncology Group study. *Proc Am Soc Clin Oncol* 9:156, 1990.

121. **McGuire WP, Hoskins WJ, Brady MF, et al:** A phase III trial comparing cisplatin/cytoxan (PC) and cisplatin/taxol (PT) in advanced ovarian cancer. *Proc Am Soc Clin Oncol* 29:808, 1993.

122. **Manetta A, MacNeill C, Lyter JA, et al:** Hexamethylamelamine as a second-line agent in ovarian cancer. *Gynecol Oncol* 36:93, 1990.

123. **Ozols RF, Ostchega Y, Curt G, Young RC:** High-dose carboplatin in refractory ovarian cancer patients. *J Clin Oncol* 5:197, 1987.

124. **Markman M, Rothman R, Hakes J, et al:** Second-line platinum therapy in patients with ovarian cancer previously treated with cisplatin. *J Clin Oncol* 9:389, 1991.

125. **Advanced Ovarian Cancer Trialists Group:** Chemotherapy in advanced ovarian cancer: an overview of randomized clinical trials. *Br Med J* 303:884, 1991.

126. **Young RC, Chabner BA, Hubbard SP, et al:** Advanced ovarian adenocarcinoma: a prospective clinical trial of melphalan (L-PAM) versus combination chemotherapy. *N Engl J Med* 299:1261, 1978.

127. **Lambert HE, Berry RJ:** High dose cisplatin compared with high dose cyclophosphamide in the management of advanced epithelial ovarian cancer (FIGO Stages III and IV): report from the North Thames Cooperative Group. *Br Med J* 290:889, 1985.

128. **Greco FA, Julian CG, Richardson RL:** Advanced ovarian cancer: brief intensive combination chemotherapy and second-look laparotomy. *Obstet Gynecol* 58:202, 1981.

129. **Neijt JP, van der Burg ME, Vriesendorp R, et al:** Randomized trial comparing two combination chemotherapy regions (Hexa-CAF vs. CHAP-5) in advanced ovarian carcinoma. *Cancer* 2:594, 1984.

130. **Ehrlich EC, Einhorn L, Williams SD, et al:** Chemotherapy for stage III-IV epithelial ovarian cancer with cis-dichlorodiamineplatinum (II), Adriamycin, and cyclophosphamide: a preliminary report. *Cancer Treat Rep* 63:281, 1979.

131. **Neijt JP, ten Bokkel Huinink WW, van der Burg MET, et al:** Randomized trial comparing two combination chemotherapy regimens (CHAP-5 versus CP) in advanced ovarian carcinoma: a randomized trial of the Netherlands joint study group for ovarian cancer. *J Clin Oncol* 5:1157, 1987.

132. **Edmonson JH, McCormack GW, Weiand HS:** Late emerging survival differences in a comparative study of HCAP versus CP in stage III-IV ovarian carcinoma. In Salmon S (ed): *Adjuvant Therapy of Cancer.* Philadelphia, WB Saunders, 1990, pp 512–521.

133. **Hainsworth JD, Grosh WW, Burnett LS, et al:** Advanced ovarian cancer: long term results of treatment with intensive cisplatin based chemotherapy of brief duration. *Ann Intern Med* 108:165, 1988.

134. **Omura G, Bundy B, Berek JS, et al:** Randomized trial of cyclophosphamide plus cisplatin with or without doxorubicin in ovarian carcinoma: a Gynecologic Oncology Group study. *J Clin Oncol* 7:457, 1989.

135. **Bertelsen K, Jacobsen A, Andersen JE, et al:** A randomized study of cyclophosphamide and cisplatin with or without doxorubicin in advanced ovarian cancer. *Gynecol Oncol* 28:161, 1987.

136. **Conte PF, Brazzone M, Chiara S, et al:** A randomized trial comparing cisplatin plus cyclophosphamide versus cisplatin, doxorubicin and cyclophosphamide in advanced ovarian cancer. *J Clin Oncol* 4:965, 1986.

137. **Gruppo Interegionale Cooperativo Oncologico Ginecologia:** Randomized comparison of cisplatin with cyclophosphamide/cisplatin with cyclophosphamide/doxorubicin/cisplatin in advanced ovarian cancer. *Lancet* 2:353, 1987.

138. **Ovarian Cancer Meta-Analysis Project:** Cyclophosphamide plus cisplatin versus cyclophosphamide, doxorubicin, and cisplatin chemotherapy of ovarian carcinoma: a meta-analysis. *J Clin Oncol* 9:1668, 1991.

139. **McGuire WP, Hoskins WJ, Brady MS, et al:** A phase III trial of dose-intensive versus standard dose cisplatin and Cytoxan in advanced ovarian cancer. *Proc Int Gynecol Cancer Soc* 3:35, 1991.

140. **Kaye SB, Lewis CR, Paul J, et al:** Randomized study of two doses of cisplatin with cyclophosphamide in epithelial ovarian cancer. *Lancet* 340:329, 1992.

141. **ten Bokkel Huinink WW, van der Burg MET, van Oosterom AT, et al:** Carboplatin in combination therapy for ovarian cancer. *Cancer Treat Rev* 15:9, 1988.

142. **Calvert AH, Newall DR, Gumbrell LA, et al:** Carboplatin dosage: prospective evaluation of a simple formula based on renal function. *J Clin Oncol* 7:1748, 1989.

143. **Alberts DS, Green S, Hannigan EV, et al:** Improved therapeutic index of carboplatin plus cyclophosphamide versus cisplatin plus cyclophosphamide: final report by the Southwest Oncology Group of a phase III randomized trial in stages III (suboptimal) and IV ovarian cancer. *J Clin Oncol* 10:706, 1992.

144. **Swenerton K, Jeffrey J, Stuart G, et al:** Cisplatin-cyclophosphamide versus carboplatin-cyclophosphamide in advanced ovarian cancer: a randomized phase III study of the National Cancer Institute of Canada Clinical Trials Group. *J Clin Oncol* 10:718, 1992.

145. **Sarosy G, Kohn E, Stone DA, et al:** Phase I study of Taxol and granulocyte colony-stimulating factor in patients with refractory ovarian cancer. *J Clin Oncol* 10:1165, 1992.

146. **Reed E, Janik J, Bookman MA, et al:** High-dose carboplatin and recombinant granulocyte–macrophage colony-stimulating factor in advanced-stage recurrent ovarian cancer. *J Clin Oncol* 11:2118, 1993.

147. **Rothenberg ML, Ozols RF, Glatstein E, et al:** Dose-intensive induction therapy with cyclophosphamide, cisplatin and consolidative abdominal radiation in advanced stage epithelial cancer. *J Clin Oncol* 10:727, 1992.

148. **Rendina GM, Donadio C, Giovanni M:** Steroid receptors and progestinic therapy in ovarian endometrioid carcinoma. *Eur J Gynaecol Oncol* 3:241, 1982.

149. **Berek JS, Hacker NF, Lagasse LD, et al:** Second-look laparotomy in stage III epithelial ovarian cancer: clinical variables associated with disease status. *Obstet Gynecol* 64:207, 1984.

150. **Schwartz PE, Smith JP:** Second-look operation in ovarian cancer. *Am J Obstet Gynecol* 138:1124, 1980.

151. **Webb MJ, Snyder JA, Williams TJ, et al:** Second-look laparotomy in ovarian cancer. *Gynecol Oncol* 14:285, 1982.

152. **Cohen CJ, Goldberg JD, Holland JF, et al:** Improved therapy with cisplatin regimens for patients with ovarian carcinoma (FIGO stages III and IV) as measured by surgical end-staging (second-look operation). *Am J Obstet Gynecol* 145:955, 1983.

153. **Barnhill DR, Hoskins JW, Heller PB, Park RC:** The second-look surgical reassessment for epithelial ovarian carcinoma. *Gynecol Oncol* 19:148, 1984.

154. **Podratz KC, Malkasian GD, Hilton JF, et al:** Second-look laparotomy in ovarian cancer: evaluation of pathologic variables. *Am J Obstet Gynecol* 152:230, 1985.

155. **Copeland LJ, Gershenson DM, Wharton JT, et al:** Microscopic disease at second-look laparotomy in advanced ovarian cancer. *Cancer* 55:472, 1985.

156. **Gershenson DM, Copeland LJ, Wharton JT, et al:** Prognosis of surgically determined complete responders in advanced ovarian cancer. *Cancer* 55:1129, 1985.

157. **Smira LR, Stehman FB, Ulbright TM, et al:** Second-look laparotomy after chemotherapy in the management of ovarian malignancy. *Am J Obstet Gynecol* 152:661, 1985.

158. **Freidman JB, Weiss NS:** Second thoughts about second-look laparotomy in advanced ovarian cancer. *N Engl J Med* 322:1079, 1990.

159. **Berek JS:** Second-look versus second-nature. *Gynecol Oncol* 44:1, 1992.

160. **Rubin SC, Hoskins WJ, Hakes TB, et al:** Recurrence after negative second-look laparotomy for ovarian cancer: analysis of risk factors. *Am J Obstet Gynecol* 159:1094, 1988.

161. **Berek JS, Griffith CT, Leventhal JM:** Laparoscopy for second-look evaluation in ovarian cancer. *Obstet Gynecol* 58:192, 1981.

162. **Berek JS, Hacker NF:** Laparoscopy in the management of patients with ovarian carcinoma. In DiSaia P (ed): *The Treatment of Ovarian Cancer.* London, WB Saunders, 1983, pp 213–222.

163. **Lele S, Piver MS:** Interval laparoscopy prior to second-look laparotomy in ovarian cancer. *Obstet Gynecol* 68:345, 1986.

164. **Berek JS, Knapp RC, Malkasian GD, et al:** CA 125 serum levels correlated with second-look operations among ovarian cancer patients. *Obstet Gynecol* 67:685, 1986.

165. **Lavin PT, Knapp RC, Malkasian GD, et al:** CA 125 for the monitoring of ovarian carcinoma during primary therapy. *Obstet Gynecol* 69:223, 1987.

166. **Brenner DE, Shaft MI, Jones HW, et al:** Abdominopelvic computed tomography: evaluation in patients undergoing second-look laparotomy for ovarian carcinoma. *Obstet Gynecol* 65:715, 1985.

167. **Berek JS, Hacker NF, Lagasse LD, et al:** Survival of patients following secondary cytoreductive surgery in ovarian cancer. *Obstet Gynecol* 61:189, 1983.

168. **Hoskins WJ, Rubin SC, Dulaney E, et al:** Influence of secondary cytoreduction at the time of second-look laparotomy on the survival of patients with epithelial ovarian carcinoma. *Gynecol Oncol* 34:365, 1989.

169. **Ozols RF, Ostchega Y, Myers CE:** High dose cisplatin in hypertonic saline in refractory ovarian cancer. *J Clin Oncol* 3:1246, 1985.

170. **Gershenson DM, Kavanagh JJ, Copeland LJ, et al:** Retreatment of patients with recurrent epithelial ovarian cancer with cisplatin-based chemotherapy. *Obstet Gynecol* 73:798, 1989.

171. **Ozols RF, Ostchega Y, Curt G, et al:** High dose carboplatin in refractory ovarian cancer patients. *J Clin Oncol* 5:197, 1987.

172. **Markman M, Rothman R, Hakes T, et al:** Second-line platinum therapy in patients with ovarian cancer previously treated with cisplatin. *J Clin Oncol* 9:389, 1991.

173. **Gore ME, Fryatt I, Wiltshaw E, Dawson T:** Treatment of relapsed carcinoma of the ovary with cisplatin or carboplatin following initial treatment with these compounds. *Gynecol Oncol* 36:207, 1990.

174. **Sutton GP, Blessing JA, Homesley HD, et al:** Phase II trial of ifosfamide and mesna in advanced ovarian carcinoma: a Gynecologic Oncology Group study. *J Clin Oncol* 7:1672, 1989.

175. **Markman M, Howell SB:** Intraperitoneal chemotherapy for ovarian cancer. In Alberts DS, Surwit EA (eds): *Ovarian Cancer.* Boston, Martinus Nijhoff, 1985, pp 179–212.

176. **Hacker NF, Berek JS, Pretorius G, et al:** Intraperitoneal cisplatin as salvage therapy in persistent epithelial ovarian cancer. *Obstet Gynecol* 70:759, 1987.

177. **Markman M, Howell SB, Lucas WE, et al:** Combination intraperitoneal chemotherapy with cisplatin, cytarabine, and doxorubicin for refractory ovarian carcinoma and other malignancies principally confined to the peritoneal cavity. *J Clin Oncol* 2:1312, 1984.

178. **King ME, Pfeiffe CE, Howell SB:** Intraperitoneal cytosine arabinoside therapy in ovarian carcinoma. *J Clin Oncol* 2:662, 1984.

179. **Howell SB, Pfeiffe CE, Wung WE, et al:** Intraperitoneal cisplatin with systemic thiosulfate protection. *Ann Intern Med* 97:845, 1982.

180. **Howell SB, Kirmani S, Lucas WE, et al:** A phase II trial of intraperitoneal cisplatin and etoposide for primary treatment of ovarian epithelial cancer. *J Clin Oncol* 8:137, 1990.

181. **Kirmani S, Lucas WE, Kim S, et al:** A phase II trial of intraperitoneal cisplatin and etoposide as salvage treatment for minimal residual ovarian carcinoma. *J Clin Oncol* 9:649, 1991.

182. **Markman M, Hakes T, Reichman B, et al:** Phase II trial of weekly or biweekly intraperitoneal mitoxantrone in epithelial ovarian cancer. *J Clin Oncol* 9:978, 1991.

183. **Howell SB, Zimm S, Markman M, et al:** Long-term survival of advanced refractory ovarian carcinoma patients with small-volume disease treated with intraperitoneal chemotherapy. *J Clin Oncol* 5:1607, 1987.

184. **Berek JS, Hacker NF, Lichtenstein A, et al:** Intraperitoneal recombinant alpha$_2$ interferon for salvage epithelial ovarian cancer immunotherapy in Stage III: a Gynecologic Oncology Group study. *Cancer Res* 45:4447, 1985.

185. **Willemse PHB, De Vries EGE, Mulder NH, et al:** Intraperitoneal human recombinant interferon alpha-2b in minimal residual ovarian cancer. *Eur J Cancer* 26:353, 1990.

186. **Nardi M, Lognetti F, Pallera F, et al:** Intraperitoneal alpha-2-interferon alternating with cisplatin as salvage therapy for minimal residual disease ovarian cancer: a phase II study. *J Clin Oncol* 6:1036, 1990.

187. **Bezwoda WR, Golombick T, Dansey R, Keeping J:** Treatment of malignant ascites due to recurrent/refractory ovarian cancer: the use of interferon-alpha or interferon-alpha plus chemotherapy. In vivo and in vitro observations. *Eur J Cancer* 27:1423, 1991.

188. **Pujade-Lauraine E, Guastella JP, Colombo N, et al:** Intraperitoneal recombinant human interferon gamma (IFNg) in residual ovarian cancer: efficacy is independent of previous response to chemotherapy. *Proc Am Soc Clin Oncol* 713:225, 1991.

189. **Steis RG, Urba WJ, Vandermolen LA, et al:** Intraperitoneal lymphokine-activated killer cell and interleukin 2 therapy for malignancies limited to the peritoneal cavity. *J Clin Oncol* 10:1618, 1990.

190. **Markman M, Berek JS, Blessing JA, et al:** Characteristics of patients with small-volume residual ovarian cancer unresponsive to cisplatin-based ip chemotherapy: lessons learned from a Gynecologic Oncology Group phase II trial of ip cisplatin and recombinant α-interferon. *Gynecol Oncol* 45:3, 1992.

191. **Ozols RF:** Intraperitoneal therapy in ovarian cancer: time's up. *J Clin Oncol* 9:197, 1991.

192. **Hacker NF, Berek JS, Juillard G, et al:** Whole abdominal radiation as salvage therapy for epithelial ovarian cancer. *Obstet Gynecol* 65:50, 1985.

193. **Shea TC, Flaherty M, Elias A, et al:** A phase I clinical pharmacokinetic study of carboplatin and autologous bone marrow support. *J Clin Oncol* 7:651, 1989.

194. **Stoppa A, Maraninchi D, Viens P, et al:** High doses of melphalan and autologous marrow rescue in advanced common epithelial ovarian carcinomas: a retrospective analysis in 35 patients. In Nicke K, Spitzer G, Zander A (eds): *Autologous Bone Marrow Transplantation: Proceedings of the Fourth International Symposium.* University of Texas Cancer Center, MD Anderson Hospital, Houston, 1989, pp 125–134.

195. **Shpall EJ, Clarke-Pearson D, Soper JT, et al:** High-dose alkylating agent chemotherapy with autologous bone marrow support in patients with stage III/IV epithelial ovarian cancer. *Gynecol Oncol* 38:386, 1990.

196. **Castaldo TW, Petrilli ES, Ballon SC, et al:** Intestinal operations in patients with ovarian carcinoma. *Am J Obstet Gynecol* 139:80, 1981.

197. **Krebs HB, Goplerud DR:** Surgical management of bowel obstruction in advanced ovarian cancer. *Obstet Gynecol* 61:237, 1983.

198. **Tunca JC, Buchler DA, Mack EA, et al:** The management of ovarian cancer caused bowel obstruction. *Gynecol Oncol* 12:186, 1981.

199. **Piver MS, Barton JJ, Lele SB, Frank A:** Survival after ovarian cancer induced intestinal obstruction. *Gynecol Oncol* 13:44, 1982.

200. **Clarke-Pearson D, DeLong EL, Chin N, et al:** Intestinal obstruction in patients with ovarian cancer: variables associated with surgical complications and survival. *Arch Surg* 123:42, 1988.

201. **Fernandes JR, Seymour RJ, Suissa S:** Bowel obstruction in patients with ovarian cancer: a search for prognostic factors. *Am J Obstet Gynecol* 158:244, 1988.

202. **Rubin SC, Hoskins WJ, Benjamin I, Lewis JJ:** Palliative surgery for intestinal obstruction in advanced ovarian cancer. *Gynecol Oncol* 34:16, 1989.

203. **Malone JJ, Koonce T, Larson DM, et al:** Palliation of small bowel obstruction by percutaneous gastrostomy in patients with progressive ovarian carcinoma. *Obstet Gynecol* 68:43, 1986.

204. **Bolis G, Marsoni S, Belloni C, et al:** Randomized comparison of cisplatin with cyclophosphamide/cisplatin and with cyclophosphamide/doxorubicin/cisplatin in advanced ovarian cancer. *Lancet* 8555:353, 1987.

375

10

Nonepithelial Ovarian and Fallopian Tube Cancers

Jonathan S. Berek
Neville F. Hacker

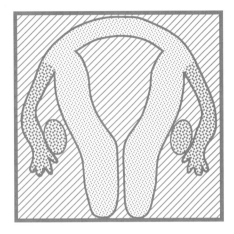

Compared with epithelial ovarian cancers, other malignant tumors of the female genital adnexal structures are uncommon. Nonepithelial ovarian cancers include malignancies of germ cell origin, sex cord-stromal cell origin, metastatic carcinomas to the ovary, and a variety of extremely rare ovarian cancers (e.g., sarcomas, lipoid cell tumors). Fallopian tube carcinomas and sarcomas are also rare.

Nonepithelial malignancies of the ovary account for about 10% of all ovarian cancers (1, 2). Although there are many similarities in the presentation, evaluation, and management of these patients, these tumors also have many unique qualities that require a special approach.

Germ Cell Malignancies

Germ cell tumors are derived from the primordial germ cells of the ovary. Their incidence is only about one-tenth the incidence of malignant germ cell tumors of the testis, so most of the advances in the management of these tumors have been extrapolations from experience with the corresponding testicular tumors. Although malignant germ cell tumors can arise in extragonadal sites such as the mediastinum and the retroperitoneum, the majority of germ cell tumors arise in the gonad from the undifferentiated germ cells. The variation in the site of these cancers is explained by the embryonic migration of the germ cells from the caudal part of the yolk sac to the dorsal mesentery before their incorporation into the sex cords of the developing gonads (3).

Classification

A histologic classification of ovarian germ cell tumors is presented in Table 10.1 (4). Both α-fetoprotein (AFP) and human chorionic gonadotropin (hCG) are secreted by some germ cell malignancies; therefore, the presence of circulating

377

Table 10.1   Histologic Typing of Ovarian Germ Cell Tumors

1. *Dysgerminoma*

2. *Teratoma*
   A. Immature
   B. Mature
       (1) Solid
       (2) Cystic
           a. Dermoid cyst (mature cystic teratoma)
           b. Dermoid cyst with malignant transformation
   C. Monodermal and highly specialized
       (1) Struma ovarii
       (2) Carcinoid
       (3) Struma ovarii and carcinoid
       (4) Others

3. *Endodermal sinus tumor*

4. *Embryonal carcinoma*

5. *Polyembryoma*

6. *Choriocarcinoma*

7. *Mixed forms*

Reproduced, with permission, from Serov SF, Scully RE, Robin IH: Histological Typing of Ovarian Tumors: *International Histological Classification of Tumors*, No. 9, Geneva, World Health Organization, 1973.

hormones can be clinically useful in the diagnosis of a pelvic mass and in monitoring the course of a patient after surgery. Placental alkaline phosphatase (PLAP) and lactate dehydrogenase (LDH) are commonly produced by dysgerminomas and may be useful for monitoring the disease. α-1-antitrypsin (AAT) can be detected rarely in association with germ cell tumors. When the histologic and immunohistologic identification of these substances in tumors is correlated, a classification of germ cell tumors emerges (Fig. 10.1) (5).

In this scheme, embryonal carcinoma, which is a cancer composed of undifferentiated cells, synthesizes both hCG and AFP, and this lesion is the progenitor of several other germ cell tumors (3, 5). More differentiated germ cell tumors, such as the endodermal sinus tumor, which secretes AFP, and the choriocarcinoma, which secretes hCG, are derived from the extraembryonic tissues; the immature teratomas derived from the embryonic cells have lost the ability to secrete these substances. Pure germinomas do not secrete these markers.

Epidemiology

Although 20–25% of all benign and malignant ovarian neoplasms are of germ cell origin, only about 3% of these tumors are malignant (1). Germ cell malignancies account for fewer than 5% of all ovarian cancers in Western countries. Germ cell malignancies represent up to 15% of ovarian cancers in Oriental and black societies, where epithelial ovarian cancers are much less common.

In the first two decades of life, almost 70% of ovarian tumors are of germ cell origin, and one-third of these are malignant (1, 2). Germ cell tumors account for two-thirds of the ovarian malignancies in this age group. Germ cell cancers also are seen in the third decade, but thereafter they become quite rare.

Clinical Features

Symptoms

In contrast to the relatively slow-growing epithelial ovarian tumors, germ cell malignancies grow rapidly and often are characterized by subacute pelvic pain

378

related to capsular distention, hemorrhage, or necrosis. The rapidly enlarging pelvic mass may produce pressure symptoms on the bladder or rectum, and menstrual irregularities also may occur in menarchal patients. Some young patients may misinterpret the early symptoms of a neoplasm as those of pregnancy, and this can lead to a delay in the diagnosis. Acute symptoms associated with torsion or rupture of the adnexa can develop. These symptoms may be confused

Figure 10.1   Relationship between examples of pure malignant germ cell tumors and their secreted marker substances.

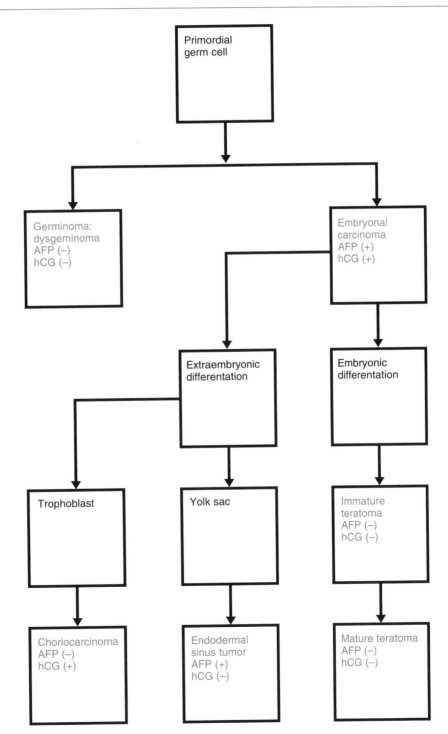

with acute appendicitis. In more advanced cases, ascites may develop, and the patient can have abdominal distention (3).

Signs

In patients with a palpable adnexal mass, the evaluation can proceed as outlined in Chapter 9. Some patients with germ cell tumors will be premenarchal and may require examination under anesthesia. If the lesions are principally solid or a combination of solid and cystic, as might be noted on an ultrasonographic evaluation, a neoplasm is probable and a malignancy is possible (Fig. 10.2). The remainder of the physical examination should search for signs of ascites, pleural effusion, and organomegaly.

Diagnosis

Adnexal masses measuring 2 cm or larger in premenarchal girls or 8 cm or larger in other premenopausal patients will usually require surgical exploration (Fig. 10.3). In young patients, blood tests should include serum hCG and AFP titers, a complete blood count, and liver function tests. A radiograph of the chest is important because germ cell tumors can metastasize to the lungs or mediastinum. A karyotype should be obtained preoperatively on all premenarchal girls because of the propensity of these tumors to arise in dysgenetic gonads. A preoperative computed tomography (CT) scan or magnetic resonance imaging (MRI) may document the presence and extent of retroperitoneal lymphadenopathy or liver metastases; however, because these patients require surgical exploration, such extensive and time-consuming evaluation is unnecessary. If postmenarchal pa-

Figure 10.2 Dysgerminoma of the ovary. Note that the lesion is principally solid with some cystic areas.

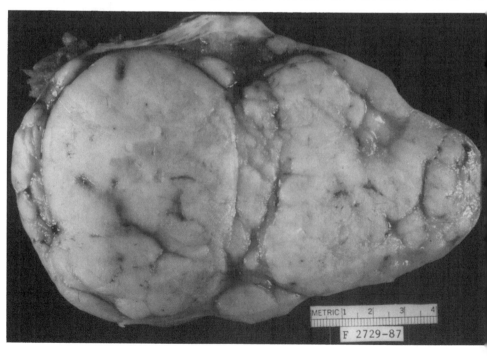

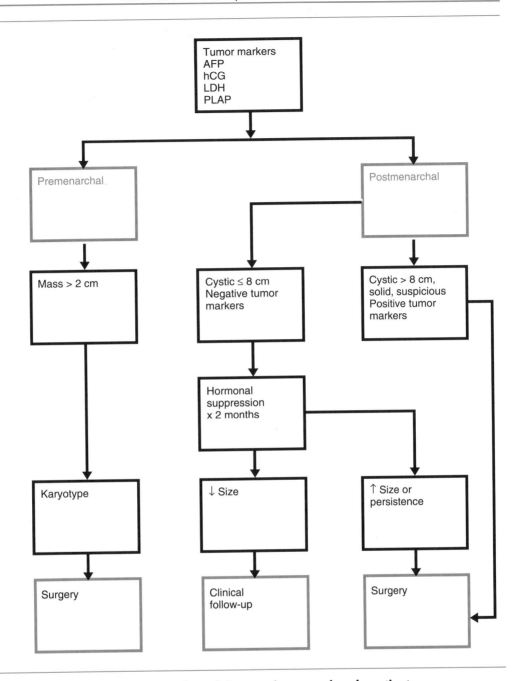

Figure 10.3 Evaluation of a pelvic mass in young female patients.

tients have predominantly cystic lesions up to 8 cm in diameter, they may undergo a trial of hormonal suppression for two cycles (6).

Dysgerminoma

The dysgerminoma is the most common malignant germ cell tumor, accounting for about 30–40% of all ovarian cancers of germ cell origin (2, 5). The tumors represent only 1–3% of all ovarian cancers, but they represent as many as 5–10% of ovarian cancers in patients younger than 20 years of age. Seventy-five percent of dysgerminomas occur between the ages of 10 and 30 years, 5% occur under the age of 10 years, and they rarely occur over the age of 50 years (1, 3). Because these malignancies occur in young women, 20–30% of ovarian malignancies associated with pregnancy are dysgerminomas.

Approximately 5% of dysgerminomas are discovered in phenotypic females with abnormal gonads (1). This malignancy can be associated with patients who have pure gonadal dysgenesis (46XY, bilateral streak gonads), mixed gonadal dysgenesis (45X/46XY, unilateral streak gonad, contralateral testis), and the androgen insensitivity syndrome (46XY, testicular feminization). Therefore, in premenarchal patients with a pelvic mass the karyotype should be determined.

In most patients with gonadal dysgenesis, dysgerminomas arise in gonadoblastomas, which are benign ovarian tumors that are composed of germ cells and sex cord stroma. If gonadoblastomas are left *in situ* in patients with gonadal dysgensis, more than 50% will develop into ovarian malignancies (7).

About 75% of dysgerminomas are Stage I (i.e., confined to one or both ovaries) at diagnosis (8–11). About 85–90% of Stage I tumors are confined to one ovary; 10–15% are bilateral. In fact, dysgerminoma is the only germ cell malignancy that has this significant rate of bilaterality, other germ cell tumors being rarely bilateral.

In patients whose contralateral ovary has been preserved, disease can develop in 5–10% of the retained gonads over the next 2 years (1). This figure includes those not given additional therapy, as well as patients with gonadal dysgenesis.

In the 25% of patients who present with metastatic disease, the tumor most commonly spreads via the lymphatics. It can also spread hematogenously or by direct extension through the capsule of the ovary with exfoliation and dissemination of cells throughout the peritoneal surfaces. Metastases to the contralateral ovary may be present when there is no other evidence of spread. An uncommon site of metastatic disease is bone; and when metastasis to this site occurs, the lesions are seen principally in the lower vertebrae. Metastases to the lungs, liver, and brain are seen most often in patients with long-standing or recurrent disease. Metastasis to the mediastinum and supraclavicular lymph nodes is usually a late manifestation of disease.

Treatment

The treatment of patients with early dysgerminoma is primarily surgical, including resection of the primary lesion and proper surgical staging. Chemotherapy and/or radiation is administered to patients with metastatic disease. Because the disease principally affects young females, special consideration must be given to the preservation of fertility whenever possible. An algorithm for the management of ovarian dysgerminoma is presented in Figure 10.4.

Surgery

The minimum operation for ovarian dysgerminoma is a unilateral oophorectomy. If there is a desire to preserve fertility, the contralateral ovary, fallopian tube, and uterus should be left *in situ*, even in the presence of metastatic disease, because of the sensitivity of the tumor to chemotherapy. If fertility need not be preserved, it may be appropriate to perform a total abdominal hysterectomy and bilateral salpingo-oophorectomy in patients with advanced disease. In patients whose karyotype analysis reveals a Y chromosome, both ovaries should be removed, although the uterus may be left *in situ* for possible future embryo transfer. While cytoreductive surgery is of unproven value, bulky disease that can be readily resected (e.g., an omental cake) should be removed at the initial operation.

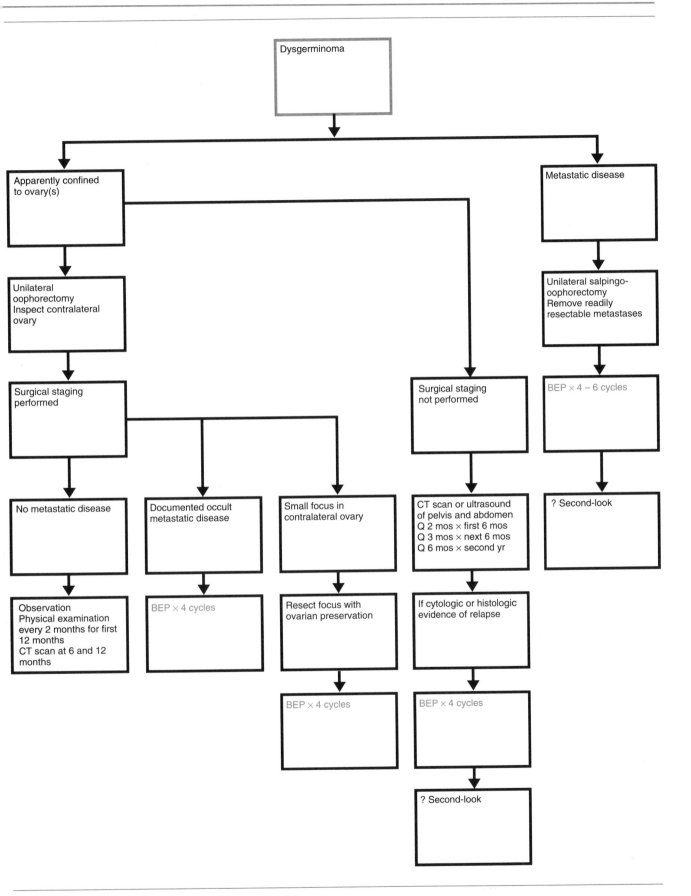

Figure 10.4   Management of dysgerminoma of the ovary.

In patients in whom the neoplasm appears on inspection to be confined to the ovary, a careful staging operation should be undertaken to determine the presence of any occult metastatic disease. All peritoneal surfaces should be inspected and palpated, and any suspicious lesions should be biopsied. Unilateral pelvic lymphadenectomy and at least careful palpation and biopsy of enlarged para-aortic nodes are particularly important parts of the staging. These tumors often metastasize to the para-aortic nodes around the renal vessels. Dysgerminoma is the only germ cell tumor that tends to be bilateral, and not all of the bilateral lesions have obvious ovarian enlargement. Therefore bisection of the contralateral ovary and excisional biopsy of any suspicious lesion are desirable (8, 9). If a small contralateral tumor is found, it may be possible to resect it and preserve some normal ovary.

Radiation

Dysgerminomas are very sensitive to radiation therapy, and doses of 2500–3500 cGy may be curative, even for gross metastatic disease. Loss of fertility is a problem with radiation therapy, however, so radiation should rarely be used as first-line treatment (12).

Chemotherapy

Many patients with a dysgerminoma will have a tumor that is apparently confined to one ovary and will be referred after unilateral salpingo-oophorectomy without surgical staging. The options for such patients are repeat laparotomy for surgical staging, regular pelvic and abdominal surveillance with CT scans, and adjuvant chemotherapy. As these are rapidly growing tumors, our preference is to perform regular CT surveillance. Tumor markers (AFP and βhCG) should also be monitored in case occult mixed germ cell elements are present (Figure 10.1).

There have been numerous reports of successful control of metastatic dysgerminomas with systemic chemotherapy, and this should now be regarded as the treatment of choice (12–19). **The obvious advantage is the preservation of fertility** (15).

The most frequently used chemotherapeutic regimens for germ cell tumors are BEP (bleomycin, etoposide, and cisplatin), VBP (vinblastine, bleomycin, and cisplatin), and VAC (vincristine, actinomycin, and Cytoxan) (14–20) (Table 10.2). The Gynecologic Oncology Group (GOG) is currently studying 3 cycles of carboplatin (400 mg/M^2 intravenously on day 1 every 4 weeks) and etoposide (120 mg/M^2 intravenously on days 1, 2, and 3 every 4 weeks) for patients with completely resected ovarian dysgerminoma, Stages Ib, Ic, II, or III (19).

For patients with advanced, incompletely resected germ cell tumors, the GOG studied cisplatin-based chemotherapy on two consecutive protocols. In the first study, patients received 4 cycles of vinblastine (12 mg/M^2 every 3 weeks), bleomycin (20 units/M^2 intravenously every week for 12 weeks), and cisplatin (20 mg/M^2/day intravenously for 5 days every 3 weeks). Patients with persistent or progressive disease at second-look laparotomy were treated with 6 cycles of VAC. In the second ongoing trial, patients received 3 cycles of BEP initially, followed by consolidation with VAC, which was later discontinued in patients with dysgerminomas (17). The VAC consolidation after BEP in patients with tumors other than dysgerminoma is still being investigated, but VAC does not appear to improve the outcome of the BEP regimen (20). A total of 20 evaluable

Table 10.2   Combination Chemotherapy for Germ Cell Tumors of the Ovary

Regimen & Drugs	Dose & Schedule*
BEP	
Bleomycin	15 units/M²/week × 5; then on day 1 of course 4
Etoposide	100 mg/M²/day × 5 days every 3 weeks
Cisplatin	20 mg/M²/day × 5 days, or 100 mg/M²/day × 1 day every 3 weeks
VBP	
Vinblastine	0.15 mg/kg days 1 and 2 every 3 weeks
Bleomycin	15 units/M²/week × 5; then on day 1 of course 4
Cisplatin	100 mg/M² on day 1 every 3 weeks
VAC	
Vincristine	1–1.5 mg/M² on day 1 every 4 weeks
Actinomycin-D	0.5 mg/day × 5 days every 4 weeks
Cytoxan	150 mg/M²/day × 5 days every 4 weeks

*All doses given intravenously.

patients with Stage III and IV dysgerminoma were treated in these two protocols, and 19 are alive and free of disease after 6 to 68 months (median = 26 months) (17). Fourteen of these patients had a second-look laparotomy, and all findings were negative. Another study at M.D. Anderson Hospital (18) used BEP in 14 patients with residual disease, and all patients were free of disease with long-term follow-up. These results suggest that patients with advanced-stage, incompletely resected dysgerminoma have an excellent prognosis when treated with cisplatin-based combination chemotherapy. The optimal regimen is unknown, but 3–4 cycles of BEP seems sufficient.

There appears to be no need to perform a second-look laparotomy in patients with dysgerminoma whose macroscopic disease has all been resected at the primary operation (12). In patients with macroscopic residual disease at the start of chemotherapy, we prefer to perform a second-look operation because second-line therapy is available and the earlier persistent disease is identified, the better the prognosis should be.

Recurrent Disease

About 75% of recurrences occur within the first year after initial treatment (3), the most common sites being the peritoneal cavity and the retroperitoneal lymph nodes. These patients should be treated with either radiation or chemotherapy, depending on their primary treatment. Patients with recurrent disease who have had no therapy other than surgery should be treated with chemotherapy. If prior chemotherapy with BEP has been given, POMB-ACE may be used (Table 10.3), and consideration should be given to the use of high-dose chemotherapy (e.g., with carboplatin and etoposide) and autologous bone marrow transplantation. Alternatively, radiation therapy is effective for this disease, with the major disadvantage being loss of fertility if pelvic and abdominal radiation is required.

Pregnancy

Because dysgerminomas tend to occur in young patients, they may coexist with pregnancy. When a Stage Ia cancer is found, the tumor can be removed intact and the pregnancy continued. In patients with more advanced disease, continuation of the pregnancy will depend on gestational age. Chemotherapy can be given in the second and third trimesters in the same dosages as given for the nonpregnant patient without apparent detriment to the fetus (14).

385

Table 10.3   POMB/ACE Chemotherapy For Germ Cell Tumors of the Ovary

POMB	
Day 1	Vincristine 1 mg/M² intravenously; methotrexate 300 mg/M² as a 12 hr infusion
Day 2	Bleomycin 15 mg as a 24 hr infusion: folinic acid rescue started at 24 hrs after the start of methotrexate in a dose of 15 mg every 12 hrs for 4 doses
Day 3	Bleomycin infusion 15 mg by 24 hr infusion
Day 4	Cisplatin 120 mg/M² as a 12 hr infusion, given together with hydration and 3 g magnesium sulfate supplementation
ACE	
Days 1–5	Etoposide (VP16-213) 100 mg/M², days 1 to 5
Day 3, 4, 5	Actinomycin D 0.5 mg IV, days 3, 4, and 5
Day 5	Cyclophosphamide 500 mg/M² IV, day 5
OMB	
Day 1	Vincristine 1 mg/M² intravenously; methotrexate 300 mg/M² as a 12 hr infusion
Day 2	Bleomycin 15 mg by 24 hr infusion; folinic acid rescue started at 24 hrs after start of methotrexate in a dose of 15 mg every 12 hrs for 4 doses
Day 3	Bleomycin 15 mg by 24 hr infusion

The sequence of treatment schedules is two courses of POMB followed by ACE. POMB is then alternated with ACE until patients are in biochemical remission as measured by hCG and AFP, PLAP and LDH. The usual number of courses of POMB is three to five. Following biochemical remission, patients alternate ACE with OMB until remission has been maintained for approximately 12 weeks. The interval between courses of treatment is kept to the minimum (usually 9 to 11 days). If delays are caused by myelosuppression after courses of ACE, the first 2 days of etoposide are omitted from subsequent courses of ACE. (Reproduced, with permission, from Newlands ES, et al: In Williams CJ, et al: *Textbook of Uncommon Cancer.* New York, John Wiley & Sons, 1988.)

Prognosis

In patients whose initial disease is Stage Ia (i.e., a unilateral encapsulated dysgerminoma), unilateral oophorectomy alone results in a 5-year disease-free survival rate of greater than 95% (11–14, 19). The features that have been associated with a higher tendency to recurrence include lesions larger than 10–15 cm in diameter, age younger than 20 years, and a microscopic pattern that includes numerous mitoses, anaplasia, and a medullary pattern (2, 11).

Although in the past surgery for advanced disease followed by pelvic and abdominal radiation resulted in a 5-year survival rate of 63–83%, cure rates of 85–90% for this same group of patients are now being reported with the use of VBP or BEP combination chemotherapy (16–20).

Immature Teratomas

Immature teratomas contain elements that resemble tissues derived from the embryo. Immature teratomatous elements may occur in combination with other germ cell tumors as mixed germ cell tumors. The pure immature teratoma accounts for fewer than 1% of all ovarian cancers, but it is the second most common germ cell malignancy. This lesion represents 10–20% of all ovarian malignancies seen in females under 20 years of age and 30% of the deaths from ovarian cancer in this age group (1). About 50% of pure immature teratomas of the ovary occur between the ages of 10 and 20 years, and they rarely occur in postmenopausal women. Immature teratomas are classified according to a grading system (grades 1–3) that is based on the degree of differentiation and the quantity of immature tissue (21).

Diagnosis

The preoperative evaluation and differential diagnosis are the same as for patients with other germ cell tumors. Some of these lesions will contain calcifications

386

similar to mature teratomas, and this can be detected by a radiograph of the abdomen or by ultrasonography. Rarely, they are associated with the production of steroid hormones and can be accompanied by *sexual pseudoprecosity* (3). Tumor markers are negative unless a mixed germ cell tumor is present.

Treatment

Surgery

In a premenopausal patient whose lesion appears confined to a single ovary, unilateral oophorectomy and surgical staging should be performed. In postmenopausal patients a total abdominal hysterectomy and bilateral salpingo-oophorectomy may be performed. Contralateral involvement is rare, and routine resection or wedge biopsy of the contralateral ovary is unnecessary (21). Any lesions on the peritoneal surfaces should be sampled and submitted for histologic evaluation. The most frequent site of dissemination is the peritoneum and, much less commonly, the retroperitoneal lymph nodes. Blood-borne metastases to organ parenchyma, such as the lungs, liver, or brain, are uncommon. When present, they are usually seen in patients with late or recurrent disease and most often in tumors that are poorly differentiated (i.e., grade 3) (3).

Chemotherapy

Patients with Stage Ia, grade 1, tumors have an excellent prognosis, and no adjuvant therapy is required. In patients whose tumors are Stage Ia, grades 2 or 3, adjuvant chemotherapy should be used (3, 22). Chemotherapy is also indicated in patients who have ascites regardless of tumor grade.

The most frequently used combination chemotherapeutic regimen in the past has been VAC (14, 19, 23–26). However, in a GOG study, the relapse-free survival rate in patients with incompletely resected disease was only 75% (3, 25).

The newer approach has been to incorporate cisplatin into the primary treatment of these tumors, and most of the experience has been with the VBP and BEP regimens (16, 19, 20). No direct comparison of these regimens with VAC has been reported, but the BEP combination can save some patients who have persistent or recurrent disease after VAC (20, 26, 27).

The GOG has been prospectively studying three courses of BEP therapy in patients with completely resected Stage I, II, and III ovarian germ cell tumors (28). Overall, the toxicity has been acceptable, and all 38 patients with nondysgerminomatous tumors treated (19 immature teratomas, 10 mixed, and 9 endodermal sinus tumors) are clinically free of disease. Thus the BEP regimen, which is used more extensively for testicular cancer, appears to be superior to the VAC regimen in the treatment of completely resected nondysgerminomatous germ cell tumors of the ovary. Because some patients can progress rapidly, treatment should be initiated as soon as possible after surgery, preferably within 7 to 10 days (19).

The switch from VBP to BEP has been prompted by the experience in patients with testicular cancer, where the replacement of vinblastine with etoposide has been associated with a better therapeutic index (i.e., equivalent efficacy and lower morbidity), especially less neurologic and gastrointestinal toxicity. Furthermore, the use of bleomycin appears to be important in this group of patients. In a randomized study of three cycles of etoposide plus cisplatin with

387

or without bleomycin (EP versus BEP) in 166 patients with germ cell tumors of the testes, the BEP regimen had a relapse-free survival rate of 84% compared with 69% for the EP regimen ($p = 0.03$) (29). **In addition, cisplatin may be slightly better than carboplatin in the setting of metastatic germ cell tumors.** One hundred ninety-two patients with germ cell tumors of the testes were entered into a study of 4 cycles of etoposide plus cisplatin (EP) versus 4 cycles of etoposide plus carboplatin (EC). There have been three relapses with the EP regimen versus seven with the EC regimen, although the overall survival of the two groups is identical thus far (30). **In view of these results, BEP is the preferred treatment regimen for patients with gross residual disease and is replacing the VAC regimen for patients with completely resected disease.**

Immature teratomas with malignant squamous elements appear to have a poorer prognosis than those tumors without these elements (31). The treatment in these patients is identical (i.e., chemotherapy with BEP regimen).

Radiation

Radiation therapy is generally not used in the primary treatment of patients with immature teratomas. Furthermore, there is no evidence that the combination of chemotherapy and radiation has a higher rate of disease control than chemotherapy alone. Radiation should be reserved for patients with localized persistent disease after chemotherapy (14, 21).

Second-Look Laparotomy   The need for a second-look operation has been questioned (3). It seems not to be justified in patients who have received chemotherapy in an adjuvant setting (i.e., Stage Ia, grades 2 and 3), because chemotherapy in these patients is so effective. We continue to prefer second-look laparotomy in patients with macroscopic residual disease at the start of chemotherapy, because there are no reliable tumor markers for this disease and such patients are at higher risk of failure (19, 32).

If a second-look operation is performed, careful sampling of any peritoneal lesions should be performed and the retroperitoneal lymph nodes should be evaluated carefully. If only mature elements are found at the second look, chemotherapy should be discontinued. If persistent immature elements are documented, alternative chemotherapy should be employed. An enlarged contralateral ovary may contain a benign cyst or a mature cystic teratoma, which may be managed with an ovarian cystectomy (3).

Prognosis   The most important prognostic feature of the immature teratoma is the grade of the lesion (1, 13, 33). In addition, the stage of disease and the extent of tumor at the initiation of treatment also have an impact on the curability of the lesion. Patients whose tumors have been incompletely resected before treatment have a significantly lower probability of 5-year survival than those whose lesions have been completely resected (i.e., 94% versus 50%) (3). Overall, the 5-year survival rate for patients with all stages of pure immature teratomas is 70–80%, and it is 90–95% for patients with surgical Stage I lesions (19–22).

The degree or grade of immaturity generally predicts the metastatic potential and curability. The 5-year survival rates have been reported to be 82%, 62%, and

30% for patients with grades 1, 2, and 3, respectively (21). Occasionally, these tumors are associated with mature or low-grade glial elements that have implanted throughout the peritoneum, and such patients usually have a favorable long-term survival (3).

Endodermal Sinus Tumor

Endodermal sinus tumors (EST) have also been referred to as "yolk sac carcinomas," because they are derived from the primitive yolk sac (2). These lesions are the third most frequent malignant germ cell tumors of the ovary.

Endodermal sinus tumors have a median age of 18 years (3). About one-third of the patients are premenarchal at the time of initial presentation. Abdominal and/or pelvic pain is the most frequent presenting symptom, occurring in about 75% of patients, whereas an asymptomatic pelvic mass is documented in 10% of patients (18).

Most EST lesions secrete α-fetoprotein (AFP), and rarely they may elaborate detectable α-1-antitrypsin (AAT). There is a good correlation between the extent of disease and the level of AFP, although discordance also has been observed. The serum level of these markers, particularly AFP, is useful in monitoring the patient's response to treatment (33, 34).

Treatment

Surgery

The treatment of the EST consists of surgical exploration, unilateral salpingo-oophorectomy, and a frozen section for diagnosis. The addition of a hysterectomy and contralateral salpingo-oophorectomy does not alter outcome (3, 12). Any gross metastases should be removed if possible, but thorough surgical staging is not indicated because all patients need chemotherapy. At surgery, the tumors tend to be solid and large, ranging in size from 7–28 cm (median = 15 cm) in the GOG series (3, 26, 32). Bilaterality is not seen in these lesions, and the other ovary is involved with metastatic disease only when there are other metastases in the peritoneal cavity. Most patients have early-stage disease: 71% Stage I, 6% Stage II, and 23% Stage III (23).

Chemotherapy

All patients with endodermal sinus tumors are treated with either adjuvant or therapeutic chemotherapy. Prior to the routine use of combination chemotherapy for this disease, the 2-year survival rate was only about 25%. After the introduction of the VAC regimen, this rate improved to 60–70%, indicating the chemosensitivity of the majority of these tumors (23, 24). Furthermore, with conservative surgery and adjuvant chemotherapy, fertility can be preserved as with other germ cell tumors.

VBP is a more effective regimen in the treatment of EST, particularly in the treatment of measurable or incompletely resected tumors (24, 25). In the GOG series, only about 20% of patients with residual metastatic disease responded completely to the VAC regimen, whereas about 60% of those treated with VBP had a complete response (20). In addition, this regimen may save some patients in whom VAC therapy has failed.

Workers at the Charing Cross Hospital in London have developed the POMB-ACE regimen for high-risk germ cell tumors of any histologic type (35) (Table

389

10.3). This protocol introduces seven drugs into the initial management, which is intended to minimize the chances of developing drug resistance. This is particularly relevant in patients with massive metastatic disease, and we use the POMB-ACE regimen as primary therapy for such cases as well as in patients with liver or brain metastases. The POMB schedule is only moderately myelosuppressive, so the intervals between each course can be kept to a maximum of 14 days (usually 9–11 days), thereby minimizing the time for tumor regrowth between courses. When bleomycin is given by a 48-hour infusion, pulmonary toxicity is reduced. With a maxmimum of 9 years of follow-up, the Charing Cross group has seen no long-term side effects in patients treated with POMB-ACE. Children have developed normally, menstruation has been physiologic, and several have completed normal pregnancies.

Therefore **cisplatin-containing combination chemotherapy, preferably BEP or POMB-ACE, should be used as primary chemotherapy for EST**. The optimal number of treatment cycles has not been established. The GOG protocols have used 3–4 treatment cycles given every 4 weeks (17, 19, 20). Our policy has been to give 3 cycles for patients with Stage I and completely resected disease and 2 further cycles after negative tumor marker status for patients with macroscopic residual disease prior to chemotherapy.

Second-Look Laparotomy

The value of a second-look operation has yet to be established in patients with EST. It appears that it is reasonable to omit the operation in patients with pure low-stage lesions and in patients whose AFP values return to normal and remain normal for the balance of their treatment (19, 32). There have been reported cases in which the AFP has returned to normal in spite of persistent measurable disease; some of these cases have been mixed germ cell tumors (32). In patients whose AFP titers do not return to normal, persistent disease can be assumed and alternative chemotherapy (e.g., POMB-ACE) offered.

Embryonal Carcinoma

Embryonal carcinoma of the ovary is an extremely rare tumor that is distinguished from a choriocarcinoma of the ovary by the absence of syncytiotrophoblastic and cytotrophoblastic cells. The patients are very young, their ages ranging between 4 and 28 years (median = 14 years) in two series (1, 33). Embryonal carcinomas may secrete estrogens, with the patient exhibiting symptoms and signs of precocious pseudopuberty or irregular bleeding (1). The presentation is otherwise similar to that of the EST. The primary lesions tend to be large, and about two-thirds are confined to one ovary at the time of presentation. These lesions frequently secrete AFP and hCG, which are useful for following the response to subsequent therapy (34).

The treatment of embryonal carcinomas is the same as for the EST (i.e., a unilateral oophorectomy followed by combination chemotherapy with BEP) (14, 17–19). Radiation does not appear to be useful for primary treatment.

Choriocarcinoma of the Ovary

Pure nongestational choriocarcinoma of the ovary is an extremely rare tumor. Histologically, it has the same appearance as gestational choriocarcinoma metastatic to the ovaries (1). The majority of patients with this cancer are younger than 20 years. The presence of hCG can be useful in monitoring the patient's response to treatment. In the presence of high hCG levels, isosexual precocity has been seen, occurring in about 50% of patients whose lesions appear before menarche.

There are only a few limited reports on the use of chemotherapy for these non-gestational choriocarcinomas, but complete responses have been reported to the MAC regimen (methotrexate, actinomycin D, and Cytoxan) used in a manner described for gestational trophoblastic disease (36) (see Chapter 13). Alternatively, the BEP regimen can be used (19, 28). The prognosis for ovarian choriocarcinomas has been poor, with the majority of patients having metastases to organ parenchyma at the time of initial diagnosis (1, 37).

Polyembryoma

Polyembryoma of the ovary is another extremely rare tumor, which is composed of "embryoid bodies." This tumor replicates the structures of early embryonic differentiation (i.e., the three somatic layers: endoderm, mesoderm, and ectoderm) (1, 5). The lesion tends to occur in very young, premenarchal girls with signs of pseudopuberty and elevated AFP and hCG titers. Anecdotally, the VAC chemotherapeutic regimen has been reported to be effective (14).

Mixed Germ Cell Tumors

Mixed germ cell malignancies of the ovary contain two or more elements of the lesions described above. In one series (38), the most common component of a mixed malignancy was dysgerminoma, which occurred in 80%, followed by EST in 70%, immature teratoma in 53%, choriocarcinoma in 20%, and embryonal carcinoma in 16%. The most frequent combination was a dysgerminoma and an EST. The mixed lesions may secrete either AFP, hCG, both, or neither, depending on the components.

These lesions should be managed with combination chemotherapy, preferably BEP. The serum marker, if positive initially, may become negative during chemotherapy, but this may reflect regression of only a particular component of the mixed lesion. Therefore in these patients a second-look laparotomy may be indicated to determine the precise response to therapy if macroscopic disease was present at initiation of chemotherapy.

The most important prognostic features are the size of the primary tumor and the relative amount of its most malignant component (38). In Stage Ia lesions smaller than 10 cm, survival is 100%. Tumors composed of less than one-third EST, choriocarcinoma, or grade 3 immature teratoma also have an excellent prognosis, but it is less favorable when these components comprise the majority of the mixed lesions.

Sex Cord-Stromal Tumors

Sex cord-stromal tumors of the ovary account for about 5–8% of all ovarian malignancies (1–3, 34). This group of ovarian neoplasms is derived from the sex cords and the ovarian stroma or mesenchyme. The tumors usually are composed of various combinations of elements, including the "female" cells (i.e., granulosa and theca cells), and "male" cells (i.e., Sertoli and Leydig cells), as well as morphologically indifferent cells. A classification of this group of tumors is presented in Table 10.4.

Granulosa-Stromal Cell Tumors

Granulosa-stromal cell tumors include granulosa cell tumors, thecomas, and fibromas. The granulosa cell tumor is a low-grade malignancy; rarely thecomas and fibromas have morphologic features of malignancy and then may be referred to as *fibrosarcomas*.

Table 10.4   Sex Cord-Stromal Tumors

1. *Granulosa-stromal cell tumors*
   A. Granulosa cell tumor
   B. Tumors in thecoma-fibroma group
      (1) Thecoma
      (2) Fibroma
      (3) Unclassified

2. *Androblastromas; Sertoli-Leydig cell tumors*
   A. Well-differentiated
      (1) Sertoli cell tumor
      (2) Sertoli-Leydig cell tumor
      (3) Leydig cell tumor; hilus cell tumor
   B. Moderately differentiated
   C. Poorly differentiated (sarcomatoid)
   D. With heterologous elements

3. *Gynandroblastoma*

4. *Unclassified*

Modified and reprinted, with permission, from Young RE, Scully RE: Ovarian sex cord-stromal tumors: recent progress. *Int J Gynecol Pathol* 1:153, 1980.

Granulosa cell tumors, which secrete estrogen, are seen in women of all ages. They are found in prepubertal girls in 5% of cases; the remainder are distributed throughout the reproductive and postmenopausal years (29). They are bilateral in only 2% of patients.

Of the rare prepubertal lesions, 75% are associated with sexual pseudoprecocity because of the estrogen secretion (39). In the reproductive age group, most patients have menstrual irregularities or secondary amenorrhea, and cystic hyperplasia of the endometrium is frequently present. In postmenopausal women, abnormal uterine bleeding is frequently the presenting symptom. Indeed, the estrogen secretion in these patients can be sufficient to stimulate the development of endometrial cancer. **Endometrial cancer occurs in association with granulosa cell tumors in at least 5% of cases and 25%-50% are associated with endometrial hyperplasia** (1, 39–41).

The other symptoms and signs of granulosa cell tumors are nonspecific and the same as most ovarian malignancies. Ascites is present in about 10% of cases, and rarely a pleural effusion is present (39–41). Granulosa tumors tend to be hemorrhagic: occasionally they rupture and produce a hemoperitoneum (41).

Granulosa cell tumors are usually Stage I at diagnosis but may recur 5–30 years after initial diagnosis (40). The tumors may also spread hematogenously, and metastases can develop in the lungs, liver, and brain years after initial diagnosis. When they do recur, they can progress quite rapidly. Malignant thecomas are extremely rare, and their presentation, management, and outcome are similar to those of the granulosa cell tumors (39–43). Inhibin has been reported to be secreted by some granulosa cell tumors and may be a useful marker for the disease (44).

Treatment

The treatment of granulosa cell tumors depends on the age of the patient and the extent of disease. For most patients, surgery alone is sufficient primary therapy, with radiation and chemotherapy reserved for the treatment of recurrent or metastatic disease (41–43).

Surgery

Because granulosa cell tumors are bilateral in only about 2% of patients, a unilateral salpingo-oophorectomy is appropriate therapy for Stage Ia tumors in children or in women of reproductive age (40). At the time of laparotomy, if a granulosa cell tumor is identified by frozen section, a staging operation is performed, including an assessment of the contralateral ovary. If the opposite ovary appears enlarged, it should be biopsied. In perimenopausal and postmenopausal women for whom ovarian preservation is not important, a hysterectomy and bilateral salpingo-oophorectomy should be performed. In premenopausal patients in whom the uterus is left *in situ*, a dilatation and curettage of the uterus should be performed, because of the possibility of a coexistent adenocarcinoma of the endometrium (38).

Radiation

There is no evidence to support the use of adjuvant radiation therapy for granulosa cell tumors (39), although pelvic radiation may help to palliate isolated pelvic recurrences (40).

Chemotherapy

There is no evidence that adjuvant chemotherapy will prevent recurrence of disease. Metastatic lesions and recurrences have been treated with a variety of different antineoplastic drugs. There has been no consistently effective regimen in these patients, although complete responses have been reported anecdotally in patients treated with a single agent, Cytoxan or melphalan, as well as in those treated with the combinations, VAC (vincristine, Adriamycin, Cytoxan) and PAC (cisplatin, Adriamycin, Cytoxan) (3). The AcFuCy regimen (actinomycin D, 5-FU, and Cytoxan) was used by the GOG and produced only a 20% partial response rate (3, 42). The use of hormonal agents such as progestins or antiestrogens has been suggested, but there are no data available to suggest effectiveness (40).

Prognosis

Granulosa cell tumors have a prolonged natural history and a tendency toward late relapse, reflecting their low-grade biology. As such, 10-year survival rates of about 90% have been reported, with 20-year survival rates dropping to 75% (39–43). Most histologic types have the same prognosis, but the more poorly differentiated diffuse or sarcomatoid type tends to do worse (39).

The DNA ploidy of the tumors has recently been correlated with survival. Holland and colleagues (45) reported DNA aneuploidy in 13 of 37 patients (35%) with primary granulosa cell tumors. The presence of residual disease was found to be the most important predictor of progression-free survival, but DNA ploidy was an independent prognostic factor. **Patients with residual-negative DNA diploid tumors had a 10-year progression-free survival of 96%.**

Sertoli-Leydig Tumors

Sertoli-Leydig tumors occur most frequently in the third and fourth decades, with 75% of the lesions seen in women younger than 40 years. These lesions are extremely rare and account for less than 0.2% of ovarian cancers (1). Sertoli-Leydig cell tumors are most frequently low-grade malignancies, although occasionally a poorly differentiated variety may behave more aggressively.

The tumors typically produce androgens, and clinical virilization is noted in 70–85% of patients (3). Signs of virilization include oligomenorrhea followed by amenorrhea, breast atrophy, acne, hirsutism, clitoromegaly, a deepening voice, and a receding hairline. Measurement of plasma androgens may reveal elevated testosterone and androstenedione, with normal or slightly elevated dehydroepiandrosterone sulphate (1). Rarely, the Sertoli-Leydig tumor can be associated with manifestations of estrogenization (i.e., isosexual precocity, irregular or postmenopausal bleeding).

Treatment

Because these low-grade lesions are only rarely bilateral (< 1%), the usual treatment is unilateral salpingo-oophorectomy and evaluation of the contralateral ovary in patients who are in their reproductive years (46). In older patients, hysterectomy and bilateral salpingo-oophorectomy are appropriate.

There are insufficient data to document the utility of radiation or chemotherapy in patients with persistent disease, but some responses in patients with measurable disease have been reported with pelvic radiation and the VAC chemotherapy regimen (3, 32).

Prognosis

The 5-year survival rate is 70–90%, and recurrences thereafter are uncommon (3, 36). Poorly differentiated lesions comprise the majority of fatalities.

Uncommon Ovarian Cancers

There are several varieties of malignant ovarian tumors, which together comprise only 0.1% of ovarian malignancies (1). Two of these lesions are the lipoid (or lipid) cell tumors and the primary ovarian sarcomas.

Lipoid Cell Tumors

Lipoid cell tumors are thought to arise in adrenal cortical rests that reside in the vicinity of the ovary. More than 100 cases have been reported, and bilaterality has been noted in only a few (1). Most are associated with virilization, and occasionally with obesity, hypertension, and glucose intolerance reflecting glucocorticoid secretion. Rare cases of estrogen secretion and isosexual precocity have been reported.

The majority of these tumors have a benign or low-grade behavior, but about 20%, most of which are initially larger than 8 cm in diameter, develop metastatic lesions. Metastases are usually in the peritoneal cavity but rarely occur at distant sites (5). The primary treatment is surgical extirpation of the primary lesion. There are no data regarding radiation or chemotherapy for this disease.

Sarcomas

Malignant mixed mesodermal sarcomas of the ovary are extremely rare; only about 100 cases have been reported. Most lesions are heterologous, and 80% occur in postmenopausal women. The presentation is similar to that of most ovarian malignancies. These lesions are biologically aggressive, and the majority of patients have evidence of metastases.

There is no effective treatment for ovarian sarcomas, and most patients die within 2 years. Adriamycin, with or without Cytoxan, has produced an occasional partial response, and cisplatin is currently undergoing clinical trials (47). In patients in whom all macroscopic disease can be resected, we have observed disease-free survival of more than 3 years in two patients treated with 6 cycles of cisplatin and epirubicin.

Metastatic Tumors

About 5–6% of ovarian tumors are metastatic from other organs, most frequently from the female genital tract, the breast, or the gastrointestinal tract (48). The metastases may occur from direct extension of another pelvic neoplasm, by hematogenous spread, lymphatic spread, or transcoelomic dissemination, with surface implantation of tumors that spread in the peritoneal cavity.

Gynecologic

Nonovarian cancers of the genital tract can spread by direct extension or they may metastasize to the ovaries. Tubal carcinoma involves the ovaries secondarily in 13% of cases (49), usually by direct extension. Under some circumstances, it is difficult to know whether the tumor originates in the tube or in the ovary when both are involved. Cervical cancer spreads to the ovary only in rare cases (< 1%), and most of these are of an advanced clinical stage or are adenocarcinomas (50). Although adenocarcinoma of the endometrium can spread and implant directly onto the surface of the ovaries in as many as 5% of cases, two synchronous primary tumors probably occur with greater frequency. In these cases, an endometrioid carcinoma of the ovary is usually associated with the adenocarcinoma of the endometrium.

Nongynecologic

The frequency of metastatic breast carcinoma to the ovaries varies according to the method of determination, but the phenomenon is common. **In autopsy data of women who die of metastatic breast cancer, the ovaries are involved in 24% of cases and 80% of the involvement is bilateral** (51, 52). Similarly, when ovaries are removed to palliate advanced breast cancer, about 20–30% of the cases reveal ovarian involvement, 60% bilaterally (52). The involvement of ovaries in early-stage breast cancer appears to be considerably lower, but precise figures are not available. In almost all cases, either ovarian involvement is occult or a pelvic mass is discovered after other metastatic disease becomes apparent.

Krukenberg Tumor

The Krukenberg tumor, which can account for 30–40% of metastatic cancers to the ovaries, arises in the ovarian stroma and has characteristic mucin-filled, signet-ring cells (53). The primary tumor is most frequently the stomach, but less commonly the colon, breast, or biliary tract. Rarely, the cervix or the bladder may be the primary site (1). Krukenberg tumors can account for about 2% of ovarian cancers at some institutions, and they are usually bilateral. The lesions are usually not discovered until the primary disease is advanced, and therefore most patients die of their disease within a year (53). In some cases, a primary tumor is not found.

Other Gastrointestinal

In other cases of metastasis from the gastrointestinal tract to the ovary, the tumor does not have the classic histologic appearance of a Krukenberg tumor; most of these are from the colon and, less commonly, the small intestine. As many as 1–2% of women with intestinal carcinomas will develop metastases to the ovaries during the course of their disease (46). Prior to exploration for an adnexal tumor in a woman more than 40 years of age, a barium enema is indicated to exclude a primary gastrointestinal carcinoma with metastases to the ovaries, particularly if there are any gastrointestinal symptoms. Metastatic colon cancer can mimic a mucinous cystadenocarcinoma of the ovary histologically (53, 54).

Carcinoid

Metastatic carcinoid tumors are rare, representing fewer than 2% of metastatic lesions to the ovaries (50). Conversely, only about 2% of primary carcinoids have evidence of ovarian metastasis, and only 40% of these patients have the carcinoid syndrome at the time of discovery of the metastatic carcinoid. However, in peri-menopausal and postmenopausal women explored for an intestinal carcinoid, it is reasonable to remove the ovaries to prevent subsequent ovarian metastasis. Furthermore, the discovery of an ovarian carcinoid should prompt a careful search for a primary intestinal lesion (55).

Lymphoma and Leukemia

Lymphomas and leukemia can involve the ovary. When they do, the involvement is usually bilateral (46, 56). About 5% of patients with Hodgkin's disease will have lymphomatous involvement of the ovaries, but this occurs typically with advanced-stage disease. **With Burkitt's lymphoma, ovarian involvement is very common (57). Other types of lymphoma involve the ovaries much less frequently, and leukemic infiltration of the ovaries is uncommon.** Sometimes the ovaries can be the only apparent site of involvement of the abdominal or pelvic viscera with a lymphoma, and if this circumstance is found a careful surgical exploration may be necessary. An intraoperative consultation with a hematologist-oncologist should be obtained to determine the need for these procedures if frozen section of a solid ovarian mass reveals a lymphoma. In general, most lymphomas no longer require extensive surgical staging, although enlarged lymph nodes should generally be biopsied. In some cases of Hodgkin's disease, a more extensive evaluation may be necessary. Treatment involves that of the lymphoma or leukemia in general. Removal of a large ovarian mass may improve patient comfort and facilitate a response to subsequent radiation or chemotherapy.

Fallopian Tube Cancer

Carcinoma of the fallopian tube accounts for 0.3% of all cancers of the female genital tract (2, 49, 58). In histologic features and behavior, fallopian tube carcinoma is similar to ovarian cancer; thus the evaluation and treatment are also essentially the same. The fallopian tubes are frequently involved secondarily from other primary sites, most often the ovaries, endometrium, gastrointestinal tract, or breast. They may also be involved in primary peritoneal carcinomatosis. The criteria for distinguishing primary from metastatic tubal cancer are discussed in Chapter 4. Almost all cancers are of "epithelial" origin, most frequently of serous histology. Rarely, sarcomas have also been reported.

Clinical Features

Tubal cancers are seen most frequently in the fifth and sixth decades, with a mean age of 55 to 60 years (2, 49). There are no known predisposing factors.

Symptoms and Signs

The classic triad of symptoms and signs associated with fallopian tube cancer is (1) a prominent watery vaginal discharge, i.e., *hydrops tubae profluens*;

(2) pelvic pain; and (3) a pelvic mass. However, this triad is noted in fewer than 15% of patients (49).

Either vaginal discharge or bleeding is the most common symptom reported by patients with tubal carcinoma and is documented in more than 50% of patients (39). Lower abdominal or pelvic pressure and pain also are noted in many patients. However, the presentation may be rather vague and nonspecific. In perimenopausal and postmenopausal women with an unusual, unexplained, or persistent vaginal discharge, even in the absence of bleeding, the clinician should be concerned about the possibility of an occult tubal cancer. Fallopian tube cancer is often found incidentally in asymptomatic women at the time of abdominal hysterectomy and bilateral salpingo-oophorectomy.

On examination, a pelvic mass is present in about 60% of patients, and ascites may be present if advanced disease exists. Patients with tubal carcinoma will have a negative dilatation and curettage (58), although abnormal or adenocarcinomatous cells may be seen in cytologic specimens obtained from the cervix in 10% of patients.

Spread Pattern

Tubal cancers spread in much the same manner as epithelial ovarian malignancies, principally by the transcoelomic exfoliation of cells that implant throughout the peritoneal cavity. In about 80% of the patients with advanced disease, metastases are confined to the peritoneal cavity at the time of diagnosis (59).

The fallopian tube is richly permeated with lymphatic channels, and spread to the para-aortic and pelvic lymph nodes is common. Metastases to the para-aortic lymph nodes have been documented in at least 33% of the patients with all stages of disease (60).

Staging

Although there is no official International Federation of Gynecology and Obstetrics (FIGO) staging for tubal cancer, the ovarian staging system has been adapted to apply to fallopian tube disease (59). Thus staging is based on the surgical findings at laparotomy (Table 10.5). According to this system, about 20–25% of patients have Stage I disease, 20–25% have Stage II, 40–50% have Stage III, and 5–

Table 10.5 Surgical Stage of Fallopian Tube Cancer		
Stage I	Carcinoma confined to fallopian tube(s)	
	Stage Ia	Unilateral disease; no ascites
	Stage Ib	Bilateral disease; no ascites
	Stage Ic	Either a or b with ascites and/or neoplastic cells in peritoneal washings
Stage II	Carcinoma extends beyond fallopian tube(s) but confined to pelvis	
	Stage IIa	Extension to uterus and/or ovary
	Stage IIb	Extension to other pelvic organs
	Stage IIc	Either a or b with ascites and/or neoplastic cells in peritoneal washings
Stage III	Carcinoma extends beyond pelvis but confined to abdominal cavity	
	Stage IIIa	Tumor microscopic only
	Stage IIIb	Tumor metastasis ≤ 2 cm
	Stage IIIc	Tumor metastasis > 2 cm
Stage IV	Carcinoma extends beyond abdominal cavity	

Modified, with permission, from Podratz KC, Podczaski ES, Gaffey TA, et al.: Primary carcinoma of the fallopian tube. *Am J Obstet Gynecol* 154:1319, 1986.

10% have Stage IV (59). A somewhat lower incidence of advanced disease is seen in these patients than in patients with epithelial ovarian carcinomas, presumably because of the earlier occurrence of symptoms, particularly vaginal bleeding or unusual vaginal discharge.

Treatment

The treatment of this disease is similar to that of epithelial ovarian cancer (58–61). Exploratory laparotomy is necessary to remove the primary tumor, to stage the disease, and to resect metastases. After surgery, the most frequently employed treatment is now combination chemotherapy, although radiation is also used in selected cases.

Surgery

Patients with tubal carcinoma should undergo total abdominal hysterectomy and bilateral salpingo-oophorectomy (2). If there is no evidence of gross tumor spread, a staging operation is performed. The retroperitoneal lymph nodes should be adequately evaluated, and peritoneal cytologic studies and biopsies should be performed, along with an infracolic omentectomy.

In patients with metastatic disease, an effort should be made to remove as much tumor bulk as possible. The role of cytoreductive surgery in this disease is unclear, but extrapolation from the experience with epithelial ovarian cancer indicates that significant benefit might be expected, particularly if all macroscopic disease can be resected.

Chemotherapy

The most active single agents appear to be alkylating agents and cisplatin. Recent experience with cisplatin given in combination with Cytoxan (PC) or Adriamycin and Cytoxan (PAC) indicates that complete responses can be obtained (61). It appears justifiable, therefore, to employ the same protocols that are used for epithelial ovarian cancer in patients with epithelial tubal malignancies.

Data on well-staged lesions are scarce. Therefore it is unclear whether patients with disease confined to the fallopian tube (i.e., a Stage Ia, grade 1 or 2 carcinoma), benefit from additional therapy.

Radiation

Whereas the majority of patients with tubal cancers have been treated with radiation in the past, the role of radiation in the management of the disease remains unclear, because patients have not been treated in any consistent manner and the small numbers treated preclude any meaningful conclusions (58). Pelvic radiation alone was once popular, but this approach seems inappropriate when the pattern of spread of this disease to the upper abdomen is considered (57, 59, 60). Intraperitoneal ^{32}P has also been used, but these data are limited. More recently, whole-abdominal radiation with a pelvic boost has been used in patients with no evidence of gross disease in the abdomen (i.e., completely resected disease or microscopic metastases only). As with epithelial ovarian cancer, there may be a role in properly selected patients (59).

Prognosis

The overall 5-year survival for patients with epithelial tubal carcinomas is about 40%. This number is higher than for patients with ovarian cancer and reflects

398

the somewhat higher proportion of patients with early-stage disease. The outlook is clearly related to the stage of disease, but the available data relate to patients who have not been surgically staged. Thus the reported 5-year survival rate for patients with Stage I disease is only about 65%. The 5-year survival rate for patients with Stage II disease is 50–60%, but it is only 10–20% for patients with Stages III and IV (49, 58, 59).

Tubal Sarcomas

Tubal sarcomas, particularly malignant mixed mesodermal tumors, have been described but are rare. They occur mainly in the sixth decade and are typically advanced at the time of diagnosis. If all gross disease can be resected, cisplatin-based combination chemotherapy should be tried. However, survival is generally poor, and most patients die of their disease within 2 years (47).

References

1. **Scully RE:** Tumors of the ovary and maldeveloped gonads. In *Atlas of Tumor Pathology*, Fascicle 16, Washington, D.C., Armed Forces Institute of Pathology, 1979.

2. **Berek JS, Hacker NF:** Ovarian and fallopian tubes. In Haskell CM (ed): *Cancer Treatment*, ed 3, Philadelphia, WB Saunders, 1990, pp 295.

3. **Slayton RE:** Management of germ cell and stromal tumors of the ovary. *Semin Oncol* 11:299, 1984.

4. **Serov SF, Scully RE, Robin IH:** Histological typing of ovarian tumors: *International Histological Classification of Tumors*. No. 9, Geneva, World Health Organization, 1973.

5. **Kurman RJ, Scardino PT, Waldmann TA, et al:** Malignant germ cell tumors of the ovary and testis: an immunologic study of 69 cases. *Ann Clin Lab Sci* 9:462, 1979.

6. **Spanos WJ:** Preoperative hormonal therapy of cystic adnexal masses. *Am J Obstet Gynecol* 116:551, 1973.

7. **Kurman RJ, Norris HJ:** Germ cell tumors of the ovary. *Hum Pathol* 1:291, 1978.

8. **Asadourian L, Taylor H:** Dysgerminoma. *Obstet Gynecol* 33:370, 1969.

9. **Malkasian G, Symmonds R:** Treatment of the unilateral encapsulated ovarian dysgerminoma. *Am J Obstet Gynecol* 90:379, 1964.

10. **Freel JH, Cassir JF, Pierce VK, et al:** Dysgerminoma of the ovary. *Cancer* 43:798, 1979.

11. **Gordon A, Lipton D, Woodruff JD:** Dysgerminoma: a review of 158 cases from the Emil Novak Ovarian Tumor Registry. *Obstet Gynecol* 58:497, 1981.

12. **Thomas GM, Dembo AJ, Hacker NF, DePetrillo AD:** Current therapy for dysgerminoma of the ovary. *Obstet Gynecol* 70:268, 1987.

13. **Gershenson DM, Wharton JT, Kline RC, et al:** Chemotherapeutic complete remission in patients with metastatic ovarian dysgerminoma. *Cancer* 58:2594, 1986.

14. **Gershenson DM, Wharton JT:** Malignant germ cell tumors of the ovary. In Albert DS, Surwit EA (eds): *Ovarian Cancer*. Boston, Martinus Nijhoff, 1985, pp 227–269.

15. **Gershenson DM:** Menstrual and reproductive function after treatment with combination chemotherapy for malignant ovarian germ cell tumors. *J Clin Oncol* 6:270, 1988.

16. **Williams SD, Birch R, Einhorn LH, et al:** Disseminated germ cell tumors: chemotherapy with cisplatin plus bleomycin plus either vinblastine or etoposide. *N Engl J Med* 316:1435, 1987.

17. **Williams SD, Blessing JA, Hatch K, Homesley HD:** Chemotherapy of advanced ovarian dysgerminoma: trials of the Gynecologic Oncology Group. *J Clin Oncol* 9:1950, 1991.

18. **Gershenson DM, Morris M, Cangir A, et al:** Treatment of malignant germ cell tumors of the ovary with bleomycin, etoposide, and cisplatin. *J Clin Oncol* 8:715, 1990.

19. **Williams SD:** Germ cell tumors. In Ozols RF (eds): *Ovarian Cancer*. Philadelphia, WB Saunders, 1992, pp 967–974.

20. **Williams SD, Blessing JA, Moore DH, et al:** Cisplatin, vinblastine, and bleomycin in advanced and recurrent ovarian germ-cell tumors. *Ann Intern Med* 111:22, 1989.

21. **Norris HJ, Zirken HJ, Benson WL:** Immature (malignant) teratoma of the ovary: a clinical and pathologic study of 58 cases. *Cancer* 37:2359, 1976.

22. **Curry SL, Smith JP, Gallagher HS:** Malignant teratoma of the ovary: prognostic factors and treatment. *Am J Obstet Gynecol* 131:845, 1978.

23. **Cangir A, Smith J, VanEys J:** Improved prognosis in children with ovarian cancers following modified VAC (vincristine sulfate, dactinomycin, and cyclophosphamide) chemotherapy. *Cancer* 42:1234, 1978.

24. **Slayton RE, Hreshchyshyn MM, Silverberg SC, et al:** Treatment of malignant ovarian germ cell tumors: response to vincristine, dactinomycin and cyclophosphamide. *Cancer* 42:390, 1978.

25. **Slayton RE, Park RC, Silverberg SC, et al:** Vincristine, dactinomycin, and cyclophosphamide (VAC) in the treatment of malignant germ cell tumors of the ovary: a Gynecologic Oncology Group study (a final report). *Cancer* 56:243, 1985.

26. **Creasman WJ, Soper JT:** Assessment of the contemporary management of germ cell malignancies of the ovary. *Am J Obstet Gynecol* 153:828, 1985.

27. **Taylor MH, DePetrillo AD, Turner AR, et al:** Vinblastine, bleomycin and cisplatinum in malignant germ cell tumors of the ovary. *Cancer* 56:1341, 1985.

28. **Williams SD, Blessing JA, Slayton R, et al:** Ovarian germ cell tumors: adjuvant trials of the Gynecologic Oncology Group. *J Clin Oncol* 12:1994.

29. **Loehrer PJ, Elson P, Johnson DH, et al:** A randomized trial of cisplatin plus etoposide with or without bleomycin in favorable prognosis disseminated germ cell tumors: an ECOG study. *Proc Am Soc Clin Oncol* 10:540, 1991.

30. **Bajorin DF, Sarosdy MF, Bosl GJ, et al:** A randomized trial of etoposide plus carboplatin versus etoposide plus cisplatin in patients with metastatic germ cell tumors. *J Clin Oncol* 11:598, 1993.

31. **Loehrer PJ Sr, Hui S, Clark S, et al:** Teratoma following cisplatin-based combination chemotherapy for nonseminomatous germ cell tumors: a clincopathological correlation. *J Urol* 135:1183, 1986.

32. **Gershenson DM, Copeland JL, Del Junco G, et al:** Second-look laparotomy in the management of malignant germ cell tumors of the ovary. *Obstet Gynecol* 67:789, 1986.

33. **Kurman RJ, Norris HJ:** Endodermal sinus tumor of the ovary: a clinical and pathological analysis of 71 cases. *Cancer* 38:2404, 1976.

34. **Talerman A, Haije WG, Baggerman L:** Serum alpha-fetoprotein (AFP) in patients with germ cell tumors of the gonads and extragonadal sites: correlation between endodermal sinus (yolk sac) tumors and raised serum AFP. *Cancer* 46:380, 1980.

35. **Newlands ES, Southall PJ, Paradinas FJ, Holden L:** Management of ovarian germ cell tumours. In Williams CJ, Krikorian JG, Green MR, Ragavan D (eds): *Textbook of Uncommon Cancer*. New York, John Wiley & Sons Ltd., 1988, pp 37–53.

36. **Kurman RJ, Norris HJ:** Embryonal carcinoma of the ovary: a clinicopathologic entity distinct from endodermal sinus tumor resembling embryonal carcinoma of the adult testis. *Cancer* 38:2420, 1976.

37. **Gerbie MV, Brewer JI, Tamimi U:** Primary choriocarcinoma of the ovary. *Obstet Gynecol* 46:720, 1975.

38. **Kurman RJ, Norris HJ:** Malignant mixed germ cell tumors of the ovary: a clinical and pathologic analysis of 30 cases. *Obstet Gynecol* 48:579, 1976.

39. **Young RE, Scully RE:** Ovarian sex cord-stromal tumors: recent progress. *Int J Gynecol Pathol* 1:153, 1980.

40. **Bjorkholm E, Pettersson F:** Granulosa-cell and thecacell tumors: the clinical picture and long-term outcome for the Radiumhemmet series. *Acta Obstet Gynecol Scand* 59:278, 1983.

41. **Fox H, Agarical K, Langley FA:** A clinicopathologic study of 92 cases of granulosa cell tumors of the ovary with special reference to the factors influencing prognosis. *Cancer* 35:231, 1975.

42. **Slayton RE, Johnson G, Brady L, Blessing J:** Radiotherapy and chemotherapy in malignant tumors of the ovarian stroma: a Gynecologic Oncology Group study. *Proc Am Soc Clin Oncol* C444, 1980.

43. **Norris HJ, Taylor HB:** Prognosis of granulosa-theca tumors of the ovary. *Cancer* 21:255, 1968.

44. **Lappohn RE, Burger HG, Bouma J, et al:** Inhibin as a marker for granulosa-cell tumors. *N Engl J Med* 321:826, 1989.

45. **Holland DR, LeRiche J, Swenerton KD, et al:** Flow cytometric assessment of DNA ploidy is a useful prognostic factor for patients with granulosa cell ovarian tumors. *Int J Gynecol Cancer* 1:227, 1991.

46. **Roth LM, Anderson MC, Govan AD, et al:** Sertoli-Leydig cell tumors: a clinicopathologic study of 34 cases. *Cancer* 48:187, 1981.

47. **Berek JS, Hacker NF:** Sarcomas of the female genital tract. In Eilber FR, Morton DL, Sondak VK, Economou JS (eds). *The Soft Tissue Sarcomas*. Orlando, Grune & Stratton, 1987, pp 229–238.

48. **Fox H, Langley FA:** *Tumors of the Ovary.* Chicago, Year Book, 1976.

49. **Sedlis A:** Carcinoma of the fallopian tube. *Surg Clin North Am* 58:121, 1978.

50. **Woodruff JD, Murthy YS, Bhaskar JN, et al:** Metastatic ovarian tumors. *Am J Obstet Gynecol* 107:202, 1970.

51. **Kasilag FB, Rutledge FN:** Metastatic breast carcinoma to the ovary. *Am J Obstet Gynecol* 74:989, 1957.

52. **Lee YN, Hori JM:** Significance of ovarian metastasis in therapeutic oophorectomy for advanced breast cancer. *Cancer* 27:1374, 1971.

53. **Woodruff JD, Novak ER:** The Krukenberg tumor: study of 48 cases from the Emil Novak Ovarian Tumor Registry. *Obstet Gynecol* 15:351, 1960.

54. **Webb MJ, Decker DG, Mussey E:** Cancer metastatic to the ovary: factors influencing survival. *Obstet Gynecol* 45:391, 1975.

55. **Robboy SJ, Scully RE, Norris HJ:** Carcinoid metastatic to the ovary: a clinicopathologic analysis 35 cases. *Cancer* 33:798, 1974.

56. **Freeman C, Berg JW, Cutler SJ:** Occurrence and prognosis of extranodal lymphomas. *Cancer* 29:252, 1972.

57. **Arseneau JC, Canellos GP, Banks DM, et al:** American Burkitt's lymphoma: a clinicopathologic study of 30 cases. I. Clinical factors relating to prolonged survival. *Am J Med* 58:314, 1975.

58. **Podczaski E, Herbst Al:** Cancer of the vagina and fallopian tube. In Knapp RC, Berkowitz RS (eds). *Gynecologic Oncology,* New York, MacMillan, 1986, pp 394–424.

59. **Podratz KC, Podczaski ES, Gaffey TA, et al:** Primary carcinoma of the fallopian tube. *Am J Obstet Gynecol* 254:1319, 1986.

60. **Tamimi HK, Figge DC:** Adenocarcinoma of the uterine tube: potential for lymph node metastases. *Am J Obstet Gynecol* 141:132, 1981.

61. **Deppe G, Bruckner HW, Cohen CJ:** Combination chemotherapy for advanced carcinoma of the fallopian tube. *Obstet Gynecol* 56:530, 1980.

11 Vulvar Cancer

Neville F. Hacker

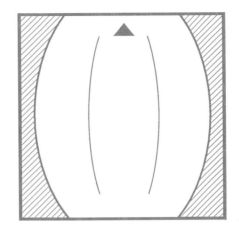

Vulvar cancer is uncommon, representing about 4% of malignancies of the female genital tract. Squamous cell carcinomas account for about 90% of the cases, whereas melanomas, adenocarcinomas, basal cell carcinomas, and sarcomas are much less common. **The incidence of *in situ* vulvar cancer nearly doubled between the mid 1970s and the mid 1980s, whereas the rate of invasive squamous cell carcinoma has remained stable** (1).

In the early part of this century, patients commonly presented with advanced disease, and surgical techniques were poorly developed; thus the 5-year survival for vulvar cancer was 20–25% (2, 3). Basset (4), in France, was the first to suggest an *en bloc* dissection of the vulva, groin, and iliac lymph nodes, although he performed the operation only on cadavers. Taussig (5), in the United States, and Way (6), in Great Britain, pioneered the radical *en bloc* dissection for vulvar cancer and reported 5-year survival rates of 60–70%. Postoperative morbidity was high after these procedures, with wound breakdown, infection, and prolonged hospitalization the norm. For patients with disease involving the anus, rectum, or proximal urethra, pelvic exenteration was often combined with radical vulvectomy.

Over the past 15 years, a number of significant advances have been made in the management of vulvar cancer. These changes include:

1. Individualization of treatment for all patients with invasive disease (7, 8)

2. Vulvar conservation for patients with unifocal tumors, and an otherwise normal vulva (7–11)

3. Omission of the groin dissection for patients with T_1 tumors and ≤ 1 mm of stromal invasion (7, 8)

4. Elimination of routine pelvic lymphadenectomy (12–16)

403

5. The use of separate groin incisions for the groin dissection to improve wound healing (17, 18)

6. Omission of the contralateral groin dissection in patients with lateral T lesions and negative ipsilateral nodes (8, 19)

7. The use of preoperative radiation therapy to obviate the need for exenteration in patients with advanced disease (20, 21)

8. The use of postoperative radiation to decrease the incidence of groin recurrence in patients with multiple positive groin nodes (16)

With careful selection of patients, a more conservative surgical approach to vulvar cancer is possible without compromising patient survival.

Etiology

No specific etiologic factor has been identified for vulvar cancer, and the relationship of the invasive disease to vulvar dystrophy and to vulvar intraepithelial neoplasia remains unclear. Chronic pruritus is usually an important antecedent phenomenon in patients with invasive vulvar cancer (22). In addition, carcinoma *in situ* of the vulva, which does not appear to have the same malignant potential as its counterpart in the cervix, is most likely to progress to invasive disease if the patient is elderly or immunosuppressed (23).

Vulvar cancer has been reported to be more common in patients who are obese, hypertensive, diabetic, or nulliparous (24, 25), but a recent case-control study of vulvar cancer was unable to confirm any of these as risk factors (26).

A second primary malignancy, usually invasive or preinvasive cervical cancer, has been reported in up to 22% of cases (19, 27). The common association between cervical, vaginal, and vulvar cancer suggests a common pathogen, and the case-control study by Brinton et al. found a significantly increased risk in association with multiple sexual partners, a history of genital warts, and smoking (26). Human papillomavirus (HPV) DNA has been reported in 20–60% of patients with invasive vulvar cancer (28). The HPV-positive group has been characterized by a younger mean age, more tobacco use, and the presence of vulvar intraepithelial neoplasia (VIN) in association with the invasive component (29–31).

Most of these studies deal with small numbers of patients, but they do suggest two different etiologic types of vulvar cancer. **One type is seen mainly in younger patients, is related to HPV and smoking, and is commonly associated with VIN. The more common type is seen mainly in elderly patients, is unrelated to smoking or HPV infection, and concurrent VIN is uncommon.**

Other diseases known to be associated with vulvar cancer include syphilis and nonluetic granulomatous venereal disease, particularly lymphogranuloma venereum and granuloma inguinale *(Donovanosis)*. In approximately 5% of patients with vulvar cancer a serologic test for syphilis is positive; these patients develop the disease at an earlier age and have more poorly differentiated lesions (24, 25). Antecedent chronic granulomatous disease has been reported in 66% of black patients with vulvar cancer in Jamaica (32), but such diseases are not seen commonly in Western countries.

Preinvasive Disease

"Vulvar Dystrophies"

In the past, a number of terms have been used to denote disorders of epithelial growth and differentiation that produce a variety of nonspecific macroscopic vulvar changes. These terms included "leukoplakia," "lichen sclerosis et atrophicus," "primary atrophy," "sclerotic dermatosis," "atrophic and hyperplastic vulvitis," and "kraurosis vulvae" (33).

In 1966, Jeffcoate (34) suggested that these terms did not refer to separate disease entities, because their macroscopic and microscopic appearances were variable and interchangeable. He assigned the generic term *chronic vulvar dystrophy* to the entire group of lesions.

Several classifications of vulvar diseases have been subsequently proposed, and this has been confusing for clinicians and pathologists alike. The most recent recommendation from the International Society for the Study of Vulvar Disease (ISSVD) is that the old "dystrophy" terminology should be replaced by a new classification under the pathologic heading "nonneoplastic epithelial disorders of skin and mucosa." The classification is shown in Table 11.1. Diagnosis in all cases requires biopsy of suspicious lesions, which are best detected by careful inspection of the vulva in a bright light, aided if necessary by a magnifying glass (35).

The malignant potential of these nonneoplastic epithelial disorders is low, particularly now that the lesions with atypia are classified as VIN. However, patients with lichen sclerosis and concomitant hyperplasia may be at particular risk. Rodke and colleagues reported the development of vulvar carcinoma in 3 of 18 such cases (17%) postulating that the areas of hyperplasia were superimposed on a background of lichen sclerosis because of chronic irritation and trauma (36).

Table 11.1 Classification of Vulvar Diseases

Nonneoplastic epithelial disorders of skin and mucosa
    Lichen sclerosus (as before)
    Squamous hyperplasia, not otherwise specified (formerly "hyperplastic dystrophy without
       atypia")
    Other dermatoses

Mixed nonneoplastic and neoplastic epithelial disorders

Intraepithelial neoplasia
    Squamous intraepithelial neoplasia (formerly "dystrophies with atypia")
       VIN 1
       VIN 2
       VIN 3 (severe dysplasia or carcinoma *in situ*)
    Nonsquamous intraepithelial neoplasia
       Paget's disease
       Tumors of melanocytes, noninvasive

Invasive tumors

From Committee on Terminology, International Society for the Study of Vulvar Disease. New nomenclature for vulvar disease. *Int J Gynecol Pathol* 8:83, 1989.

Vulvar Intraepithelial Neoplasia

As with the vulvar dystrophies, there has been confusion in the past over the nomenclature for vulvar intraepithelial neoplasia. Four major terms were used. "erythroplasia of Queyrat," "Bowen's disease," "carcinoma *in situ* simplex," and "Paget's disease." In 1976 the ISSVD decreed that the first three lesions were merely gross variants of the same disease process and that all should be included under the umbrella term "squamous cell carcinoma *in situ*" (Stage 0) (33). In 1986, they recommended the term "vulvar intraepithelial neoplasia (VIN)," carcinoma *in situ* of the vulva being VIN 3 (Table 11.1).

The term *bowenoid papulosis* has been used by some dermatologists to refer to cases of VIN associated with multiple papule formations (37). Use of the terms *bowenoid papulosis* or *bowenoid dysplasia* is not recommended by the ISSVD for either clinical or pathologic use. Treatment of VIN is discussed in Chapter 6.

Paget's Disease of the Vulva

Extramammary Paget's disease of the vulva (*adenocarcinoma in situ*) was first described in 1901 (38), 27 years after the description by Sir James Paget of the mammary lesion that now bears his name. Unlike its counterpart in the breast, which is invariably associated with an underlying ductal carcinoma, only about 20% of patients with vulvar Paget's disease have an underlying adenocarcinoma.

Clinical Features The disease predominantly affects postmenopausal white women, and the presenting symptoms are usually pruritus and vulvar soreness. The lesion has an eczematoid appearance macroscopically and usually begins on the hair-bearing portions of the vulva. It may extend to involve the mons pubis, thighs, and buttocks. Extension to involve the mucosa of the rectum, vagina, or urinary tract also has been described (39). The more extensive lesions are usually raised and velvety in appearance. Persistent weeping, which may necessitate the constant protection of a napkin, is a distressing feature of extensive Paget's disease.

A second synchronous or metachronous primary neoplasm is associated with extramammary Paget's disease in about 30% of patients (40). Associated carcinomas have been reported in the cervix, colon, bladder, gallbladder, and breast. When the anal mucosa is involved, there is usually an underlying rectal adenocarcinoma (41).

Treatment **Unlike squamous cell carcinoma *in situ*, where the histologic extent of disease usually correlates closely with the macroscopic lesion, Paget's disease usually extends well beyond the gross lesion** (42). This results in positive surgical margins and frequent local recurrence unless a wide local excision is performed. It is desirable to check the surgical margins with frozen sections to ensure complete removal of the disease (41). **Underlying adenocarcinomas are usually clinically apparent, but this is not invariable and thus the underlying dermis should be removed for adequate histologic evaluation.** For this reason, laser therapy is unsatisfactory for primary Paget's disease. If an underlying invasive carcinoma is present, it should be treated in the same manner as a squamous vulvar cancer. This will usually require radical vulvectomy and at least an ipsilateral inguinal-femoral lymphadenectomy.

Recurrent lesions are almost always *in situ*, although there has been at least one case report of an underlying adenocarcinoma in recurrent Paget's disease (40).

In general, it is reasonable to treat recurrent lesions with surgical excision or laser therapy.

Invasive Vulvar Cancer

Squamous Cell Carcinoma

Squamous cell carcinoma of the vulva is predominantly a disease of postmenopausal women, the mean age at diagnosis being about 65 years.

Clinical Features

Most patients present with a vulvar lump or mass, although there is often a long history of pruritus, which may be due to an associated vulvar dystrophy. Less common presenting symptoms include vulvar bleeding, discharge, or dysuria. Occasionally a large metastatic mass in the groin may be the initial presenting symptom. This is much less common than in the past, as women are now more likely to present with earlier-stage disease.

On physical examination, the lesion is usually raised and may be fleshy, ulcerated, leukoplakic, or warty in appearance. There is an increasing incidence of warty carcinoma of the vulva, and such lesions account for about 20% of all cases (43). These warty carcinomas may occur at any age after adolescence and are multifocal in about one-third of the cases (43). They are often initially diagnosed as condylomata acuminata.

Most squamous carcinomas of the vulva occur on the labia majora, but the labia minora, clitoris, and perineum also may be primary sites. Approximately 10% of the cases are too extensive to determine a site of origin, and about 5% of the cases are multifocal.

As part of the clinical assessment, the groin lymph nodes should be evaluated carefully and a complete pelvic examination performed. A Pap smear should be taken from the cervix, and colposcopy of the cervix and vagina should be performed because of the common association with other squamous intraepithelial neoplasms of the lower genital tract.

Diagnosis

Diagnosis requires a wedge biopsy specimen, which usually can be taken in the office with the patient under local anesthesia. The biopsy specimen should include some surrounding skin and some underlying dermis and connective tissue so that the pathologist can adequately evaluate the depth and nature of the stromal invasion. If the lesion is only about 1 cm in diameter, excisional biopsy is preferable.

Physician delay is a common problem in the diagnosis of vulvar cancer, particularly if the lesion has a warty appearance. Although isolated condylomata do not require histologic confirmation for diagnosis, any confluent warty lesion should be biopsied before medical or ablative therapy is initiated.

Routes of Spread

Vulvar cancer spreads by the following routes:

1. Direct extension, to involve adjacent structures such as the vagina, urethra, and anus

407

2. Lymphatic embolization to regional lymph nodes

3. Hematogenous spread to distant sites, including the lungs, liver, and bone

Lymphatic metastases may occur early in the disease. Initially, spread is usually to the inguinal lymph nodes, which are located between Camper's fascia and the fascia lata (9). From these superficial groin nodes, the disease will spread to the femoral nodes, which are located along the femoral vessels (Fig. 11.1). *Cloquet's node*, situated beneath the inguinal ligament, is the most cephalad of the femoral node group. **Metastases to the femoral nodes without involvement of the inguinal nodes have been reported** (44–47).

From the inguinal-femoral nodes, the cancer spreads to the pelvic nodes, particularly the external iliac group. Although direct lymphatic pathways from the clitoris and Batholin gland to the pelvic nodes have been described, these channels seem to be of minimal clinical significance (12, 48, 49).

Since 1970, the overall incidence of lymph node metastases is reported to be about 30% (Table 11.2). This incidence is much lower than the 61% reported by Way (6) in 1960 and reflects the trend toward earlier diagnosis and smaller lesions. The incidence of nodal metastases is related to lesion size, stage of disease, and depth of invasion. The incidence in relation to lesion size is as follows: ≤ 1 cm, 5%; 1–2 cm, 16%; 2–4 cm, 33%; > 4 cm, 53% (56). The incidence in relation

Figure 11.1 Inguinal-femoral lymph nodes. (Reproduced, with permission, from Hacker NF, Vulvar Cancer. In Hacker NF, Moore JG (eds): *Essentials of Obstetrics and Gynecology*, Second ed. Philadelphia, WB Saunders, 1992, p 618).

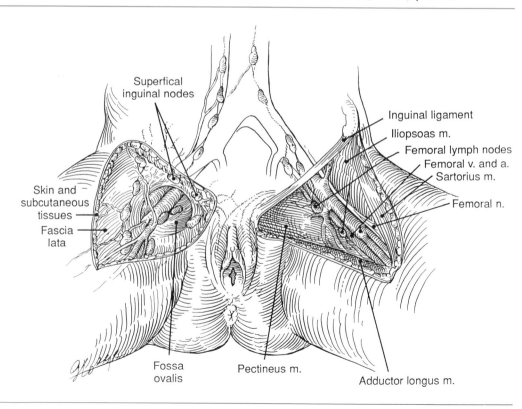

Table 11.2 Incidence of Lymph Node Metastases in Operable Vulvar Cancer

Author	No. of Cases	Positive Nodes	Percent
Rutledge et al., 1970 (50)	110	40	36.4
Green et al., 1978 (51)	142	54	38.0
Krupp and Bohm, 1978 (52)	195	40	20.5
Benedet et al., 1979 (53)	120	34	28.3
Curry et al., 1980 (12)	191	57	29.8
Iversen et al., 1980 (54)	268	86	32.1
Hacker et al., 1983 (13)	113	31	27.4
Podratz et al., 1983 (55)	175	59	33.7
Monaghan and Hammond, 1984 (14)	134	37	27.6
Total	**1448**	**438**	**30.2**

Table 11.3 Incidence of Lymph Node Metastases in Relation to Clinical Stage of Disease

Stage	No. of Cases	Positive Nodes	Percent
I	140	15	10.7
II	145	38	26.2
III	137	88	64.2
IV	18	16	88.9

Data compiled from Green et al., 1978 (51); Iversen et al., 1980 (54); and Hacker et al., 1983 (13).

Table 11.4 Nodal Status in T_1 Squamous Cell Carcinoma of the Vulva Versus Depth of Stromal Invasion

Depth of Invasion	No.	Positive Nodes	Nodes
< 1 mm	163	0	0
1.1–2 mm	145	11	7.7
2.1–3 mm	131	11	8.3
3.1–5 mm	101	27	26.7
> 5 mm	38	13	34.2
Total	**578**	**62**	**10.7**

Data compiled from Parker, 1975 (45); Magrina, 1979 (58); Iversen, 1981 (7); Wilkinson, 1982 (59); Hoffman, 1983 (57); Hacker, 1984 (8); Boice, 1984 (60); Ross, 1987 (61); Rowley, 1988 (62); Struyk, 1989 (63).

to clinical stage of disease is shown in Table 11.3, and that in relation to depth of invasion is shown in Table 11.4.

Metastases to pelvic nodes are uncommon, reported frequencies ranging from 2–12% (14, 27, 51). The overall reported frequency is about 9% (64). Pelvic nodal metastases are rare in the absence of clinically suspicious (N_2) groin nodes (13) and three or more positive groin nodes (12, 13, 54). About 20% of patients with positive groin nodes have positive pelvic nodes (64).

Hematogenous spread usually occurs late in the course of vulvar cancer and is rare in the absence of lymph node metastases. As shown in Table 11.5, distant metastases are very uncommon in patients with one or two positive groin nodes, but they are more common in patients with three or more positive nodes (13).

Staging

A clinical staging system based on the TNM classification was adopted by the International Federation of Gynecology and Obstetrics (FIGO) in 1969 (Table 11.6). The staging was based on a clinical evaluation of the primary tumor and regional lymph nodes and a limited search for distant metastases.

Clinical evaluation of the groin lymph nodes is inaccurate in about 25–30% of the cases (6, 14, 65). Microscopic metastases may be present in nodes that are not clinically suspicious, and suspicious nodes may be enlarged because of inflammation only. **When compared with surgical staging of vulvar cancer, the percentage of error in clinical staging increases from 18% for Stage I disease to 44% for Stage IV disease** (55).

These factors led the Cancer Committee of FIGO to introduce a surgical staging for vulvar cancer in 1988 (Table 11.7). Most available data are still based on the 1969 FIGO staging, which is appropriate because the new staging system requires further modification. There are two major problems with the staging system as presently proposed. First, patients with negative lymph nodes have a very good prognosis, regardless of the size of the primary tumor (13, 66), so survival for both Stages I and II should be better than 80%. Second, survival is dependent on the number of lymph nodes (12, 13, 55, 66). Therefore, Stage III represents a very heterogeneous group of patients, ranging from those with negative nodes and involvement of the distal urethra or vagina, who should have an excellent prognosis, to those with multiple positive groin nodes, who have a very poor prognosis.

Treatment

After the pioneering work of Taussig (5) in the United States and Way (3, 6) in Great Britain, *en bloc* radical vulvectomy and bilateral dissection of the groin and pelvic nodes became the standard treatment for most patients with operable vulvar cancer. If the disease involved the anus, rectovaginal septum, or proximal urethra, some type of pelvic exenteration was combined with the above dissection.

Table 11.5 Recurrence Site in Relation to the Number of Positive Unilateral Groin Nodes

Nodal Status	Vulva (%)	Groin (%)	Pelvis (%)	Systemic (%)
1–2 positive	6/104 (5.8)	3/104 (2.9)	0/104 (0)	4/104 (3.8)
≥ 3 positive	3/9 (33)	3/9 (33)	4/9 (44)	6/9 (66)

Reproduced, with permission, from the American College of Obstetricians and Gynecologists, Hacker NF, Berek JS, Lagasse LD, et al.: Management of regional lymph nodes and their prognostic influence in vulvar cancer. *Obstet Gynecol* 61:408, 1983.

Table 11.6   Clinical Staging of Carcinoma of the Vulva

FIGO Stage	TNM	Clinical Findings
Stage 0		Carcinoma *in situ*, e.g., VIN 3, noninvasive Paget's disease
Stage I	$T_1N_0M_0$ $T_1N_1M_0$	Tumor confined to the vulva, 2 cm or less in largest diameter, and no suspicious groin nodes
Stage II	$T_2N_0M_0$ $T_2N_1M_0$	Tumor confined to the vulva more than 2 cm in diameter, and no suspicious groin nodes
Stage III	$T_3N_0M_0$ $T_3N_1M_0$ $T_3N_2M_0$ $T_1N_2M_0$ $T_2N_2M_0$	Tumor of any size with: (1) adjacent spread to the urethra and/or the vagina, the perineum, and the anus, and/or (2) clinically suspicious lymph nodes in either groin
Stage IV	$T_xN_3M_0$ $T_4N_0M_0$ $T_4N_1M_0$ $T_4N_2M_0$ $T_xN_xM_{1a}$ $T_xN_xM_{1b}$	Tumor of any size: (1) infiltrating the bladder mucosa, or the rectal mucosa, or both, including the upper part of the urethral mucosa, and/or (2) fixed to the bone and/or (3) other distant metastases.

TNM Classification

T:	Primary Tumor	N:	Regional Lymph Nodes
T_1	Tumor confined to the vulva, 2 cm in largest diameter	N_0	No nodes palpable
T_2	Tumor confined to the vulva, > 2 cm in diameter	N_1	Nodes palpable in either groin, not enlarged, mobile (not clinically suspicious for neoplasm)
T_3	Tumor of any size with adjacent spread to the urethra and/or vagina and/or perineum and/or anus	N_2	Nodes palpable in either or both groins, enlarged, firm and mobile (clinically suspicious for neoplasm)
T_4	Tumor of any size infiltrating the bladder mucosa and/or the rectal mucosa or including the upper part of the urethral mucosa and/or fixed to the bone	N_3	Fixed or ulcerated nodes
		M:	Distant Metastases
		M_0	No clinical metastases
		M_{1a}	Palpable deep pelvic lymph nodes
		M_{1b}	Other distant metastases

x = any T or N category.

Although the survival improved markedly with this aggressive surgical approach, several factors have led to modifications of this "standard" treatment plan during the past 15 years. These factors may be summarized as follows:

1. An increasing proportion of patients with early-stage disease—up to 50% of patients in many centers—have T_1 tumors.

2. Concern about the postoperative morbidity and associated long-term hospitalization common with the *en bloc* radical dissection.

3. Increasing awareness of the psychosexual consequences of radical vulvectomy.

Management of Early Vulvar Cancer (T_1N_{0-1})

The modern approach to the management of patients with T_1 carcinoma of the vulva should be individualized (7, 8). There is no "standard" operation

411

Table 11.7   Revised FIGO Staging for Vulvar Cancer

1988 FIGO Stage	TNM	Clinical/Pathological Findings
Stage 0	T_{is}	Carcinoma *in situ,* intraepithelial carcinoma
Stage I	$T_1N_0M_0$	Tumor confined to the vulva or perineum, < 2 cm in greatest dimension, nodes are negative
Stage II	$T_2N_0M_0$	Tumor confined to the vulva and/or perineum, > 2 cm in greatest dimension, nodes are negative
Stage III	$T_3N_0M_0$ $T_3N_1M_0$ $T_1N_1M_0$ $T_2N_1M_0$	Tumor of any size with 1. Adjacent spread to the lower urethra or the anus 2. Unilateral regional lymph-node metastasis
Stage IVA	$T_1N_2M_0$ $T_2N_2M_0$ $T_3N_2M_0$ T_4 any N M_0	Tumor invades any of the following: Upper urethra, bladder mucosa, rectal mucosa, pelvic bone or bilateral regional node metastasis
Stage IVB	Any T, any N M_1	Any distant metastasis including pelvic lymph nodes

TNM Classification

T:	Primary Tumor	N:	Regional Lymph Nodes
T_x	Primary tumor cannot be assessed		Regional lymph nodes are the femoral and inguinal nodes
T_0	No evidence of primary tumor	N_x	Regional lymph nodes cannot be assessed
T_{is}	Carcinoma *in situ* (pre-invasive carcinoma)	N_0	No lymph node metastasis
T_1	Tumor confined to the vulva and/or perineum 2 cm or less in greatest dimension	N_1	Unilateral regional lymph node metastasis
T_2	Tumor confined to the vulva and/or perineum more than 2 cm in greatest dimension	N_2	Bilateral regional lymph node metastasis
T_3	Tumor involves any of the following: lower urethra, vagina, anus	**M:**	**Distant Metastasis**
T_4	Tumor involves any of the following: bladder mucosa, rectal mucosa, upper urethra, pelvic bone	M_x	Presence of distant metastasis cannot be assessed
		M_0	No distant metastasis
		M_1	Distant metastasis (Pelvic lymph node metastasis is M1)

applicable to every patient, and emphasis is on performing the most conservative operation that is consistent with cure of the disease.

In considering the appropriate operation, it is necessary to determine independently the appropriate management of:

1. The primary lesion

2. The groin lymph nodes

Prior to any surgery, all patients should have colposcopy of the cervix, vagina, and vulva, because preinvasive (and rarely invasive) lesions may be present at other sites along the lower genital tract.

Management of the Primary Lesion   The two factors to take into account in determining the management of the primary tumor are:

1. The condition of the remainder of the vulva

2. The patient's age

Although radical vulvectomy has been regarded as the standard treatment for the primary vulvar lesion, this operation is associated with significant disturbances of sexual function and body image. DiSaia et al. (9) regarded the psychosexual disturbances as the major long-term morbidity associated with the treatment of vulvar cancer. Andersen and Hacker (67) reported that sexual arousal was reduced to the 8th percentile and body image to the 4th percentile in women who had undergone vulvectomy, when compared with healthy adult women.

Over the past 15 years, several investigators have advocated a radical local excision rather than a radical vulvectomy for the primary lesion in patients with T_1 tumors (7–10, 66). Traditionally, vulvar cancer has been considered to be a "diffuse disease involving the entire vulva" (25). Anything less than radical vulvectomy has been considered inadequate local treatment that is likely to result in local recurrence. In addition, there has been concern that without an *en bloc* resection, intervening tissue left between the primary tumor and the regional lymph nodes may contain microscopic tumor foci in draining lymphatics. However, squamous carcinomas spread by embolization, not permeation (68), and experience with a separate incision technique for node dissection has confirmed that metastases rarely occur in the skin bridge in patients without clinically suspicious (N_2) nodes in the groin (18).

Regardless of whether a radical vulvectomy or a radical local excision is performed, the surgical margins adjacent to the tumor will be the same, and an analysis of the available literature indicates that the incidence of local invasive recurrence after radical local excision is not higher than that after radical vulvectomy (Table 11.8). This suggests that in the presence of an otherwise normal-appearing vulva, radical local excision is a safe surgical option, regardless of the depth of invasion. Local recurrences reflect the biologic behavior of the disease, not the inadequacies of the surgical resection.

There has been uncertainty regarding the surgical margins that must be obtained to prevent local recurrence, but a recent review of 135 patients from UCLA with all stages of disease revealed that a 1 cm tumor-free surgical margin on the vulva resulted in a very high rate of local control (72). Neither clinical tumor size nor the presence of coexisting benign vulvar pathology correlated with local recurrence.

Table 11.8 Incidence of Local Invasive Recurrence after Radical Local Excision and Radical Vulvectomy for T_1 Squamous Cell Carcinoma of the Vulva

	No.	*Recurrence*	*DOD*
Radical local excision	165	12 (7.2%)	1 (0.6%)
Radical vulvectomy	365	23 (6.3%)	2 (0.6%)

DOD = Dead of disease
$P = 0.85$.
Data compiled from Parker, 1975 (45); Di Saia, 1979 (9); Iversen, 1981 (7); Wilkinson, 1982 (59); Chu, 1982 (70); Hacker, 1984 (8); Boice, 1984 (60); Ross, 1987 (61); Rowley, 1988 (62); Berman, 1989 (71); Struyk, 1989 (62).
Only in papers 7, 8, and 59 are all patients with T_1 lesions included. In the other papers, some type of selection was made (e.g. only tumors with < 5mm of invasion, only unifocal lesions, only tumors ≤ 1 cm in diameter). Length of follow-up ranged from > 12 months (62) to > 63 months (60).

413

When vulvar cancer arises in the presence of VIN or some nonneoplastic epithelial disorder, treatment will be influenced by the patient's age. Elderly patients who have often had many years of chronic itching are not disturbed by the prospect of a radical vulvectomy. In younger women, it will be desirable to conserve as much of the vulva as possible; thus radical local excision should be performed for the invasive disease and the associated disease should be treated in the most appropriate manner. For example, topical steroids may be required for squamous hyperplasia, whereas VIN may require superficial local excision and primary closure.

Radical local excision is most appropriate for lesions on the lateral or posterior aspects of the vulva (Fig. 11.2), where preservation of the clitoris is feasible. For anterior lesions that involve the clitoris or that are in close proximity to it, any type of surgical excision will have psychosexual consequences, particularly in younger patients. In addition, marked edema of the posterior vulva may occur. In young patients with periclitoral lesions, consideration should be given to treating the primary lesion with a small field of radiation therapy. Small vulvar lesions will respond very well to about 5000 cGy external radiation, and biopsy can be performed after therapy to confirm the absence of any residual disease.

Technique for Radical Local Excision Radical local excision implies a wide and deep excision of the primary tumor. The surgical margins should be at least 1 cm. The incision should be carried down to the inferior fascia of the urogenital diaphragm, which is coplanar with the fascia lata and the fascia over the pubic symphysis. The surgical defect is closed in two layers. For perineal lesions, close

Figure 11.2 Small (T1) vulvar carcinoma at the posterior fourchette.

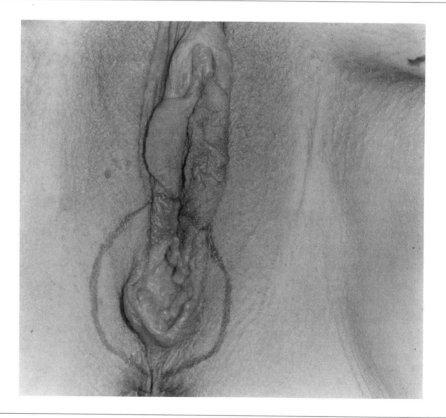

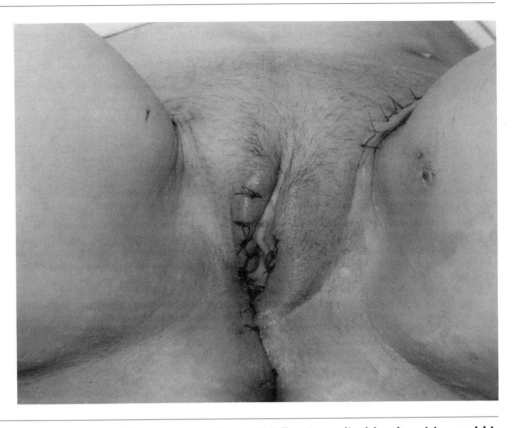

Figure 11.3   Satisfactory cosmetic result following radical local excision and bilateral groin dissection (for the small posterior vulvar carcinoma shown in Figure 11.2).

proximity to the anus may preclude adequate surgical margins, and consideration should be given to preoperative or postoperative radiation in such cases. For periurethral lesions, the distal 1 cm of urethra may be resected without loss of continence. Figure 11.3 shows the satisfactory cosmetic result achieved in the treatment of the lesion shown in Figure 11.2.

Management of the Groin Lymph Nodes   Groin dissection is associated with postoperative wound infection and breakdown and chronic leg edema (49). Although the incidence of wound breakdown is reduced significantly when separate incisions are used for the groin dissection (18), chronic leg edema remains a major problem.

The early papers on early vulvar cancer suggested that it was reasonable to omit the groin dissection in most patients with clinical Stage I disease, provided the depth of stromal invasion was < 5 mm (45, 73). On the basis of these reports, the groin dissection was omitted in many such patients. However, with an increasing number of reports in the literature, two facts have become clear:

1. **The only patients without risk of lymph node metastases are those whose tumor invades the stroma to ≤ 1 mm** (Table 11.4).

2. **Patients who develop recurrent disease in an undissected groin have a very high mortality** (Table 11.9).

415

Table 11.9 Death From Recurrence in an Undissected Groin

Author	Recurrence	Death from Disease
Rutledge et al., 1970 (50)	4	3
Magrina et al., 1979 (58)	4	3
Hoffman et al., 1983 (57)	4	4
Hacker et al., 1984 (8)	3	3
Monaghan and Hammond, 1984 (14)	4	4
Lingard et al., 1992 (74)	7	7
Total	**26**	**24 (92%)**

In 1984 the ISSVD stated that the current definition of microinvasion was misleading and dangerous and should be dropped (75). They recommended that the term "Stage Ia carcinoma of the vulva" be adopted for a single lesion:

1. 2 cm or less in diameter, and

2. 1 mm or less of stromal invasion

Appropriate groin dissection is the single most important factor in decreasing the mortality for early vulvar cancer. All patients with > 1 mm of stromal invasion require inguinal-femoral lymphadenectomy. A wedge biopsy specimen of the primary tumor should be obtained, and the depth of invasion should be determined. If it is < 1 mm on the wedge biopsy specimen, the entire lesion should be locally excised and analyzed histologically to determine the depth of invasion. If there is still no invasive focus > 1 mm, groin dissection may be omitted. Although an occasional patient with < 1 mm of stromal invasion has had documented groin node metastases (76), the incidence is so low that it is of no practical significance. In frail, elderly patients with up to 3 mm of invasion, it may be reasonable to omit groin dissection, provided there is no vascular space invasion, the tumor is not poorly differentiated, and the tumor does not have a "spray" pattern of infiltration.

If groin dissection is indicated in patients with early vulvar cancer, it should be a thorough inguinal-femoral lymphadenectomy. The GOG recently reported six groin recurrences among 121 patients with T_1N_{0-1} tumors after a superficial (inguinal) dissection, even though the inguinal nodes were negative (77). Whether all these recurrences were in the femoral nodes is unclear, but this larger multi-institutional study does indicate that modification of the groin dissection will increase groin recurrences and, therefore, mortality.

From the accumulated experience now available in the literature, it is clear that it is not necessary to perform a bilateral groin dissection if the primary lesion is unilateral (Table 11.10), although lesions involving the anterior labia minora should have bilateral dissection because of the more frequent contralateral lymph flow from this region (78).

Measurement of Depth of Invasion The Nomenclature Committee of the International Society of Gynecological Pathologists has recommended that depth of invasion should be measured from the most superficial dermal papilla adjacent to the tumor to the deepest focus of invasion. This method was originally proposed by Wilkinson et al. (59). Tumor thickness is also commonly measured (58, 79), and Fu and Reagan (80) estimated that the average difference between tumor thickness and depth of invasion as determined by the Wilkinson method was 0.3 mm.

Technique for Groin Dissection   An ellipse of skin is removed 1 cm below and parallel to the groin crease (Fig. 11.4). The incision is carried through the subcutaneous tissues to the superficial fascia. The latter is incised, grasped with artery forceps to place it on traction, and the fatty tissue between it and the fascia lata is removed over the femoral triangle. The dissection is carried 2 cm above the inguinal ligament to include all the inguinal nodes. The saphenous vein is tied off at the apex of the femoral triangle and at its point of entry into the femoral vein. **To avoid skin necrosis, all subcutaneous tissue above the superficial fascia must be preserved.**

The fascia lata is then split longitudinally over the proximal femoral vein, and the fatty tissue containing the femoral lymph nodes is removed. **The femoral lymph nodes are only one to three in number, and they are always situated medial to the femoral vein within the opening of the fossa ovalis** (81). Hence, there is no need to remove the fascia lata lateral to the femoral vessels and no need to perform a sartorius muscle transposition. The node of Cloquet is not consistently present but should be checked for by retraction of the inguinal ligament cephalad over the femoral canal. At the conclusion of the dissection, a suction drain is placed in the groin and the wound is closed in two layers.

Management of a Patient with Positive Groin Nodes   No additional treatment is recommended if one microscopically positive groin node is found. The prognosis for this group of patients is excellent (13), and only careful observation is required. Even if a unilateral groin dissection has been performed for a lateral lesion, there seems to be no indication for dissection of the other groin, as

Table 11.10   Incidence of Positive Contralateral Nodes in Patients with Lateral T₁ Squamous Cell Vulvar Carcinomas and Negative Ipsilateral Nodes

Author	Unilateral Lesions	Contalateral Nodes Positive	Percent
Wharton et al., 1974 (73)	25	0	0
Parker et al., 1975 (45)	41	0	0
Magrina et al., 1979 (58)	77	2	2.6
Iversen et al., 1981 (7)	112	0	0
Buscema et al., 1981 (69)	38	0	0
Hoffman et al., 1983 (57)*	70	0	0
Hacker et al., 1984 (8)	60	0	0
Struyk et al., 1989 (63)	53	0	0
Total	**476**	**2**	**0.4**

*Information not contained in reference but obtained from personal communication.

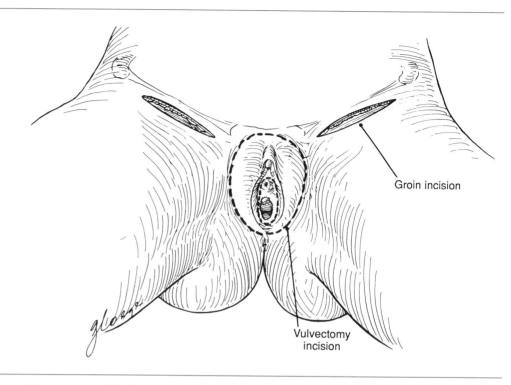

Figure 11.4 Skin incision for groin dissection through a separate incision. A line is drawn 1 cm below and parallel to the groin crease, and a narrow ellipse of skin is removed.

contralateral lymph node involvement is likely only if there are multiple ipsilateral inguinal node metastases (16, 82).

If two or more positive groin nodes are found, which is unusual in patients with T_1 vulvar cancer, the patient is at increased risk of groin and pelvic recurrence and should receive postoperative groin and pelvic radiation (16).

Management of Patients with T_2 and Early T_3 Tumors and N_{0-1} Nodes

In general, the management of patients with T_2 and early T_3 tumors consists of radical vulvectomy and bilateral inguinal-femoral lymphadenectomy. If the disease involves the distal urethra or vagina, partial resection of these organs will be required. Alternatively, it may be preferable to give preoperative radiation therapy to allow a less radical resection.

There are two basic surgical approaches that can be used:

1. The *en bloc* approach through a trapezoid or butterfly incision (65, 83) (Fig. 11.5).

2. The separate-incision approach, involving three separate incisions, one for the radical vulvectomy and one for each groin dissection (17, 18) (Fig. 11.4). This technique leaves a skin bridge between the primary tumor and the draining lymph nodes, but examination of these intervening tissues in patients with early nodal metastases has failed to reveal tumor in connecting lymphatic channels (68).

In general, there is a greater likelihood of primary healing with the separate-incision technique, and it is being used increasingly.

Technique for* En Bloc *Radical Vulvectomy and Groin Dissection   The operation is usually performed with the patient in the low lithotomy position, and groin and vulvar dissections can proceed simultaneously with two teams of surgeons if appropriate. The skin incision has been significantly modified from the original Stanley Way technique to allow primary skin closure (Figure 11.5). The groin dissection is accomplished initially, the abdominal incision being carried down to the aponeurosis of the external oblique muscle, about 2 cm above the inguinal ligament. A skin flap is raised over the femoral triangle, with preservation of the subcutaneous fat above the superficial (Camper's) fascia. The technique for groin dissection has been described earlier.

The vulvar incision is carried posteriorly along each labiocrural fold, or within a 1 cm margin of the primary lesion. The technique for vulvectomy is described below.

Technique for Radical Vulvectomy   If the radical vulvectomy is performed through a separate incision, the lateral incision is basically elliptical. Each lateral incision should commence on the mons pubis anteriorly and extend through the fat and superficial fascia to the fascia over the pubic symphysis. Then it is easy to bluntly develop the plane immediately above the pubic symphysis and fascia lata. The skin incision is extended posteriorly along the labiocrural folds to the

Figure 11.5   Incision used for *en bloc* radical vulvectomy and bilateral groin dissection.

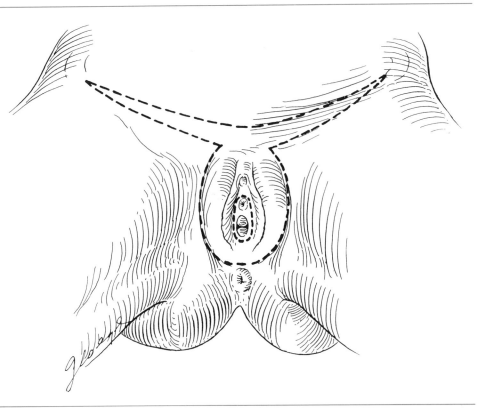

perianal area and carried down to the fascia lata. The medial incision is usually placed around the introitus, just anterior to the external urethral meatus. However, either incision may need to be modified to clear the primary tumor with surgical margins of at least 1 cm. If necessary, the distal half of the urethra may be resected without compromising continence. If the tumor is close to the urethra or the vagina, dissection around the tumors will be facilitated by transection of the vulva, thereby improving exposure of the involved area.

The specimen will include the bulbocavernosus muscles and the vestibular bulb. Because of the vascularity, it is desirable to perform most of the dissection by diathermy after the initial skin incision. In addition, the vessels supplying the clitoris should be clamped and tied, as should the internal pudendal vessels posterolaterally.

Closure of Large Defects It is usually possible to close the vulvar defect without tension. However, if a more extensive dissection has been required because of a large primary lesion, a number of options are available to repair the defect. These include the following:

1. An area may be left open to granulate, which it will usually do over a period of 6 to 8 weeks (84).

2. Full-thickness skin flaps may be devised (85, 86). An example is the rhomboid flap, which is best suited for covering large defects of the posterior vulva (87).

3. Unilateral or bilateral gracilis myocutaneous grafts may be developed. These are most useful when an extensive area from the mons pubis to the perianal area has been resected. Because the graft brings a new blood supply to the area, it is particularly applicable if the vulva is poorly vascularized from prior surgical resection or radiation (88).

4. If extensive defects exist in the groin and vulva, the tensor fascia lata myocutaneous graft is applicable (89).

The technique for these grafts is discussed in Chapter 15.

Vulvar Conservation for T_2 and Early T_3 Tumors In recent years, the indications for vulvar conservation have been extended by some surgeons to selected patients with T_2 and early T_3 tumors. Although the reported experience is limited (10, 11, 90), a recent study at UCLA suggests that the local recurrence rate for patients with conservatively treated Stage II tumors is identical to that for patients with Stage I tumors (91) as long as surgical margins of at least 1 cm are obtained. The tumor-free margin should be the same, whether or not a radical vulvectomy or a radical local excision is performed, so it would seem to be both feasible and desirable to extend the indications for vulvar conservation, particularly in younger patients. Tumors most suitable for a more conservative resection are those involving the posterior half of the vulva, where preservation of the clitoris and mon pubis is feasible.

Management of the Pelvic Lymph Nodes In the past, pelvic lymphadenectomy has been considered to be part of the routine surgery for invasive vulvar cancer. However, the incidence of pelvic node metastases is $< 10\%$, so a more selective approach is justified.

420

Most authors (19, 50, 65) suggest that pelvic lymphadenectomy should be reserved for patients with positive groin nodes, unless the primary tumor involves the clitoris or Bartholin gland. It has been demonstrated that even with clitoral (12, 50) and Bartholin gland carcinomas (48), pelvic node metastases are rare in the absence of inguinal-femoral metastases, so there is no reason to make an exception for these tumors.

In a review of the UCLA data, Hacker et al. (13) reported that **pelvic nodal metastases did not occur unless the patient had:**

1. **Clinically suspicious (N_2) groin nodes,** or

2. **Three or more positive unilateral groin nodes**

All positive pelvic nodes were located on the same side as the multiple positive groin nodes. A similar experience has been reported from the M.D. Anderson Hospital (12), the Mayo Clinic (55), and the University of Michigan (15).

In 1977, the Gynecologic Oncology Group (GOG) initiated a prospective trial in which patients with positive groin nodes were randomized to either ipsilateral pelvic node dissection or bilateral pelvic plus groin irradiation (16). Radiation therapy consisted of 4500–5000 cGy to the midplane of the pelvis at a rate of 180–200 cGy per day. Survival for the radiation group (68% at 2 years) was significantly better than the survival for the pelvic lymphadenectomy group (54% at 2 years) ($P = 0.03$). The survival advantage was limited to patients with clinically evident groin nodes or more than one positive groin node. Groin recurrence occurred in 3 of 59 patients (5%) treated with radiation, compared with 13 of 55 (23.6%) treated with lymphadenectomy ($P = 0.02$). Four patients who received radiation had a pelvic recurrence, compared with one who had lymphadenectomy. These data indicate no benefit from pelvic irradiation compared with pelvic lymphadenectomy for the prevention of pelvic recurrence, but they do highlight the value of prophylactic groin irradiation in preventing groin recurrence in patients with multiple positive groin nodes.

From the above observations, it would seem that patients with one microscopically positive groin node require no further therapy. Patients with two or more positive groin nodes are best treated with pelvic and groin irradiation.

Postoperative Management   In spite of the age and general medical condition of most patients with vulvar cancer, the surgery is usually remarkably well tolerated. However, a postoperative mortality rate of about 2% can be expected, usually as a result of pulmonary embolism or myocardial infarction. Patients should be able to commence a low-residue diet on the first postoperative day. Bed rest is advisable for 3–5 days to allow immobilization of the wounds to foster healing. Pneumatic calf compression or subcutaneous heparin should be given to help prevent deep venous thrombosis, and active, non-weight-bearing leg movements are to be encouraged. Frequent wound dressings and perineal swabs are given. Suction drainage of each groin is continued for about 10 days to help decrease the incidence of groin seromas. A Foley catheter is left in the bladder until the patient is walking around. When the patient is fully mobilized, Sitz baths or whirlpool therapy are helpful, followed by drying of the perineum with a hair dryer.

Early Postoperative Complications The major immediate morbidity is related to groin wound infection, necrosis, and breakdown, and this has been reported in up to 85% of patients having an *en bloc* operation (55). With the separate-incision approach, the incidence of wound breakdown can be reduced to about 44%, with major breakdown occurring in about 14% of patients (18). With debridement and wound dressings, the area will granulate and reepithelialize over the next few weeks and may be managed with home nursing. Whirlpool therapy is effective for areas of extensive breakdown.

Other early postoperative complications include urinary tract infection, seromas in the femoral triangle, deep venous thrombosis, pulmonary embolism, myocardial infarction, hemorrhage, and, rarely, osteitis pubis. Seromas occur in about 10–15% of cases and should be managed by periodic sterile aspiration. Anesthesia of the anterior thigh from femoral nerve injury is common and usually resolves slowly.

Late Complications The major late complication is chronic leg edema, which has been reported in up to 69% of patients (55). Recurrent lymphangitis or cellulitis of the leg occurs in about 10% of patients and usually responds to erythromycin tablets. Urinary stress incontinence, with or without genital prolapse, occurs in about 10% of patients and may require corrective surgery. Introital stenosis can lead to dyspareunia and may require a vertical relaxing incision, which is sutured transversely. An uncommon late complication is femoral hernia, which can usually be prevented intraoperatively by closure of the femoral canal with a suture from the inguinal ligament to Cooper's ligament. Pubic osteomyelitis and rectovaginal or rectoperineal fistulas are rare late complications.

Advanced Disease

Vulvar cancer may be considered to be advanced on the basis of a large T_3 or a T_4 primary tumor or the presence of bulky, positive groin nodes. As with early vulvar cancer, management needs to be individualized.

Management of Patients with a Large T_3 or a T_4 Primary Tumor When the primary disease involves the anus, rectum, rectovaginal septum, or proximal urethra, adequate surgical clearance of the primary tumor is possible only by pelvic exenteration combined with radical vulvectomy and bilateral groin dissection. Such radical surgery is often inappropriate for these elderly patients, and even in suitable surgical candidates psychological morbidity is high (67, 92). In addition, operative mortality is about 10%, and the postoperative physical morbidity is significant. Nevertheless, a 5-year survival rate of about 50% can be expected with this approach (93–96). Surgery alone is rarely curative for patients with fixed or ulcerated (N_3) groin nodes.

Radiation therapy traditionally has been considered to have a limited role in the management of patients with vulvar cancer. In the orthovoltage era, local tissue tolerance was poor and vulvar necrosis was common, but, with megavoltage therapy, tolerance has improved significantly.

Boronow (20) was the first to suggest a combined radiosurgical approach as an alternative to pelvic exenteration for patients with advanced vulvar cancer. In his initial report, he recommended intracavitary radium, with or without external irradiation, to eliminate the internal genital disease and subsequent surgery, usu-

422

ally radical vulvectomy and bilateral groin dissection, to treat the external genital disease.

In 1984, Hacker et al. (21) reported the use of preoperative teletherapy in patients with advanced vulvar cancer; brachytherapy was reserved for patients with persistent disease that would otherwise necessitate exenteration. Rather than radical vulvectomy for all patients, only the tumor bed was resected, on the assumption that any microscopic foci originally present in the vulva would have been sterilized by the radiation. In specimens from one-half of the patients, there was no residual disease. Long-term morbidity was low with the predominant use of teletherapy, and no patient developed a fistula. Two patients whose primary tumor was fixed to bone were long-term survivors (21). Backstrom et al. (97) from the Radiumhemmet reported cure of only 4 of 19 patients (21%) with advanced vulvar cancer when external radiation alone was used, emphasizing the need for a combined radiosurgical approach.

In 1987, Boronow et al. (98) updated their experience with preoperative radiation for locally advanced vulvovaginal cancer, reporting 37 primary cases and 11 cases of recurrent disease. The 5-year survival rate for the primary cases was 75.6%, whereas the recurrent cases had a 5-year survival rate of 62.6%. Seventeen of 40 vulvectomy specimens (42.5%) contained no residual disease. Eight patients (17%) had a local recurrence, and five patients (10.4%) developed a fistula.

As the experience of these investigators has evolved, their approach has been refined. They now recommend external beam therapy for all cases, with more selective use of brachytherapy. The radicality of the surgery has also been significantly modified. A more limited vulvar resection is now advocated, and bulky N_2 and N_3 nodes are resected without full groin dissection in order to avoid the leg edema associated with groin dissection and radiation.

In 1989, Thomas et al. (99) reported on the use of radiation with concurrent infusional *5-fluorouracil*, with or without *mitomycin C*, for 33 patients with vulvar cancer. Median follow-up was 16 months. Of 9 patients who received primary chemoradiation, 6 had an initial complete response in the vulva, but 3 of the 6 subsequently had a local recurrence. This suggests that chemoradiation should always be combined with excision of the tumor bed. Berek et al. (100) treated 12 patients with preoperative chemoradiation using *cisplatin* and *5-fluorouracil* as the radiation sensitizers. The 3-year survival rate was 83%. Using preoperative radiation alone, Rotmensch et al. (101) reported a 45% survival rate for 13 patients with advanced vulvar cancer.

With the experience now accrued, preoperative radiation, with or without concurrent chemotherapy, should be regarded as the treatment of first choice for patients with advanced vulvar cancer who would otherwise require some type of pelvic exenteration.

Management of Patients with Bulky Positive Groin Nodes   In the past, such patients would have undergone a pelvic lymphadenectomy after full groin dissection. The GOG study showed the advantage of postoperative pelvic and groin irradiation in decreasing the incidence of groin recurrence and improving survival for patients with bulky, positive groin nodes (16). However, the incidence of pelvic recurrence was higher in the group receiving pelvic radiation, possibly because of the inability of external beam therapy to sterilize bulky positive pelvic nodes. In addition, our experience is that full groin dissection combined with groin irradiation often produces quite severe leg edema.

In view of these considerations, our current approach to patients with N_2 or N_3 groin nodes is as follows:

1. A preoperative CT scan or ultrasonogram of the pelvis is obtained to determine whether there are any enlarged pelvic nodes.

2. All enlarged groin nodes are removed through a separate-incision approach and sent for frozen section diagnosis. If metastatic disease is confirmed, full lymphadenectomy is not carried out.

3. Any enlarged pelvic nodes seen on CT scan or ultrasonogram are removed via an extraperitoneal approach.

4. Full pelvic and groin irradiation is given as soon as the groin incisions are healed.

5. If the frozen section reveals no metastatic disease in the removed nodes, full groin dissection is performed.

Role of Radiation

Radiation therapy, with or without the addition of concurrent chemotherapy, is likely to have an increasingly important role in the management of patients with vulvar cancer. The indications for radiation therapy in patients with this disease are still evolving. At present, radiation seems to be clearly indicated in the following situations:

1. Preoperatively, in patients with advanced disease who would otherwise require pelvic exenteration (20, 21).

2. Postoperatively, to treat the pelvic lymph nodes and groin in patients with two or more positive groin nodes (16).

Possible roles for radiation therapy include the following:

1. Postoperatively, to help prevent local recurrences in patients with involved or close surgical margins (< 5 mm) (102, 103).

2. As primary therapy for patients with small primary tumors, particularly clitoral or periclitoral lesions in young and middle-aged women, in whom surgical resection would have significant psychological consequences.

Groin irradiation has been proposed as an alternative to groin dissection in patients with N_0 lymph nodes. However, the GOG recently reported the results of a phase III trial in which patients with T_1, T_2, or T_3 tumors and N_{0-1} groin nodes were randomized between surgical resection (and postoperative irradiation for patients with positive groin nodes) and primary groin irradiation (104). Patients with N_1 nodes were allowed fine needle aspiration cytology of the nodes and exclusion from the trial if findings were positive. The study was closed prematurely because 5 of 26 patients in the groin-irradiation arm of the study had recurrences in the groin. Of 23 patients undergoing groin dissection, 5 showed groin node metastases, but no groin recurrences occurred after postoperative irradiation. The dose of radiation was 5000 cGy given in daily 200 cGy fractions to a depth of 3 cm below the anterior skin surface.

Recurrent Vulvar Cancer

Recurrence of vulvar cancer correlates most closely with the number of positive groin nodes (13). Patients with fewer than three positive nodes, particularly if the nodes are only microscopically involved, have a low incidence of recurrence at any site, whereas patients with three or more positive nodes have a high incidence of local, regional, and systemic recurrences (13, 16).

Local vulvar recurrences are most likely in patients with primary lesions larger than 4 cm in diameter (102) and are usually amenable to further surgical excision, often with a gracilis myocutaneous graft to cover the defect. If this is the only site of recurrence, most patients can be saved (18, 105). Radiation therapy, particularly a combination of external beam therapy plus interstitial needles, has also been used to treat vulvar recurrences. Hoffman et al. (106) recently reported on 10 patients treated in this manner, and 9 were still alive with a mean follow-up of 28 months. However, 6 of the 10 developed severe radionecrosis at a median of 8.5 months after radiation, and the authors concluded that, although this treatment was highly effective, it was also highly morbid.

Regional and distant recurrences are difficult to manage (102). Radiation therapy may be used in conjunction with surgery for groin recurrence, whereas chemotherapeutic agents that have activity against squamous carcinomas may be offered for distant metastases. The most active agents are cisplatin, methotrexate, Cytoxan, bleomycin, and mitomycin C, but response rates are low and the duration of response is usually disappointing. Long-term survival is very uncommon with regional or distant recurrence (102).

Prognosis

With appropriate management, the prognosis for vulvar cancer is generally good, the overall 5-year survival rate in operable cases being about 70%. Survival correlates with the FIGO clinical stage of disease (Table 11.11) and also with lymph node status. Patients with negative lymph nodes have a 5-year survival rate of about 90% (Table 11.12), but this falls to about 50% for patients with positive nodes (Table 11.13).

Table 11.11 Five-Year Survival Versus Stage for Patients Treated with Curative Intent

Clinical FIGO Stage	No.	Dead of Disease	Corrected 5-Year Survival (%)
I	376	36	90.4
II	310	71	77.1
III	238	116	51.3
IV	111	91	18.0
Total	**1035**	**314**	**69.7**

Data compiled from Rutledge et al., 1970 (50), Boutselis, 1972 (107), Morley, 1976 (65), Japeze et al., 1977 (108), Benedet et al., 1979 (53), Hacker et al., 1983 (13), Cavanagh et al., 1986 (95).

Table 11.12 Five-Year Survival for Patients with Negative Lymph Nodes

Author	No.	Dead of Disease	5-Year Survival (%)
Rutledge et al., 1970 (50)	53	0	100.0
Morley, 1976 (65)	118	9	92.4
Green, 1978 (51)	63	3	95.2
Hacker et al., 1983 (13)	82	5	93.9
Podratz et al., 1983 (55)	115	12	90.0
Monaghan and Hammond, 1984 (14)	95	9	90.0
Cavanagh et al., 1986 (109)	96	16	83.0
Total	**622**	**54**	**91.3**

Table 11.13 Five-Year Survival for Patients with Positive Lymph Nodes Treated with Curative Intent

Author	No.	Dead of Disease	5-Year Survival (%)
Rutledge et al., 1970 (50)	28	15	46.4
Morley, 1976 (65)	62	38	38.7
Green, 1978 (51)	46	18	60.8
Benedet et al., 1979 (53)	34	16	52.9
Curry et al., 1980 (12)	52	30	42.3
Hacker et al., 1983 (13)	31	10	67.7
Cavanagh et al., 1986 (109)	58	36	37.9
Total	**311**	**163**	**52.4**

The number of positive groin nodes is the single most important prognostic variable (13, 15, 16, 55). Patients with one microscopically positive node have a good prognosis, regardless of the stage of disease (13, 15), but patients with three or more positive nodes have a poor prognosis. Because the number of positive nodes correlates with the clinical status of the groin nodes (13), survival also correlates significantly with this variable. In the GOG study, patients with N_0 or N_1 nodes had a 2-year survival rate of 78%, compared with 52% for patients with N_2 nodes and 33% for patients with N_3 nodes ($P = 0.01$) (16). The survival rate for patients with positive pelvic nodes is about 11% (64).

As discussed earlier, the recently proposed FIGO surgical staging is flawed, and it is hoped that it will be revised. However, the GOG staged 588 patients with vulvar cancer by the new criteria, and reported 5-year survival rates of 98%, 85%, 74%, and 31% for Stages I, II, III, and IV, respectively (66).

Recently, workers at the Norwegian Radium Hospital evaluated DNA ploidy for its prognostic significance in 118 squamous cell carcinomas of the vulva (110). The 5-year crude survival rate was 62% for the diploid and 23% for the aneuploid tumors ($p < 0.001$). Aneuploid tumors without lymph node metastases had a 5-year cancer-related survival rate of 44% as compared with 58% for the diploid tumors with lymph node metastases. In a multivariate Cox regression analysis, the most important independent prognostic parameters were

1. Lymph node involvement ($p < 0.0001$)

2. Tumor ploidy ($p = 0.0001$)

3. Tumor size ($p = 0.0039$)

Melanoma

Vulvar melanomas are rare, although they are the second most common vulvar malignancy. Most arise *de novo* (111), but they may arise from a preexisting junctional nevus. They occur predominantly in postmenopausal white women, most commonly on the labia minora or the clitoris (Fig. 11.6). The incidence of cutaneous melanomas worldwide is increasing significantly.

Most patients with a vulvar melanoma have no symptoms except for the presence of a pigmented lesion that may be enlarging. Some patients have itching or bleeding, and a few present with a groin mass.

There are three basic histologic types. The most common is the *superficial spreading melanoma*, which tends to remain relatively superficial early in its development. The *lentigo maligna melanoma* is a flat freckle, which may become quite extensive but also tends to remain superficial. The most aggressive lesion is the

Figure 11.6 Melanoma of the vulva involving the right labium minus.

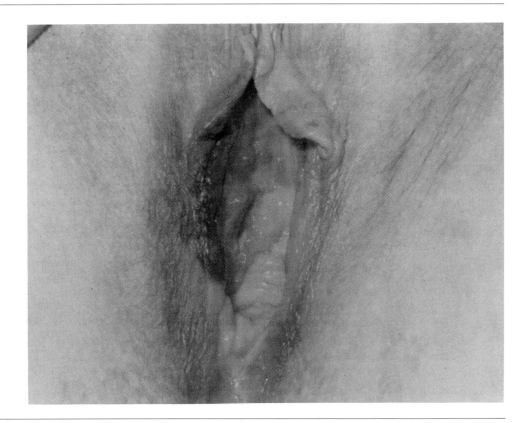

nodular melanoma, which is a raised lesion that penetrates deeply and may metastasize widely. Amelanotic varieties occasionally occur. Any pigmented lesion on the vulva should be excised or biopsied, unless it is known to have been present and unchanged for some years.

Staging

The FIGO staging used for squamous lesions is not applicable for melanomas, because these lesions are usually much smaller and the prognosis is related to the depth of penetration rather than to the diameter of the lesion (112–114). The leveling system established by Clark et al. (115) for cutaneous melanomas is less readily applicable to vulvar lesions because of the different skin morphology. Chung et al. (112) proposed a modified system that retained Clark's definitions for levels I and V but arbitrarily defined levels II, III, and IV, using measurements in millimeters. Breslow (116) measured the thickest portion of the melanoma from the surface of intact epithelium to the deepest point of invasion. A comparison of these systems is shown in Table 11.14.

Treatment

With better understanding of the prognostic significance of the microstage, some individualization of treatment has developed. **Lesions with less than 1 mm of invasion may be treated with radical local excision alone** (112, 113). With more invasive lesions, *en bloc* resection of the primary tumor and regional groin nodes is required. In line with trends toward more conservative surgery for cutaneous melanomas (117, 118), there is a trend toward more conservative resection for vulvar melanomas (119–121). Radical vulvectomy is being performed less frequently, and survival does not appear to be compromised. Davidson et al. (120) reported on 32 patients with vulvar melanoma who underwent local excision ($N = 14$), simple vulvectomy ($N = 7$), or radical resection ($N = 11$). No group had a superior survival, although the overall survival rate at 5 years was only 25%. More recently, Trimble et al. (121) reported on 59 patients who underwent radical vulvectomy and 19 who underwent more conservative resections. Survival was not improved by the more radical approach, and they recommended radical local excision for the primary tumor, with groin dissection for tumors with a thickness > 1 mm.

As melanomas commonly involve the clitoris and labia minora, the vaginourethral margin of resection is a common site of failure, and care should be taken to obtain an adequate "inner" resection margin (122). Podratz et al. (114) demonstrated a 10-year survival rate of 61% for lateral lesions, compared with 37% for medial lesions ($p = 0.027$).

Pelvic node metastases do not occur in the absence of groin node metastases (122–124). In addition, the prognosis for patients with positive pelvic nodes is so poor that there appears to be no value in performing pelvic lymphadenectomy for this disease.

Table 11.14 Microstaging of Vulvar Melanomas

	Clark's Levels (90)	*Chung (87)*	*Breslow (91)*
I	Intraepithelial	Intraepithelial	< 0.76 mm
II	Into papillary dermis	≤ 1 mm from granular layer	0.76–1.50 mm
III	Filling dermal papillae	1.1–2 mm from granular layer	1.51–2.25 mm
IV	Into reticular dermis	> 2 mm from granular layer	2.26–3.0 mm
V	Into subcutaneous fat	Into subcutaneous fat	> 3 mm

Chemotherapy and immunotherapy for vulvar melanoma are disappointing. Estrogen receptors have been demonstrated in human melanomas (125), and responses to tamoxifen have been reported (126, 127).

Prognosis

The behavior of melanomas can be quite unpredictable, but the overall prognosis is poor. The mean 5-year survival rate for reported cases of vulvar melanoma ranges from 21.7% (111) to 54% (114). Patients with lesions invading to 1 mm or less have an excellent prognosis, but as depth of invasion increases, prognosis worsens. Chung et al. (112) reported a corrected 5-year survival rate of 100% for patients with level II lesions, 40% for level III or IV lesions, and 20% for level V lesions. Tumor volume has been reported to correlate with prognosis; patients whose lesions have a volume under 100 mm^3 have an excellent prognosis (124).

Bartholin Gland Carcinoma

Primary carcinoma of the Bartholin gland accounts for about 5% of vulvar malignancies. Because of its rarity, individual experience with the tumor is limited, and recommendations for management must be based on literature reviews. To date, about 280 cases have been reported (48, 128).

The bilateral Bartholin glands are greater vestibular glands situated posterolaterally in the vulva. Their main duct is lined with stratified squamous epithelium, which changes to transitional epithelium as the terminal ducts are reached. As tumors may arise from the gland or the duct, a variety of histologic types may occur, including adenocarcinomas, squamous carcinomas, and, rarely, transitional cell, adenosquamous, and adenoid cystic carcinomas.

Classification of a vulvar tumor as a Bartholin gland carcinoma has typically required that it fulfill *Honan's criteria*, which are:

1. The tumor is in the correct anatomic position.

2. The tumor is located deep in the labium majus.

3. The overlying skin is intact.

4. There is some recognizable normal gland present.

Strict adherence to these criteria will result in underdiagnosis of some cases. Large tumors may ulcerate through the overlying skin and obliterate the residual normal gland. Although transition between normal and malignant tissue is the best criterion, some cases will be diagnosed on the basis of their histologic characteristics and anatomic location.

A history of preceding inflammation of the Bartholin gland may be obtained in about 10% of patients, and malignancies may be mistaken for benign cysts or abscesses. Hence delay of diagnosis is common, particularly in premenopausal patients. The differential diagnosis of any pararectovaginal neoplasm should include cloacogenic carcinoma and secondary neoplasm (128).

Treatment

Traditionally treatment has been by radical vulvectomy, with bilateral groin and pelvic node dissection (129). However, there seems to be no indication for dissection of the pelvic nodes in the absence of positive groin nodes, and Copeland et al. (128) at the M.D. Anderson Hospital have reported good results with hemivulvectomy or radical local excision for the primary tumor. Because these lesions are deep in the vulva, extensive dissection is required in the ischiorectal fossa, and, even then, surgical margins are often close. Postoperative radiation to the vulva decreased the likelihood of local recurrence in Copeland's series from 27% (6 of 22) to 7% (1 of 14). If the ipsilateral groin nodes are positive, bilateral groin and pelvic radiation may decrease regional recurrence. If the tumor is fixed to the inferior pubic ramus or involving adjacent structures, such as the anal sphincter or rectum, preoperative radiation is preferable to avoid exenterative surgery and permanent colostomy.

Prognosis

Because of the deep location of the gland, cases tend to be more advanced than squamous carcinomas at the time of diagnosis, but stage for stage, the prognosis is similar.

The *adenoid cystic* variety is less likely to metastasize to lymph nodes and carries a somewhat better prognosis. Local recurrences are common, however, and they may metastasize, particularly to the lungs. The slowly progressive nature of these tumors is reflected in the disparity between progression-free interval and survival curves (130).

Other Adenocarcinomas

Adenocarcinomas of the vulva usually arise in a Bartholin gland or occur in association with Paget's disease. They may rarely arise from the skin appendages, paraurethral glands, minor vestibular glands, aberrant breast tissue, endometriosis, or a misplaced cloacal remnant (80).

A particularly aggressive type is the *adenosquamous carcinoma*. This tumor has a number of synonyms, including cylindroma, pseudoglandular squamous cell carcinoma, and adenoacanthoma of the sweat gland of Lever. The tumor has a propensity for perineural invasion, early lymph node metastasis, and local recurrence. Underwood et al. (131) reported a crude 5-year survival rate of 5.5% (1 of 18) for adenosquamous carcinoma of the vulva, compared with 62.3% (48 of 77) for patients with squamous cell carcinoma. Treatment should be by radical vulvectomy and bilateral groin dissection, and postoperative radiation may be appropriate.

Basal Cell Carcinoma

Basal cell carcinomas represent about 2% of vulvar cancers. As with other basal cell carcinomas, vulvar lesions commonly appear as a "rodent ulcer" with rolled edges, although nodules and macules are other morphologic varieties. Most lesions are smaller than 2 cm in diameter and are usually situated on the anterior labia majora. Giant lesions occasionally occur (132). They usually affect postmenopausal white women and are locally aggressive. Radical local excision is generally adequate treatment. Metastasis to regional lymph nodes has been reported but is rare (133–135). The local recurrence rate is about 20% (136).

About 3–5% of basal cell carcinomas contain a malignant squamous component, the so-called *basosquamous carcinoma*. These lesions are more aggressive and should be treated as squamous carcinomas (135). Another subtype of basal cell carcinoma is the *adenoid basal cell carcinoma*, which must be differentiated from the more aggressive adenoid cystic carcinoma arising in a Bartholin gland or the skin (135).

Verrucous Carcinoma

Verrucous carcinoma is a variant of squamous cell carcinoma and has distinctive clinical and pathologic characteristics (137). Although most commonly found in the oral cavity, verrucous lesions may be found on any moist membrane composed of squamous epithelium (138).

Grossly, the tumors have a "cauliflower-like" appearance; microscopically, they contain multiple papillary fronds that lack the central connective tissue core that characterizes condylomata acuminata. The gross and microscopic features of a verrucous carcinoma are very similar to those of the *giant condyloma of Buschke-Loewenstein*, and they probably represent the same disease entity (80). Adequate biopsy from the base of the lesion is required to differentiate a verrucous carcinoma from a benign condyloma acuminatum or a squamous cell carcinoma with a verrucous growth pattern.

Clinically, verrucous carcinomas usually occur in postmenopausal women, and they are slowly growing but locally destructive lesions. Even bone may be invaded. Metastasis to regional lymph nodes is rare but has been reported (139). Radical local excision is the basic treatment, although if there are palpably suspicious groin nodes, these should be evaluated with fine needle aspiration cytology or excisional biopsy. Usually, enlarged nodes will be due to inflammatory hypertrophy (140). If the nodes contain metastases, radical vulvectomy and bilateral inguinal-femoral lymphadenectomy is indicated.

Radiation therapy is contraindicated, as it may induce anaplastic transformation with subsequent regional and distant metastasis (141). Japaze et al. (140) reported a corrected 5-year survival rate of 94% for 17 patients treated with surgery alone, compared with 42% for 7 patients treated with surgery and radiation. If there is a recurrence, further surgical excision is the treatment of choice. This may occasionally necessitate some type of exenteration.

Vulvar Sarcomas

Sarcomas represent 1–2% of vulvar malignancies and comprise a heterogenous group of tumors. Leiomyosarcomas are the most common, and other histologic types include fibrosarcomas, neurofibrosarcomas, liposarcomas, rhabdomyosarcomas, angiosarcomas, epithelioid sarcomas, and malignant schwannomas (80).

Leiomyosarcomas usually appear as enlarging, often painful masses, usually in the labium majus. In a review of 32 smooth muscle tumors of the vulva, Tavassoli and Norris (142) reported that recurrence was associated with three main determinants: diameter > 5 cm, infiltrating margins, ≥ 5 mitotic figures per 10 high-power fields. Neoplasms with these three features should be regarded as sarcomas. The absence of one, or even all, of these features does not guarantee that recurrence will not occur (142). Lymphatic metastases are uncommon, and radical local excision is the usual treatment.

Epithelioid sarcomas characteristically develop in the soft tissues of the extremities of young adults but may rarely occur on the vulva. Ulbright et al. (143) described two cases and reviewed three other reports. They concluded that these tumors may mimic a Bartholin cyst, thus leading to inadequate initial treatment. They also believed that vulvar epithelioid sarcomas behave more aggressively than their extragenital counterparts, with four of the five patients dying of met-

431

astatic disease. They suggested that early recognition and wide excision should improve the prognosis.

Rhabdomyosarcomas are the most common soft tissue sarcomas in childhood, and 20% involve the pelvis or genitourinary tract (144). Dramatic gains have been made in the treatment of these tumors over the past 20 years. Previously, radical pelvic surgery was the standard approach, but results were poor. More recently, a multimodality approach has evolved and survival rates have improved significantly, with a corresponding decrease in morbidity.

Hays et al. (145) reported the experience of the Intergroup Rhabdomyosarcoma Study I and II (1972–1984) with primary tumors of the female genital tract (145). Nine patients 1 to 19 years of age had primary vulvar tumors, and these were often regarded as a form of Bartholin gland infection prior to biopsy. They were all managed with chemotherapy (*vincristine, Dactinomycin ± Cytoxan ± Adriamycin*), with or without radiotherapy. Wide local excision of the tumor, with or without inguinal-femoral lymphadenectomy, was carried out before or after the chemotherapy. Seven of the nine patients were free of disease 4 years or more from diagnosis, one patient was free of disease when lost to follow-up at 5 years, and one patient was alive with disease.

Rare Vulvar Malignancies

Other than the tumors mentioned above, a number of malignancies more commonly seen in other areas of the body may rarely present as isolated vulvar tumors. These include the following:

Lymphomas   The genital tract may be involved primarily by malignant lymphomas, but more commonly involvement is a manifestation of systemic disease. In the lower genital tract, the cervix is most commonly involved, followed by the vulva and the vagina (80). Most patients are in their third to sixth decade of life, and about three-fourths of the cases involve diffuse large cell or histiocytic non-Hodgkin's lymphomas. The remainder are nodular or Burkitt's lymphomas (146). Treatment is by surgical excision followed by chemotherapy and/or radiation, and the overall 5-year survival rate is about 70% (146).

Endodermal Sinus Tumor   There have been four case reports of endodermal sinus tumor of the vulva, and three of the four patients died of distant metastases (80, 147). All patients were in their third decade of life, but none were treated with modern chemotherapy.

Merkel Cell Carcinoma   Merkel cell carcinomas are primary small cell carcinomas of the skin, which resemble oat cell carcinomas of the lung. They metastasize widely and have a very poor prognosis (148, 149). They should be locally excised and treated with cisplatinum-based chemotherapy.

Dermatofibrosarcoma Protuberans   This is a rare, low-grade cutaneous malignancy, which occasionally involves the vulva. It has a marked tendency for local recurrence but a low risk of systemic spread (150). Radical local excision should be sufficient treatment.

Malignant Schwannoma   Five cases of malignant schwannoma in the vulvar region have been reported. The patients ranged in age from 25 to 45 years. Four of the five were free of tumor from 1 to 9 years after radical surgery, and the fifth patient died of multiple pulmonary metastases (80).

Secondary Vulvar Tumors

Eight percent of vulvar tumors are metastatic (80). The most common primary site is the cervix, followed by the endometrium, kidney, and urethra. Most patients who develop vulvar metastases have advanced primary tumors at presentation, and in about one-fourth of the patients the primary lesion and the vulvar metastasis are diagnosed simultaneously (151).

References

1. **Sturgeon SR, Brinton LA, Devesa SS, Kurman RJ:** In situ and invasive vulvar cancer incidence trends (1973 to 1987). *Am J Obstet Gynecol* 166:1482, 1992.

2. **Blair-Bell W, Datnow MM:** Primary malignant diseases of the vulva, with special reference to treatment by operation. *J Obstet Gynaecol Br Emp* 43:755, 1936.

3. **Way S:** The anatomy of the lymphatic drainage of the vulva and its influence on the radical operation for carcinoma. *Ann R Coll Surg Engl* 3:187, 1948.

4. **Basset A:** Traitement chirurgical operatoire de l'epithelioma primitif du clitoris: indications—technique—results. *Rev Chir* 46:546, 1912.

5. **Taussig FJ:** Cancer of the vulva: an analysis of 155 cases. *Am J Obstet Gynecol* 40:764, 1940.

6. **Way S:** Carcinoma of the vulva. *Am J Obstet Gynecol* 79:692, 1960.

7. **Iversen T, Abeler V, Aalders J:** Individualized treatment of stage I carcinoma of the vulva. *Obstet Gynecol* 57:85, 1981.

8. **Hacker NF, Berek JS, Lagasse LD, et al:** Individualization of treatment for stage I squamous cell vulvar carcinoma. *Obstet Gynecol* 63:155, 1984.

9. **DiSaia PJ, Creasman WT, Rich WM:** An alternative approach to early cancer of the vulva. *Am J Obstet Gynecol* 133:825, 1979.

10. **Burke TW, Stringer CA, Gershenson DM, et al:** Radical wide excision and selective inguinal node dissection for squamous cell carcinoma of the vulva. *Gynecol Oncol* 38:328, 1990.

11. **Burrell MO, Franklin EW III, Campion MJ, et al:** The modified radical vulvectomy with groin dissection. An eight-year experience. *Am J Obstet Gynecol* 159:715, 1988.

12. **Curry SL, Wharton JT, Rutledge F:** Positive lymph nodes in vulvar squamous carcinoma. *Gynecol Oncol* 9:63, 1980.

13. **Hacker NF, Berek JS, Lagasse LD, et al:** Management of regional lymph nodes and their prognostic influence in vulvar cancer. *Obstet Gynecol* 61:408, 1983.

14. **Monaghan JM, Hammond IG:** Pelvic node dissection in the treatment of vulval carcinoma—is it necessary? *Br J Obstet Gynaecol* 91:270, 1984.

15. **Hoffman JS, Kumar NB, Morley GW:** Prognostic significance of groin lymph node metastases in squamous carcinoma of the vulva. *Obstet Gynecol* 66:402, 1985.

16. **Homesley HD, Bundy BN, Sedlis A, Adcock L:** Radiation therapy versus pelvic node resection for carcinoma of the vulva with positive groin nodes. *Obstet Gynecol* 68:733, 1986.

17. **Byron RL, Mishell DR, Yonemoto RH:** The surgical treatment of invasive carcinoma of the vulva. *Surg Gynecol Obstet* 121:1243, 1965.

18. **Hacker NF, Leuchter RS, Berek JS, et al:** Radical vulvectomy and bilateral inguinal lymphadenectomy through separate groin incisions. *Obstet Gynecol* 58:574, 1981.

19. **Figge CD, Gaudenz R:** Invasive carcinoma of the vulva. *Am J Obstet Gynecol* 119:382, 1974.

20. **Boronow RC:** Therapeutic alternative to primary exenteration for advanced vulvo-vaginal cancer. *Gynecol Oncol* 1:223, 1973.

21. **Hacker NF, Berek JS, Juillard GJF, Lagasse LD:** Preoperative radiation therapy for locally advanced vulvar cancer. *Cancer* 54:2056, 1984.

22. **Zacur H, Genandry R, Woodruff JD:** The patient-at-risk for development of vulvar cancer. *Gynecol Oncol* 9:199, 1980.

23. **Buscema J, Woodruff JD, Parmley TH, et al:** Carcinoma in situ of the vulva. *Obstet Gynecol* 55:225, 1980.

24. **Franklin EW, Rutledge FD:** Epidemiology of epidermoid carcinoma of the vulva. *Obstet Gynecol* 39:165, 1972.

25. **Green TH Jr, Ulfelder H, Meigs JV:** Epidermoid carcinoma of the vulva: An analysis of 238 cases. Parts I and II. *Am J Obstet Gynecol* 73:834, 1958.

26. **Brinton LA, Nasca PC, Mallin K, et al:** Case control study of cancer of the vulva. *Obstet Gynecol* 75:859, 1990.

27. **Collins CG, Lee FY, Roman-Lopez JJ:** Invasive carcinoma of the vulva with lymph node metastases. *Am J Obstet Gynecol* 109:446, 1971.

28. **Rusk D, Sutton GP, Look KY, Roman A:** Analysis of invasive squamous cell carcinoma of the vulva and vulvar intraepithelial neoplasia for the presence of human papillomavirus DNA. *Obstet Gynecol* 77:918, 1991.

29. **Bloss JD, Liao SY, Wilczynski SP, et al:** Clinical and histologic features of vulvar carcinomas analysed for human papillomavirus status: evidence that squamous cell carcinoma of the vulva has more than one etiology. *Hum Pathol* 22:711, 1991.

30. **Toki T, Kurman RJ, Park JS, et al:** Probable nonpapillomavirus etiology of squamous cell carcinoma of the vulva in older women: a clinicopathologic study using *in situ* hybridization and polymerase chain reaction. *Int J Gynecol Pathol* 10:107, 1991.

31. **Nuovo GJ, Delvenne P, MacConnel P, et al:** Correlation of histology and detection of human papillomavirus DNA in vulvar cancers. *Gynecol Oncol* 43:275, 1991.

32. **Hay DM, Cole FM:** Primary invasive carcinoma of the vulva in Jamaica. *J Obstet Gynaecol Br Commonw* 76:821, 1969.

33. **Gardner HL, Friedrich EG Jr, Kaufman RH, Woodruff JD:** The vulvar dystrophies, atypias, and carcinoma in situ. An invitational symposium. *J Reprod Med* 17:131, 1976.

34. **Jeffcoate TNA:** Chronic vulval dystrophies. *Am J Obstet Gynecol* 95:61, 1966.

35. **Committee on Terminology, International Society for the Study of Vulvar Disease:** New nomenclature for vulvar disease. *Int J Gynecol Pathol* 8:83, 1989.

36. **Rodke G, Friedrich EG, Wilkinson EJ:** Malignant potential of mixed vulvar dystrophy (lichen slerosis associated with squamous cell hyperplasia). *J Reprod Med* 33:545, 1988.

37. **Wade TR, Kopf AW, Ackerman AB:** Bowenoid papulosis of the penis. *Cancer* 42:1890, 1978.

38. **Dubreuilh W:** Pigmentation of the skin due to demodex folliculorum. *Br J Dermatol* 13:403, 1901.

39. **Lee RA, Dahlin DC:** Paget's disease of the vulva with extension into the urethra, bladder, and ureters: a case report. *Am J Obstet Gynecol* 140:834, 1981.

40. **Hart WR, Millman RB:** Progression of intraepithelial Paget's disease of the vulva to invasive carcinoma. *Cancer* 40:2333, 1977.

41. **Stacy D, Burrell MO, Franklin EW III:** Extramammary Paget's disease of the vulva and anus: use of intraoperative frozen-section margins. *Am J Obstet Gynecol* 155:519, 1986.

42. **Gunn RA, Gallager HS:** Vulvar Paget's disease: a topographic study. *Cancer* 46:590, 1980.

43. **Rastkar G, Okagaka T, Twiggs LB, Clark BA:** Early invasive and in situ warty carcinoma of the vulva: clinical, histologic, and electron microscopic study with particular reference to viral association. *Am J Obstet Gynecol* 143:814, 1982.

44. **Hacker NF, Nieberg RK, Berek JS, et al:** Superficially invasive vulvar cancer with nodal metastases. *Gynecol Oncol* 15:65, 1983.

45. **Parker RT, Duncan I, Rampone J, et al:** Operative management of early invasive epidermoid carcinoma of the vulva. *Am J Obstet Gynecol* 123:349, 1975.

46. **Chu J, Tamimi HK, Figge DC:** Femoral node metastases with negative superficial inguinal nodes in early vulvar cancer. *Am J Obstet Gynecol* 140:337, 1981.

47. **Podczaski E, Sexton M, Kaminski P, et al:** Recurrent carcinoma of the vulva after conservative treatment for "microinvasive" disease. *Gynecol Oncol* 39:65, 1990.

48. **Leuchter RS, Hacker NF, Voet RL, et al:** Primary carcinoma of the Bartholin gland: a report of 14 cases and a review of the literature. *Obstet Gynecol* 60:361, 1982.

49. **Piver MS, Xynos FP:** Pelvic lymphadenectomy in women with carcinoma of the clitoris. *Obstet Gynecol* 49:592, 1977.

50. **Rutledge F, Smith JP, Franklin EW:** Carcinoma of the vulva. *Am J Obstet Gynecol* 106:1117, 1970.

51. **Green TH Jr:** Carcinoma of the vulva: a reassessment. *Obstet Gynecol* 52:462, 1978.

52. **Krupp PJ, Bohm JW:** Lymph gland metastases in invasive squamous cell cancer of the vulva. *Am J Obstet Gynecol* 130:943, 1978.

53. **Benedet JL, Turko M, Fairey RN, et al:** Squamous carcinoma of the vulva: results of treatment, 1938 to 1976. *Am J Obstet Gynecol* 134:201, 1979.

54. **Iversen T, Aalders JG, Christensen A, et al:** Squamous cell carcinoma of the vulva: a review of 424 patients, 1956–1974. *Gynecol Oncol* 9:271, 1980.

55. **Podratz KC, Symmonds RE, Taylor WF, et al:** Carcinoma of the vulva: analysis of treatment and survival. *Obstet Gynecol* 61:63, 1983.

56. **Hacker NF, Berek JS:** Vulva. In Haskell CM (ed): *Cancer Treatment.* Third ed. Philadelphia, WB Saunders Company, 1990, pp 351–361.

57. **Hoffman JS, Kumar NB, Morley GW:** Microinvasive squamous carcinoma of the vulva: Search for a definition. *Obstet Gynecol* 61:615, 1983.

58. **Magrina JF, Webb MJ, Gaffey TA, et al:** Stage I squamous cell cancer of the vulva. *Am J Obstet Gynecol* 134:453, 1979.

59. **Wilkinson EJ, Rico MJ, Pierson KK:** Microinvasive carcinoma of the vulva. *Int J Gynaecol Pathol* 1:29, 1982.

60. **Boice CR, Seraj IM, Thrasher T, King A:** Microinvasive squamous carcinoma of the vulva: present status and reassessment. *Gynecol Oncol* 18:71, 1984.

61. **Ross M, Ehrmann RL:** Histologic prognosticators in stage I squamous cell carcinoma of the vulva. *Obstet Gynecol* 70:774, 1987.

62. **Rowley K, Gallion HH, Donaldson ES, et al:** Prognostic factors in early vulvar cancer. *Gynecol Oncol* 31:43, 1988.

63. **Struyk APHB, Bouma JJ, van Lindert ACM, et al:** Early stage cancer of the vulva: a pilot investigation on cancer of the vulva in gynecologic oncology centers in the Netherlands. *Proc Int Gynecol Cancer Soc* 2:303, 1989.

64. **van der Velden J, Hacker NF:** Update on vulvar carcinoma. In Rothenberg ML (ed). *Gynecologic Oncology. Controversies and new developments.* Boston, Kluwer Academic Publishers, 1994, pp 101–119.

65. **Morley GW:** Infiltrative carcinoma of the vulva: results of surgical treatment. *Am J Obstet Gynecol* 124:874, 1976.

66. **Homesley HD, Bundy BN, Sedlis A, et al:** Assessment of current International Federation of Gynecology and Obstetrics staging of vulvar carcinoma relative to prognostic factors for survival (a Gynecologic Oncology Group study). *Am J Obstet Gynecol* 164:997, 1991.

67. **Andersen BL, Hacker NF:** Psychological adjustment after vulvar surgery. *Obstet Gynecol* 62:457, 1983.

68. **Willis RA:** *The Spread of Tumours in the Human Body,* ed 3. London, Butterworth, 1973, pp 19–30.

69. **Buscema J, Stern JL, Woodruff JD:** Early invasive carcinoma of the vulva. *Am J Obstet Gynecol* 140:563, 1981.

70. **Chu J, Tamimi HK, Ek M, Figge DC:** Stage I vulvar cancer: criteria for microinvasion. *Obstet Gynecol* 59:716, 1982.

71. **Berman ML, Soper JT, Creasman WT, et al:** Conservative surgical management of superficially invasive stage I vulvar carcinoma. *Gynecol Oncol* 35:352, 1989.

72. **Heaps JM, Fu YS, Montz FJ, et al:** Surgical-pathologic variables predictive of local recurrence in squamous cell carcinoma of the vulva. *Gynecol Oncol* 38:309, 1990.

73. **Wharton JT, Gallager S, Rutledge RN:** Microinvasive carcinoma of the vulva. *Am J Obstet Gynecol* 118:159, 1974.

74. **Lingard D, Free K, Wright RG, Battistutta D:** Invasive squamous cell carcinoma of the vulva: behaviour and results in the light of changing management regimes. *Aust N Z J Obstet Gynaecol* 32:137, 1992.

75. **Microinvasive cancer of the vulva:** Report of the ISSVD task force. *J Reprod Med* 29:454, 1984.

76. **Atamdede F, Hoogerland D:** Regional lymph node recurrence following local excision for microinvasive vulvar carcinoma. *Gynecol Oncol* 34:125, 1989.

77. **Stehman FB, Bundy BN, Droretsky PM, Creasman WT:** Early stage I carcinoma of the vulva treated with ipsilateral superficial inguinal lymphadenectomy and modified radical hemivulvectomy: a prospective study of the Gynecologic Oncology Group. *Obstet Gynecol* 79:490, 1992.

78. **Iversen T, Aas M:** Lymph drainage from the vulva. *Gynecol Oncol* 16:179, 1983.

79. **Sedlis A, Homesley H, Bundy BN, et al:** Positive groin lymph nodes in superficial squamous cell vulvar cancer. *Am J Obstet Gynecol* 156:1159, 1987.

80. **Fu YS, Reagan JW:** Benign and malignant epithelial tumors of the vulva. In *Fu YS, Reagan JW: Pathology of the Uterine Cervix, Vagina, and Vulva.* Philadelphia, WB Saunders, 1989, pp 138–192.

81. **Micheletti L, Borgno G, Barbero M, et al:** Deep femoral lymphadenectomy with preservation of the fascial lata. *J Reprod Med* 35:1130, 1990.

82. **Dvoretsky PM, Bonfiglio TA, Helmkamp F, et al:** The pathology of superficially invasive thin vulvar squamous cell carcinoma. *Int J Gynecol Pathol* 3:331, 1984.

83. **Abitbol MM:** : Carcinoma of the vulva: improvements in the surgical approach. *Am J Obstet Gynecol* 117:483, 1973.

84. **Simonsen E, Johnsson JE, Tropé C:** Radical vulvectomy with warm-knife and open-wound techniques in vulvar malignancies. *Gynecol Oncol* 17:22, 1984.

85. **Trelford JD, Deer DA, Ordorica E, et al:** Ten-year prospective study in a management change of vulvar carcinoma. *Am J Obstet Gynecol* 150:288, 1984.

86. **Julian CG, Callinson J, Woodruff JD:** Plastic management of extensive vulvar defects. *Obstet Gynecol* 38:193, 1971.

87. **Barnhill DR, Hoskins WJ, Metz P:** Use of the rhomboid flap after partial vulvectomy. *Obstet Gynecol* 62:444, 1983.

88. **Ballon SC, Donaldson RC, Roberts JA:** Reconstruction of the vulva using a myocutaneous graft. *Gynecol Oncol* 7:123, 1979.

89. **Chafe W, Fowler WC, Walton LA, Currie JL:** Radical vulvectomy with use of tensor fascia lata myocutaneous flap. *Am J Obstet Gynecol* 145:207, 1983.

90. **Hacker NF:** Surgery for malignant tumors of the vulva. In Gershenson DM, Curry S (eds): *Operative Gynecology.* Philadelphia, WB Saunders, 1993.

91. **Farias-Eisner R, Cirisano F, Grouse D, et al:** Conservative and individualized surgery for early squamous carcinoma of the vulva: the treatment of choice for stages I and II (T_{1-2}, N_{0-1}, M_0) disease. *Gynecol Oncol* 52: 1994.

92. **Andersen BL, Hacker NF:** Psychosexual adjustment following pelvic exenteration. *Obstet Gynecol* 61:457, 1983.

93. **Kaplan AL, Kaufman RH:** Management of advanced carcinoma of the vulva. *Gynecol Oncol* 3:220, 1975.

94. **Phillips B, Buchsbaum JH, Lifshitz S:** Pelvic exenteration for vulvovaginal carcinoma. *Am J Obstet Gynecol* 141:1038, 1981.

95. **Cavanagh D, Shepherd JH:** The place of pelvic exenteration in the primary management of advanced carcinoma of the vulva. *Gynecol Oncol* 13:318, 1982.

96. **Grimshaw RN, Aswad SG, Monaghan JM:** The role of anovulvectomy in locally advanced carcinoma of the vulva. *Int J Gynecol Cancer* 1:15, 1991.

97. **Backstrom A, Edsmyr F, Wicklund H:** Radiotherapy of carcinoma of the vulva. *Acta Obstet Gynecol* 51:109, 1972.

98. **Boronow RC, Hickman BT, Reagan MT, et al:** Combined therapy as an alternative to exenteration for locally advanced vulvovaginal cancer. II. Results, complications and dosimetric and surgical considerations. *Am J Clin Oncol* 10:171, 1987.

99. **Thomas G, Dembo A, DePetrillo A, et al:** Concurrent radiation and chemotherapy in vulvar carcinoma. *Gynecol Oncol* 34:263, 1989.

100. **Berek JS, Heaps JM, Fu YS, et al:** Concurrent cisplatin and 5-fluorouracil chemotherapy and radiotherapy for advanced stage squamous carcinoma of the vulva. *Gynecol Oncol* 42:197, 1991.

101. **Rotmensch J, Rubin SJ, Sutton HG, et al:** Preoperative radiotherapy followed by radical vulvectomy with inguinal lymphadenectomy for advanced vulvar carcinomas. *Gynecol Oncol* 36:181, 1990.

102. **Podratz KC, Symmonds RE, Taylor WF:** Carcinoma of the vulva: analysis of treatment failures. *Am J Obstet Gynecol* 143:340, 1982.

103. **Malfetano J, Piver MS, Tsukada Y:** Stage III and IV squamous cell carcinoma of the vulva. *Gynecol Oncol* 23:192, 1986.

104. **Stehman F, Bundy B, Bell J, et al:** Groin dissection versus groin radiation in carcinoma of the vulva: a Gynecologic Oncology Group study. *Int J Radiat Oncol Biol Phys* 24:389, 1992.

105. **Hopkins MP, Reid GC, Morley GW:** The surgical management of recurrent squamous cell carcinoma of the vulva. *Obstet Gynecol* 75:1001, 1990.

106. **Hoffman M, Greenberg S, Greenberg H, et al:** Interstitial radiotherapy for the treatment of advanced or recurrent vulvar and distal vaginal malignancy. *Am J Obstet Gynecol* 162:1278, 1990.

107. **Boutselis JG:** Radical vulvectomy for invasive sqaumous cell carcinoma of the vulva. *Obstet Gynecol* 39:827, 1972.

108. **Japeze H, Garcia-Bunuel R, Woodruff JD:** Primary vulvar neoplasia: a review of in situ and invasive carcinoma, 1935–1972. *Obstet Gynecol* 49:404, 1977.

109. **Cavanagh D, Roberts WS, Bryson SCP, et al:** Changing trends in the surgical treatment of invasive carcinoma of the vulva. *Surg Gynecol Obstet* 162:164, 1986.

110. **Kaern J, Iversen T, Tropé C, et al:** Flow cytometric DNA measurements in squamous cell carcinoma of the vulva: an important prognostic method. *Int J Gynecol Cancer* 2:169, 1992.

111. **Blessing K, Kernohan NM, Miller ID, Al Nafussi AI:** Malignant melanoma of the vulva: clinicopathological features. *Int J Gynecol Oncol* 1:81, 1991.

112. **Chung AF, Woodruff JW, Lewis JL Jr:** Malignant melanoma of the vulva: a report of 44 cases. *Obstet Gynecol* 45:638, 1975.

113. **Phillips GL, Twiggs LB, Okagaki T:** Vulvar melanoma: a microstaging study. *Gynecol Oncol* 14:80, 1982.

114. **Podratz KC, Gaffey TA, Symmonds RE, et al:** Melanoma of the vulva: an update. *Gynecol Oncol* 16:153, 1983.

115. **Clark WH, From L, Bernardino EA, Mihm MC:** The histogenesis and biologic behavior of primary human malignant melanomas of the skin. *Cancer Res* 29:705, 1969.

116. **Breslow A:** Thickness, cross-sectional area and depth of invasion in the prognosis of cutaneous melanoma. *Ann Surg* 172:902, 1970.

117. **Aitkin DR, Clausen K, Klein JP, et al:** The extent of primary melanoma excision—a re-evaluation. How wide is wide? *Ann Surg* 198:634, 1983.

118. **Day CL, Mihm MC, Sober AJ, et al:** Narrower margins for clinical stage I malignant melanoma. *N Engl J Med* 306:479, 1982.

119. **Rose PG, Piver MS, Tsukada Y, Lau T:** Conservative therapy for melanoma of the vulva. *Am J Obstet Gynecol* 159:52, 1988.

120. **Davidson T, Kissin M, Wesbury G:** Vulvovaginal melanoma—should radical surgery be abandoned? *Br J Obstet Gynecol* 94:473, 1987.

121. **Trimble EL, Lewis JL Jr, Williams LL, et al:** Management of vulvar melanoma *Gynecol Oncol* 45:254, 1992.

122. **Morrow CP, Rutledge FN:** Melanoma of the vulva. *Obstet Gynecol* 39:745, 1972.

123. **Jaramillo BA, Ganjei P, Averette HE, et al:** Malignant melanoma of the vulva. *Obste Gynecol* 66:398, 1985.

124. **Beller U, Demopoulos RI, Beckman EM:** Vulvovaginal melanoma: a clinicopathologic study. *J Reprod Med* 31:315, 1986.

125. **Fischer RI, Neifeld JP, Lippman ME:** Oestrogen receptors in human malignant melanoma. *Lancet* 2:337, 1976.

126. **Masiel A, Buttrick P, Bitran J:** Tamoxifen in the treatment of malignant melanoma *Cancer Treat Rep* 65:531, 1981.

127. **Nesbit RA, Woods RL, Tattersall MH, et al:** Tamoxifen in malignant melanoma. *N Engl J Med* 301:1241, 1979.

128. **Copeland LJ, Sneige N, Gershenson DM, et al:** Bartholin gland carcinoma. *Obste Gynecol* 67:794, 1986.

129. **Barclay DL, Collins CG, Macey HB:** Cancer of the Bartholin gland: a review and report of 8 cases. *Obstet Gynecol* 24:329, 1964.

130. **Copeland LJ, Sneige N, Gershenson DM, et al:** : Adenoid cystic carcinoma of Bartholin gland. *Obstet Gynecol* 67:115, 1986.

131. **Underwood JW, Adcock LL, Okagaki T:** Adenosquamous carcinoma of skin appendages (adenoid squamous cell carcinoma, pseudoglandular squamous cell carcinoma adenoacanthoma of sweat gland of Lever) of the vulva: a clinical and ultrastructural study. *Cancer* 42:1851, 1978.

132. **Dudzinski MR, Askin FB, Fowler WC:** Giant basal cell carcinoma of the vulva. *Obste Gynecol* 63:575, 1984.

133. **Jimenez HT, Fenoglio CM, Richart RM:** Vulvar basal cell carcinoma with metastasis a case report. *Am J Obstet Gynecol* 121:285, 1975.

134. **Sworn MJ, Hammond GT, Buchanan R:** Metastatic basal cell carcinoma of the vulva a case report. *Br J Obstet Gynaecol* 86:332, 1979.

135. **Hoffman MS, Roberts WS, Ruffolo EH:** Basal cell carcinoma of the vulva with inguinal lymph node metastases. *Gynecol Oncol* 29:113, 1988.

136. **Palladino VS, Duffy JL, Bures GJ:** Basal cell carcinoma of the vulva. *Cancer* 24:460, 1969.

137. **Isaacs HJ:** Verrucous carcinoma of the female genital tract. *Gynecol Oncol* 4:259, 1976.

138. **Partridge EE, Murad R, Shingleton HM, et al:** Verrucous lesions of the female genitalia. II. Verrucous carcinoma *Am J Obstet Gynecol* 137:419, 1980.

139. **Gallousis S:** Verrucous carcinoma: report of three vulvar cases and a review of the literature. *Obstet Gynecol* 40:502, 1972.

140. **Japaze H, Dinh TV, Woodruff JD:** Verrucous carcinoma of the vulva: study of 24 cases. *Obstet Gynecol* 60:462, 1982.

141. **Demian SDE, Bushkin FL, Echevarria RA:** Perineural invasion and anaplastic transformation of verrucous carcinoma. *Cancer* 32:395, 1973.

142. **Tavassoli FA, Norris HJ:** Smooth muscle tumors of the vulva. *Obstet Gynecol* 53:213, 1979.

143. **Ulbright TM, Brokaw SA, Stehman FB, Roth LM:** Epithelioid sarcoma of the vulva. *Cancer* 52:1462, 1983.

144. **Bell J, Averette H, Davis J, Toledano S:** Genital rhabdomyosarcoma: current management and review of the literature. *Obstet Gynecol Surv* 41:257, 1986.

145. **Hays DM, Shimada H, Raney RB, et al:** Clinical staging and treatment results in rhabdomyosarcoma of the female genital tract among children and adolescents. *Cancer* 61:1893, 1988.

146. **Harris NL, Scully RE:** Malignant lymphoma and granulocytic sarcoma of the uterus and vagina. *Cancer* 53:2530, 1984.

147. **Dudley AG, Young RH, Lawrence WD, Scully RE:** Endodermal sinus tumour of the vulva in an infant. *Obstet Gynecol* 61:765, 1983.

148. **Bottles K, Lacy CG, Goldberg J, et al:** Merkel cell carcinoma of the vulva. *Obstet Gynecol* 63:61S, 1984.

149. **Husseinzadeh N, Wesseler T, Newman N, et al:** Neuroendocrine (Merkel cell) carcinoma of the vulva. *Gynecol Oncol* 20:105, 1988.

150. **Bock JE, Andreasson B, Thorn A, Holck S:** Dermatofibromasarcoma protuberans of the vulva. *Gynecol Oncol* 20:129, 1985.

151. **Dehner LP:** Metastatic and secondary tumors of the vulva. *Obstet Gynecol* 42:47, 1973.

Vaginal Cancer

Neville F. Hacker

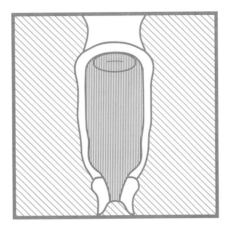

Primary cancer of the vagina constitutes 1–2% of malignant neoplasms of the female genital tract. It represents one of the most challenging therapeutic problems in gynecologic oncology, and until the late 1930s the disease was generally considered to be incurable. With improved techniques for radiation therapy and radical surgery, cure of even advanced cases has been well documented. However, although vaginal cancer appears to behave biologically in a way similar to cervical cancer (1), overall cure rates remain generally much lower and morbidity from treatment is relatively high. In spite of the opportunity for early diagnosis with routine vaginal examinations and Papanicolaou (Pap) smears, the disease has spread beyond the vagina by the time most patients are seen.

Most vaginal malignancies are metastatic (2), usually from the cervix or the vulva. This is partly related to the International Federation of Gynecology and Obstetrics (FIGO) classification and staging of malignant tumors of the female pelvis. The staging requires that a tumor that has extended to the portio and reached the area of the external os should be regarded as a carcinoma of the cervix, whereas a tumor that involves the vulva and vagina should be classified as a vulvar carcinoma. Endometrial carcinomas and choriocarcinomas commonly metastasize to the vagina, whereas tumors from the bladder or rectum may invade the vagina directly.

Primary Vaginal Tumors

The histologic types of primary vaginal tumor are shown in Table 12.1 (1, 3–12). Squamous cell carcinomas are the most common, although adenocarcinomas, melanomas, and sarcomas are also seen. Sarcomas occasionally follow radiotherapy for cervical cancer.

Squamous Cell Carcinoma

Squamous cell carcinoma is the most common vaginal cancer. The mean age of the patients is about 60 years, although the disease occasionally is seen in the

Table 12.1   Primary Vaginal Cancer: Reported Incidence of Histologic Types

Histologic Type	No.	Per Cent
Squamous cell	698	83.4
Adenocarcinoma	74	8.9
Sarcoma	26	3.1
Melanoma	21	2.5
Undifferentiated	8	1.0
Small cell	5	.6
Adenosquamous	2	.2
Lymphoma	2	.2
Carcinoid	1	.1
Total	**837**	**100.0**

Data compiled from Dunn and Napier, 1966 (1), Rutledge, 1967 (3), Perez et al., 1974 (4), Pride and Buchler, 1979 (5), Ball and Berman, 1982 (6), Houghton and Iversen, 1982 (7), Benedet et al., 1983 (8), Peters et al., 1985 (9), Rubin et al., 1985 (10), Sulak et al., 1988 (11), Eddy et al., 1991 (12).

third and fourth decades of life (3, 4, 7, 10). Perez et al. (4) reported that 76% of patients were older than 50 years.

Etiology

The cause of squamous cell carcinoma of the vagina is unknown, although interest has focused on the association between human papillomavirus infection and multifocal carcinoma of the lower female genital tract (13). Vaginal intraepithelial neoplasia (VAIN) has been the subject of increasing attention as a precursor of vaginal cancer (14), although the true malignant potential of VAIN is not known. Benedet and Saunders (15) reviewed 136 cases of carcinoma *in situ* of the vagina seen over a 30-year period. Four cases (3%) progressed to invasive vaginal cancer in spite of various methods of treatment. Lenehan et al. (14) reported invasive vaginal cancer after treatment for VAIN in 3 of 59 patients (5%). Chronic local irritation from long-term use of a pessary may be of significance (3), although pessaries are used less commonly in modern gynecology.

Up to 30% of patients with primary vaginal carcinoma have a history of *in situ* or invasive cervical cancer treated at least 5 years earlier (8–10). In a recent report from the University of South Carolina, a past history of invasive cervical cancer was present in 20% of the cases and of cervical intraepithelial neoplasia (CIN) in 7% (12). The median interval between the diagnosis of cervical cancer and the diagnosis of vaginal cancer was 14 years, with a range of 5 years 8 months to 28 years. Sixteen percent of the patients had a history of prior pelvic irradiation.

There are three possible mechanisms for the occurrence of vaginal cancer after cervical neoplasia:

1. Occult residual disease

2. New primary disease arising in an "at risk" lower genital tract

3. Radiation carcinogenicity

442

In the first instance, extension of intraepithelial neoplasia from the cervix to the upper vagina is not appreciated and an adequate vaginal cuff is not taken because vaginal colposcopy was not performed before surgical management of the cervical tumor. Surgical margins of the upper vaginal resection usually show carcinoma *in situ*, and these persistent foci eventually progress to invasive disease. In the second instance, vaginal colposcopy is normal, and the surgical margins of resection are free of disease. In such circumstances, **any new vaginal carcinoma developing at least 5 years after the cervical cancer should be considered a new primary lesion.** Prior pelvic radiation therapy has been considered a possible cause of vaginal carcinoma (5), and this may be particularly important in young patients who live long enough to develop a second neoplasm in the irradiated vagina (16).

Screening

For screening to be cost-effective, the incidence of the disease must be sufficient to justify the cost of screening. In the United States, the age-adjusted incidence of vaginal cancer is 0.6 per 100,000, making routine screening of all patients inappropriate (17). However, women with a history of cervical intraepithelial or invasive neoplasia are at increased risk and should be followed carefully with Pap smears.

Up to 59% of patients with vaginal cancer have had a prior hysterectomy (6), and some authors have suggested that all patients who have had a hysterectomy should be followed routinely with Pap smears (18, 19). When vaginal cancer occurs in patients who have had a hysterectomy because of benign disease, it is usually more advanced at presentation (18), presumably because these patients have not been under gynecologic surveillance. However, **when age and prior cervical disease are controlled for, there is no increased risk of vaginal cancer in women who have had a hysterectomy for benign disease** (20).

Symptoms and Signs

Most patients with vaginal cancer present with painless vaginal bleeding and discharge. The bleeding is usually postmenopausal but may be postcoital. Because the bladder neck is close to the vagina, bladder pain and frequency of micturition occur earlier than with cervical cancer (3). Posterior tumors may produce tenesmus. About 5% of patients present with pelvic pain because of extension of disease beyond the vagina, and about 5–10% of patients have no symptoms, the disease being detected on routine pelvic examination and Pap smear.

Most lesions are situated in the upper one-third of the vagina, usually on the posterior wall. Macroscopically, the lesions are usually exophytic (fungating, polyploid), but they may be endophytic. Surface ulceration usually occurs late in the course of the disease.

Diagnosis

The diagnosis of carcinoma of the vagina is often missed on first examination, particularly if the lesion is small and situated in the lower two-thirds of the vagina, where it may be covered by the blades of the speculum. Frick et al. (21) reported that at least 10 of 52 cases (19%) in their series were missed on initial examination. Definitive diagnosis is usually made by biopsy of a gross lesion, which can often be performed in the office without anesthesia. Particularly in elderly patients or in those with some degree of vaginal stenosis, examination while the patient is under anesthesia may be desirable to allow adequate biopsy and clinical staging. The latter may require cystoscopy or proctoscopy, depending on the location of the tumor.

In patients with an abnormal Pap smear and no gross abnormality, careful vaginal colposcopy and the liberal use of Lugol's iodine to stain the vagina will be necessary. This should be performed with the patient under regional or general anesthesia to allow the removal of wide biopsy specimens of colposcopically abnormal lesions. **For definitive diagnosis of early vaginal carcinoma, it may be necessary to resect the entire vaginal vault and submit it for careful histologic evaluation, as the lesion may be partially buried by closure of the vaginal vault at the time of hysterectomy.** Inadvertent cystotomy may occur occasionally, and it requires immediate repair.

Hoffman et al. (22) at the University of South Florida recently reported on 32 patients who underwent upper vaginectomy for VAIN 3. Occult invasive carcinoma was found in 9 patients (28%). In 5 cases the invasion was < 2 mm, but in 4 cases invasion ranged from 3.5 mm to full-thickness involvement.

Staging

The FIGO staging for vaginal carcinoma is shown in Table 12.2. The staging is clinical and is based on the findings at general physical and pelvic examination, cystoscopy, proctoscopy, chest radiographs, and skeletal radiographs, if the latter are indicated because of bone pain.

Because it is difficult to determine accurately the spread into subvaginal tissues, particularly of anterior or posterior lesions, differences in observations are common. This is reflected in the wide range of stage distributions reported and the wide range of survival within a given stage. The distribution by FIGO stage from eight recent series is shown in Table 12.3 (5–10, 12, 23). Fewer than one-third of patients present with disease confined to the vagina.

Surgical staging for vaginal cancer has been used less commonly than for cervical cancer, but in selected premenopausal patients, a pretreatment laparotomy may allow better definition of the extent of disease, excision of any grossly enlarged lymph nodes, and placement of an ovary up into the paricolic gutter beyond the radiation field.

Peters et al. (24) suggested criteria for microinvasive carcinoma of the vagina: focal invasion associated with VAIN 3, no lymph-vascular invasion, free margins

Table 12.2 FIGO Staging of Vaginal Cancer	
Stage 0	Carcinoma *in situ*, intraepithelial carcinoma.
Stage I	The carcinoma is limited to the vaginal wall.
Stage II	The carcinoma has involved the subvaginal tissue but has not extended to the pelvic wall.
Stage III	The carcinoma has extended to the pelvic wall.
Stage IV	The carcinoma has extended beyond the true pelvis or has involved the mucosa of the bladder or rectum.
Stage IVa	Spread of the growth to adjacent organs.
Stage IVb	Spread to distant organs.

Table 12.3   Primary Vaginal Carcinoma: Distribution by Stage of Disease

Stage	No.	Per Cent
I	226	25.8
II	294	33.6
III	220	25.1
IV	136	15.5
Total	**876**	**100.0**

Data compiled from Pride and Buchler, 1977 (5), Ball and Berman, 1982 (6), Houghton and Iversen, 1982 (7), Benedet et al., 1983 (8), Peters et al., 1985 (9), Rubin et al., 1985 (10), Eddy et al., 1991 (12), Kucera et al., 1985 (23).

on partial or total vaginectomy, and maximum depth of invasion < 2.5 mm, measured from the overlying surface. However, Eddy et al. (25) reported six patients who met these criteria and were treated by either partial or total vaginectomy. In one of the six a bladder recurrence developed at 35 months.

Patterns of Spread

Vaginal cancer spreads by the following routes:

1. *Direct extension* to the pelvic soft tissues, pelvic bones, and adjacent organs (bladder and rectum).

2. *Lymphatic dissemination* to the pelvic and later the para-aortic lymph nodes. Lesions in the lower one-third of the vagina metastasize directly to the inguinal-femoral lymph nodes, with the pelvic nodes being involved secondarily.

3. *Hematogenous dissemination* to distant organs, including lungs, liver, and bone. Hematogenous dissemination is a late phenomenon in vaginal cancer, the disease usually remaining confined to the pelvis for most of its course.

There is little information available on the incidence of lymph node metastases in vaginal cancer, because most patients are treated with radiation therapy. Rubin et al. (10) reported that 16 of 38 patients (42%) with all stages of disease had abnormal lymphangiograms, but many of these abnormalities were not confirmed histologically. Al-Kurdi and Monaghan (26) performed lymph node dissections on 35 patients and reported positive pelvic nodes in 10 patients (28.6%). Positive inguinal nodes were present in 6 of 19 patients (31.6%), with disease involving the lower vagina.

Preoperative Evaluation

Apart from the standard staging investigations, a computed tomography (CT) scan of the pelvis and abdomen is useful for evaluation of the status of the primary tumor, liver, pelvic and para-aortic lymph nodes, and ureters.

Treatment

There is no consensus as to the proper management of primary vaginal cancer; this is related in part to the rarity of the disease. Most gynecologic oncology centers in the United States see only two to five new cases per year, and even in

445

some European centers, where referral of oncology cases tends to be more centralized, only about one new case per month can be expected (23). Therapy must be individualized and will vary, depending on the stage of disease and the site of vaginal involvement, further limiting individual experience.

Anatomic factors and psychologic considerations place significant constraints on treatment planning. The close proximity of the vagina to the rectum, bladder, and urethra limits the dose of radiation that can be delivered and restricts the surgical margins that can be attained unless an exenterative procedure is performed. For most patients, maintenance of a functional vagina is an important factor in the planning of therapy.

Surgery

Surgery has a limited role in the management of patients with vaginal cancer, but in selected cases satisfactory results can be achieved (6, 26). Surgery may be useful in the following circumstances:

1. *In patients with Stage I disease involving the upper posterior vagina;* if the uterus is still *in situ*, these patients require radical hysterectomy, partial vaginectomy, and bilateral pelvic lymphadenectomy. If the patient has had a hysterectomy, radical upper vaginectomy and pelvic lymphadenectomy can be performed after development of the paravesicle and pararectal spaces and dissection of each ureter out to its point of entry into the bladder.

2. *In young patients who require radiation therapy;* pretreatment laparotomy in such patients may allow ovarian transposition, surgical staging, and resection of any enlarged lymph nodes.

3. *In patients with Stage IVa disease, particularly if a rectovaginal or vesicovaginal fistula is present;* primary pelvic exenteration is a suitable treatment option for such patients, provided they are medically fit. Eddy et al. (25) recently reported a 5-year disease-free survival in three of six patients with Stage IVa disease treated with preoperative radiation followed by anterior or total pelvic exenteration. In sexually active patients, vaginal reconstruction should be performed simultaneously, preferably with the use of Gracilis myocutaneous grafts (27).

4. *In patients with a central recurrence after radiation therapy;* surgical resection, which will frequently necessitate pelvic exenteration, is the only option for this group of patients.

Radiation Therapy

Radiation therapy is the treatment of choice for all patients except those listed above and comprises an integration of teletherapy and intracavitary/interstitial therapy (4, 23). Small superficial lesions can be treated adequately with intracavitary radiation alone (28). For larger lesions, treatment is usually started with about 5000 cGy external irradiation to shrink the primary tumor and treat the pelvic lymph nodes. **If the lower one-third of the vagina is involved, the groin nodes should also be treated or dissected.** Intracavitary treatment

446

follows. If the uterus is intact and the lesion involves the upper vagina, an intrauterine tandem and ovoids can be used. If the uterus has been previously removed, a Bloedorn type of applicator or vaginal cylinder may be used. If the lesion is more deeply invasive (thicker than 0.5 cm), interstitial irradiation, alone or in conjunction with the intracavitary therapy, will improve the dose distribution. Extended-field radiation has rarely been used for patients with vaginal cancer, but if positive para-aortic nodes are documented after either surgical staging or CT scanning and fine needle aspiration cytology, this treatment should be given.

Similarly, there is no reported experience with chemoradiation for vaginal cancer. However, in view of the problem with control of the central tumor, consideration should be given to the concurrent use of *5-fluorouracil (5-FU)* and/or *cisplatin* with the radiation therapy, as is being done in some centers for other squamous carcinomas.

Complications of Therapy

Major complications of therapy are usually reported in 10–15% of patients treated for primary vaginal cancer, whether the treatment is by surgery or radiation. The close proximity of the rectum, bladder, and urethra predisposes these structures to injury, and radiation cystitis, rectovaginal or vesicovaginal fistulas, and rectal strictures or ulceration may occur. Radiation necrosis of the vagina occasionally occurs, and radiation-induced fibrosis and subsequent vaginal stenosis are a constant concern. Patients who are sexually active must be encouraged to continue regular intercourse, but those who are not sexually active or for whom intercourse is temporarily too painful should be encouraged to use topical estrogen and a vaginal dilator every second night. There is inadequate documentation of the adequacy of vaginal function after either surgery or radiation therapy.

Prognosis

The overall 5-year survival rate for vaginal cancer is about 42%, which is about 15% poorer than that for carcinoma of the cervix or vulva and reflects the difficulties involved in treating this disease (7, 8, 10, 12, 23, 29) (Table 12.4). Even for patients with Stage I disease, the 5-year survival rate is under 70%. Most recurrences are in the pelvis, so improved radiation therapy, which may include chemoradiation and/or increasing experience with interstitial techniques, may improve the results. Because of the rarity of the disease, these patients should be referred centrally to a limited number of radiation oncology centers so that increasing experience can be gained in such centers.

Table 12.4   Primary Vaginal Carcinoma: 5-Year Survival

Stage	No.	5-Year Survival	Per Cent
I	172	118	68.6
II	236	108	45.8
III	203	62	30.5
IV	114	20	17.5
Total	**725**	**308**	**42.5**

Data compiled from Houghton and Iversen, 1982 (7), Benedet et al., 1983 (8), Rubin et al., 1985 (10), Eddy et al., 1991 (12), Kucera et al., 1985 (23), Pride et al., 1979 (29).

447

Adenocarcinoma

About 9% of primary vaginal carcinomas are adenocarcinomas, and they affect a younger population of women, regardless of whether exposure to diethylstilbestrol (DES) *in utero* has occurred (30). Adenocarcinomas may arise in areas of vaginal adenosis, particularly in patients exposed to DES *in utero*, but they probably also arise in wolffian rest elements, periurethral glands (21), and foci of endometriosis. Secondary tumors from such sites as the colon, endometrium, or ovary should be considered when vaginal adenocarcioma is diagnosed.

DES Exposure *In Utero*

In 1970 Herbst and Scully (31) initially reported on seven women aged 15 to 22 years with clear cell adenocarcinoma of the vagina, seen over a 4-year period. Subsequently, Herbst et al. (32) reported an association with maternal DES ingestion during pregnancy in six of these seven cases. A Registry for Research on Hormonal Transplacental Carcinogenesis was established by Herbst and Scully in 1971 to investigate the clinical, pathologic, and epidemiologic aspects of clear cell adenocarcinoma of the vagina and cervix occurring in females born after 1940 (i.e., during the years when DES was used to maintain high-risk pregnancies). Such high-risk situations included diabetic and twin pregnancies in women with a history of spontaneous abortion. The use of DES for pregnant patients was discontinued in the United States in 1971.

More than 500 cases of clear cell carcinoma of the vagina or cervix have been reported to the Registry, although only about two-thirds of the completely investigated cases have a history of prenatal exposure to DES. In all instances, the mother had been treated in the first half of the pregnancy (33). An additional 10% of the mothers received some unknown medication, but in 25% of the cases there was no indication of maternal hormone ingestion.

These cancers become most frequent after the age of 14 years, and the peak age at diagnosis is 19 years. The oldest reported DES-exposed patient with vaginal clear cell carcinoma is 33 years. The estimated risk of clear cell adenocarcinoma in an exposed offspring is 1:1000 or less. Approximately 70% of vaginal adenocarcinomas are Stage I at diagnosis.

Although DES exposure *in utero* rarely leads to vaginal adenocarcinoma, vaginal adenosis occurs in about 45% of such patients, and about 25% of exposed females have structural changes to the cervix and vagina. Such changes include a transverse vaginal septum, a cervical collar, a cockscomb (a raised ridge, usually on the anterior cervix), or cervical hypoplasia. The occurrence of these abnormalities is related to the dosage of medication given and the time of first exposure, the risk being insignificant if administration is begun after the 22nd week.

Two types of cells have been described in vaginal adenosis and cervical ectropion: the mucinous cell, which resembles the endocervical epithelium, and the tuboendometrial cell. Robboy et al. (34) reported foci of atypical tuboendometrial epithelium in 16 of 20 (80%) cases of clear cell adenocarcinoma of the cervix or vagina. The foci were almost immediately adjacent to the tumor, and they suggested that atypical vaginal adenosis and atypical cervical ectropion of the tuboendometrial type may be precursors of clear cell adenocarcinoma. In 1980 Sandberg and Christian (35) reported the appearance of cervicovaginal clear cell

448

adenocarcinoma in only one of a genetically identical (monozygotic) pair of twins, simultaneously exposed to DES *in utero*. Benign teratologic changes were present in both twins. This discordance suggests that factors other than embryonic exposure to DES may be operative in tumorigenesis.

Areas of vaginal adenosis and cervical ectropion are progressively covered with metaplastic squamous epithelium as the individual matures, and areas of adenosis may disappear completely and be replaced by normally glycogenated squamous epithelium. Structural abnormalities (e.g., cervical hoods) also tend to disappear progressively (36). During the process of squamous metaplasia, colposcopic examination will reveal mosaicism and punctation, changes commonly associated with squamous dysplasia (37). Women exposed *in utero* to DES may have twice the incidence of CIN and VAIN as unexposed women, although the reason for this increased risk is not clear (38).

In addition to benign changes in the lower genital tract, a number of other abnormalities have been reported in DES-exposed female offspring. Kaufman et al. (39) reported abnormalities of the hysterosalpingogram in 185 of 267 (69%) exposed women. The most common abnormality was a T-shaped uterus, with or without a small cavity; less common abnormalities included constriction rings, uterine filling defects, synechia, diverticula, and uterus unicornis or bicornis. These abnormalities translate into an impaired reproductive experience for DES-exposed offspring, with the incidence of primary infertility, ectopic pregnancy, spontaneous abortion, and premature delivery being increased (40).

It is recommended that a young woman exposed to DES *in utero* should be initially seen when she begins to menstruate, or at about the age of 14 years. The most important aspects of the examination are careful inspection and palpation of the entire vagina and cervix and cytologic sampling by direct scraping of the vagina and cervix. Colposcopy is not essential if clinical and cytologic evaluation are normal, but staining with half-strength Lugol's iodine will delineate areas of adenosis.

Treatment

In general, these tumors may be treated in a way similar to squamous carcinomas, except that in these young patients every effort should be made to preserve vaginal and ovarian function. For early-stage tumors, particularly those involving the upper vagina, radical hysterectomy, pelvic lymphadenectomy, vaginectomy, and replacement of the vagina with a split-thickness skin graft have been successful in a high percentage of cases. A combination of wide local excision, retroperitoneal lymphadenectomy, and local irradiation can be effective therapy for Stage I tumors (41). Local surgical excision alone for small primary tumors is associated with a higher incidence of local and regional recurrence. About 16% of patients with Stage I disease have positive pelvic nodes (42). If radiation alone is used, a pretreatment staging laparotomy to allow pelvic lymphadenectomy and ovarian transposition will facilitate an optimal functional outcome.

Prognosis

The overall 5-year survival rate for Registry patients, regardless of the mode of therapy, is 78%. Survival correlates well with stage of disease: 87% for patients with Stage I disease, 76% for patients with Stage II, and 30% for those with Stage III (33).

449

Verrucous Carcinoma

Verrucous carcinomas of the vagina are rare, but their clinical and pathologic features are similar to their vulvar counterparts (43). They are large, warty tumors that are locally aggressive but have a minimal tendency to metastasize. Wide surgical excision of the tumor is the treatment of choice. Regional lymphadenectomy is not required, provided there is no suspicious lymphadenopathy. Radiation therapy has been implicated in the rapid transformation of such lesions to a more malignant tumor (44).

Vaginal Melanoma

Malignant melanomas of the vagina are rare, with only about 130 reported cases (45). They presumably arise from melanocytes that are present in the vagina in 3% of normal women (46). The average age of the patients is 58 years, but vaginal melanomas have been reported from the third to the ninth decades of life (47). Almost all cases occur in white women (45).

Clinically, most patients are seen with vaginal bleeding, a vaginal mass, or discharge. The lesions most commonly arise in the distal part of the vagina, particularly on the anterior wall (45, 48). They may be nonpigmented and are frequently ulcerated, making them easily confused with squamous carcinomas. Most are deeply invasive. Expressed in terms of Chung's level of invasion (as defined for vulvar melanomas (49), Chung et al. (48) reported that 13 of 15 vaginal melanomas were at level IV. About 60% of the cases exhibit spread of melanocytic cells into the adjacent epithelium, and in about 30% of the cases the lateral spread is extensive (48).

Radical surgery has been the mainstay of treatment, and this has often involved anterior, posterior, or total pelvic exenteration, depending on the location of the lesion. Small upper vaginal lesions may be treated with radical hysterectomy, subtotal vaginectomy, and pelvic lymphadenectomy; small distal vaginal lesions may be amenable to partial vaginectomy, total or partial vulvectomy, and bilateral inguinal-femoral lymphadenectomy. If vaginal mucosa is left, frozen sections should be obtained to exclude lateral superficial spread, as the most common site of initial recurrence is the vagina (45, 48). More conservative operations (e.g., wide local excision) have also been used, and Reid et al. (45) reported that there was no significant benefit in terms of survival or disease-free interval for radical versus conservative surgery. Radiation therapy, particularly a combination of external and interstitial radiation, may be effective in selected patients. High-dose fractions (> 400 cGy) may yield better response rates than conventional or low-dose fractions (50). Chemotherapy (e.g., with methyl-CCNU or dacarbazine [DTIC]) is disappointing.

The overall prognosis for patients with vaginal melanoma is poor, as most patients have deeply penetrating lesions at the time of diagnosis. Reid et al. (45) reviewed the literature and reported that only 14 of 130 patients (10.8%) survived for 5 years or longer. Six of the 14 patients were treated with radical operative procedures, 4 with radiation, and 4 with wide local excision. Using life-table survival curves, they estimated an actuarial 2-year survival rate of 33.8% and a 5-year survival rate of 17.5%. The mean disease-free interval was 15.2 months. Three of 4 reported patients with tumor thickness < 2 mm were alive and free of disease at 18 to 153 months. Once a recurrence is noted, prognosis is extremely poor, with a mean survival time of 8.5 months.

Vaginal Sarcomas

Vaginal sarcomas, such as *fibrosarcomas* and *leiomyosarcomas*, are rare tumors. They are usually bulky lesions and occur most commonly in the upper vagina. Tavassoli and Norris (51) reported 60 smooth muscle tumors of the vagina, only five of which recurred. All recurrences were seen in tumors > 3 cm in diameter with moderate to marked cytologic atypia and > 5 mitoses per 10 high-power fields.

Surgical excision is the mainstay of treatment. If the lesion is well differentiated and the surgical margins are not involved, as is likely with tumors of low malignant potential, the likelihood of cure is good. For frankly malignant lesions, lymphatic and hematogenous dissemination is common. The value of adjuvant chemotherapy and/or pelvic radiation for such tumors is not known.

Embryonal Rhabdomyosarcoma

Embryonal rhabdomyosarcoma is a malignant tumor of the rhabdomyoblasts characterized by two structural variants—a solid form and a multicystic grapelike form referred to as *sarcoma botryoides*. Sarcoma botryoides is a highly malignant tumor. **Within the female genital tract, sarcoma botryoides is usually found in the vagina during infancy and early childhood, in the cervix during the reproductive years, and in the corpus uteri during the postmenopausal period.** Hilgers et al. (52) reported a peak incidence of vaginal sarcoma botryoides at around 3 years of age, and these lesions may rarely be present at birth.

The term "botryoides" comes from the Greek work "botrys," which means "grapes," and, grossly, the tumor usually appears as a polyploid mass extruding from the vagina and resembling a bunch of grapes. Microscopically, the characteristic feature is the presence of cross-striated rhabdomyoblasts (strap cells).

In the past, exenterative surgery was usually performed for these tumors, but survival was poor. More recently, conservative surgery has been used in conjunction with preoperative or postoperative chemotherapy and radiation, with significantly improved survival (53, 54). The usual chemotherapy has consisted of vincristine, actinomycin D, and Cytoxan (VAC). If the tumor is small and can be resected with organ preservation, surgery should be the initial treatment. If the lesion is bulky, preoperative chemotherapy or radiation should be given (55). Permanent local control with drugs alone occurs in fewer than 15% of cases (56).

Endodermal Sinus Tumor (Yolk Sac Tumor)

These rare germ cell tumors are occasionally found in extragonadal sites such as the vagina. Leverger et al. (57) recently reported 11 such cases from the Institut Gustave-Roussy. The average age of the patients was 10 months, and the presenting symptom was vaginal bleeding. Diagnosis was made by examination and biopsy with the patient under anesthesia. All children had high serum α-fetoprotein levels. Since 1977, six of eight children have been cured, with an average follow-up of 3 years. Treatment consisted of primary chemotherapy to reduce the tumor volume, followed by either partial colpectomy, radiotherapy, or both.

Carcinoma of the Urethra

Primary carcinoma of the female urethra is a rare malignancy, accounting for fewer than 0.1% of all female genital malignancies (58). The disease has been reported from the third to the ninth decades of life, with a median age of about 65 years. The most common presenting symptoms are urethral bleeding, hematuria, dysuria, urinary obstruction, urinary frequency, and a mass at the introitus. Uncommon presenting symptoms include urinary incontinence, perineal pain, and dyspareunia.

Most tumors involve the anterior or distal urethra and may be confused with a urethral caruncle or mucosal prolapse. Histologically, these distal lesions are usually squamous cell carcinomas. Tumors involving the posterior or proximal urethra are usually adenocarcinomas or transitional cell carcinomas. The relative frequency of the various histologic variants is shown in Table 12.5 (58–61). Urethral carcinomas occasionally arise in a urethral diverticulum (61).

There is no FIGO staging for the disease, and several staging classifications have been suggested (60, 62, 63). The TNM staging system is shown in Table 12.6. Distal tumors spread to the lymph nodes of the groin, whereas proximal tumors spread to pelvic nodes, and treatment planning should take this into consideration. Bladder neck involvement is a common cause of local recurrence, and examination under anesthesia, endoscopic evaluation, and biopsy of the bladder neck should be undertaken as part of the pretreatment work-up.

The treatment of urethral cancer must be individualized (58). Radiation therapy is generally considered to be the treatment of choice, although, when used for urethral cancer, it may cause complications such as urinary stricture, fistula, or total incontinence. Surgery is used in conjunction with radiation for more advanced lesions (60). Interstitial radiation may be satisfactory for early lesions, but for more advanced lesions, preoperative external pelvic radiation followed by anterior exenteration and, if necessary, vulvectomy should be performed (59). For lesions involving the distal half of the urethra, bilateral inguinal-femoral lymphadenectomy should be performed for all but the most superficial lesions. The distal half of the urethra can be excised without loss of urinary continence.

The main cause of treatment failure is local recurrence. In an attempt to improve local control in advanced cases, two approaches have been suggested: chemoradiation and ultraradical surgery. Klein et al. (64) from Memorial Sloan-Kettering reported on five women who were treated with preoperative radiation followed by anterior exenteration combined with resection of the inferior pubic rami. Two died with distant metastases, and one died of surgical complications at 1 month. Only one patient treated with chemoradiation has been reported (65). However,

Table 12.5 Histology of Urethral Carcinomas

Type	No.	Per Cent
Squamous cell	97	53.6
Transitional cell	38	21.0
Adenocarcinoma	35	19.3
Undifferentiated	8	4.4
Melanoma	3	1.7
Total	**181**	**100.0**

Data compiled from Weghaupt et al., 1984 (58), Bracken et al., 1976 (59), Prempree et al., 1984 (60), Benson et al., 1982 (61).

Table 12.6 Staging for Urethral Cancer

Stage	TNM		
Stage 0$_a$	T$_a$	N$_0$	M$_0$
Stage 0$_{is}$	T$_{is}$	N$_0$	M$_0$
Stage I	T$_1$	N$_0$	M$_0$
Stage II	T$_2$	N$_0$	M$_0$
Stage III	T$_1$	N$_1$	M$_0$
	T$_2$	N$_1$	M$_0$
	T$_3$	N$_0$	M$_0$
	T$_3$	N$_1$	M$_0$
Stage IV	T$_4$	N$_0$	M$_0$
	T$_4$	N$_1$	M$_0$
	Any T	N$_2$	M$_0$
	Any T	N$_3$	M$_0$
	Any T	Any N	M$_1$

TNM Classification

T:	Primary Tumor	M:	Distant Metastases
T$_{is}$	Carcinoma *in situ*	M$_x$	Presence of distant metastasis cannot be assessed
T$_1$	Tumor invades subepithelial connective tissue	M$_0$	No distant metastasis
T$_2$	Tumor invades the periurethral muscle	M$_1$	Distant metastasis
T$_3$	Tumor invades the anterior vagina or bladder neck	**Histopathologic Type**	
T$_4$	Tumor invades other adjacent organs		Cell types can be divided into transitional, squamous, and glandular.
N:	**Regional Lymph Nodes**	**G:**	**Histopathologic Grade**
N$_x$	Regional lymph nodes cannot be assessed	G$_x$	Grade cannot be assessed
N$_0$	No regional lymph node metastasis	G$_1$	Well-differentiated
N$_1$	Metastasis in a single lymph node, 2 cm or less in greatest dimension	G$_2$	Moderately differentiated
N$_2$	Metastasis in a single lymph node, more than 2 cm but not more than 5 cm in greatest dimension; or multiple lymph nodes, none more than 5 cm in greatest dimension	G$_{3-4}$	Poorly differentiated or undifferentiated
N$_3$	Metastasis in a lymph node more than 5 cm in greatest dimension		

in view of the experience with other primary sites, this would seem to be an acceptable initial approach for locally advanced cases.

Bracken et al. (59) from the M.D. Anderson Hospital reported an overall 5-year survival of only 32% for 81 cases of carcinoma of the female urethra (59).

References

1. **Dunn LJ, Napier JG:** Primary carcinoma of the vagina. *Am J Obstet Gynecol* 96:1112, 1966.

2. **Gompel C, Silverberg SC:** *Pathology in Gynecology and Obstetrics.* Philadelphia, JB Lippincott, 1977.

3. **Rutledge F:** Cancer of the vagina. *Am J Obstet Gynecol* 97:635, 1967.

4. **Perez CA, Arneson AN, Dehner LP, et al:** Radiation therapy in carcinoma of the vagina. *Obstet Gynecol* 44:862, 1974.

5. **Pride GL, Buchler DA:** Carcinoma of vagina 10 or more years following pelvic irradiation therapy. *Am J Obstet Gynecol* 127:513, 1977.

6. **Ball HG, Berman ML:** Management of primary vaginal carcinoma. *Gynecol Oncol* 14:154, 1982.

7. **Houghton CRS, Iversen T:** Squamous cell carcinoma of the vagina: a clinical study of the location of the tumor. *Gynecol Oncol* 13:365, 1982.

8. **Benedet JL, Murphy KJ, Fairey RN, et al:** Primary invasive carcinoma of the vagina. *Obstet Gynecol* 62:715, 1983.

9. **Peters WA III, Kumar NB, Morley GW:** Carcinoma of the vagina. *Cancer* 55:892, 1985.

10. **Rubin SC, Young J, Mikuta JJ:** Squamous carcinoma of the vagina: treatment, complications, and long-term follow-up. *Gynecol Oncol* 20:346, 1985.

11. **Sulak P, Barnhill D, Heller P, et al:** Nonsquamous cancer of the vagina. *Gynecol Oncol* 29:309, 1988.

12. **Eddy GL, Marks RD, Miller MC III, Underwood PB Jr:** Primary invasive vaginal carcinoma. *Am J Obstet Gynecol* 165:282, 1991.

13. **Weed JC, Lozier C, Daniel SJ:** Human papilloma virus in multifocal, invasive female genital tract malignancy. *Obstet Gynecol* 62:832, 1983.

14. **Lenehan PM, Meffe F, Lickrish GM:** Vaginal intraepithelial neoplasia: biologic aspects and management. *Obstet Gynecol* 68:333, 1986.

15. **Benedet JL, Saunders BH:** Carcinoma in situ of the vagina. *Am J Obstet Gynecol* 148:695, 1984.

16. **Choo YC, Anderson DG:** Neoplasms of the vagina following cervical carcinoma. *Gynecol Oncol* 14:125, 1982.

17. **Cramer DW, Cutler SJ:** Incidence and histopathology of malignancies of the female genital organs in the United States. *Am J Obstet Gynecol* 118:443, 1974.

18. **Stuart GCE, Allen HH, Anderson RJ:** Squamous cell carcinoma of the vagina following hysterectomy. *Am J Obstet Gynecol* 139:311, 1981.

19. **Bell J, Sevin BU, Averette H, et al:** Vaginal cancer after hysterectomy for benign disease: value of cytologic screening. *Obstet Gynecol* 64:699, 1984.

20. **Herman JM, Homesley HD, Dignan MB:** Is hysterectomy a risk factor for vaginal cancer? *JAMA* 256:601, 1986.

21. **Frick HC, Jacox HW, Taylor HC:** Primary carcinoma of the vagina. *Am J Obstet Gynecol* 101:695, 1968.

22. **Hoffman MS, De Cesare SL, Roberts WS, et al:** Upper vaginectomy for *in situ* and occult superficially invasive carcinoma of the vagina. *Am J Obstet Gynecol* 166:30, 1992.

23. **Kucera H, Langer M, Smekal G, et al:** Radiotherapy of primary carcinoma of the vagina: management and results of different therapy schemes. *Gynecol Oncol* 21:87, 1985.

24. **Peters WA III, Kumar NB, Morley GW:** Microinvasive carcinoma of the vagina: a distinct clinical entity? *Am J Obstet Gynecol* 153:505, 1985.

25. **Eddy GL, Singh KP, Gansler TS:** Superficially invasive carcinoma of the vagina following treatment for cervical cancer: a report of six cases. *Gynecol Oncol* 36:376, 1990.

26. **Al-Kurdi M, Monaghan JM:** Thirty-two years experience in management of primary tumors of the vagina. *Br J Obstet Gynaecol* 88:1145, 1981.

27. **Berek JS, Hacker NF, Lagasse LD:** Vaginal reconstruction performed simultaneously with pelvic exenteration. *Obstet Gynecol* 63:318, 1984.

28. **Reddy S, Lee MS, Graham JE, et al:** Radiation therapy in primary carcinoma of the vagina. *Gynecol Oncol* 26:19, 1987.

29. **Pride GL, Schultz AE, Chuprevich TW, et al:** Primary invasive squamous carcinoma of the vagina. *Obstet Gynecol* 53:218, 1979.

30. **Ballon SC, Lagasse LD, Chang NH, et al:** Primary adenocarcinoma of the vagina. *Surg Gynecol Obstet* 149:233, 1979.

31. **Herbst AL, Scully RE:** Adenocarcinoma of the vagina in adolescence. *Cancer* 25:745, 1970.

32. **Herbst AL, Ulfelder H, Poskanzer DC:** Adenocarcinoma of the vagina: association of maternal stilbestrol therapy with tumor appearance in young women. *N Engl J Med* 284:878, 1971.

33. **Herbst AL, Cole P, Norusis MJ, et al:** Epidemiologic aspects and factors related to survival in 384 Registry cases of clear cell adenocarcinoma of the vagina and cervix. *Am J Obstet Gynecol* 135:876, 1979.

34. **Robboy SJ, Young RH, Welch WR, et al:** Atypical vaginal adenosis and cervical ectropion. *Cancer* 54:869, 1984.

35. **Sandberg EC, Christian JC:** Diethylstilbestrol-exposed monozygotic twins discordant for cervicovaginal clear cell adenocarcinoma. *Am J Obstet Gynecol* 137:220, 1980.

36. **Antonioli DA, Burke L, Friedman EA:** Natural history of diethylstilbestrol associated genital tract lesions: cervical ectopy and cervicovaginal hood. *Am J Obstet Gynecol* 137:847, 1980.

37. **Robboy SJ, Szyfelbein WM, Goellner J, et al:** Dysplasia and cytologic findings in 4589 young women enrolled in diethylstilbestrol-adenosis (DESAD) project. *Am J Obstet Gynecol* 140:579, 1981.

38. **Bornstein J, Adam E, Adler-Storthz K, Kaufman RH:** Development of cervical and vaginal squamous cell neoplasia as a late consequence of in utero exposure to diethyl-stilbestrol. *Obstet Gynecol Surv* 43:15, 1988.

39. **Kaufman RH, Adam E, Binder GL, et al:** Upper genital tract changes and pregnancy outcome in offspring exposed in utero to diethylstilbestrol. *Am J Obstet Gynecol* 137:299, 1980.

40. **Herbst AL, Hubby MM, Aziz F, et al:** Reproductive and gynecologic surgical experience in diethylstilbestrol-exposed daughters. *Am J Obstet Gynecol* 141:1019, 1981.

41. **Senekjian EK, Frey KW, Anderson D, Herbst Al:** Local therapy in stage I clear cell adenocarcinoma of the vagina. *Cancer* 60:1319, 1987.

42. **Herbst Al, Robboy SJ, Scully RE, et al:** Clear-cell adenocarcinoma of the vagina and cervix in girls: analysis of 170 Registry cases. *Am J Obstet Gynecol* 119:713, 1974.

43. **Isaacs JH:** Verrucous carcinoma of the female genital tract. *Gynecol Oncol* 4:259, 1976.

44. **Gallousis S:** Verrucous carcinoma: report of three vulvar cases and review of the literature. *Obstet Gynecol* 40:502, 1972.

45. **Reid GC, Schmidt RW, Roberts JA, et al:** Primary melanoma of the vagina: A clinico-pathologic analysis. *Obstet Gynecol* 74:190, 1989.

46. **Nigogosyam G, De La Pava S, Pickren JW:** Melanoblasts in vaginal mucosa. *Cancer* 17:912, 1964.

47. **Morrow CP, DiSaia PJ:** Malignant melanoma of the female genitalia: a clinical analysis. *Obstet Gynecol Surv* 31:233, 1976.

48. **Chung AF, Casey MJ, Flannery JT, et al:** Malignant melanoma of the vagina—report of 19 cases. *Obstet Gynecol* 55:720, 1980.

49. **Chung AF, Woodruff JW, Lewis JL Jr:** Malignant melanoma of the vulva: a report of 44 cases. *Obstet Gynecol* 45:638, 1975.

50. **Harwood AR, Cumming BJ:** Radiotherapy for mucosal melanoma. *Int J Radiat Oncol Biol Phys* 8:1121, 1982.

51. **Tavassoli FA, Norris HJ:** Smooth muscle tumors of the vagina. *Obstet Gynecol* 53:689, 1979.

52. **Hilgers RD, Malkasian GD, Soule EH:** Embryonal rhabdomyosarcoma (botryoid type) of the vagina: a clinicopathologic review. *Am J Obstet Gynecol* 107:484, 1970.

53. **Kumar APM, Wrenn EL, Fleming ID, et al:** Combined therapy to prevent complete pelvic exenteration for rhabdomyosarcoma of the vagina or uterus. *Cancer* 37:118, 1976.

54. **Dewhurst J:** *Practical Pediatric and Adolescent Gynecology.* New York, Marcel Dekker, 1980.

55. **Friedman M, Peretz BA, Nissenbaum M, Paldi E:** Modern treatment of vaginal embryonal rhabdomyosarcoma. *Obstet Gynecol Surv* 41:614, 1986.

56. **Chavimi F, Herr H, Exelby PR:** Treatment of genitourinary rhabdomyosarcoma in children. *J Oncol* 132:313, 1984.

57. **Leverger G, Flamant F, Gerbaulet A, et al:** Tumors of the vitelline sac located in the vagina in children. *Arch Fr Pediatr* 40:85, 1983.

58. **Weghaupt K, Gerstner GJ, Kucera H:** Radiation therapy for primary carcinoma of the female urethra: a survey over 25 years. *Gynecol Oncol* 17:58, 1984.

59. **Bracken RB, Johnson DE, Miller LS, et al:** Primary carcinoma of the female urethra. *J Urol* 116:188, 1976.

60. **Prempree T, Amornmarn R, Patanphan V:** Radiation therapy in primary carcinoma of the female urethra. *Cancer* 54:729, 1984.

61. **Benson RC, Tunca JC, Buchler DA, et al:** Primary carcinoma of the female urethra. *Gynecol Oncol* 14:313, 1982.

62. **Ampil FL:** Primary malignant neoplasms of the female urethra. *Obstet Gynecol* 66:799, 1985.

63. **Grabstald H, Hilaris B, Henschke U, et al:** Cancer of the female urethra. *JAMA* 197:835, 1966.

64. **Klein FA, Whitmore WF, Herr HW, et al:** Inferior pubic rami resection with en bloc radical excision for invasive proximal urethral carcinoma. *Cancer* 51:1238, 1983.

65. **Shah A, Kalra J, Silber L, et al:** Squamous cell carcinoma of the female urethra: successful treatment with chemoradiotherapy. *Urology* 25:284, 1985.

13 Gestational Trophoblastic Neoplasia

Ross S. Berkowitz
Donald P. Goldstein

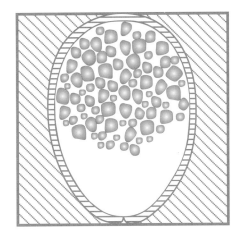

Gestational trophoblastic neoplasia (GTN) is among the rare human malignancies that can be cured even in the presence of widespread metastases (1–3). GTN includes a spectrum of interrelated tumors, including hydatidiform mole, invasive mole, placental-site trophoblastic tumor, and choriocarcinoma, that have varying propensities for local invasion and metastasis. Although persistent GTN most commonly ensues after a molar pregnancy, it may follow any gestational event, including therapeutic or spontaneous abortion and ectopic or term pregnancy. Dramatic advances have been made in the diagnosis, treatment, and follow-up of patients with GTN since the introduction of chemotherapy in 1956.

Hydatidiform Mole

Complete Versus Partial Hydatidiform Mole

Hydatidiform moles may be categorized as either complete or partial moles on the basis of gross morphology, histopathology, and karyotype (Table 13.1).

Complete Hydatidiform Mole

Pathology Complete moles lack identifiable embryonic or fetal tissues, and the chorionic villi exhibit generalized hydatidiform swelling and diffuse trophoblastic hyperplasia.

Chromosomes **Cytogenetic studies have demonstrated that complete hydatidiform moles usually have a 46XX karyotype, and the molar chromosomes are entirely of paternal origin** (4). Complete moles appear to arise from an ovum that has been fertilized by a haploid sperm, which then duplicates its own chromosomes, and the ovum nucleus may be either absent or inactivated (5). Although most complete moles have a 46XX chromosomal pattern, about 10%

457

Table 13.1 Features of Complete and Partial Hydatidiform Moles

	Complete Mole	Partial Mole
Fetal or embryonic tissue	Absent	Present
Hydatidiform swelling of chorionic villi	Diffuse	Focal
Trophoblastic hyperplasia	Diffuse	Focal
Scalloping of chorionic villi	Absent	Present
Trophoblastic stromal inclusions	Absent	Present
Karyotype	46XX; 46XY	69XXY; 69XYY

Reproduced, with permission, from Berkowitz RS, Goldstein DP: The management of molar pregnancy and gestational trophoblastic tumors. In Knapp RC, Berkowitz RS (eds): *Gynecologic Oncology*. New York, MacMillan, p 425.

have a 46XY karyotype (6). Chromosomes in a 46XY complete mole also appear to be entirely of paternal origin.

Partial Hydatidiform Mole

Pathology Partial hydatidiform moles are characterized by the following pathologic features (7):

1. Chorionic villi of varying size with focal hydatidiform swelling and cavitation

2. Marked villous scalloping

3. Focal trophoblastic hyperplasia with or without atypia

4. Prominent stromal trophoblastic inclusions

5. Identifiable embryonic or fetal tissues

Chromosomes Partial moles generally have a triploid karyotype (69 chromosomes), with the extra haploid set of chromosomes usually derived from the father (8). When a fetus is present in conjunction with a partial mole, it generally exhibits the stigmata of triploidy, including growth retardation and multiple congenital malformations.

Clinical Features

The presenting symptoms and signs of patients with complete and partial molar pregnancy are presented in Table 13.2 (9, 10).

Complete Hydatidiform Mole

Vaginal Bleeding Vaginal bleeding is the most common presenting symptom in patients with complete molar pregnancy and occurs in 97% of cases. Molar tissues may separate from the decidua and disrupt maternal vessels, and large volumes of retained blood may distend the endometrial cavity. As intrauterine clots undergo oxidation and liquefaction, "prune juice"–like fluid may leak into the vagina. Because vaginal bleeding may be considerable and prolonged, half of these patients present with anemia (hemoglobin < 10 g/100 ml) (11).

458

Excessive Uterine Size Excessive uterine enlargement relative to gestational age is one of the classic signs of a complete mole, although it is present in only about half of the patients. The endometrial cavity may be expanded by both chorionic tissue and retained blood. Excessive uterine size is generally associated with markedly elevated levels of human chorionic gonadotropin (hCG), because uterine enlargement results in part from exuberant trophoblastic growth (11).

Toxemia Preeclampsia is observed in 27% of patients with a complete hydatidiform mole. Although preeclampsia is often associated with hypertension, proteinuria, and hyperreflexia, eclamptic convulsions rarely occur. Toxemia develops almost exclusively in patients with excessive uterine size and markedly elevated hCG levels. Curry et al. (12) observed that 81% of their patients with molar pregnancy and preeclampsia had excessive uterine enlargement. The diagnosis of hydatidiform mole should be considered whenever preeclampsia develops early in pregnancy.

Hyperemesis Gravidarum Hyperemesis requiring antiemetic and/or intravenous replacement therapy occurs in one-fourth of the patients with a complete mole, particularly those with excessive uterine size and markedly elevated hCG levels. Severe electrolyte disturbances may develop occasionally and require treatment with parenteral fluids.

Hyperthyroidism Clinically evident hyperthyroidism is observed in 7% of patients with a complete molar gestation. These patients may present with tachycardia, warm skin, and tremor, and the diagnosis can be confirmed by detection of elevated serum levels of free thyroxine (T_4) and triiodothyronine (T_3).

Laboratory evidence of hyperthyroidism is commonly detected in asymptomatic patients with hydatidiform moles. Galton et al. (13) reported 11 patients whose thyroid function test values were elevated before molar evacuation, and the thyroid function test values rapidly returned to normal in all patients after evacuation.

If hyperthyroidism is suspected, it is important to administer β-adrenergic blocking agents before the induction of anesthesia for molar evacuation because anesthesia or surgery may precipitate a thyroid storm. The latter may be manifested

Table 13.2 **Presenting Symptoms and Signs in Patients with Complete and Partial Molar Pregnancy**

Sign	*Complete Mole* N = 307 (%)*	*Partial Mole** N = 81 (%)*
Vaginal bleeding	97	73
Excessive uterine size	51	4
Prominent ovarian theca lutein cysts	50	0
Toxemia	27	3
Hyperemesis	26	0
Hyperthyroidism	7	0
Trophoblastic emboli	2	0

Adapted from Berkowitz RS et al: *Pathobiol Annu 11:391, 1981, and **Obstet Gynecol 66:667, 1985.

by hyperthermia, delirium, convulsions, atrial fibrillation, high-output heart failure or cardiovascular collapse. Administration of β-adrenergic blocking agents prevents or rapidly reverses many of the metabolic and cardiovascular complications of a thyroid storm.

Some investigators have suggested that hCG is the thyroid stimulator in patients with a hydatidiform mole, because positive correlations between serum hCG and total T_4 or T_3 concentrations have sometimes been observed. However, Amir et al. (14) measured thyroid function in 47 patients with a complete mole and reported no correlation between serum hCG levels and serum levels of free T_4 index or free T_3 index. Thus the identity of a thyrotropic factor in hydatidiform mole has not been clearly delineated. Although some investigators have speculated about a separate chorionic thyrotropin, this substance has not yet been isolated.

Trophoblastic Embolization **Respiratory distress develops in 2% of patients with a complete mole. These patients may have chest pain, dyspnea, tachypnea, and tachycardia and may experience severe respiratory distress after molar evacuation.** Auscultation of the chest usually reveals diffuse rales, and the chest radiograph may demonstrate bilateral pulmonary infiltrates. The signs and symptoms of respiratory distress usually resolve within 72 hours with cardiopulmonary support. Respiratory insufficiency may result not only from trophoblastic embolization but also from the cardiopulmonary complications of thyroid storm, toxemia, and massive fluid replacement.

Theca Lutein Ovarian Cysts **Prominent theca lutein ovarian cysts (> 6 cm in diameter) develop in about half the patients with a complete mole** (11). These cysts contain amber-colored or serosanguineous fluid and are usually multilocular. Their formation may be related to increased serum levels of hCG and prolactin (15). Ovarian enlargement occurs almost exclusively in patients with markedly elevated hCG values. Because the uterus may also be excessively enlarged, theca lutein cysts may be difficult to palpate on physical examination; however, ultrasonography can accurately document their presence and size. After molar evacuation, theca lutein cysts normally regress spontaneously within 2–4 months.

Prominent theca lutein cysts frequently cause symptoms of marked pelvic pressure, and they may be decompressed by laparoscopic or transabdominal aspiration to relieve such symptoms. If acute pelvic pain develops, laparoscopy should be performed to assess possible cystic torsion or rupture, and laparoscopic manipulation may successfully manage incomplete ovarian torsion or cystic rupture (16).

Partial Hydatidiform Mole

Patients with a partial hydatidiform mole usually do not have the clinical features characteristic of complete molar pregnancy. **In general, these patients present with the signs and symptoms of incomplete or missed abortion, and the diagnosis of partial mole may be made only after histologic review of the curettings** (17).

The main presenting sign among 81 patients with a partial mole seen at the New England Trophoblastic Disease Center (NETDC) was vaginal bleeding that occurred in 59 patients (72.8%). There was absence of a fetal heart beat in 12 patients (15.1%) (9). Excessive uterine enlargement and preeclampsia were present in only 3 (3.7%) and 2 (2.5%) patients, respectively. No patient presented with theca lutein ovarian cysts, hyperemesis, or hyperthyroidism. The presenting clinical diagnosis was incomplete or missed abortion in 74 patients (91.3%) and hydatidiform mole in only five patients (6.2%). Preevacuation hCG levels were measured in 30 patients and were > 100,000 mIU/ml in only two.

Natural History

Complete Hydatidiform Mole

Complete moles are well recognized to have a potential for local invasion and distant spread. **After molar evacuation, local uterine invasion occurs in 15% of patients and metastases in 4%** (10).

A review of 858 patients with complete hydatidiform mole (11) revealed that two-fifths of the patients had the following signs of marked trophoblastic proliferation at the time of presentation:

1. Human chorionic gonadotropin level > 100,000 mIU/ml

2. Excessive uterine enlargement

3. Theca lutein cysts > 6 cm in diameter

Patients with any one of these signs were considered at high risk. The sequelae of 858 patients with low- and high-risk complete hydatidiform moles are shown in Table 13.3. After molar evacuation, local uterine invasion occurred in 31%, and metastases developed in 8.8% of the 352 high-risk patients. For the 506 low-risk patients, local invasion was found in only 3.4% and metastases developed in 0.6%.

Patients more than 40 years of age are also at increased risk of postmolar GTN. Tow (18) reported that 37% of such women developed persistent GTN.

Partial Hydatidiform Mole

About 4% of patients with a partial mole develop persistent nonmetastatic GTN and require chemotherapy to achieve remission (19). Those patients who develop persistent disease have no distinguishing clinical or pathologic characteristics. To

Table 13.3 Sequelae of Low- and High-Risk Complete Hydatidiform Moles

Outcome	No. of Patients (%)			
	Low-Risk		High-Risk	
Normal involution	486/506	(96)	212/352	(60.2)
Persistent GTN				
Nonmetastatic	17/506	(3.4)	109/352	(31.0)
Metastatic	3/506	(0.6)	31/352	(8.8)
Totals	**506/858**	**(59)**	**352/858**	**(41)**

Reproduced, with permission, from Goldstein DP, Berkowitz RS, Bernstein MR: Management of molar pregnancy. *J Reprod Med* 26:208, 1981.
All patients managed by evacuation without prophylactic chemotherapy.

date, there have been no reported cases of choriocarcinoma after partial molar pregnancy.

Diagnosis

Ultrasonography is a reliable and sensitive technique for the diagnosis of complete molar pregnancy. Because the chorionic villi exhibit diffuse hydatidiform swelling, complete moles produce a characteristic vesicular sonographic pattern, usually referred to as a "snowstorm" pattern.

Ultrasonography may also contribute to the diagnosis of partial molar pregnancy by demonstrating focal cystic spaces in the placental tissues and an increase in the transverse diameter of the gestational sac (20).

Treatment

After molar pregnancy is diagnosed, the patient should be evaluated carefully for the presence of associated medical complications, including preeclampsia, hyperthyroidism, electrolyte imbalance, and anemia. After the patient has been stabilized, a decision must be made concerning the most appropriate method of evacuation.

Hysterectomy

If the patient desires surgical sterilization, a hysterectomy may be performed with the mole *in situ*. The ovaries may be preserved at the time of surgery, even though theca lutein cysts are present. Prominent ovarian cysts may be decompressed by aspiration. Although hysterectomy eliminates the risks associated with local invasion, it does not prevent distant spread.

Suction Curettage

Suction curettage is the preferred method of evacuation, regardless of uterine size, in patients who desire to preserve fertility. It involves the following steps:

1. *Oxytocin infusion* This is begun in the operating room before the induction of anesthesia.

2. *Cervical dilatation* As the cervix is being dilated, the surgeon frequently encounters increased uterine bleeding. Retained blood in the endometrial cavity may be expelled during cervical dilatation. However, active uterine bleeding should not deter the prompt completion of cervical dilatation.

3. *Suction curettage* Within a few minutes of commencing suction curettage, the uterus may decrease dramatically in size and the bleeding is generally well controlled. If the uterus is > 14 weeks in size, one hand may be placed on top of the fundus and the uterus massaged to stimulate uterine contraction and reduce the risk of perforation.

4. *Sharp curettage* When suction evacuation is thought to be complete, sharp curettage with a large Reynolds curette is performed to remove any residual molar tissue.

The specimens obtained on suction and sharp curettage should be submitted separately for pathologic review.

Prophylactic Chemotherapy

The use of prophylactic chemotherapy at the time of molar evacuation is controversial (21). The debate concerns the wisdom of exposing all patients to potentially toxic treatment when only about 20% are at risk of developing persistent GTN.

In a study of 247 patients with complete molar pregnancy who received a single course of actinomycin D prophylactically at the time of evacuation, local uterine invasion subsequently developed in only 10 patients (4%), and in no case did metastases occur (Table 13.4).

Furthermore, all 10 patients with local invasion achieved remission after only one additional course of chemotherapy. Prophylactic chemotherapy, therefore, not only prevented metastases; it also reduced the incidence and morbidity of local uterine invasion. Kim et al. (22) performed a prospective randomized study of prophylactic chemotherapy in patients with a complete mole and observed a significant decrease in persistent GTN in patients with high-risk mole who received prophylactic chemotherapy. Therefore **prophylaxis may be particularly useful in the management of high-risk molar pregnancy, especially when hormonal follow-up is unavailable or unreliable.**

Follow-Up

Human Chorionic Gonadotropin

Human chorionic gonadotropin is a predictable secretory product of the trophoblastic cell. Like the other glycoprotein hormones—luteinizing hormone (LH), follicle-stimulating hormone (FSH), and thyroid-stimulating hormone (TSH)—hCG is composed of two polypeptide chains (alpha and beta) attached to a carbohydrate moiety. There is considerable cross-reactivity between hCG and LH because they share indistinguishable alpha chains. Each of the β-chains of these four glycoprotein hormones is biochemically unique and confers biologic and immunologic specificity. The β-subunit radioimmunoassay is the most reliable assay currently available for the management of patients with GTN and is particularly useful in quantitating low levels of hCG without substantial interference from physiologic levels of LH.

After molar evacuation, patients should be followed by weekly determinations of β-subunit hCG levels until these are normal for 3 consecutive weeks and then by monthly determinations until the levels are normal for 6 consecu-

Table 13.4   Prophylactic Actinomycin D (Act-D) After Evacuation or Hysterectomy for Molar Pregnancy

Outcome	No. of Patients (%)			
	Act-D		No Act-D	
Normal involution	237	(96)	698	(81.4)
Persistent GTN				
Nonmetastatic	10	(4)	126	(14.6)
Metastatic	0	(0)	34	(4.0)
Totals	**247**	**(100)**	**858**	**(100)**

Reproduced, with permission, from Goldstein DP, Berkowitz RS, Bernstein MR: Management of molar pregnancy. *J Reprod Med* 26:208, 1981.

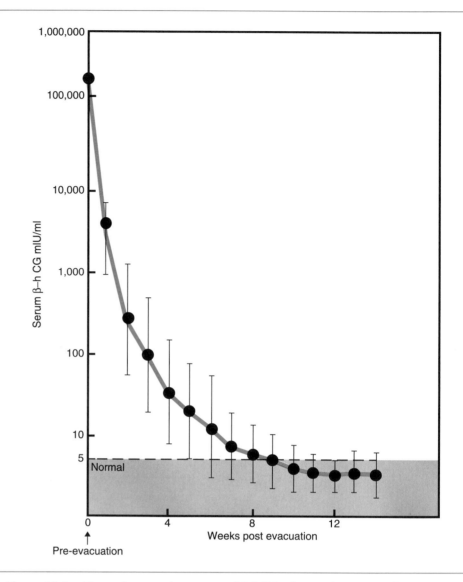

Figure 13.1 Normal regression curve of β-hCG after molar evacuation. (Reprinted, with permission, from Morrow CP, et al: Clinical and laboratory correlates of molar pregnancy and trophoblastic disease. *Am J Obstet Gynecol* 128:428, 1977.)

tive months. The normal postmolar β-hCG regression curve is presented in Figure 13.1.

Contraception

Patients are encouraged to use effective contraception during the entire interval of gonadotropin follow-up. Intrauterine devices should not be inserted until the patient achieves a normal hCG level, because of the potential risk of uterine perforation. If the patient does not desire surgical sterilization, the choice is to use either oral contraceptives or barrier methods.

The incidence of postmolar GTN has been reported to be increased among patients who used oral contraceptives before gonadotropin remission (23). However, data from both the NETDC and the Gynecologic Oncology Group (GOG) indicate that these agents do not increase the risk of postmolar trophoblastic disease (24, 25). Postmolar GTN developed in 14.3% of the patients who used barrier methods and in 18.9% of those who used oral contraceptives ($P > 0.10$) (24). In addition, the contraceptive method did not influence the mean hCG regression time. It appears that oral contraceptives may be safely prescribed after molar evacuation during the entire interval of hormonal follow-up.

Malignant Gestational Trophoblastic Neoplasia

Nonmetastatic Disease   Locally invasive GTN develops in 15% of patients after molar evacuation and infrequently after other gestations (10). These patients usually present clinically with the following:

1. Irregular vaginal bleeding

2. Theca lutein cysts

3. Uterine subinvolution or asymmetric enlargement

4. Persistently elevated serum hCG levels

The trophoblastic tumor may perforate through the myometrium, causing intraperitoneal bleeding, or erode into uterine vessels, causing vaginal hemorrhage. Bulky, necrotic tumor may involve the uterine wall and serve as a nidus for infection. Patients with uterine sepsis may have a purulent vaginal discharge and acute pelvic pain.

After molar evacuation, persistent GTN may exhibit the histologic features of either hydatidiform mole or choriocarcinoma. After a nonmolar pregnancy, however, persistent GTN always has the histologic pattern of choriocarcinoma. Histologically, choriocarcinoma is characterized by sheets of anaplastic syncytiotrophoblast and cytotrophoblast with no preserved chorionic villous structure.

Placental-Site Trophoblastic Tumor   Placental-site trophoblastic tumor is an uncommon but important variant of GTN that consists predominantly of intermediate trophoblast and a few syncytial elements (26). These tumors produce small amounts of hCG and human placental lactogen relative to their mass and tend to remain confined to the uterus and metastasize late in their course. In contrast to other trophoblastic tumors, placental-site tumors are relatively insensitive to chemotherapy, so surgical resection of disease is important.

Metastatic Disease   Metastatic GTN occurs in 4% of patients after molar evacuation and is infrequent after other pregnancies (10). Metastasis is usually associated with choriocarcinoma, which has a tendency toward early vascular invasion with widespread dissemination. Because trophoblastic tumors are often perfused by a network of fragile vessels, they are frequently hemorrhagic. Symptoms of metastases may result from spontaneous bleeding at metastatic foci. Sites of metastatic spread are shown in Table 13.5.

Pulmonary   At the time of presentation, 80% of the patients with metastatic GTN show lung involvement on chest radiographs. Patients with pulmonary metastases may have chest pain, cough, hemoptysis, dyspnea, or an asymptomatic lesion on chest radiographs. Respiratory symptoms may be of acute onset, or they may be protracted over many months.

465

Table 13.5   Relative Incidence of Common Metastatic Sites

Lungs	80%
Vagina	30%
Pelvis	20%
Brain	10%
Liver	10%
Bowel, kidney, spleen	< 5%
Other	< 5%
Undetermined*	< 5%

Reproduced, with permission, from Berkowitz RS, Goldstein DP: Pathogenesis of gestational trophoblastic neoplasms. *Pathobiol Annu* 11:391, 1981.
*Persistent hCG titer after hysterectomy.

GTN may produce four principal radiographic patterns in the lungs:

1. An alveolar or "snowstorm" pattern

2. Discrete rounded densities

3. Pleural effusion

4. An embolic pattern caused by pulmonary arterial occlusion

Because respiratory symptoms and radiographic findings may be dramatic, the patient may be thought to have primary pulmonary disease. Some patients with extensive pulmonary involvement have minimal or no gynecologic symptoms because the reproductive organs may be free of trophoblastic tumor. Regrettably the diagnosis of GTN may be confirmed only after thoracotomy has been performed, particularly in patients with a nonmolar antecedent pregnancy.

Pulmonary hypertension may develop in patients with GTN secondary to pulmonary arterial occlusion by trophoblastic emboli. Although patients with pulmonary hypertension may have many symptoms, the chest film may reveal only minimal changes.

Vaginal   Vaginal metastases are present in 30% of the patients with metastatic tumor. These lesions are usually highly vascular and may appear reddened or violaceous. They can bleed vigorously when biopsy specimens are removed, so attempts at histologic confirmation of the diagnosis should be resisted. Metastases to the vagina may occur in the fornices or suburethrally and may produce irregular bleeding or a purulent discharge.

Hepatic   Liver metastases occur in 10% of the patients with disseminated trophoblastic tumor. Hepatic involvement is encountered almost exclusively in patients with protracted delays in diagnosis and extensive tumor burdens. Epigastric or right upper quadrant pain may develop if metastases stretch Glisson's capsule. Hepatic lesions may be hemorrhagic and friable and may cause hepatic rupture and exsanguinating intraperitoneal bleeding.

Central Nervous System   Ten percent of metastatic trophoblastic disease involves the brain. Cerebral involvement is generally seen in patients with far advanced disease; virtually all patients with brain metastases have concurrent pulmonary and/or vaginal involvement. Because cerebral lesions may undergo spontaneous hemorrhage, patients may develop acute focal neurologic deficits.

Staging

An anatomic staging system for GTN has been adopted by the International Federation of Gynecology and Obstetrics (FIGO) (Table 13.6). It is hoped that this staging system will encourage the objective comparison of data among various centers.

Stage I **includes all patients with persistently elevated hCG levels and tumor confined to the uterine corpus.**

Stage II **comprises all patients with metastases to the vagina and/or pelvis.**

Stage III **includes all patients with pulmonary metastases with or without uterine, vaginal, or pelvic involvement.** The diagnosis is based on a rising hCG level in the presence of pulmonary lesions on a chest film.

Stage IV **patients have far advanced disease with involvement of the brain, liver, kidneys, or gastrointestinal tract.** These patients are in the highest risk category, because they are most likely to be resistant to chemotherapy. Most have the histologic pattern of choriocarcinoma, and their disease commonly follows a nonmolar pregnancy.

Prognostic Scoring System

In addition to anatomic staging, it is important to consider other variables to predict the likelihood of drug resistance and to assist in selection of appropriate chemotherapy (2). A prognostic scoring system, based on one developed by Bagshawe, has been proposed by the World Health Organization and reliably predicts the potential for resistance to chemotherapy (Table 13.7).

When the prognostic score is ≥ 8, the patient is categorized as high-risk and requires intensive combination chemotherapy to achieve remission. Patients with Stage I disease usually have a low-risk score, and those with Stage IV disease have a high-risk score, so that the distinction between low and high risk applies mainly to patients with Stage II or III disease.

Diagnostic Evaluation

Optimal management of persistent GTN requires a thorough assessment of the extent of the disease prior to the initiation of treatment. All patients with persistent GTN should undergo a careful pretreatment evaluation, including:

1. A complete history and physical examination

2. Measurement of the serum hCG value

Table 13.6   Staging of Gestational Trophoblastic Neoplasia

Stage I	Confined to uterine corpus
Stage II	Metastases to pelvis and vagina
Stage III	Metastases to lung
Stage IV	Distant metastases

Table 13.7 Scoring System Based on Prognostic Factors

	Score			
	0	*1*	*2*	*4*
Age (years)	< 39	> 39		
Antecedent pregnancy	H. mole	Abortion	Term	
Interval between end of antecedent pregnancy and start of chemotherapy (months)	< 4	4-6	7-12	> 12
hCG (IU/liter)	< 10_3	10^3-10^4	10^4-10^5	>10^5
ABO groups		O or A	B or AB	
Largest tumor, including uterine (cm)	< 3	3-5	> 5	
Site of metastases		Spleen Kidney	GI tract Liver	Brain
Number of metastases		1-3	4-8	> 8
Prior chemotherapy			1 drug	≥ 2 drugs

Reproduced, with permission, from Bagshawe KD: Treatment of high-risk choriocarcinoma. *J Reprod Med* 29:813, 1984.
The total score for a patient is obtained by adding the individual scores for each prognostic factor. Total score: < 4 = low-risk; 5-7 = middle-risk; ≥ 8 = high risk.

3. Hepatic, thyroid, and renal function tests

4. Determination of baseline peripheral white blood cell and platelet counts

The metastatic work-up should include:

1. A chest radiograph

2. An ultrasonogram or a computed tomographic (CT) scan of the abdomen and pelvis

3. A computed tomographic scan of the head

4. Measurement of cerebrospinal fluid hCG level if any metastatic disease is present and the head CT scan is negative

5. Selective angiography of abdominal and pelvic organs if indicated

Liver ultrasonography and CT scanning of the liver will document most hepatic metastases in patients with abnormal liver function tests. Computed tomography of the head has facilitated the early diagnosis of asymptomatic cerebral lesions (27).

In patients with choriocarcinoma and/or metastatic disease, hCG levels should be measured in the cerebrospinal fluid (CSF) to exclude cerebral involvement if the CT scan of the brain is normal. The plasma/CSF hCG ratio tends to be < 60 in the presence of cerebral metastases (28). However, a single plasma/CSF hCG ratio may be misleading, because rapid changes in plasma hCG levels may not be promptly reflected in the CSF.

Stool guaiac tests should also be routinely performed in patients with persistent GTN. If the guaiac test is positive or if the patient reports gastrointestinal symptoms, a complete radiographic evaluation of the gastrointestinal tract should be undertaken.

Pelvic ultrasonography appears to be useful in detecting extensive trophoblastic uterine involvement and may also aid in identifying sites of resistant uterine tumor (29). Because ultrasonography can accurately and noninvasively detect extensive uterine tumor, it may help to select patients who will benefit from hysterectomy. When the uterus contains large amounts of tumor, hysterectomy may substantially reduce the tumor burden and limit the exposure to chemotherapy needed to induce remission (30).

Management of Malignant GTN

Stage 1

The NETDC protocol for the management of Stage I disease is presented in Table 13.8. The selection of treatment is based primarily on whether or not the patient desires to retain fertility.

Hysterectomy Plus Chemotherapy

If the patient no longer wishes to preserve fertility, hysterectomy with adjuvant single-agent chemotherapy may be performed as primary treatment. Adjuvant chemotherapy is administered for three reasons:

1. To reduce the likelihood of disseminating viable tumor cells at surgery.

2. To maintain a cytotoxic level of chemotherapy in the bloodstream and tissues in case viable tumor cells are disseminated at surgery.

3. To treat any occult metastases that may already be present at the time of surgery.

Chemotherapy can be administered safely at the time of hysterectomy without increasing the risk of bleeding or sepsis. At the NETDC, 28 patients were treated with primary hysterectomy and a single course of adjuvant chemotherapy, and all have achieved complete remission with no additional therapy.

Hysterectomy is also performed in all patients with a *placental-site trophoblastic tumor*. Because placental-site tumors are resistant to chemotherapy, hysterectomy for presumed nonmetastatic disease is the only curative treatment. To date, rare

Table 13.8 Protocol for Treatment of Stage I GTN	
Initial	MTX-FA; if resistant, switch to Act-D or hysterectomy with adjuvant chemotherapy
Resistant	Combination chemotherapy or hysterectomy with adjuvant chemotherapy; local uterine resection; pelvic intra-arterial infusion
Follow-up hCG	Weekly until normal for 3 weeks, then monthly until normal for 12 months
Contraception	12 consecutive months of normal hCG values

Modified, with permission, from Goldstein DP, Berkowitz RS (eds): *Gestational Trophoblastic Neoplasms—Clinical Principles of Diagnosis and Management.* Philadelphia, WB Saunders, 1982.
MTX = methotrexate; Act-D = actinomycin D; FA = folinic acid.

469

patients with a metastatic placental-site tumor have been reported to be in sustained remission as a result of chemotherapy (31).

Chemotherapy Alone

Single-agent chemotherapy is the preferred treatment in patients with Stage I disease who desire to retain fertility. Primary single-agent chemotherapy was administered at the NETDC to 368 patients with Stage I GTN, and 347 (94.3%) achieved complete remission. The remaining 21 resistant patients subsequently attained remission after a change of chemotherapy or surgical intervention.

When patients are resistant to single-agent chemotherapy and desire to preserve fertility, combination chemotherapy should be administered. If the patient is resistant to both single-agent and combination chemotherapy and wants to retain fertility, local uterine resection may be considered. When local resection is planned, a preoperative ultrasonogram and/or arteriogram may help to define the site of the resistant tumor.

Follow-Up

All patients with Stage I lesions should be followed with:

1. Weekly measurement of hCG levels until they are normal for 3 consecutive weeks

2. Monthly hCG values until levels are normal for 12 consecutive months

3. Effective contraception during the entire interval of hormonal follow-up

---

Stages II and III

Low-risk patients are treated with primary single-agent chemotherapy, and high-risk patients are managed with primary intensive combination chemotherapy. A protocol for the management of patients with Stage II and III disease is presented in Table 13.9.

All 26 patients with Stage II disease treated at the NETDC achieved remission. Single-agent chemotherapy induced complete remission in 16 (88.9%) of 18 low-risk patients. Two patients with resistant disease were cured with local resection.

Table 13.9 Protocol for Treatment of Stages II and III GTN	
Low-risk*	
Initial	MTX-FA; if resistant, switch to Act-D
Resistant to both single agents	Combination chemotherapy
High-risk*	
Initial	Combination chemotherapy
Resistant	Second-line combination chemotherapy
Follow-up hCG	Weekly until normal for 3 weeks, then monthly until normal for 12 months
Contraception	Until there have been 12 consecutive months of normal hCG values

Modified, with permission, from Goldstein DP, Berkowitz RS (eds): *Gestational Trophoblastic Neoplasms—Clinical Principles of Diagnosis and Management.* Philadelphia, WB Saunders, 1982.
MTX = methotrexate; FA = folinic acid; ACT-D = actinomycin D.
*Local resection optional.

In contrast, only two of eight high-risk patients achieved remission with single-agent treatment, the others requiring combination chemotherapy and local resection.

Vaginal Metastasis

Vaginal metastases may bleed profusely because they are highly vascular and friable. When bleeding is substantial, it may be controlled by packing of the hemorrhagic lesion or by wide local excision. Infrequently, arteriographic embolization of the hypogastric arteries may be required to control hemorrhage from vaginal metastases.

Pulmonary Metastasis

Of 121 patients with Stage III disease managed at the NETDC, 120 (99%) attained complete remission. Gonadotropin remission was induced with single-agent chemotherapy in 67 of 79 (85%) patients with low-risk disease. All patients who were resistant to single-agent treatment subsequently achieved remission with combination chemotherapy and/or local pulmonary resection.

Thoracotomy   Thoracotomy has a limited role in the management of Stage III disease. However, if a patient has a persistent viable pulmonary metastasis despite intensive chemotherapy, thoracotomy may be attempted to excise the resistant focus. A thorough metastatic work-up should be performed before surgery to exclude other sites of persistent disease. Fibrotic pulmonary nodules may persist indefinitely on radiographs of the chest, even after complete gonadotropin remission has been attained. In patients undergoing thoracotomy for resistant disease, chemotherapy should be administered postoperatively to treat potential occult sites of micrometastases.

Hysterectomy

Hysterectomy may be required in patients with metastatic GTN to control uterine hemorrhage or sepsis. Furthermore, in patients with extensive uterine tumor, hysterectomy may substantially reduce the trophoblastic tumor burden and thereby limit the need for multiple courses of chemotherapy.

Follow-Up

Follow-up monitoring for patients with Stage II and III disease is the same as for patients with Stage I disease.

Stage IV

A protocol for the management of Stage IV disease is presented in Table 13.10. These patients are at greatest risk of developing rapidly progressive and unresponsive tumors despite intensive multimodal therapy. They should all be referred to centers with special expertise in the management of trophoblastic disease.

All patients with Stage IV disease should be treated with primary intensive combination chemotherapy and the selective use of radiation therapy and surgery. Before 1975, only 6 of 20 patients (30%) with Stage IV disease treated at the NETDC attained complete remission. Since 1975, however, 14 of 18 patients (77.8%) with Stage IV tumors have achieved gonadotropin remission. This gratifying improvement in survival has resulted from the use of primary combination chemotherapy in conjunction with radiation and surgical treatment.

Table 13.10 Protocol for Treatment of Stage IV GTN	
Initial	Combination chemotherapy
Brain	Whole-head irradiation (3000 rads)
	Craniotomy to manage complications
Liver	Resection to manage complications
Resistant*	Second-line combination chemotherapy
	Hepatic arterial infusion
Follow-up hCG	Weekly until normal for 3 weeks, then monthly until normal for 24 months
Contraception	Until there have been 24 consecutive months of normal hCG values

Modified, with permission, from Goldstein DP, Berkowitz RS (eds): *Gestational Trophoblastic Neoplasms—Clinical Principles of Diagnosis and Management*. Philadelphia, WB Saunders, 1982.
*Local resection optional.

Hepatic Metastasis

The management of hepatic metastases is particularly challenging and problematic. If a patient is resistant to systemic chemotherapy, hepatic arterial infusion of chemotherapy may induce complete remission in selected cases. Hepatic resection may also be required to control acute bleeding or to excise a focus of resistant tumor.

Cerebral Metastasis

If cerebral metastases are diagnosed, whole-brain irradiation (3000 rads in 10 fractions) should be instituted promptly. The risk of spontaneous cerebral hemorrhage may be lessened by the concurrent use of combination chemotherapy and brain irradiation, because irradiation may be both hemostatic and tumoricidal (32).

Craniotomy   Craniotomy may be required to provide acute decompression or to control bleeding and should be performed to manage life-threatening complications in the hope that the patient ultimately will be cured with chemotherapy. Hammond et al. (30) performed craniotomy in six patients to control bleeding, and three of these patients ultimately achieved complete remission. Infrequently, cerebral metastases that are resistant to chemotherapy may be amenable to local resection. Fortunately, patients with cerebral metastases who achieve sustained remission generally have no residual neurologic deficits (33).

Follow-Up

Patients with Stage IV disease should be followed with:

1. Weekly determination of hCG levels until they are normal for 3 consecutive weeks.

2. Monthly determination of hCG levels until they are normal for 24 consecutive months.

These patients require prolonged gonadotropin follow-up because they are at increased risk of late recurrence.

An algorithm for the management of gestational trophoblastic neoplasia is presented in Figure 13.2.

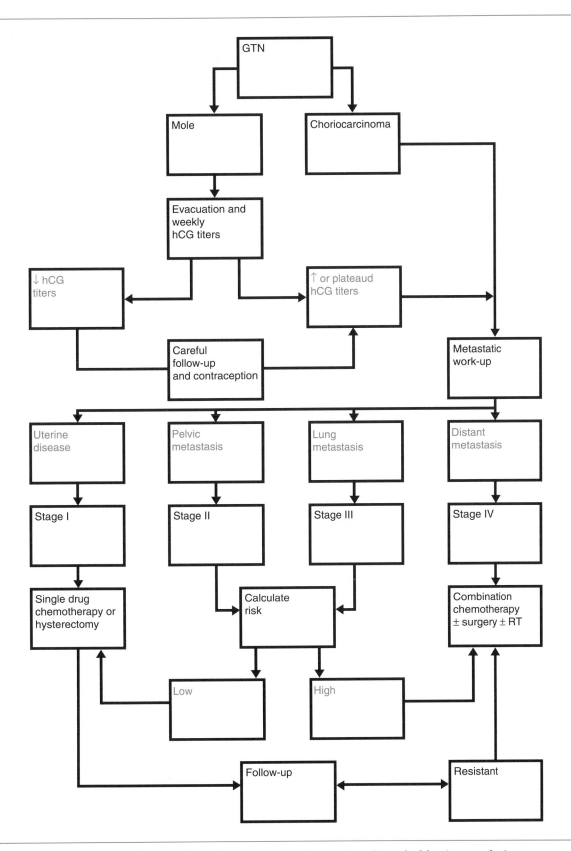

Figure 13.2   Management of gestational trophoblastic neoplasia.

Chemotherapy

Single-Agent Chemotherapy

Single-agent chemotherapy with either actinomycin D (Act-D) or methotrexate (MTX) has achieved comparable and excellent remission rates in both nonmetastatic and low-risk metastatic GTN (34). There are several protocols available for the treatment of patients with Act-D or MTX (Table 13.11).

Act-D can be given every other week in a 5-day regimen or in a pulse fashion, and MTX can be given similarly in a 5-day regimen or weekly in a pulse fashion. No study has compared all of these protocols with regard to success, but the morbidity is comparable. The selection of chemotherapy should be influenced by the associated systemic toxicity. An optimal regimen should maximize response rate while minimizing morbidity.

In 1964, Bagshawe and Wilde (35) first reported the administration of methotrexate with folinic acid (MTX-FA) in GTN to limit systemic toxicity, and subsequently it has been confirmed that MTX-FA is both effective and safe in the management of GTN (36) (Table 13.12).

MTX-FA has been the preferred single-agent regimen in the treatment of GTN at the NETDC since 1974. An evaluation of 185 patients treated in this manner between 1974 and 1984 revealed that complete remission was achieved in 162 patients (87.6%), and 132 patients (81.5%) required only one course of MTX-FA to attain remission (36). MTX-FA induced remission in 147 of 163 patients (90.2%) with Stage I GTN and in 15 of 22 patients (68.2%) with low-risk Stages II and III GTN. Resistance to therapy was more common in patients with choriocarcinoma, metastases, and pretreatment serum hCG levels > 50,000 mIU/ml. After treatment with MTX-FA, thrombocytopenia, granulocytopenia, and hepatotoxicity developed in only 3 (1.6%), 11 (5.9%), and 26 (14.1%) patients, respectively. MTX-FA therefore achieved an excellent therapeutic outcome with minimal toxicity and attained this goal with limited exposure to chemotherapy.

Rustin et al. (37) investigated the incidence of second tumors after cytotoxic chemotherapy in 457 long-term survivors treated for GTN. MTX was adminis-

---

Table 13.11   Single Drug Treatment

I. Actinomycin D treatment
  A. *5-Day actinomycin D*
    Actinomycin D 12 micrograms/kg IV daily for 5 days
    CBC, platelet count, SGOT daily
    With response, retreat at the same dose
    Without response, add 2 μg/kg to the initial dose or switch to methotrexate protocol
  B. *Pulse Actinomycin D*
    Actinomycin D 1.25 mg/M^2 every 2 weeks

II. Methotrexate treatment
  A. *5-Day methotrexate*
    Methotrexate 0.4 mg/kg IV or IM daily for 5 days
    CBC, platelet count daily
    With response, retreat at the same dose
    Without response, increase dose to 0.6 mg/kg or switch to actinomycin D protocol
  B. *Pulse methotrexate*
    Methotrexate 40 mg/M^2 IM weekly

CBC = complete blood count; SGOT = serum glutamic-oxaloacetic transaminase.

Table 13.12   Protocol for Therapy with Methotrexate and Folinic Acid "Rescue"

Day	Time	Follow-up Tests and Therapy
1	8 AM 4 PM	CBC, platelet count, SGOT Methotrexate, 1.0 mg/kg
2	4 PM	Folinic acid, 0.1 mg/kg
3	8 AM 4 PM	CBC, platelet count, SGOT Methotrexate, 1.0 mg/kg
4	4 PM	Folinic acid, 0.1 mg/kg
5	8 AM 4 PM	CBC, platelet count, SGOT Methotrexate, 1.0 mg/kg
6	4 PM	Folinic acid, 0.1 mg/kg
7	8 AM 4 PM	CBC, platelet count, SGOT Methotrexate, 1.0 mg/kg
8	4 PM	Folinic acid, 0.1 mg/kg

Reproduced, with permission, from Berkowitz RS, Goldstein DP, Bernstein MR: Ten years' experience with methotrexate and folinic acid as primary therapy for gestational trophoblastic disease. *Gynecol Oncol* 23:111, 1986.

tered to all but two patients, and 261 (57%) also received other cytotoxic drugs. **There was no increase in second tumors after cytotoxic chemotherapy for GTN.**

Administration of Single-Agent Treatment

The serum hCG level is measured weekly after each course of chemotherapy, and the hCG regression curve serves as the primary basis for determining the need for additional treatment.

After the first treatment:

1. Further chemotherapy is withheld as long as the hCG level is falling progressively.

2. Additional single-agent chemotherapy is not administered at any predetermined or fixed time interval.

A second course of chemotherapy is administered under the following conditions:

1. If the hCG level plateaus for more than 3 consecutive weeks or begins to rise again.

2. If the hCG level does not decline by 1 log within 18 days after completion of the first treatment.

If a second course of MTX-FA is required, the dosage of MTX is unaltered if the patient's response to the first treatment was adequate. **An adequate response is defined as a fall in the hCG level by one log after a course of chemotherapy.** If the response to the first treatment is inadequate, the dosage of MTX is increased from 1.0 mg/kg/day to 1.5 mg/kg/day for each of the four treatment days. If the response to two consecutive courses of MTX-FA is inadequate, the patient is considered to be resistant to MTX, and Act-D is promptly substituted in patients with nonmetastatic and low-risk metastatic GTN. If the hCG titers do not decline by 1 log after treatment with Act-D, the patient is also considered resistant to Act-D as a single agent. She must then be treated intensively with combination chemotherapy to achieve remission.

Combination Chemotherapy

MAC III

The preferred combination drug regimen at the NETDC used to be MAC III (triple therapy) protocol, which included MTX-FA, Act-D, and cytoxan (CTX) (38). However, triple therapy is inadequate as an initial treatment in patients with metastases and a high-risk prognostic score. Collectively, data from the GOG, M.D. Anderson, and the NETDC indicate that triple therapy induced remission in only 21 (49%) of 43 patients with metastases and a high-risk score (score > 8) (39–41).

EMA-CO

Etoposide, has been reported to induce complete remission in 56 (93%) of 60 patients with nonmetastatic and low-risk metastatic GTN (42). In 1984, Bagshawe (43) first described a new combination regimen that included etoposide, MTX, Act-D, CTX, and vincristine (EMA-CO), (Table 13.13) and reported an 83% remission in patients with metastases and a high-risk score (43). Importantly, Bolis et al. (44) confirmed that primary EMA-CO induced complete remission in 76% of the patients with metastatic GTN and a high-risk score. Furthermore, Rustin et al. (45) reported an EMA-CO remission in 13 (86%) of 15 patients with brain metastases.

The EMA-CO regimen is generally well tolerated, and treatment seldom has to be suspended because of toxicity.

The EMA-CO regimen may now be the preferred primary treatment in patients with metastases and a high-risk prognostic score. However, the optimal combination drug protocol in GTN has not yet been clearly defined. Surwit

Table 13.13   EMA-CO Regimen for GTN Patients

	Regimen
Course 1 (EMA)	
Day 1	VP-16, 100 mg/M², IV infusion in 200 ml of saline over 30 minutes Actinomycin D, 0.5 mg, IV push Methotrexate, 100 mg/M², IV push, followed by a 200 mg/M², IV infusion over 12 hours
Day 2	VP-16, 100 mg/M², IV infusion in 200 ml of saline over 30 minutes Actinomycin D, 0.5 mg, IV push Folinic Acid, 15 mg, IM or orally every 12 hours for 4 doses beginning 24 hours after start of methotrexate
Course 2 (CO)	
Day 8	Vincristine, 1.0 mg/M², IV push Cytoxan, 600 mg/M², IV in saline

Reproduced, with permission, from Bagshawe KD: Treatment of high-risk choriocarcinoma. *J Reprod Med* 29:813, 1984.
This regimen consists of two courses: (1) course 1 is given on days 1 and 2; (2) course 2 is given on day 8. Course 1 might require overnight hospital stay; course 2 does not. These courses can usually be given on days 1 and 2, 8, 15, and 16, 22, etc., and the intervals should not be extended without cause.

and Childers (46) have proposed a modification of the EMA-CO regimen wherein cisplatin and etoposide are substituted on day 8 (46). The optimal combination drug protocol will most likely include etoposide, MTX, and Act-D and perhaps other agents, administered in the most dose-intensive manner. Vinblastine, bleomycin, and cisplatin also effectively induced remission in four of seven patients who were resistant to triple therapy (47).

Duration of Therapy

Patients who require combination chemotherapy must be treated intensively to attain remission. Combination chemotherapy should be given as often as toxicity permits until the patient achieves three consecutive normal hCG levels. After normal hCG levels are attained, at least two additional courses of chemotherapy are undertaken to reduce the risk of relapse.

Subsequent Pregnancies

Pregnancies After Hydatidiform Mole

Patients with hydatidiform moles can anticipate normal reproduction in the future (48). From 1965 to 1989, patients who were treated at the NETDC for complete molar gestation had 1162 subsequent pregnancies that resulted in 803 full-term live births (69.1%), 84 premature deliveries (7.2%), nine ectopic pregnancies (0.8%), six stillbirths (0.5%), and 15 repeat molar pregnancies (1.3%). First- and second-trimester spontaneous abortions occurred in 208 pregnancies (17.9%). There were 37 therapeutic abortions (3.2%). Major and minor congenital malformations were detected in 35 infants (3.9%). Primary cesarean section was performed in 49 of 288 (17.0%) term or premature births from 1979 to 1989. **Patients with a complete molar pregnancy therefore should be reassured that in later pregnancies they are at no increased risk of obstetric complications, either prenatally or intrapartum. Although data concerning subsequent pregnancies after a partial mole are limited, the information is reassuring.**

When a patient has had a hydatidiform mole, she is at increased risk of molar pregnancy in subsequent conceptions (48). About 1 in 100 patients has at least two molar gestations. Later molar pregnancies are characterized by worsening histology and increased risk of postmolar GTN. Furthermore, the probability of a normal subsequent term pregnancy after two prior hydatidiform moles is low.

Therefore, for any subsequent pregnancy, it seems prudent to:

1. Obtain a pelvic ultrasonogram during the first trimester to confirm normal gestational development.

2. Obtain a thorough histologic review of the placenta or products of conception.

3. Obtain an hCG measurement 6 weeks after completion of the pregnancy to exclude occult trophoblastic neoplasia.

Pregnancies After Persistent GTN

Patients with GTN who are treated successfully with chemotherapy can expect normal reproduction in the future. Patients who were treated with chemotherapy at the NETDC from 1965 to 1989 had 385 subsequent pregnancies that resulted in 275 term live births (71.4%), 14 premature deliveries (3.6%), 4 ectopic pregnancies (1.0%), 6 stillbirths (1.5%), and only 1 repeat molar pregnancy (0.3%) (48). First- and second-trimester spontaneous abortions occurred in 65 pregnancies (17.0%). There were 20 therapeutic abortions (5.2%). Major and minor congenital anomalies were detected in only 6 infants (2%). Primary cesarean section was performed in 28 (14.8%) of 189 subsequent term and premature births from 1979 to 1989. It is particularly reassuring that the frequency of congenital malformations is not increased, although chemotherapeutic agents are known to have teratogenic and mutagenic potential.

References

1. **Berkowitz RS, Goldstein DP:** The management of molar pregnancy and gestational trophoblastic tumors. In Knapp RC, Berkowitz RS (eds): *Gynecologic Oncology*, ed 2. New York, MacMillan, 1993, pp 328–338.

2. **Goldstein DP, Berkowitz RS:** *Gestational Trophoblastic Neoplasms—Clinical Principles of Diagnosis and Management*. Philadelphia, WB Saunders, 1982, p 1.

3. **Bagshawe KD:** Risks and prognostic factors in trophoblastic neoplasia. *Cancer* 38:1373, 1976.

4. **Kajii T, Ohama K:** Androgenetic origin of hydatidiform mole. *Nature* 268:633, 1977.

5. **Yamashita K, Wake N, Araki T, et al:** Human lymphocyte antigen expression in hydatidiform mole: androgenesis following fertilization by a haploid sperm. *Am J Obstet Gynecol* 135:597, 1979.

6. **Pattillo RA, Sasaki S, Katayama KP, et al:** Genesis of 46,XY hydatidiform mole. *Am J Obstet Gynecol* 141:104, 1981.

7. **Szulman AE, Surti U:** The syndromes of hydatidiform mole. I. Cytogenetic and morphologic correlations. *Am J Obstet Gynecol* 131:665, 1978.

8. **Lawler SD, Fisher RA, Dent J:** A prospective genetic study of complete and partial hydatidiform moles. *Am J Obstet Gynecol* 164:1270, 1991.

9. **Berkowitz RS, Goldstein DP, Bernstein MR:** Natural history of partial molar pregnancy. *Obstet Gynecol* 66:677, 1985.

10. **Berkowitz RS, Goldstein DP:** Pathogenesis of gestational trophoblastic neoplasms. *Pathobiol Annu* 11:391, 1981.

11. **Goldstein DP, Berkowitz RS, Bernstein MR:** Management of molar pregnancy. *J Reprod Med* 26:208, 1981.

12. **Curry SL, Hammond CB, Tyrey L, et al:** Hydatidiform mole: diagnosis, management and long-term follow-up of 347 patients. *Am J Obstet Gynecol* 45:1, 1975.

13. **Galton VA, Ingbar SH, Jimenez-Fonseca J, Hershman JM:** Alterations in thyroid hormone economy in patients with hydatidiform mole. *J Clin Invest* 50:1345, 1971.

14. **Amir SM, Osathanondh R, Berkowitz RS, Goldstein DP:** Human chorionic gonadotropin and thyroid function in patients with hydatidiform mole. *Am J Obstet Gynecol* 150:723, 1984.

15. **Osathanondh R, Berkowitz RS, de Cholnoky C, et al:** Hormonal measurements in patients with theca lutein cysts and gestational trophoblastic disease. *J Reprod Med* 31:179, 1986.

16. **Berkowitz RS, Goldstein DP, Bernstein MR:** Laparoscopy in the management of gestational trophoblastic neoplasms. *J Reprod Med* 24:261, 1980.

17. **Szulman AE, Surti U:** The clinicopathologic profile of the partial hydatidiform mole. *Obstet Gynecol* 59:597, 1982.

18. **Tow WSH:** The influence of the primary treatment of the hydatidiform mole on its subsequent course. *J Obstet Gynaecol Br Commonw* 73:545, 1966.

19. **Berkowitz RS, Goldstein DP, Bernstein MR:** Advances in management of partial molar pregnancy. *Contemp Obstet Gynecol* 36:33, 1991.

20. **Fine C, Bundy AL, Berkowitz RS, et al:** Sonographic diagnosis of partial hydatidiform mole. *Obstet Gynecol* 73:414, 1989.

21. **Goldstein DP:** Prevention of gestational trophoblastic disease by use of actinomycin-D in molar pregnancies. *Obstet Gynecol* 43:475, 1974.

22. **Kim DS, Moon H, Kim KT, et al:** Effects of prophylactic chemotherapy for persistent trophoblastic disease in patients with complete hydatidiform mole. *Obstet Gynecol* 67:690, 1986.

23. **Stone M, Dent J, Kardana A, Bagshawe KD:** Relationship of oral contraception to development of trophoblastic tumour after evacuation of a hydatidiform mole. *Br J Obstet Gynaecol* 83:913, 1976.

24. **Berkowitz RS, Goldstein DP, Marean AR, Bernstein MR:** Oral contraceptives and postmolar trophoblastic disease. *Obstet Gynecol* 58:474, 1981.

25. **Curry SL, Schlaerth JB, Kohorn EI, et al:** Hormonal contraception and trophoblastic sequelae after hydatidiform mole (a Gynecologic Oncology Group study). *Am J Obstet Gynecol* 160:805, 1989.

26. **Finkler NJ, Berkowitz RS, Driscoll SD, et al:** Clinical experience with placental site trophoblastic tumors at the New England Trophoblastic Disease Center. *Obstet Gynecol* 71:854, 1988.

27. **Athanassiou A, Begent RHJ, Newlands ES, et al:** Central nervous system metastases of choriocarcinoma: 23 years' experience at Charing Cross Hospital. *Cancer* 52:1728, 1983.

28. **Bagshawe KD, Harland S:** Immunodiagnosis and monitoring of gonadotropin-producing metastases in the central nervous system. *Cancer* 38:112, 1976.

29. **Berkowitz RS, Birnholz J, Goldstein DP, Bernstein MR:** Pelvic ultrasonography and the management of gestational trophoblastic disease. *Gynecol Oncol* 15:403, 1983.

30. **Hammond CB, Weed JC Jr, Currie JL:** The role of operation in the current therapy of gestational trophoblastic disease. *Am J Obstet Gynecol* 136:844, 1980.

31. **Dessau R, Rustin GJS, Dent J, et al:** Surgery and chemotherapy in the management of placental site tumor. *Gynecol Oncol* 39:56, 1990.

32. **Yordan EL Jr, Schlaerth J, Gaddis O, Morrow CP:** Radiation therapy in the management of gestational choriocarcinoma metastatic to the central nervous system. *Obstet Gynecol* 69:627, 1987.

33. **Weed JC Jr, Hammond CB:** Cerebral metastatic choriocarcinoma: intensive therapy and prognosis. *Obstet Gynecol* 55:89, 1980.

34. **Osathanondh R, Goldstein DP, Pastorfide GB:** Actinomycin D as the primary agent for gestational trophoblastic disease. *Cancer* 36:863, 1975.

35. **Bagshawe KD, Wilde CE:** Infusion therapy for pelvic trophoblastic tumors. *J Obstet Gynaecol Br Commonw* 71:565, 1964.

36. **Berkowitz RS, Goldstein DP, Bernstein MR:** Ten years' experience with methotrexate and folinic acid as primary therapy for gestational trophoblastic disease. *Gynecol Oncol* 23:111, 1986.

37. **Rustin GJS, Rustin F, Dent J, et al:** No increase in second tumors after cytotoxic chemotherapy for gestational trophoblastic tumors. *N Engl J Med* 308:473, 1983.

38. **Berkowitz RS, Goldstein DP, Bernstein MR:** Modified triple chemotherapy in the management of high-risk metastatic gestational trophoblastic tumors. *Gynecol Oncol* 19:173, 1984.

39. **Curry SL, Blessing JA, DiSaia PJ, et al:** A prospective randomized comparison of methotrexate, dactinomycin and chlorambucil versus methotrexate, dactinomycin, cyclophosphamide, doxorubicin, melphalan, hydroxyurea and vincristine in "poor prognosis" metastatic gestational trophoblastic disease: a Gynecologic Oncology Group study. *Obstet Gynecol* 73:357, 1989.

40. **Gordon AN, Gershenson DM, Copeland LJ, et al:** High-risk metastatic gestational trophoblastic disease: further stratification into clinical entities. *Gynecol Oncol* 34:54, 1989.

41. **DuBeshter B, Berkowitz RS, Goldstein DP, et al:** Metastatic gestational trophoblastic disease: Experience at the New England Trophoblastic Disease Center, 1965–1985. *Obstet Gynecol* 69:390, 1987.

42. **Wong LC, Choo YC, Ma HK:** Primary oral etoposide therapy in gestational trophoblastic disease: an update. *Cancer* 58:14, 1986.

43. **Bagshawe KD:** Treatment of high-risk choriocarcinoma. *J Reprod Med* 29:813, 1984.

44. **Bolis G, Bonazzi C, Landoni F, et al:** EMA-CO regimen in high-risk gestational trophoblastic tumor (GTT). *Gynecol Oncol* 31:439, 1988.

45. **Rustin GJS, Newlands ES, Begent RHJ, et al:** Weekly alternating etoposide, methotrexate, actinomycin D/vincristine and cyclophosphamide chemotherapy for the treatment of CNS metastases of choriocarcinoma. *J Clin Oncol* 7:900, 1989.

46. **Surwit EA, Childers JM:** High-risk metastatic gestational trophoblastic disease: a new dose-intensive, multiagent chemotherapeutic regimen. *J Reprod Med* 36:45, 1991.

47. **DuBeshter B, Berkowitz RS, Goldstein DP, et al:** Vinblastine, cisplatin and bleomycin as salvage therapy for refractory high-risk metastatic gestational trophoblastic disease. *J Reprod Med* 34:189, 1989.

48. **Berkowitz RS, Goldstein DP, Bernstein MR:** Reproductive experience after complete and partial molar pregnancy and gestational trophoblastic tumors. *J Reprod Med* 36:3, 1991.

14 Breast Disease

Armando E. Giuliano

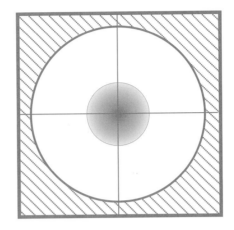

An understanding of the pathophysiology of breast disorders, skill at detecting and diagnosing breast cancer, and an appreciation of the numerous options for treating breast cancer are essential for the practicing gynecologist. Common benign conditions that mimic malignancy, as well as the diagnosis and management of invasive and preinvasive cancer of the breast, are discussed.

Detection

Physical Examination

Breast tumors, particularly cancerous ones, are usually asymptomatic and are discovered only by physical examination or screening mammography. It is important to record the physical findings of routine breast examination in the medical record for future reference.

Inspection

Inspection is done initially while the patient is seated comfortably with her arms relaxed at her sides. The breasts can be compared for symmetry, contour, and skin appearance. Edema or erythema can be identified easily, and skin dimpling or nipple retraction can be demonstrated by having the patient raise her arms above her head, then press her hands on her hips, thereby contracting the pectoralis muscles. Tumors that distort Cooper's ligaments may lead to skin dimpling with these maneuvers (Fig. 14.1).

Palpation

With the patient seated, each breast should be methodically palpated. An easily reproducible method is to palpate the breast in enlarging concentric circles until the entire breast is palpated. Palpation is best performed with the flat portion of the fingers rather than the tips. While the patient is seated, the examiner may palpate the pendulous breast bimanually by placing one hand between the breast and the chest wall and gently palpating the breast between both examining hands. The axillary and supraclavicular areas should be palpated for enlarged lymph

481

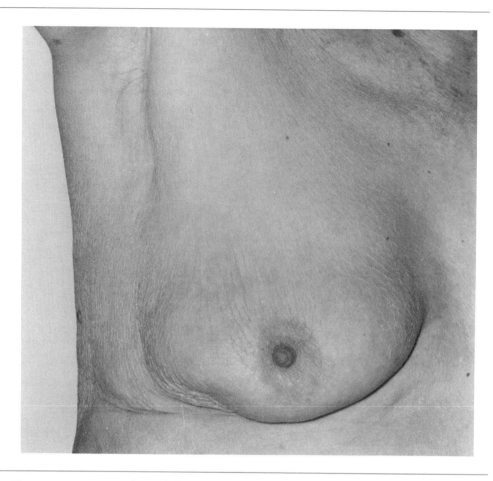

Figure 14.1 **Retraction of the skin of the lower, outer quadrant seen only upon raising the arm**. A small carcinoma was palpable.

nodes. The entire axilla, the upper outer quadrant of the breast, and the axillary tail of Spence are palpated for possible masses.

The patient is then asked to lie down and raise her arm over her head. The entire breast again is palpated methodically, with the examiner being certain to examine from the clavicle to the costal margin. Placement of a pillow or towel beneath each scapula to elevate the side being examined is important for women with large breasts, because when such women lie flat the breast tends to fall laterally, making palpation of the lateral hemisphere more difficult.

The major features to be identified on palpation of the breast are tenderness, nodularity, and dominant masses. Most patients have normally nodular breast parenchyma. The nodularity is diffuse, although predominantly in the upper, outer quadrants where there is more breast tissue. The nodules are small, similar in size, and indistinct. Breast cancer by comparison is usually a nontender, firm mass, with unclear margins, that feels distinct from the surrounding nodularity. A malignant mass may be fixed to the skin or to the underlying fascia.

In general, breast examinations are most successful 10–14 days after the onset of menses. During the premenstrual phase, most women have increased innocuous nodularity and engorgement of the breast, which can obscure an underlying lesion and make examination difficult. If the physician cannot confirm the patient's finding, the examination should be repeated again in 1 month or after her next menstrual period.

Breast Self-Examination

Self-examination of the breast has been shown to detect cancers earlier and probably results in improved survival of patients with breast carcinoma (1). Although young women have a low incidence of breast cancer, it is important to teach self-examination early so that it becomes habitual when they are older. Premenopausal women should examine their breasts monthly during the week after their menses. The reasons most women do not perform breast self-examination are complex, but reassurance, support, and patient education may encourage women to overcome psychological barriers. Patients should be told that most breast cancers are palpated first by the patient rather than by the physician.

The woman should inspect her breasts while standing or sitting before a mirror, looking for any asymmetry, skin dimpling, or nipple retraction. Elevating her arms over her head or pressing her hands against her hips to contract the pectoralis muscles will highlight any skin dimpling. While standing or sitting, she should carefully palpate her breasts with the fingers of the opposite hand. This may be performed while showering, because soap and water may increase the sensitivity of palpation. Finally, she should lie down and again palpate each quadrant of the breast, as well as the axilla.

Breast Imaging

Many imaging techniques have been used to improve the early detection of malignancy, the most common being mammography, ultrasonography, and thermography.

Mammography

The mammographic technique initially used employed industrial film and low-kilovoltage equipment, which resulted in radiation doses of almost 10 cGy to the skin (2). Theoretically, this dose may be high enough to induce a small number of cancers among women undergoing screening mammography. A large controversy ensued concerning the value of screening mammography in women who had no symptoms because, theoretically, cancer could be induced in women without medical problems. Recent improvements in film and equipment have resulted in a significantly lower dose of radiation and an improved image quality, so the risk of inducing malignancy by mammography has been virtually eliminated.

Mammography is the only reproducible method of detection for a nonpalpable breast cancer. Bilateral mammography is mandatory in the following circumstances:

1. In all patients with a dominant mass, even if biopsy is planned, to exclude disease in the opposite breast

2. In all patients with axillary or supraclavicular lymphadenopathy

3. Before cosmetic breast operations

Xeromammography Xeromammography has been used effectively for the past 20 years and produces excellent images (3). However, it results in a higher dose of radiation to the breast than the newer film screen techniques. For this reason, the technique is being used less frequently and will likely be abandoned.

Film Screen Mammography Film screen mammography can produce images as good as those seen with xeromammograms (Fig. 14.2). With a good technique and well-maintained, modern equipment, a film screen mammogram delivers only 0.02–0.03 cGy to the midbreast, with a total skin dose of 0.2–0.3 cGy (4–5).

Mammography should be performed only by radiologists who are skilled in its interpretation and who are capable of obtaining good images with good equipment. Vigorous compression of the breast is necessary to obtain good images, and patients should be forewarned that breast compression is uncomfortable.

Signs of Malignancy The most common signs of breast cancer seen on mammography are:

1. A cluster of small calcifications

2. A mass seen as an area of increased radiodensity

3. An area of breast parenchymal distortion

4. Skin thickening or edema

Figure 14.2 Bilateral film screen mammogram showing typical carcinoma in each breast, illustrating the importance of bilateral mammography in the work-up of a clinically apparent mass.

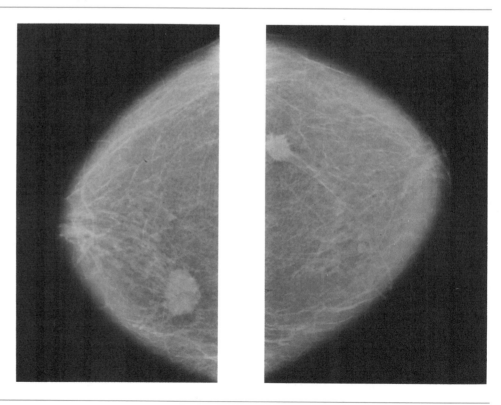

These signs may be obvious to the untrained, or they may be subtle, appreciated only by the most skilled radiologist. **The findings of malignancy can also be seen with benign lesions, leading to a false-positive rate of 15–20% (6).** False-negative mammograms occur particularly in young women with dense breast parenchyma and little fat (4, 7). If there are clinically abnormal signs, biopsy of the breast must be performed regardless of the mammographic findings (8).

Screening Mammography   Screening programs for asymptomatic women involving mammography, either alone or (preferably) combined with physical examination, have been undertaken to detect early breast cancer. In a large controlled trial conducted by the Health Insurance Plan (the "HIP" study) of New York City (9), symptom-free women undergoing screening mammography and physical examination achieved a 30% reduction in breast cancer mortality after 7 years as compared with a control group. After 14 years, the mortality was still reduced by nearly 25%. Of the 132 breast cancers detected in the screened population, 54 were detected by mammography alone, and survival overall was highest for these women. The improvement in survival was seen only in women over the age of 50, as younger women rarely had tumors that were detected solely by mammography.

The American Cancer Society and the National Cancer Institute began the Breast Cancer Detection Demonstration Project (BCDDP) in 1973 (10). Over a 5-year period, the BCDDP screened a large number of women with annual mammography and physical examination. Thermography was used initially in the study, but it was abandoned after it was deemed to be of no value. The BCDDP used mammographic equipment that was technically superior to that used in the earlier study (9). Not surprisingly, the number of cancers detected by mammography alone increased to 42%. One-third of the cancers were minimal, noninfiltrating, or smaller than 1 cm. **Patients whose tumors were found by screening had only a 20% incidence of positive axillary lymph nodes, compared with about 50% for patients with a clinically palpable mass.**

The value of mammography and physical examination as a screening technique has been supported by other studies around the world. A randomized study in Sweden, using only a single view in an attempt to lower the cost of screening mammography, showed a 31% reduction of breast cancer mortality among screened women when compared with a control group (11).

Screening Guidelines   On the basis of these studies, the American College of Radiology and the American Cancer Society recommend the following guidelines for the use of mammography in women with no symptoms (12):

1. A baseline mammogram should be obtained on all women between the ages of 35 and 40.

2. A repeat mammogram should be obtained at age 40 and every 2 years from age 40 to 49.

3. A mammogram should be performed annually from the age of 50.

High-risk women should have an annual mammogram and a biannual physical examination. The usefulness of screening mammography in young women without identifiable risk factors is not yet proven, probably because the incidence of malignancy in these women is low. **A number of recent studies have failed to show a benefit for screening mammography in women under 50 years of age. Therefore, the National Cancer Institute has recently recommended that screening should not routinely begin until age 50 years.** There are theoretical reasons why this could be true such as the radiodensity of breast parenchyma limiting the ability of mammography to detect early tumors, rapid tumor doubling time, or other factors. Several other studies, however, have shown a beneficial effect of screening mammography in younger women. Serious questions have been raised about the overall study design and the ability of small studies to demonstrate a beneficial effect of screening young women (13). An international trial has been proposed to address these issues. **Until this issue has been resolved, some organizations, including the American College of Obstetricians and Gynecologists, are recommending that the current American Cancer Society guidelines be followed.**

Ultrasonography

Both handheld and automated breast ultrasonography are popular imaging techniques. Although early reports suggested cancer-detection rates nearly as high as those achieved with x-ray mammography, repeat studies have failed to show any value for ultrasonography as a screening technique (14). Microcalcifications are not detected ultrasonographically, and masses are more difficult to detect in fatty breasts. Thus mammography is more useful in the fatty breasts of older women. In dense breasts seen typically in premenopausal women, ultrasonography may be useful in identifying noncalcified cancers.

Handheld or real-time ultrasonography is 95–100% accurate in differentiating solid masses from cysts (14). In clinical practice, this is of limited value, because a dominant mass should be studied by biopsy, and a needle aspiration can be performed on a cystic mass. Aspiration of fluid is far less expensive than ultrasonography, and when needle aspiration cytology is used handheld ultrasonography adds little to the evaluation. The primary role of handheld ultrasonography is in the evaluation of a benign-appearing, nonpalpable density identified by mammography. If such a lesion proves to be a simple cyst, no further work-up is necessary.

Thermography

Thermography is a relatively ineffective technique advocated by some for detection of both palpable and occult carcinoma (15). Thermography cannot reliably differentiate between benign and malignant breast disease. In the BCDDP study, thermography could detect 42% of all cancers, whereas physical examination alone detected 57% of cancers and mammography detected 91% (10). Thermography also gives an unacceptably high number of false-positive findings.

Benign Breast Conditions

Mammary Dysplasia

The most common breast problem seen in practice is mammary dysplasia. This term refers to a spectrum of clinical signs and symptoms and histologic changes and is not precise. The clinical significance, relationship to cancer, and management of this problem are often misunderstood. Terms such as "fibrocystic disease" and, perhaps more correctly, "fibrocystic change" have been used to label this condition. However, **most patients who are told they have "fibrocystic disease"**

have no disease at all. The essential part of the evaluation of the woman with symptoms of mammary dysplasia is to exclude malignancy, because the diagnosis of mammary dysplasia is otherwise of little clinical significance (16).

Clinical Presentation	*Symptoms and Signs* Mammary dysplasia usually appears in women between the ages of 25 and 50 years with multiple tender, palpable masses that fluctuate with the menstrual cycle. Usually the breasts are most tender and the masses largest just before the menses, and the signs and symptoms abate in the week after menstruation. Most patients with mammary dysplasia probably have a variation of the normal end-organ response to the physiologic hormonal variations during the menstrual cycle. The symptoms usually abate with menopause. More than 50% of women between the ages of 25 and 50 have clinical findings compatible with the diagnosis of mammary dysplasia (16).

Evaluation The evaluation of a woman with probable mammary dysplasia must exclude malignancy. If physical examination reveals diffuse nodularity, predominantly in the upper, outer quadrants, with no mass being dominant, a mammogram and repeat examination in the midportion of the menstrual cycle are all that is necessary. If there is a dominant mass, biopsy is imperative.

If a clear, watery, colorless, or greenish discharge is found in patients with mammary dysplasia, it should be tested for blood by means of a standard guaiac or Hemoccult test and for cytology. If the discharge is not bloody, it is most likely benign.

Pathology The histologic features of mammary dysplasia are extremely variable (18). At operation, the surgeon may see gross fluid-filled cysts or firm, fibrous tumors. A typical cyst is smooth, with blue-green or yellow fluid, and usually there are multiple cysts of varying sizes. Sometimes firm, fibrous tissue has the appearance of a malignancy. Microscopically, the histologic features are extremely pleomorphic, and almost always there is more than one histologic finding. The dominant microscopic features are cysts, sclerosing adenosis, epithelial hyperplasia, and fibrosis.

In most studies of biopsies and autopsies, 60–90% of breasts will show one or more of these histologic features (17). Probably 80% of breast biopsies will show some cyst formation. **Most of the histologic findings can be found in asymptomatic women, which lends support to the concept that mammary dysplasia or fibrocystic "disease" is not a disease.** It is, however, of value to know whether the epithelium is hyperplastic or atypical.

Cancer and Mammary Dysplasia	In the past, considerable attention was given to the increased risk of malignancy in patients with mammary dysplasia. Initial evidence was the common histologic finding of mammary dysplasia and malignancy together in the same breast (17, 19). However, inasmuch as one in every 10 women will develop breast cancer in her lifetime and as many as 80% of biopsies show mammary dysplasia, it is not surprising that these two entities frequently coexist. Other studies have shown an increased incidence of prior breast biopsies in women with cancer (20). However, the increased incidence of breast cancer in these patients may be a reflection of increased surveillance.

In a study by Dupont and Page (20) to evaluate the relationship between mammary dysplasia and breast cancer, 10,366 women who underwent biopsy from 1950 to 1968 were followed for a median of 17 years. The biopsy reports were reviewed and divided into "fibrocystic disease" with and without proliferative findings. Approximately 70% of the biopsies showed nonproliferative breast disease, whereas 30% showed proliferative breast disease. Cytologic atypia was present in 3.6% of the cases. Women with nonproliferative disease had no increased risk of breast cancer. **Women with proliferative breast disease and no atypical hyperplasia had a breast cancer risk that was approximately twice that of women with nonproliferative breast lesions. For patients whose biopsy showed atypical hyperplasia, the risk was approximately five times that of women with nonproliferative disease.**

These histologic criteria also were correlated with other risk factors. Family history added little risk for women with nonproliferative breast disease. However, a family history of breast cancer and atypia resulted in a breast cancer risk that was 11 times that for women with nonproliferative breast disease and no family history. Cysts did not increase the risk of breast cancer, but cysts and a family history of breast cancer increased the risk about threefold.

Therefore **most women with "fibrocystic disease" do *not* have an increased incidence of breast cancer. However, patients with histologic evidence of proliferative changes with or without atypia do have a significantly increased risk.**

Benign Tumors

Fibroadenoma

Fibroadenomas are the most common benign tumors of the breast. They usually occur in young women and may occur in teenagers (20). Before the age of 25, fibroadenomas are more common in the breast than are cysts. They rarely occur after menopause, although occasionally they are found, often calcified, in post-menopausal women. It is postulated that they are responsive to estrogen stimulation (20).

Symptoms and Signs Fibroadenomas may be multiple. Clinically, a young patient usually notices a mass while showering or dressing. Most masses are 2–3 cm in diameter when detected, but they can grow to an extremely large size (i.e., the giant fibroadenoma). On physical examination, they are firm, smooth, and rubbery. They do not elicit an inflammatory reaction, are freely mobile, and cause no dimpling of the skin or nipple retraction. They are often bilobed, and a groove can be palpated on examination. Mammographically, they have typical benign-appearing features with smooth, clearly defined margins. Occasionally, in older women, coarse calcifications can be seen within the fibroadenoma.

The presence of a fibroadenoma does not predispose the patient to carcinoma of the breast. Only rare cases of carcinoma developing in a fibroadenoma have been reported.

Treatment Once a fibroadenoma is suspected, its diagnosis should be confirmed by either excisional biopsy or fine needle aspiration cytology. Complete excision of a fibroadenoma with the patient under local anesthesia can treat the lesion and confirm the absence of malignancy.

Cystosarcoma Phylloides   Clinically, cystosarcomas tend to occur in older women, the mean age being the fifth to sixth decade (21). These lesions are rarely bilateral and usually appear as isolated masses that are difficult to distinguish clinically from a fibroadenoma. Numerous studies suggest that cystosarcoma phylloides may originate from a fibroadenoma, because patients often give a long history of a previously stable nodule that suddenly increased in size. However, this is unlikely. Size is not a diagnostic criterion, although cystosarcomas tend to be larger than fibroadenomas, probably because of their rapid growth. There are no good clinical criteria by which to distinguish a cystosarcoma from a fibroadenoma (22).

Pathology   The histologic distinction between fibroadenoma, "benign" cystosarcoma, and malignant cystosarcoma can be very difficult (22). Those tumors that are judged by the pathologist to be benign tend to recur locally in 15–40% of patients. Malignant cystosarcomas tend to recur locally and can metastasize to the lung. Axillary lymph node metastases are extremely unusual. Often the appearance of metastases is the first sign that a cystosarcoma is malignant.

Treatment   Treatment of cystosarcoma phylloides should consist of wide, local excision (22). Massive tumors or large tumors in relatively small breasts and those tumors with particularly infiltrative margins may require mastectomy. Mastectomy should be avoided whenever possible, however, and axillary lymph node dissection is not indicated. Typically, a patient will undergo an excisional biopsy of a mass believed to be a fibroadenoma, but histologic examination will reveal a cystosarcoma phylloides. When the pathologic diagnosis is cystosarcoma, a complete reexcision of the area should be undertaken so that the prior biopsy site and any residual tumor are excised. Some recommend radiation therapy, but the value of radiotherapy is not known and probably should be avoided. True soft tissue sarcomas occur in the breast but are rare.

Breast Cancer

Breast cancer accounts for approximately one-fourth of all cancers in women and is second only to lung cancer as the leading cause of cancer deaths in women. For 1994, it was estimated that approximately 183,000 new cases of breast cancer would be diagnosed in women, with nearly 46,300 deaths from this disease in the United States (23). Nearly one in every 10 women will have breast cancer during her lifetime. There has been a significant increase in the incidence of breast cancer in the United States during the past 50 years. The mortality rate, however, has remained stable, implying an increased cure rate.

Predisposing Factors   *Age*   The likelihood of developing breast cancer increases steadily with age. Before the age of 25, breast cancer is rare; this age group accounts for fewer than 1% of all cases of breast cancer. After the age of 30 years, there is a sharp increase in the incidence, with a small plateau between the ages of 45 and 50 years (24). Women between 40 and 50 years may have a lower mortality rate from the disease than older women (25).

Family History   Family history is a major risk factor for the development of breast cancer. Any family history of breast cancer increases the overall relative risk (26). However, women whose mothers or sisters had breast cancer after

489

menopause are not at significantly increased risk, whereas women whose mothers or sisters had bilateral premenopausal breast cancer have at least a 40–50% likelihood of developing the disease. If the patient's mother or sister had unilateral premenopausal breast cancer, the likelihood of the patient developing breast cancer is approximately 30%.

Diet and Obesity Marked differences in the incidence of breast cancer among women in different geographic areas have been correlated with mean annual per capita consumption of various nutrients. Obesity and high-fat diets in particular have been used to explain the marked differences in international incidences of breast cancer (27). However, it is not clear that obesity is a specific risk factor, because most studies have not clearly separated obesity from other known risk factors (28).

Reproductive and Hormonal Factors A number of studies have shown a relationship between early menarche, late menopause, and breast cancer (29–31). The median age at menarche is lower for women with breast cancer than for those who never develop the disease (28). However, age at menarche is probably a very minor risk factor. Either natural or artificial early menopause imparts a protective effect against the development of breast cancer (29). The incidence of breast cancer among women with menopause before the age of 40 is about three-fourths the incidence of breast cancer among women in whom menopause occurs at 45–55 years. Artificial menopause due to oophorectomy lowers the rate even further. **The longer a woman's reproductive phase, the higher the risk of developing breast cancer** (30). No clear association has been found between the risk of breast cancer and menstrual irregularity or duration of menses. Lactation does not affect the incidence of breast cancer, but childbearing definitely does (31). Women who have never been pregnant have a higher risk of breast cancer than those who are multiparous. However, it is the age at first childbirth that alters the incidence of breast cancer (31); i.e., the older primigravida has a higher incidence.

There have been conflicting reports concerning the effect of oral contraceptives and postmenopausal estrogens on the incidence of breast cancer. **A well-controlled study from the Centers for Disease Control (32) showed that oral contraceptives do not increase the risk of breast cancer, regardless of the duration of exposure to the agents, family history, or coexistence of benign breast disease.**

Studies on the use of estrogens to treat menopausal symptoms suggest that they are probably not associated with an increased risk of breast cancer. More controversy exists in this area, however, because some studies have shown that prolonged estrogen use (longer than 10 years) or higher doses of estrogen do increase the risk. In addition, continuous unopposed estrogen for postmenopausal symptoms may be associated with an increased risk of breast cancer (33). The current consensus is that postmenopausal estrogens should be given in a relatively low dose and should be either cycled or combined with progestins. Although estrogens may result in a slightly increased incidence of breast cancer, this is outweighed by the diminution of mortality from osteoporosis and heart disease.

Alcohol Alcohol consumption may increase the risk of breast cancer (34). These data are controversial, because not all studies support this observation.

Prior History of Cancer   One of the strongest single risk factors for the development of a primary breast cancer is the previous diagnosis of a contralateral breast cancer. A second microscopic breast cancer can be found in the contralateral breast of about 50% of women (35). However, clinical breast cancer can be detected in the contralateral breast in only 5–8% of patients. *Lobular carcinoma* has a higher incidence of bilaterality than does *ductal carcinoma*. A prior history of endometrial carcinoma, ovarian carcinoma, or colon cancer has also been associated with an increased risk of breast cancer (29).

Diagnosis

Breast cancer may occur anywhere in the breast, but it is most commonly found in the upper, outer quadrant, where there is more breast tissue. Extension of the "tail of Spence" into the axilla increases the likelihood that a tumor will develop in this quadrant.

Most breast cancers are discovered by the patient when she feels a painless mass. Less commonly, the tumor is found by the physician during a routine breast examination. Rarely, the patient may have an axillary mass and no obvious malignancy in the breast, or the abnormality may be found on a screening mammogram without a palpable tumor. Conversely, the findings on mammography may raise the suspicion that a palpable lesion is a breast cancer (36, 37).

Physical examination alone is quite inaccurate for the diagnosis of most breast cancers. In older women with fatty breasts in which the tumor is more obvious, the diagnosis can be made more accurately by physical examination, whereas younger women with dense, often nodular breasts are extremely difficult to examine. An area of thickening amid normal nodularity may be the only clue to an underlying malignancy. Skin dimpling, nipple retraction, or skin erosion is usually obvious, but these are late signs and, fortunately, are unusual at presentation. Algorithms for the evaluation of breast masses in premenopausal and postmenopausal women are presented in Figures 14.3 and 14.4.

A dominant breast mass in a woman of any age must be approached as a possible carcinoma. About 30–40% of lesions thought clinically to be malignant will be found to be benign on histologic examination (36). Conversely, 15–20% of lesions believed clinically to be benign will be proven malignant by open biopsy (37). Clinical judgment is insufficient to undertake definitive treatment of carcinoma.

Fine Needle Aspiration Cytology

Fine needle aspiration (FNA) cytology has been used for more than a century, and the technique is now well established for the evaluation of breast lesions. FNA is performed with a 20- or 22-gauge needle. The technique has a high diagnostic accuracy, with a 10–15% false-negative rate and a rare but persistent false-positive rate (38).

If a mass appears to be malignant on physical examination and/or mammography, the FNA cytology can aid the clinician in discussing alternatives with the patient. A negative FNA cytologic diagnosis must be followed with excisional biopsy, as it does not exclude malignancy. Most clinicians are reluctant to perform a mastectomy on the basis of FNA cytology, because of the rare false-positive diagnosis. Occasionally, an FNA cytologic diagnosis of a fibroadenoma in a young woman can be used to follow the mass safely.

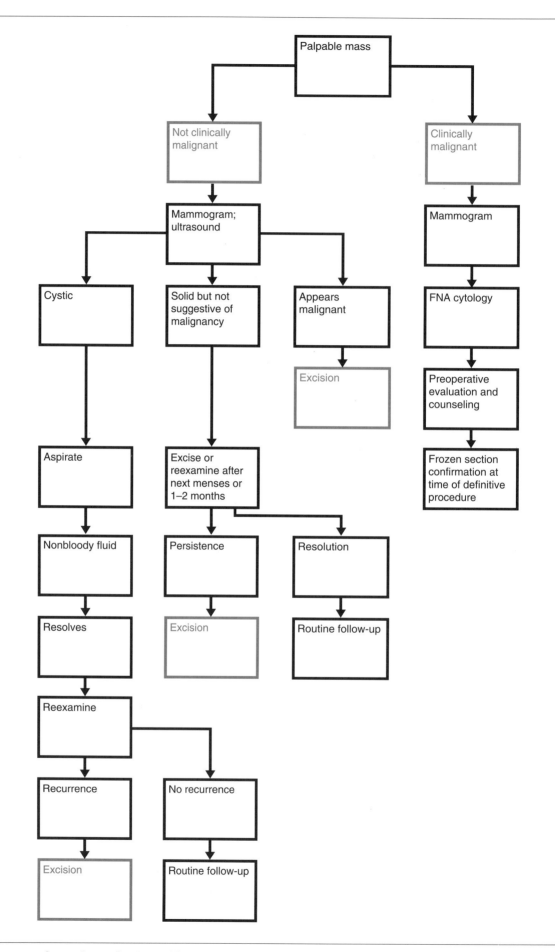

Figure 14.3 Schematic evaluation of breast masses in premenopausal women.

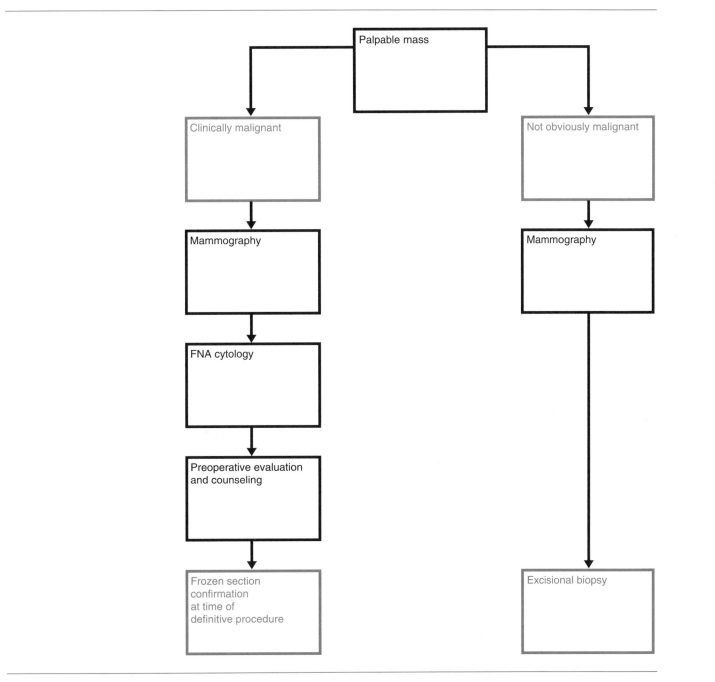

Figure 14.4   Schematic evaluation of breast masses in postmenopausal women.

Biopsy   **If FNA cytology is not performed, or if it is negative or equivocal, an open biopsy must be performed. Treatment of breast cancer should never be undertaken without an unequivocal histologic diagnosis of cancer.** Even cytologic diagnosis should not be relied on if mastectomy is contemplated. If a partial mastectomy is indicated, it can be performed and a frozen section obtained to confirm the diagnosis of cancer before the axillary dissection is started. An alternative to open biopsy is removal of a core of tissue through a Vim Silverman or Tru-Cut needle. These procedures must also be followed by open biopsy if cancer is not diagnosed.

Open biopsy can usually be performed in the office with the aid of local anesthesia. Outpatient biopsy is far less expensive and less demanding on the patient than hospitalization and biopsy with the patient under general anesthesia. The following steps are undertaken:

1. Local anesthesia is used to infiltrate the skin and subcutaneous tissue surrounding the palpable mass.

2. An incision is made directly over the mass. It should be planned to allow an ellipse of skin to be either excised with the mastectomy or placed cosmetically so that partial mastectomy can be performed through the same incision. Para-areolar incisions are best avoided, particularly if the tumor is far from the areola and would result in dragging malignant cells through a large segment of breast.

3. Once the skin and underlying tissue are incised, the mass can be gently grasped with Allys forceps or with a stay suture and delivered into the operative field.

4. The mass should be totally excised whenever possible. Large masses that are difficult to excise totally with local anesthesia can be incised. However, a frozen section should be obtained to confirm that malignant tissue has been obtained with an incisional biopsy.

5. Once the mass is excised, adequate hemostasis is achieved and the incision is closed. A cosmetically superior result will be achieved if the breast parenchyma is not reapproximated deeply. The most superficial subcutaneous fat can be reapproximated with fine, absorbable sutures. The skin is best closed with a subcuticular suture or Steri-Strips to achieve the most cosmetically pleasing result. Usually no drain is necessary.

6. At the time of initial biopsy, it is imperative to preserve a portion of the specimen for assays of estrogen and progesterone receptors (ER and PR).

Mammographically Localized Biopsy Biopsy of nonpalpable lesions seen only on mammography can be difficult, and the procedure requires cooperation of the surgeon and the mammographer. The technique relies on the mammographer's placing a needle or specialized wire into the breast parenchyma at or near the site of the suspected abnormality. Many mammographers will also inject a biologic dye to assist localization further. The surgeon then reviews the films with the mammographer and localizes the abnormality with respect to the tip of the wire or needle. An incision is made directly over this area, and that small portion of the breast that is suspected of containing the mammographic abnormality is excised. A mammogram of the surgical specimen is performed to be certain that the abnormality has been excised. Often a needle can be placed by the mammographer in the specimen at the site of the abnormality to facilitate histologic evaluation.

Two-Step Approach The two-step approach involves initial biopsy followed by subsequent definitive treatment. It has several advantages and is the preferred approach, avoiding unnecessary hospitalization of patients who do not have a

494

malignancy. In addition, women who do have cancer can discuss the alternative forms of therapy and obtain a second opinion, if desirable, before undergoing definitive treatment. Psychologically, it is preferable for the patient to be involved in the planning of her therapy rather than for her to undergo biopsy with immediate mastectomy.

For patients with obvious malignancy in whom mastectomy is the treatment of choice, it is reasonable to obtain a biopsy specimen and a frozen section, to be followed immediately with mastectomy. The treatment can be discussed in advance in such patients.

Pathology and Natural History

Numerous histologic types of breast cancer can be identified microscopically (18, 39). The malignancy arises either in the ducts or in the lobules. With some exceptions, it appears that most *lobular carcinomas* have their origin within the small terminal ducts of the lobules. *Ductal carcinomas* usually arise from the larger ducts or the intralobular ducts. However, the distinction between lobular and intraductal carcinoma is based more on the histologic appearance than on the site of origin. The cancer may be either invasive (infiltrating ductal carcinoma, infiltrating lobular carcinoma) or *in situ* (ductal carcinoma *in situ* or lobular carcinoma *in situ*). The histologic subtypes (i.e., scirrhous, tubular, medullary) often referred to by the pathologist are usually morphologic distinctions among the various patterns of infiltrating ductal carcinoma.

The most common histologic diagnosis is *infiltrating ductal carcinoma*, type not specified. This histology accounts for 60–70% of the breast cancers in the United States (39). Mammographically, it is characterized by a stellate appearance with microcalcifications. Macroscopically, there are gritty, chalky streaks within the substance of the tumor that most likely represent necrosis, whereas, microscopically, there is invasion of the surrounding fat. There is often a fibrotic response surrounding the invasive carcinoma.

Other types of infiltrating ductal carcinoma are far less common. *Medullary carcinoma* accounts for approximately 5–8% of breast carcinomas, arises from larger ducts within the breast and has a dense lymphocytic infiltrate. The tumor appears to be a slow-growing, less aggressive malignancy than the infiltrating ductal carcinoma. *Mucinous (colloid) carcinoma* accounts for fewer than 5% of all breast cancers. Grossly, the tumor may have areas that appear mucinous or gelatinous. *Infiltrating comedo carcinoma* accounts for fewer than 1% of breast malignancies and is an invasive cancer characterized by foci of necrosis, which, when cut grossly, exude a comedo, necrosis-like substance. Usually comedo carcinomas are *in situ* malignancies. *Papillary carcinoma* is used to describe a predominantly noninvasive ductal carcinoma. However, these tumors may be invasive; when invasive components are present, they should be called invasive papillary carcinomas. *Tubular carcinoma* is a well-differentiated breast cancer that accounts for fewer than 1% of all breast malignancies. *Adenoid cystic carcinomas* are extremely rare and are similar histologically to those seen in the salivary glands. They tend to be well differentiated and to metastasize late (39).

Growth Patterns

The growth potential of a breast cancer and the resistance of the individual woman to the malignancy vary widely among patients and at different stages of the disease. Estimates of the doubling time of breast cancer range from several weeks for rapidly growing tumors to months or years for slowly growing ones. If the doubling time of a breast tumor was constant and a tumor originated from one cell, a doubling time of 100 days would result in a 1 cm tumor in about 8 years (Fig. 14.5) (40). During this preclinical phase, tumor cells may be circulating throughout the body.

Because of the long preclinical tumor growth phase and the tendency of infiltrating lesions to metastasize early, many clinicians view breast cancer as a systemic disease at the time of diagnosis. Although it is true that cancer cells may be released from the tumor prior to diagnosis, variations in the tumor's ability to

Figure 14.5 Growth rate of breast cancer indicating long preclinical phase. (Reproduced, with permission, from Gullino PM: Natural history of breast cancer: progression from hyperplasia to neoplasia as predicted by angiogenesis. *Cancer* 39:2697, 1977.)

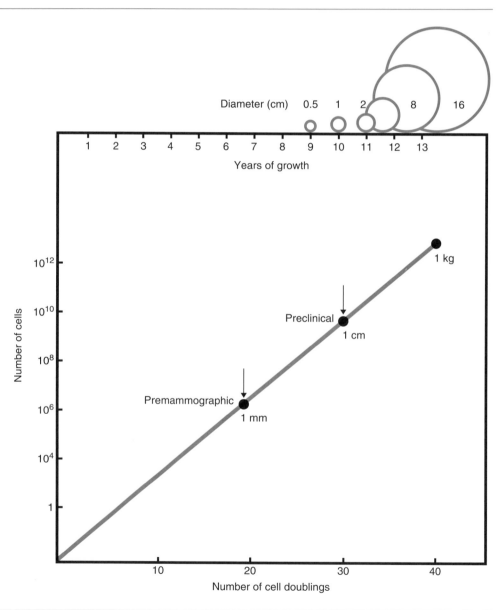

grow in other organs and the host's response to the tumor may inhibit dissemination of the disease. Indeed, many women can be treated successfully with operation alone for breast cancer, and some women have been cured even in the presence of palpable axillary disease. For this reason, a pessimistic attitude that breast cancer is systemic and incurable at the time of diagnosis is unwarranted. A more realistic approach may be to view breast cancer as a two-compartment disease: one is the primary tumor in the breast with all the inherent problems of local and regional extension and primary tumor control, and the other consists of the systemic metastases with their life-threatening consequences.

Although the natural history of breast cancer can involve metastases to any organ, 85% of women with metastatic breast cancer will have involvement of bone, lungs, or liver (41–43). If any of these sites are involved, metastases in other organs are highly likely. The use of systemic chemotherapy is altering the common sites of metastases, and more unusual metastatic sites are being seen with greater frequency. Bone metastases can give rise to pathologic fractures and/or hypercalcemia. Approximately 5–10% of women with metastatic breast cancer will develop hypercalcemia (42).

Staging

After the diagnosis of breast cancer has been established either cytologically or histologically, the clinical stage of the disease should be determined. Two clinical staging systems are currently in use. The Columbia Clinical Staging System has been widely used for many years (44), but the TNM (tumor-nodes-metastases) system has been recommended by the International Union Against Cancer (UICC) and the American Joint Committee on Cancer (45) and is presented in Tables 14.1 and 14.2. This system has the advantage of being both a preoperative clinical staging system and a postoperative or pathologic staging system. The TNM classification is becoming more widely accepted, replacing the Columbia Clinical Staging System.

Preoperative Evaluation

The extent of preoperative work-up varies with the initial stage of the disease (46). For most patients with small tumors, no palpable lymph nodes (TMN Stage I or II), and no symptoms of metastases, the preoperative evaluation should consist of:

1. Bilateral mammograms

2. Chest radiograph

3. Complete blood count

4. Screening blood chemistry tests

A routine *bone scan* and *liver scan* are not necessary unless symptoms or abnormal blood chemistry suggest bone or liver metastases, because the yield is extremely low. For patients with clinical Stage II disease, a bone scan should be obtained, but a liver scan is not necessary unless symptoms or liver function tests suggest liver metastasis. Patients with clinical Stage III or IV disease should have both a bone scan and a liver scan. A bone marrow biopsy should be performed if there is obvious bone marrow dysfunction but metastases are not evident on bone scan.

Table 14.1   TNM System for Clinical or Pathologic Staging of Breast Cancer

---

Primary Tumor (T)

TX   Minimum requirements to assess primary tumor cannot be met

T₀   No evidence of primary tumor

TIS   *In situ* cancer (*in situ* lobular, pure intraductal and Paget's disease* of the nipple without palpable tumor)

T₁   Tumor ≤ 2 cm in greatest dimension
  T_{1a} No fixation to underlying pectoral fascia or muscle
  T_{1b} Fixation to underlying pectoral fascia or muscle
    i. tumor ≤ 0.5 cm
    ii. tumor > 0.5 ≤ 1.0 cm
    iii. tumor > 1.0 ≤ 2.0 cm

T₂   Tumor > 2 cm but ≤ 5 cm in its greatest dimension
  T_{2a} No fixation to underlying pectoral fascia or muscle
  T_{2b} Fixation to underlying pectoral fascia or muscle

T₃   Tumor > 5 cm in its greatest dimension
  T_{3a} No fixation to underlying pectoral fascia or muscle
  T_{3b} Fixation to underlying pectoral fascia or muscle

T₄   Tumor of any size with direct extension to chest wall or skin (chest wall includes ribs, intercostal muscles, and serratus anterior muscle but not pectoral muscle)
  T_{4a} Fixation to chest wall
  T_{4b} Edema (including *peau d'orange*), ulceration of the skin of the breast, or satellite skin nodules confined to the same breast
  T_{4c} Both of the above

Nodal Involvement (N)

The definition of N categories varies somewhat as to time period of staging, as follows:

NX   Regional lymph nodes cannot be assessed clinically

N₀   Homolateral axillary lymph nodes not considered to contain growth

N₁   Movable homolateral axillary nodes considered to contain growth

N₂   Homolateral axillary nodes considered to contain growth and fixed to one another or to other structures

N₃   Homolateral supraclavicular or infraclavicular nodes considered to contain growth, or edema of the arm†

Definitions for Surgical-Evaluative and Postsurgical Resection-Pathologic Stage

NX   Regional lymph nodes cannot be assessed (not removed for study or previously removed)

N₀   No evidence of homolateral axillary lymph node metastasis

N₁   Metastasis to movable homolateral axillary nodes not fixed to one another or to other structure
  N_{1a} Micrometastasis ≤ 0.2 cm in lymph node(s)
  N_{1b} Gross metastasis in lymph node(s)
    I. Metastasis > 0.2 cm but < 2.0 cm in 1-3 lymph nodes
    II. Metastasis > 0.2 cm but < 2.0 cm in ≥ 4 lymph nodes
    III. Extension of metastasis beyond the lymph node capsule (< 2.0 cm in dimension
    IV. Metastasis in lymph node ≥ 2.0 cm in dimension

N₂   Metastases to homolateral axillary lymph nodes that are fixed to one another or to other structures

N₃   Metastasis to homolateral supraclavicular or infraclavicular lymph node(s)

Distant Metastasis (M)

MX   Minimum requirements to assess the presence of distant metastasis cannot be met

M₀   No (known) distant metastasis

M₁   Distant metastasis present

Reproduced, with permission, from American Joint Committee on Cancer: Beahrs OH, Myers MH (eds): *Manual for Staging of Cancer*, ed 2. Philadelphia. JB Lippincott, 1983.
*Paget's disease with a demonstrable tumor is classified according to size of the tumor. Inflammatory carcinoma should be reported separately.
†Edema of the arm may be caused by lymphatic obstruction, and lymph nodes may not then be palpable. Homolateral internal mammary nodes considered to contain growth are included in N₃, for surgical-evaluative classification and postsurgical resection-pathologic classification.

Table 14.2   Clinical-Diagnostic (cTNM), Surgical-Evaluative (sTNM) and Postsurgical Resection-Pathologic (pTNM) Staging

Stage TIS	*In situ*
Stage X	Cannot stage
Stage I	T_{1ai}, N_0, M_0
	T_{1aii}, N_0, M_0
	T_{1aiii}, N_0, M_0
	T_{1bi}, N_0, M_0
	T_{1bii}, N_0, M_0
	T_{1biii}, N_0, M_0
Stage II	T_0, N_{1a} or N_{1b}, M_0
	T_{1a} or T_{1b}, N_{1a} or N_{1b}, M_0
	T_{2a} or T_{2b}, N_0, M_0
	T_{2a} or T_{2b}, N_{1a} or N_{1b}, M_0
Stage IIIa	T_0, N_2, M_0
	T_{1a} or T_{1b}, N_2, M_0
	T_{2a} or T_{2b}, N_2, M_0
	T_{3a} or T_{3b}, N_0, M_0
	T_{3a} or T_{3b}, N_1, M_0
	T_{3a} or T_{3b}, N_2, M_0
Stage IIIb	Any T, N_3, M_0
	Any T_4, any N, M_0
Stage IV	Any T, any N, M_1

Reproduced, with permission, from American Joint Committee on Cancer: Beahrs OH, Myers MH (eds): *Manual for Staging of Cancer*, ed 2. Philadelphia, JB Lippincott, 1983.

Treatment

Mastectomy

The traditional treatment of breast cancer has been surgical, but the type of operation employed has remained a controversial and highly emotional issue. Prior to Halsted (47) in the 19th century, surgical treatment of breast cancer was haphazard, and it varied from local excision alone to total mastectomy. Halsted devised the radical mastectomy in an attempt to treat carcinoma of the breast rationally based on his understanding of breast cancer as a local infiltrative process. The radical mastectomy was planned to remove the entire breast, the underlying pectoral muscles, and the axillary lymph nodes in continuity (48) (Fig. 14.6). However, the initial operation was designed to treat patients who had palpable, axillary lymph nodes, and lesions that were at least clinical Stage III. Results of a series of more than 1000 patients treated with radical mastectomy from 1935–1972 have been reported by Haagensen and Bodian (49) and are presented in Table 14.3.

During the 20th century, extensions and modifications of the radical mastectomy were devised to remove more local and regional tissue. Supraclavicular node dissections were added to the radical mastectomy (50). In addition, supraclavicular, mediastinal, and internal mammary lymph node dissections were performed with high mortality (51).

Urban (52) added an *en bloc* internal mammary lymph node dissection to the standard radical mastectomy. This technique became popular and is the operation commonly referred to as the "extended radical mastectomy." The extended radical mastectomy has not produced an enhanced overall survival (53). Few patients

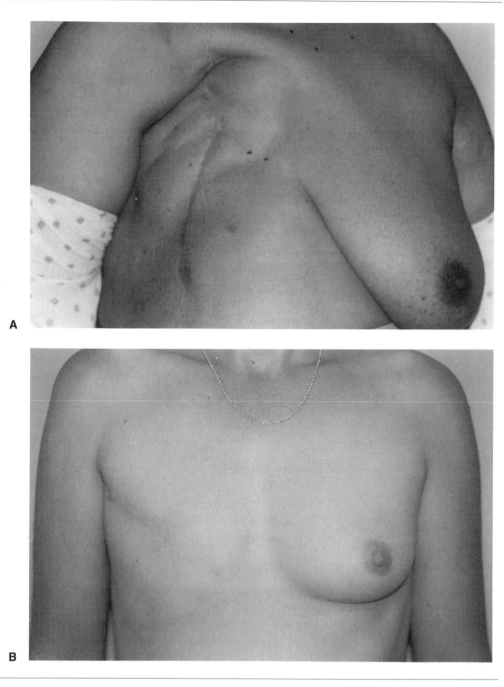

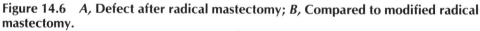

Figure 14.6 *A,* **Defect after radical mastectomy;** *B,* **Compared to modified radical mastectomy.**

without grossly involved axillary lymph nodes will have involvement of internal mammary nodes, and current understanding of the biologic behavior of breast cancer makes such locally destructive surgical endeavors unnecessary.

Modified Radical Mastectomy

In an attempt to improve the functional and cosmetic results of the radical mastectomy, a modification in which the pectoralis major muscle is preserved intact was developed (Fig. 14.6B) (54–55). The removal of the breast is similar to that

500

of the radical mastectomy; however, removal of the skin and the axillary lymph node dissection are not as extensive, and there is generally no need for skin grafting.

The advantage of the modified radical mastectomy is a better functional and cosmetic result. The radical mastectomy has been essentially replaced by the modified radical mastectomy, which remains the most common operation performed for this disease. There is no difference in survival between the two operations.(56).

Total (Simple) Mastectomy

Total mastectomy is the removal of the entire breast, nipple, and areolar complex without removal of the underlying muscles or axillary lymph nodes. In a total mastectomy, there is generally no need for skin grafts, and axillary nodes are not removed intentionally. However, the low-lying lymph nodes in the upper, outer portion of the breast and low axilla usually are included in the specimen. This form of treatment results in local control rates that are comparable to those of radical or modified radical mastectomy, but failure to examine the axillary lymph nodes microscopically makes this operation generally less desirable because the addition of adjuvant chemotherapy improves survival in certain patients with positive nodes.

Adjuvant Radiation Therapy

The combination of total mastectomy with radiation therapy was developed by McWhirter (57). Many series have advocated the use of adjuvant radiation therapy in combination with various operative procedures. Studies claiming improvements in overall survival usually are flawed by the use of historical controls and inaccurate preoperative staging. The majority of trials, both prospective randomized studies and historical control studies, show that radiation therapy, when combined with radical surgery, improves local control but does not improve survival (58–61).

A prospective randomized trial by the National Surgical Adjuvant Breast Project (NSABP) examined the role of postoperative radiation therapy (63). Patients were randomly assigned to therapy consisting either of (*1*) total mastectomy, (*2*) radical

Table 14.3   The Results of Radical Mastectomy for Carcinoma of the Breast Treated by CD Haagensen 1935-1972

Columbia Clinical Stage	Nodes Involved	No. of Patients	10-Year Survival (%)
A	0	503	78.3
	1–3	157	70.7
	4–7	35	42.9
	≥ 8	32	18.8
	Total	**727**	**52.4**
B	0	58	65.5
	1–3	63	44.4
	4–7	42	35.7
	≥ 8	45	15.6
	Total	**208**	**42.3**

Reproduced, with permission, from Haagensen CD, Bodian C: A personal experience with Halsted's radical mastectomy. *Ann Surg* 199:143, 1984.

mastectomy, or (3) total mastectomy with radiation therapy. In summary, this trial showed no difference in survival among the three groups of patients, whereas local control was improved in patients treated with total mastectomy and radiation therapy.

Conservative Surgery ± Radiation Therapy

Radiation therapy alone without excision of the tumor is associated with a high local failure rate (63–66). Veronesi et al. (67, 68) reported the first major prospective randomized trial comparing standard surgery with a combination of surgery and modern radiotherapeutic techniques. Patients were randomly assigned to either (1) quadrantectomy, axillary lymph node dissection, and postoperative radiation or (2) the standard Halsted radical mastectomy. Only patients whose tumors were < 2 cm and not centrally located and who had no clinical evidence of axillary lymph node disease ($T_1N_0M_0$) were considered for this trial. The 701 women who were randomized to either of the two groups were comparable in age, tumor size, menopausal status, and histologic involvement of the axillary lymph nodes (68). After 8 years of follow-up, there have been no statistically significant differences between the two groups in either local control or overall survival (Table 14.4).

The NSABP conducted a trial that extended these observations (69). Eligible patients could have a primary tumor ≤ 4 cm, with or without palpable axillary lymph nodes, provided that the lymph nodes were not fixed (i.e., Stage I or Stage II, T_1 or T_2, and N_0 or N_1). Patients were assigned randomly to: (a) the modified radical mastectomy; (b) segmental mastectomy (lumpectomy) and axillary lymph node dissection; or (c) segmental mastectomy, axillary lymph node dissection, and postoperative radiation therapy (Fig. 14.7). Unlike the quadrantectomy, segmental mastectomy or "lumpectomy" consists of removing only the tumor and a small rim of normal surrounding tissue. Patients were considered ineligible if they were found to have microscopic involvement of the margins. A total of 1843 women were randomized among the three treatment arms, and the groups were comparable. The lowest local recurrence rate (7.7%) was seen among patients treated with segmental mastectomy and postoperative radiation therapy, whereas it was predicted that 27.9% of the patients undergoing segmental mastectomy without radiation therapy would have a local recurrence within 5 years. Although the addition of radiation clearly improved the local control rate, no significant difference in overall survival or disease-free survival could be seen among the three treatment arms; there was a trend, however, in favor of patients who received radiation. **This NSABP study clearly shows that segmental mastectomy, axillary lymph node dissection, and postoperative radiation therapy were as**

Table 14.4 Halsted Radical Mastectomy Versus Quadrantectomy, Axillary Dissection and Radiation Therapy: Results of the Randomized Milan Trial

	Halsted % ± S.E.	Quadrantectomy + RT % ± S.E.
Number of patients	349	352
Overall survival	83 ± 2.2	85 ± 2.1
Disease-free survival	77 ± 2.4	80 ± 2.4

From Veronesi U, Zucali R, Luini A: Local control and survival in early breast cancer: the Milan trial. *Int J Radiat Oncol Biol Phys* 12:717, 1986.

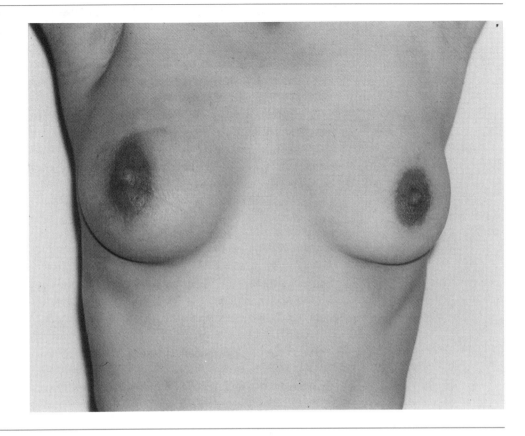

Figure 14.7   Appearance after lumpectomy, axillary dissection, and radiation therapy.

effective as modified radical mastectomy for the management of patients with Stage I and II breast cancer. The high local recurrence rate without radiation therapy makes limited surgery alone generally unacceptable, except in unusual circumstances.

Adjuvant Chemotherapy

For most patients, local-regional control of breast cancer is achieved readily with surgery and radiation therapy. More than 90% of patients will never experience a local recurrence; however, patients may still succumb to metastatic disease. The 10-year survival rate for women with positive nodes is only about 40–50%. Even when not clinically palpable, lymph node metastases portend an unfavorable course.

The goal of adjuvant systemic therapy is to eliminate occult metastases in the early postoperative period while they are theoretically most vulnerable to anti-cancer agents (70). Initial trials involved a single perioperative course of chemotherapy in an attempt to eradicate circulating tumor cells. The Nissen-Meyer study from Norway (71) showed that a single course of Cytoxan improved overall survival. Subsequently, numerous trials have shown the benefit of adjuvant chemotherapy for certain subgroups of patients (72). In the initial NSABP adjuvant trial, a 2-year course of melphalan was demonstrated to be superior to no treatment (73). Subsequent trials have shown the beneficial effect of multiple drugs and a combination of hormonal manipulation with chemotherapy in the adjuvant setting (74).

503

The most commonly used adjuvant combination chemotherapy has been Cytoxan, methotrexate, and fluorouracil (5-FU) (CMF). The original study by Bonadonna and Valagussa (77) randomized patients with positive axillary lymph nodes to receive either 12 monthly cycles of CMF or no therapy after radical mastectomy. **A statistically significant benefit was found with CMF for premenopausal patients, especially those with one to three positive nodes. A subsequent study (76) showed six cycles of CMF to be as effective as 12 cycles. However, no statistically significant effect was seen for postmenopausal women.** This was thought to be because postmenopausal women were less likely to tolerate the full course of CMF (77). The value of adjuvant chemotherapy in postmenopausal women has been controversial, and other studies have shown conflicting results (78, 79). Most recent trials confirm a beneficial effect of adjuvant therapy in premenopausal women (80).

Until recently, adjuvant systemic therapy was generally reserved for patients with involved lymph nodes. In 1988, a bulletin from the National Cancer Institute alerted clinicians to the value of adjuvant chemotherapy in patients without axillary lymph node involvement (80). In several cooperative group trials that were published simultaneously (81–86) lymph node–negative patients were randomly assigned to receive either a systemic treatment or observation. Treatment was initiated 2–6 weeks after primary therapy. **With a median follow-up of 3–4 years, these studies have shown a statistically significant improvement in disease-free survival for patients with node-negative breast cancers who received systemic chemotherapy.**

In NSABP study B-13 (81), patients with ER-negative tumors were randomly assigned to receive either no further treatment or chemotherapy with methotrexate (100 mg/m² intravenously) followed 1 hour later by 5-FU (600 mg/m² intravenously) and citrovorum factor (10 mg/m² every 6 hours for six doses commencing 24 hours after the methotrexate). The treatments were given on days 1 and 8 of each 24-day cycle for 13 3-week cycles. With a total of 741 patients entered and a median follow-up of 4 years, 80% of the chemotherapy group were alive and free of disease compared with 71% of the untreated controls ($p = 0.003$). The disease-free survival was longer for both premenopausal and postmenopausal women.

In the Intergroup Study (INT-0011) (86), a trial of adjuvant CMFP (CMF plus prednisone) versus observation alone was undertaken in patients with negative axillary nodes, ER-negative tumors of any size, and ER-positive tumors larger than 3 cm. The CMFP regimen consisted of Cytoxan (100 mg/m² orally on days 1 through 14); methotrexate (40 mg/m²; 5-FU (600 mg/m² intravenously on days 1 and 8); and prednisone (40 mg/m² orally on days 1 through 14). The chemotherapy was given every 28 days for six cycles. With a median follow-up of 3 years, the disease-free survival rate for the patients treated with CMFP was 84% compared with 67% for the control group ($p = 0.0001$). This benefit was demonstrated for patients with both ER-positive and ER-negative tumors, as well as for both premenopausal and postmenopausal patients.

In NSABP study B-14 (83), 2644 patients with ER-positive tumors and no axillary metastases were randomized, double-blind, to either tamoxifen (10 mg orally twice daily for 5 years) or a placebo control. With a 4-year median follow-up, the disease-free survival rate for the 1318 patients treated with tamoxifen was 82% compared with 77% for the 1326 patients treated with placebo

($p = 0.00001$). This advantage existed for both premenopausal and postmenopausal women.

Therefore adjuvant cytotoxic chemotherapy and/or hormonal therapy appears to affect the natural history of axillary node–negative patients with breast cancer. A 1990 consensus statement from the NIH on early-stage breast cancer (87) advised that:

1. all patients be considered for clinical trials and offered the opportunity to participate.

2. node-negative patients who are not candidates for clinical trials should be made aware of the benefits and potential risks of adjuvant systemic therapy.

In practice, oncologists are currently using systemic adjuvant therapy for most patients with early-stage breast cancer. In addition to lymph node status, other prognostic factors are being considered when they are making the decision to institute adjuvant systemic therapy. The factors that determine the patient's risk of recurrence are tumor size, estrogen and progesterone receptor status, nuclear grade, histologic type, proliferative rate, and oncogene expression (87). Table 14.5 summarizes these prognostic factors and their effect on recurrence. The assumption is made that patients with high-risk prognostic factors are more likely to benefit from adjuvant therapy, and thus these patients are generally given such therapy. Current studies are investigating whether this assumption is true, and it remains to be seen whether these patients constitute the subgroup most likely to benefit from adjuvant systemic therapy. On the basis of these new data, the current recommendations for adjuvant chemotherapy and hormonal therapy in breast cancer can be summarized as follows (Table 14.6):

1. Premenopausal women who have positive lymph nodes should be treated with adjuvant combination therapy.

2. Premenopausal women who have no evidence of axillary lymph node involvement but have other "high-risk" features also should be considered for chemotherapy.

Table 14.5   Prognostic Factors in Node-Negative Breast Cancers

Factor	*Increased Risk of Recurrence*
Size	Larger tumors
Histologic grade	High-grade tumors
DNA ploidy	Aneuploid tumors
Labeling index	High index (> 3%)
S phase fraction	High fraction (> 5%)
Lymphatic/vascular invasion	Present
Cathepsin D	High levels
HER-2/*neu* oncogene expression	High expression
Epidermal growth factor	High levels

Table 14.6 Summary of Adjuvant Chemotherapy and Hormonal Therapy for Women With Breast Cancer

Status	Nodal Involvement	Estrogen Receptors	Adjuvant Systemic Therapy
Premenopausal	Yes	Positive	Chemotherapy
	Yes	Negative	Chemotherapy
	No	Positive	Hormonal therapy, ?Chemotherapy*
	No	Negative	Chemotherapy*
Postmenopausal	Yes	Positive	Chemotherapy or hormonal therapy
	Yes	Negative	Chemotherapy*
	No	Positive	Hormonal therapy
	No	Negative	Chemotherapy*

*Consideration should be given to possible adjuvant chemotherapy in patients with "high-risk" variables, pending the definitive results of future prospective studies.

3. Postmenopausal patients who have negative lymph nodes and positive hormone receptor levels should be treated with adjuvant tamoxifen. Those with positive lymph nodes may receive tamoxifen or combination chemotherapy.

4. Postmenopausal women who have negative hormone receptor levels may be treated with adjuvant chemotherapy.

5. Adjuvant systemic therapy currently is not recommended for small non-palpable tumors, those that cannot be quantitatively tested for hormone receptors, or those with favorable DNA studies and negative axillary lymph nodes. Consideration of the hazards of chemotherapy and the effect on the quality of life must be carefully evaluated, especially in the older postmenopausal woman. Such a patient, even with axillary node involvement, may be better treated with hormonal therapy than with chemotherapy in view of the relatively few side effects of adjuvant tamoxifen.

Adjuvant Hormonal Therapy

Hormonal manipulation may improve the results of adjuvant systemic therapy, as discussed in Chapter 18. Tamoxifen has been shown to enhance the effects of melphalan and 5-FU in women whose tumors are ER positive. In an NSABP study (88), significant improvement in disease-free survival was seen only in postmenopausal women. Patients with ER-negative tumors may have a higher recurrence rate than patients with ER-positive tumors, even without axillary lymph node metastases. In NSABP study B-14 (83), both premenopausal and post-menopausal patients who had ER-positive, node-negative disease benefited from the use of adjuvant tamoxifen. Clinical studies currently are investigating the value of adjuvant hormonal therapy in women with ER-negative tumors and negative lymph nodes. The possibility of substituting tamoxifen for radiotherapy in patients with small (< 1 cm) tumors is also being studied prospectively.

The relative merits of tamoxifen plus cytotoxic chemotherapy compared with tamoxifen alone for postmenopausal patients with positive axillary lymph nodes and positive hormonal receptors remain unresolved and are the subject of current investigation. Survival benefit has yet to be established in premenopausal patients with positive axillary lymph nodes when tamoxifen is used in combination with cytotoxic chemotherapy. Trials of chemotherapy alone versus chemotherapy and tamoxifen are in progress.

Hormonal Therapy for Metastatic Disease

Metastatic disease may respond to hormonal manipulation. The latter may involve ablative surgery, drugs that block hormonal receptor sites, or drugs that block synthesis of hormones (89, 90). Hormonal manipulation should not be attempted in women with ER-negative tumors. Such patients should receive cytotoxic chemotherapy.

Premenopausal Women   In the premenopausal patient, tamoxifen has replaced bilateral oophorectomy as the primary hormonal therapy because of its ease of administration and lack of morbidity. About 60% of premenopausal patients with ER-positive tumors will respond to either tamoxifen or bilateral oophorectomy.

Patients who respond to tamoxifen should be treated with Megace if they have subsequent tumor progression. Some oncologists advocate aminoglutethimide, an inhibitor of adrenal hormonal synthesis, but its use is more complicated and it offers no therapeutic advantage. Currently, oophorectomy is rarely performed for metastatic breast cancer.

Postmenopausal Women   Primary hormonal manipulation in the postmenopausal woman should consist of tamoxifen. Tamoxifen has fewer side effects than diethylstilbestrol (DES), which was formerly the therapy of choice and appears to be just as effective. Women whose tumors respond to tamoxifen and then progress should be started on DES. Those whose tumors do not respond to tamoxifen should be treated with cytotoxic chemotherapy. Further endocrine manipulation is probably best performed with Megace. Aminoglutethimide may be tried if necessary.

Special Breast Cancers

Paget's Disease

Sir James Paget described a nipple lesion comparable to eczema and recognized that this nipple change was associated with an underlying breast malignancy (91). The erosion results from invasion of the nipple and surrounding areola by characteristic large cells with irregular nuclei, which are now called *Paget's cells.* The origin of these cells has been much debated by pathologists. However, they are probably extensions of an underlying carcinoma into the major ducts of the nipple-areolar complex. The initial invasion of the nipple may be associated with no visible changes. Often the patient will notice a nipple discharge, which is actually a combination of serum and blood from the involved ducts.

The overall prognosis for patients with Paget's disease depends on the underlying malignancy. Those cases associated with an intraductal carcinoma alone have a very favorable prognosis, whereas those with infiltrating ductal carcinoma metastatic to the regional lymph nodes do poorly. Treatment has almost always been total mastectomy and lymph node dissection, although radiotherapy is also being investigated (92).

507

Inflammatory Carcinoma

Inflammatory carcinoma of the breast initially appears to be an acute inflammation with redness and edema. The diagnosis of inflammatory cancer rather than infiltrating ductal carcinoma should be made when more than one-third of the breast is involved by erythema and edema or when biopsy of this area shows metastatic cancer in the subdermal lymphatics. There may be no distinct palpable mass, as the tumor infiltrates through the breast with ill-defined margins. There may be a dominant mass, or there may even be satellite nodules within the parenchyma. Most of the tumors are very poorly differentiated, and mammographically the breast shows skin thickening with an infiltrative process.

Surgery usually should not be used in the management of inflammatory carcinoma except for biopsy of the lesion. Mastectomy in the face of inflammatory carcinoma usually fails locally and does not improve survival. The best results are achieved with a combination of chemotherapy and radiation therapy. Mastectomy for patients who remain free of disease after initial chemotherapy and radiation may be indicated (93, 94).

In Situ Carcinomas

Both lobular carcinoma and ductal carcinoma may be confined by the basement membrane of the ducts. These carcinomas do not invade the surrounding tissue and, theoretically, lack the ability to spread. Because of their unusual natural history, they represent a special form of breast cancer and have resulted in considerable controversy.

Lobular Carcinoma In Situ (LCIS) If treated by biopsy alone, 25–30% of patients with lobular carcinoma *in situ*, also known as lobular neoplasia, will subsequently develop invasive cancer. Cancers seen in women with lobular neoplasia can occur in either breast (95).

Most women with lobular neoplasia are premenopausal. The tumor typically is not a discrete mass, but it is a multifocal lesion within one or both breasts, found incidentally at biopsy for a mass or mammographic abnormality unrelated to the LCIS. Lobular neoplasia is usually managed with excisional biopsy followed by careful observation and mammography. Patients should be informed that they have a higher risk of developing invasive breast cancer, and occasionally a patient may request bilateral prophylactic mastectomy.

Ductal Carcinoma In Situ (DCIS) DCIS is an *in situ* lesion that typically occurs in postmenopausal women. It may appear as a palpable mass that shows the typical features of an invasive ductal carcinoma, but usually it appears as a cluster of branched or Y-shaped microcalcifications. The intraductal disease does not invade beyond the basement membrane. Unlike patients with LCIS, however, when treated with excisional biopsy alone, 30–60% of patients will develop invasive cancer within the same breast (96).

Although the standard treatment for intraductal carcinoma has been modified radical mastectomy, more conservative surgery with or without radiation therapy has been performed with good results (97). The NSAPB has completed a trial comparing segmental mastectomy and axillary dissection with or without radiation therapy for intraductal carcinoma. The data from these trials have not yet been evaluated, but experience suggests that radiation and segmental mastectomy will offer excellent local control. Axillary metastases occur in fewer than 5% of

508

patients, indicating that an invasive component has been missed on biopsy. For small true DCIS, axillary dissection is not indicated. About 5% of patients whose initial biopsy shows intraductal carcinoma will be found to have infiltrating ductal carcinoma when treated with mastectomy. The incidence of contralateral breast cancer in women with intraductal carcinoma is the same as in those with invasive ductal carcinoma (i.e., 5–8%) (98).

Breast Cancer in Pregnancy

Breast cancer complicates approximately 1 in 3000 pregnancies (99–101). Initial studies suggested a significantly worse prognosis for patients with breast cancer diagnosed during pregnancy, but **more recent studies suggest that, stage for stage, the prognosis is similar to that for nonpregnant patients.**

The treatment of breast cancer in the pregnant woman must be highly individualized. Considerations include the patient's age and desire to have the child. The overall prognosis should be considered, particularly when axillary lymph nodes are involved, because adjuvant chemotherapy can be teratogenic or lethal, particularly in the first trimester. The following are recommendations:

1. Localized disease found during the first or second trimester of pregnancy is probably best treated with definitive surgery and radiation therapy, as would be used in the nonpregnant patient. Although theoretically adjuvant chemotherapy can be given after the first trimester, most oncologists prefer not to give it to pregnant women.

2. Localized tumors found in the third trimester of pregnancy must be managed on an individual basis. Initially, tumors should be excised while the patient is under local anesthesia. Early in the third trimester, one should proceed with definitive treatment. If delivery is imminent, standard therapy can be performed immediately postpartum.

3. Should the breast cancer be diagnosed during lactation, lactation should be suppressed and the cancer treated definitively.

4. Advanced, incurable cancer should be palliated and pregnancy continued or interrupted, depending on the therapy necessary and the desires of the mother.

Whether or not interruption of pregnancy improves the prognosis for patients with potentially curable breast cancer remains unknown.

Counseling regarding future childbearing for women who have had carcinoma of the breast is important. Although it has been generally assumed that subsequent pregnancies are detrimental because of the high levels of circulating estrogens, there is no clear difference in survival for women who become pregnant after the diagnosis of breast cancer (94). Theoretically, it may be that only women with ER-positive or PR-positive tumors would be affected deleteriously by subsequent pregnancy, but this has not been studied. Because most recurrences will occur within the first 2–3 years after diagnosis, patients with receptor-positive tumors probably should wait before becoming pregnant again.

Prognosis

The most reliable predictor of survival for patients with breast cancer is the stage of disease at the time of diagnosis. The overall 5-year survival for patients with breast cancer is 70–75%. Stage I patients with small tumors and no evidence of

509

Table 14.7   Five-Year Results by the Number of Pathologically Positive Axillary Nodes

Number of Positive Axillary Nodes	No. of Patients	Survival Rate (%)	Recurrence Rate (%)
0	12,299	72	19
1	2,012	63	33
2	1,338	62	40
3	842	59	43
4	615	52	44
5	478	47	54
6–10	1,261	41	63
11–15	562	29	72
16–20	301	29	75
≥ 21	225	22	82

Reproduced, with permission, from Nemato T, Vana J. Bedwam RN, et al: Management and survival of female breast cancer: results of a national survey by the American College of Surgeons. *Cancer* 45:2917, 1980.

regional spread after careful examination of the dissected lymph nodes ($T_1N_0M_0$) have the most favorable prognosis. Such patients have an 80–90% 5-year disease-free survival rate. When the axillary lymph nodes are involved with tumor (Stage II), the survival rate drops to 22–63% at 5 years. Each involved axillary lymph node imparts a diminished overall survival when large groups of women with breast cancer are studied (Table 14.7). Large lesions (T_3) or lesions with skin involvement or fixation to the underlying fascia have a 5-year survival rate of only about 20–30% (102).

Estrogen receptor status may also predict survival, although this is controversial. ER-positive tumors may be less aggressive than ER-negative tumors. Patients with T_1N_0 lesions that are ER-positive have a 5-year survival rate greater than 90%. In general, breast cancer appears to be somewhat more malignant in younger women than in older women; however, this may be because fewer younger women have ER-positive tumors. Other prognostic parameters—tumor grade, histologic type, and lymphatic or blood vessel involvement—have been proposed as important variables, but most microscopic findings other than lymph node involvement have correlated poorly with prognosis (103). Other biochemical and biologic factors such as ploidy, S-phase fraction, HER-2/neu oncogene amplification, and cathepsin D levels appear to have some prognostic significance (Table 14.5), especially in node-negative patients (104–107).

References

1. **Baines CJ:** Breast self-examination. *Cancer* 64:2661, 1989.

2. **Egan RL:** Experience with mammography in a tumor institution: evaluation of 1000 studies. *Radiology* 75:894, 1960.

3. **Wolfe JN:** Xerography of the breast. *Radiology* 91:231, 1968.

4. **Feig SA, Ehrlich SM:** Estimation of radiation risks from screening mammography: recent trends and comparison with expected benefits. *Radiology* 174:638, 1990.

5. **Dershaw DD, Masterson MA, Malik S, Cruz NM:** Mammography using an ultra high-strip-density, stationary, focused grid. *Radiology* 156:541, 1985.

6. **McLelland R:** Challenges and progress with mammography. *Cancer* 64:2664, 1989.

7. **Kopans DB, Meyer JE, Sadowsky N:** Breast imaging. *N Engl J Med* 310:960, 1984.

8. **Mann BD, Giuliano AE, Bassett LW, et al:** Delayed diagnosis of breast cancer as a result of normal mammograms. *Arch Surg* 118:23, 1983.

9. **Shapiro S, Venet W, Strax P, et al:** Ten to fourteen year effect of screening on breast cancer mortality. *J Natl Cancer Inst* 69:349, 1982.

10. **Baker LH:** The breast cancer detection demonstration projects: 5-year summary report. *CA-Cancer J Clin* 32:194, 1982.

11. **Tabar L, Gad A, Holmberg LH, et al:** Reduction in mortality from breast cancer after mass screening with mammography: randomized trial from the breast cancer screening working group of the Swedish National Board of Health and Welfare. *Lancet* 1:829, 1985.

12. **Dodd GD:** American cancer society guidelines on screening for breast cancer: an overview. *CA-A Cancer J Clin* 42:177, 1992.

13. **Fletcher SW, Black W, Harris R, et al:** Report of the international workshop on screening for breast cancer. *JNCI* 85:1644, 1993.

14. **Sickles EA, Filly RA, Callen PW:** Benign breast lesions: ultra-sound detection and diagnosis. *Radiology* 151:467, 1984.

15. **Sterns EE, Curtis AC, Miller S, Hancock JR:** Thermography in breast diagnosis. *Cancer* 50:323, 1982.

16. **Guiliano AE:** Fibrocystic disease of the breast. In Cameron J (ed): *Current Problems in Surgery*. St. Louis, CV Mosby, 1986.

17. **Maddox PR, Mansel RE:** Management of breast pain and nodularity. *World J Surg* 13:699, 1989.

18. **Azzopardi JG:** Terminology of benign diseases and the benign epithelial hyperplasias. In *Problems in Breast Pathology*. Philadelphia, WB Saunders, p 23, 1979.

19. **Page DL, Dupont WD:** Anatomic markers of human premalignancy and risk of breast cancer. *Cancer* 66:1326, 1990.

20. **Dupont DW, Page DL:** Risk factors for breast cancer in women with proliferative breast disease. *N Engl J Med* 312:146, 1985.

21. **Hart JH, Layfield LJ, Trumbull WE, et al:** Practical aspects in the diagnosis and management of cystosarcoma phyllodes. *Arch Surg* 123:1079, 1988.

22. **Naruns PL, Giuliano AE:** Sarcomas of the Breast. In Eilber FR, Morton DL, Sondak VK, Economou JS (eds): *The Soft Tissue Sarcomas*. New York, Grune & Stratton. 1987, pp 169–182.

23. **Boring CC, Squires TS, Tong T:** Cancer statistics 1994. *CA-A Cancer J Clin* 44:7, 1994.

24. **Brian DD, Melton LJ, Goellner JR, et al:** Breast cancer incidence, prevalence, mortality, and survivorship in Rochester, Minnesota, 1935–1974. *Mayo Clin Proc* 55:355, 1980.

25. **Adami HO, Malker B, Holmberg L, et al:** The relation between survival and age at diagnosis in breast cancer. *N Engl J Med* 315:559, 1986.

26. **Mesko TW, Dunlap JN, Sutherland CM:** Risk factors for breast cancer. *Compr Ther* 16:3, 1990.

27. **Van Veer P, Van Leer EM, Rietdijk A, et al:** Combination of dietary factors in relation to breast cancer occurrence. *Int J Cancer* 47:649, 1991.

28. **Hsieh CC, Trichopoulos D, Katsouyanni K, et al:** Age at menarche, age at menopause, height and obesity as risk factors for breast cancer: associations and interactions in an international case-control study. *Int J Cancer* 46:796, 1990.

29. **Brinton LA, Hoover R, Fraumeni JF:** Reproductive factors in the etiology of breast cancer. *Br J Cancer* 47:757, 1983.

30. **Pike MC, Krailo MD, Henderson BD, et al:** Hormonal risk factors, "breast tissue age" and the age incidence of breast cancer. *Nature* 303:767, 1983.

31. **Trapido EJ:** Age at first birth, parity, and breast cancer risks. *Cancer* 51:946, 1983.

32. **The Cancer and Steroid Hormone Study of the Centers for Disease Control** in the National Institute of Child Health and Human Development. Oral contraceptive use and the risk of breast cancer. *N Engl J Med* 315:405, 1986.

33. **Kaufmann DW, Miller DR, Rosenberg L, et al:** Non-contraceptive estrogen use and the risk of breast cancer. *JAMA* 252:63, 1984.

34. **Schatzkin A, Jones Y, Hoover RN, et al:** Alcohol consumption and breast cancer in the epidemiologic follow-up: study of the first national health and nutrition examination survey. *N Engl J Med* 316:1169, 1987.

35. **Nielsen M, Christensen L, Andersen J:** Contralateral cancerous breast lesions in women with clinical invasive breast carcinoma. *Cancer* 57:897, 1986.

36. **Bassett LW, Liu T, Giuliano AE, et al:** The prevalence of carcinoma in palpable vs non-palpable mammographically detected lesions. *Am J Radiol* 157:21, 1991.

37. **Miller AB, Bulbrook RD:** Screening, detection and diagnosis of breast cancer. *Lancet* 1:1109, 1982.

38. **Frable WJ:** Fine needle aspiration biopsy: a review. *Hum Pathol* 14:9, 1983.

39. **McDivitt RW, Stewart FW, Berg JW, et al:** *Atlas of Tumor Pathology Tumors of the Breast.* Second series, fascicle 2, Washington DC, Armed Forces Institute of Pathology, 1968.

40. **Tubiana M, Pejovic JM, Renaud A, et al:** Kinetic parameters and the course of the disease in breast cancer. *Cancer* 47:937, 1981.

41. **Lee Y-T:** Breast carcinoma: pattern of metastasis at autopsy. *Surg Oncol* 23:175, 1983.

42. **Hickey RC, Samaan N, Jackson GL:** Hypercalcemia in patients with breast cancer: osseous metastases, hyperplastic parathyroidism or pseudohyperparathyroidism? *Arch Surg* 116:545, 1981.

43. **Bloom HJG, Richardson MB, Harries EJ:** Natural history of untreated breast cancer (1805–1933). *Br Med J* 2:213, 1962.

44. **Haagensen CD:** *Diseases of the Breast*, ed 3. Philadelphia, WB Saunders, 1986.

45. **American Joint Committee on Cancer.** In Beahrs OH, Myers MH (eds): *Manual for Staging of Cancer*, ed 2. Philadelphia, JB Lippincott Company, 1983.

46. **Bassett LW, Giuliano AE, Gold RH:** Staging for breast carcinoma. *Am J Surg* 157:215, 1989.

47. **Halsted WS:** The results of radical operation for cure of cancer of the breast. *Ann Surg* 46:1, 1907.

48. **Meyer W:** Carcinoma of the breast; ten years experience with my method of radical operation. *JAMA* 45:297, 1905.

49. **Haagensen CD, Bodian C:** A personal experience with Halsted's radical mastectomy. *Ann Surg* 199:143, 1984.

50. **Dahl-Iversen E, Tobiassen T:** Radical mastectomy with parasternal and supraclavicular dissection for mammary carcinoma. *Ann Surg* 157:170, 1963.

51. **Lewis FJ:** Extended or super radical mastectomy for cancer of the breast. *Minn Med* 36:763, 1953.

52. **Urban JA:** Extended radical mastectomy for breast cancer. *Am J Surg* 106:399, 1963.

53. **Veronesi U, Valagussa P:** Inefficacy of internal mammary node dissection in breast cancer surgery. *Cancer* 47:170, 1981.

54. **Handley RS:** The conservative radical mastectomy of Patey: 10-year results in 425 patients. *Breast* 2:16, 1976.

55. **Maier WP, Leber D, Rosemond GP, et al:** The technique of modified radical mastectomy. *Surg Gynecol Obstet* 145:69, 1977.

56. **Robinson GN, Van Heerden JA, Payne SW, et al:** The primary surgical treatment of carcinoma of the breast: a changing trend toward modified radical mastectomy. *Mayo Clin Proc* 51:433, 1976.

57. **McWhirter R:** Should more radical treatment be attempted in breast cancer? *Am J Roentgenol* 92:3, 1964.

58. **Montague ED:** Radiation therapy in breast cancer: past, present and future. *Am J Clin Oncol* 8:455, 1985.

59. **Montague ED, Fletcher GH:** The curative value of irradiation in the treatment of nondisseminated breast cancer. *Cancer* 46:995, 1980.

60. **Wallgren A, Arner O, Bergstrom J, et al:** The value of preoperative radiotherapy in operable mammary carcinoma. *Int J Radiat Oncol Biol Phys* 6:287, 1980.

61. **Nevin JE, Baggerly JT, Laird TK:** Radiotherapy as an adjuvant in the treatment of cancer of the breast. *Cancer* 49:1194, 1982.

62. **Fisher B, Redmond C, Fisher ER, et al:** Ten-year results of a randomized clinical trial comparing radical mastectomy and total mastectomy with or without radiation. *N Engl J Med* 312:675, 1985.

63. **Keynes G:** Conservative treatment of cancer of the breast. *Br Med J* 2:643, 1937.

64. **Calle R, Pilleron JP, Schlienger P, Vilvilcoq JR:** Conservative management of operable breast cancer: ten years experience at the Foundation Curie. *Cancer* 42:2045, 1978.

65. **Prosnitz LR, Goldenberg IS, Packard RA, et al:** Radiation therapy as initial treatment for early stage cancer of the breast without mastectomy. *Cancer* 39:917, 1977.

66. **Harris JR, Hellman S, Silen W (eds):** *Conservative Management of Breast Cancer.* Philadelphia, JB Lippincott, 1983.

67. **Veronesi U, Saccozzi R, Del Veccio M, et al:** Comparing radical mastectomy with quadrantectomy, axillary dissection and radiotherapy in patients with small cancers of the breast. *N Engl J Med* 312:665, 1985.

68. **Veronesi U, Zucali R, Luini A:** Local control and survival in early breast cancer: the Milan trial. *Int J Radiat Oncol Biol Phys* 12:717, 1986.

69. **Fisher B, Bauer M, Margolese R, et al:** Five-year results of a randomized clinical trial comparing total mastectomy and segmental mastectomy with or without radiation in the treatment of cancer. *N Engl J Med* 312:665, 1985.

70. **Schabel FM Jr:** Rationale for adjuvant chemotherapy. *Cancer* 39:2875, 1977.

71. **Nissen-Meyer R:** The Scandanavian Clinical Trials. *Experientia (Suppl)* 41:571, 1982.

72. **Bonadonna G, Valagussa P:** Adjuvant systemic therapy for resectable breast cancer. *J Clin Oncol* 3:259, 1985.

73. **Fisher B, Carbone P, Economou S, et al:** L-phenylalanine mustard in the management of primary breast cancer. *N Engl J Med* 292:117, 1975.

74. **Barber Mueller C, Lesperance ML:** NSABP trials of adjuvant chemotherapy for breast cancer: a further look at the evidence. *Ann Surg* 214:206, 1991.

75. **Bonadonna G, Rossi A, Valagussa P:** Adjuvant CMF chemotherapy in operable breast cancer: ten years later. *World J Surg* 9:707, 1985.

76. **Tancine G, Bonadonna G, Valagussa P, et al:** Adjuvant CMF in breast cancer: comparative 5-year results of 12 versus 6 cycles. *J Clin Oncol* 1:2, 1983.

77. **Bonadonna G, Valagussa P:** Dose-response effective adjuvant chemotherapy in breast cancer. *N Engl J Med* 304:10, 1981.

78. **Castiglione M, Gelber RD, Goldhirsch A:** Adjuvant systemic therapy for breast cancer in the elderly: competing causes of mortality. *J Clin Oncol* 8:519, 1990.

79. **Henderson IC:** Adjuvant systemic therapy for early breast cancer: current problems. *Cancer* 11:127, 1987.

80. **Abeloff MD, Beveridge RA:** Adjuvant chemotherapy of breast cancer: the consensus development conference revisited. *Oncology* 2:21, 1988.

81. **Fisher B, Redmond C, Nikolay V, et al:** A randomized clinical trial evaluating sequential methotrexate and fluorouracil in the treatment of patients with node-negative

breast cancer who have estrogen-receptor-negative tumors. *N Engl J Med* 320:473, 1989.

82. **Mansour EG, Gray R, Shatila AH, et al:** Efficacy of adjuvant chemotherapy in high-risk node-negative breast cancer. *N Engl J Med* 320:485, 1989.

83. **Fisher B, Costantino J, Redmond C, et al:** A randomized clinical trial evaluating tamoxifen in the treatment of patients with node-negative breast cancer who have estrogen-receptor-positive tumors. *N Engl J Med* 320:479, 1989.

84. **Baum MB, Brinkley DM, Dosset JA, et al:** Control trial of tamoxifen as a single agent in the management of early breast cancer: analysis at eight years by Nolvadex adjuvant trial organization. *Br J Cancer* 57:608, 1988.

85. **Breast Cancer Trials Committee.** Scottish Cancer Trials Office (MRC) Edinburgh: Adjuvant tamoxifen in the management of operable breast cancer: the Scottish Trial. *Lancet* 2:171, 1987.

86. **Breast Cancer Study Group:** Prolonged disease-free survival after one course of perioperative adjuvant chemotherapy for node-negative breast cancer. *N Engl J Med* 320:491, 1989.

87. **National Institutes of Health Consensus Statement.** NIH consensus development conference: adjuvant chemotherapy for breast cancer. 8:16, 1990.

88. **Fisher B, Redmond C, Brown A, et al:** Treatment of primary breast cancer with chemotherapy and tamoxifen. *N Engl J Med* 305:1, 1981.

89. **Buzdar AU:** Current status of endocrine treatment of carcinoma of the breast. *Semin Surg Oncol* 6:77, 1990.

90. **Henderson IC, Garber JE, Breitmeyer JB, et al:** Comprehensive management of disseminated breast cancer. *Cancer* 66:1439, 1990.

91. **Paget J:** Disease of the mammary areola preceding cancer of the mammary gland. *St Bart Hosp Rep* 10:89, 1874.

92. **Bulens P, Vanuytsel L, Rijnders A, et al:** Breast conserving treatment of Paget's disease. *Radiother Oncol* 17:305, 1990.

93. **Droulias CA, Sewel L, McSweeney MB, et al:** Inflammatory carcinoma of the breast: a correlation of clinical radiologic and pathologic findings. *Ann Surg* 184:217, 1976.

94. **Donegan WL, Padrta B:** Combined therapy for inflammatory breast cancer. *Arch Surg* 125:578, 1990.

95. **Sunshine JA, Mosley HS, Fletcher WS, Krippachne WW:** Breast carcinoma *in situ*: a retrospective review of 112 cases with a minimum 10-year follow-up. *Am J Surg* 150:44, 1985.

96. **Page DL, Dupont WD, Rogers LW, Landenberger M:** Intraductal carcinoma of the breast: follow-up after biopsy only. *Cancer* 49:751, 1982.

97. **Stotter AT, McNeese M, Oswald MJ, et al:** The role of limited surgery with radiation and primary treatment of ductal in situ breast cancer. *Int J Radiat Ther Oncol Biol Phys* 18:283, 1990.

98. **Kinne DW, Petrek VA, Osborne MP, et al:** Breast carcinoma in situ. *Arch Surg* 124:33, 1989.

99. **Donegan WL:** Cancer and pregnancy. *CA-Cancer J Clin* 33:194, 1983.

100. **Hornstein E, Skornick Y, Rozin R:** The management of breast carcinoma in pregnancy and lactation. *J Surg Oncol* 21:179, 1982.

101. **Hoover HC:** Breast cancer during pregnancy and lactation. *Surg Clin North Am* 70:1151, 1990.

102. **Steele GD, Winchester DP, Menck HR, et al:** National cancer data base. *Annu Rev Patient Care* 1992.

103. **Fisher ER, Redmond C, Fisher B, et al:** Pathologic findings from the National Surgical Adjuvant Breast and Bowel Projects (NSABP): prognostic discriminants for eight year survival for node-negative invasive breast cancer patients. *Cancer* 65:2121, 1990.

104. **Markel DE, Osborne CK:** Prognostic factors in breast cancer. *Hematol Oncol Clin North Am* 3:641, 1989.

105. **McGuire WL, Clark GN:** Prognostic factors and treatment decisions in axillary node-negative breast cancer. *N Engl J Med* 326:1756, 1992.

106. **Tandon AK, Clark GN, Chamness GC, et al:** Cathepsin D and prognosis in breast cancer. *N Engl J Med* 322:297, 1990.

107. **Lewis WE:** Prognostic significance of flow cytometric DNA analysis in node-negative breast cancer patients. *Cancer* 65:2315, 1990.

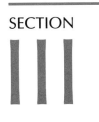

RELATED TOPICS

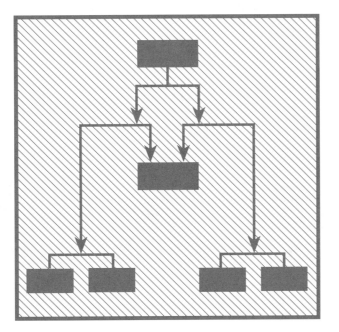

15 Surgical Techniques

Jonathan S. Berek

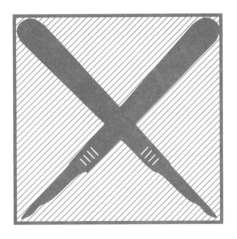

In the practice of gynecologic oncology, it is occasionally necessary to perform a number of surgical procedures that are not part of the standard training in general gynecology. These include selected operations on the intestinal and urologic tracts and plastic reconstructive operations, including the creation of a neovagina. In addition, central venous access is frequently required for hyperalimentation or chemotherapy. The surgical techniques for these nongynecologic procedures are presented.

Central Lines

Central venous-access catheters are often necessary in the critically ill gynecologic oncology patient for either central venous pressure monitoring or centrally administered hyperalimentation or chemotherapy (1). The most frequently used veins are the subclavian and the jugular. Less frequently used are the brachial and the femoral veins.

Subclavian Venous Catheter

Infraclavicular Technique Although there are many different techniques for the insertion of a central venous catheter into the subclavian vein, the *infraclavicular technique* remains the one most commonly employed and the simplest. The subclavian vein lies immediately deep to the clavicle within the costoclavicular triangle, where the vein is more commonly approached from the right side (Fig. 15.1A). The *costoclavicular-scalene triangle* is bounded by the medial end of the clavicle anteriorly, the upper surface of the first rib posteriorly, and the anterior scalene muscle laterally (1). The anterior scalene muscle separates the subclavian vein anteriorly from the subclavian artery posteriorly. Just deep to the subclavian artery are the nerves of the brachial plexus. The subclavian vein is covered by the medial 5 cm of the clavicle. Just deep to the medial head of the clavicle, the right internal jugular vein joins the right subclavian vein to form the innominate vein, which then descends into the chest, where it joins the left innominate vein to form the superior vena cava in the retrosternal space.

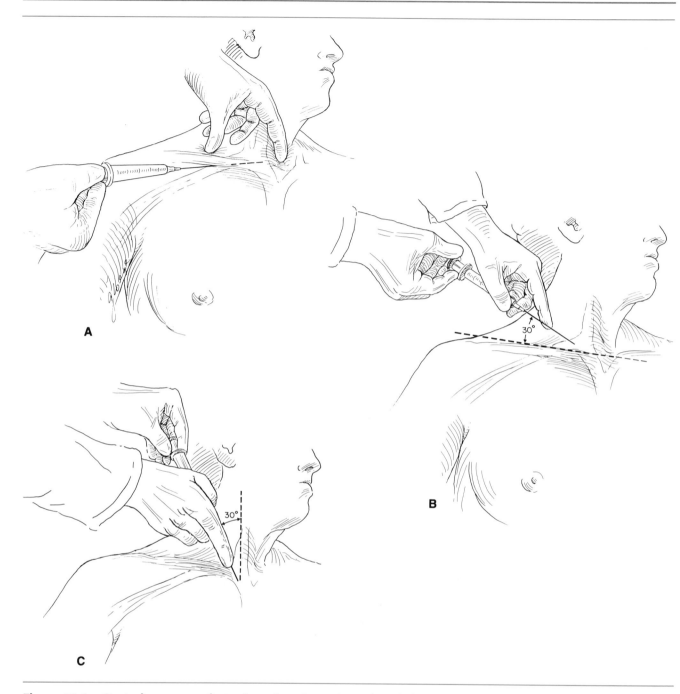

Figure 15.1   Central venous catheter insertion sites. The right subclavian and right internal jugular vein insertion sites are illustrated. The insertion sites for the subclavian venous catheter: *A*, via the infraclavicular technique; *B*, via the supraclavicular technique; *C*, the site of insertion for the internal jugular vein. The needle is directed toward the suprasternal notch.

There are several other vital structures in the scalene triangle. The phrenic nerve courses anterior to the anterior scalene muscle and therefore lies immediately deep to the subclavian vein. If the deep wall of the vein is penetrated, the phrenic nerve can be injured. If the subclavian artery is penetrated, the brachial plexus, lying just deep to the vessel, can be injured. The right lymphatic duct and the thoracic duct on the left enter their respective subclavian veins near the junction with the internal jugular veins and therefore may be injured by a misplaced needle. The most common injury is to the pleura, the apex of which is just beneath the subclavian vein at the junction of the internal jugular vein.

The technique for infraclavicular insertion of a catheter into the right subclavian vein is as follows:

1. The patient is placed in the supine position, with the foot of the bed elevated about 1 foot so that the patient is in the reverse Trendelenburg position. If possible, a bed that can be tilted into this position should be used. This position creates venous distention and increases the intraluminal pressure within the subclavian vein. The patient's head should be tilted away from the site of insertion so that the landmarks can be identified easily.

2. After careful skin preparation with povidone-iodine solution, the skin and subjacent tissues are anesthetized by means of lidocaine without epinephrine.

3. The site of insertion is located at the junction of the middle and medial thirds of the clavicle, approximately 1 cm below the bone's inferior margin.

4. Before insertion of the catheter needle, a probe needle is used to localize the subclavian vein and to identify the presence of dark venous blood. An 18-gauge needle attached to a 10 ml syringe filled with normal saline solution is used.

5. A 14-gauge Intracath needle is used to insert the catheter (Fig. 15.1A). The needle attached to the syringe is inserted into the skin with the bevel directed toward the heart. The needle should be held and directed parallel to the anterior chest wall.

6. After insertion through the skin, the needle is directed medially and advanced along the undersurface of the clavicle in the direction of the suprasternal notch.

7. The syringe is pulled gently to apply suction as the needle is inserted. The patient should exhale during insertion to avoid an air embolus.

8. After a free flow of blood has been obtained, the needle is held carefully in place, the syringe is detached, and the central venous catheter is advanced inside the lumen of the needle. The catheter should advance freely, and there should be blood returning through the catheter. The catheter is advanced into the innominate vein and then into the superior vena cava. The catheter should be aspirated, and if blood is easily withdrawn, the needle is removed.

9. While the needle is in place, the catheter should not be withdrawn because the tip can be sheared off and embolize.

10. The end of the catheter is connected to an intravenous set and the catheter is sutured to the skin.

11. The position of the catheter is verified by a chest radiograph. It should be located in the superior vena cava, not in the right atrium or ventricle, as this can result in trauma to the heart.

If central venous pressure readings are to be determined, the intravenous line is attached to a manometer, and the base of the water column is positioned at the level of the right atrium, which is about 5 cm posterior to the fourth costochondral junction when the patient is in the supine position. The normal central venous pressure should be between 5 and 12 cm of water. Because the central venous pressure may not accurately reflect left ventricular function in patients with cardiac dysfunction, a flow-directed, balloon-tipped intracardiac catheter (*Swan-Ganz*) may have to be inserted in such patients. The use of this catheter is discussed in Chapter 16.

The complication rate for central venous catheter insertion through the subclavian route is about 1–2% (1). Most serious complications are related to puncture of the pleura and lung or perforation and laceration of vessels, resulting in a pneumothorax or hemothorax. Catheter-related infection is seen in about 0.5% of patients, and the catheter should be removed if this source of infection is suspected.

Supraclavicular Insertion An alternative route of insertion into the subclavian vein is the supraclavicular route (Fig. 15.1B). Some prefer this to the infraclavicular route, but the morbidity of insertion is comparable with the two methods, and the preference is related to the technique that is most comfortable for the operator.

The technique for insertion is identical to that of the infraclavicular route, except that the needle is inserted above the clavicle, approximately 5 cm lateral to the midsternal notch. The angle of insertion is about 30 degrees from a line drawn between the two shoulders and directed caudally. The needle is aimed at the suprasternal notch.

Jugular Venous Catheterization

Another alternative for central venous access is the use of the jugular veins, either the internal or external vein. Jugular venous catheterization is frequently the method of choice when the catheter is inserted intraoperatively and the catheter is to be used primarily for acute monitoring. The advantage is that there is relatively easy access while the patient is anesthetized and draped for surgery, whereas the disadvantage is that it is more difficult to anchor the catheter because the neck is more mobile than the anterior chest wall. The location for the insertion site is illustrated in Figure 15.1C.

The technique for insertion is as follows:

1. The patient is placed in the Trendelenburg position. With the patient's head turned away from the side of insertion, the needle is inserted just above the medial head of the clavicle between the medial and middle heads of the sternocleidomastoid muscle, where a small pocket is readily apparent and helps to localize the site for insertion.

2. The angle of insertion is about 20–30 degrees from the sagittal median of the patient, and the direction is toward the heart.

3. As with subclavian catheterization, the use of a probe needle will help to localize the appropriate vessel.

4. The technique of catheter placement is the same as described above for the subclavian catheter. However, the length of catheter that must be inserted is less, as the distance to the proper location in the superior vena cava is less.

5. The position of the line inserted intraoperatively is checked with a chest radiograph obtained in the recovery room if the catheter is to be left in place.

External jugular catheters may also be used in patients who are under general anesthesia. Some patients have relatively prominent external jugular veins, and they are very easily catheterized. The external jugular is not durable, however, and this route is not useful for central hyperalimentation. The complication rate for jugular venous catheterization is essentially the same as that for the subclavian route.

Semipermanent Lines

The placement of semipermanent lines is useful in patients who require prolonged access to the central venous system, such as those with a chronic intestinal obstruction or fistula who are to receive hyperalimentation after discharge from the hospital (2).

The most common types of lines are catheters made of flexible, synthetic rubber (e.g., Broviac, Hickman, or Quinton catheters). The catheters are available in several sizes, although the adult type is used for most patients; the length is adapted by cutting the catheters as necessary. The catheters are available with either a single or double lumen. The single-lumen catheters usually are sufficient for parenteral nutrition, whereas the double-lumen ones may be necessary for patients requiring frequent bolus medication, such as intravenous pain or antibiotic medications (2).

The most common site for insertion of a semipermanent catheter is the right subclavian vein. The method of insertion is initially identical to the technique employed for the insertion of a temporary catheter, but an insertion cannula, called a Cook Introducer, can simplify and facilitate insertion of the catheter (Fig. 15.2). It is preferable to insert the catheter under fluoroscopic guidance.

The technique is as follows:

1. After the patient has been properly positioned and the anterior chest and clavicular areas prepared, the subclavian vein is identified in the manner described above.

2. A premade kit is available for the Cook Introducer. An 18-gauge needle is used to introduce a guide wire into the subclavian vein, and the guide wire is passed into the superior vena cava under fluoroscopy (Fig. 15.2A).

3. The proper position of the guide wire is documented, and the Cook Introducer is fed over the guide wire and advanced into the subclavian vein (Fig. 15.2B).

4. The introducer has an inner catheter and an outer sheath. After insertion of the entire apparatus, the central cannula is removed (Fig. 15.2C) and

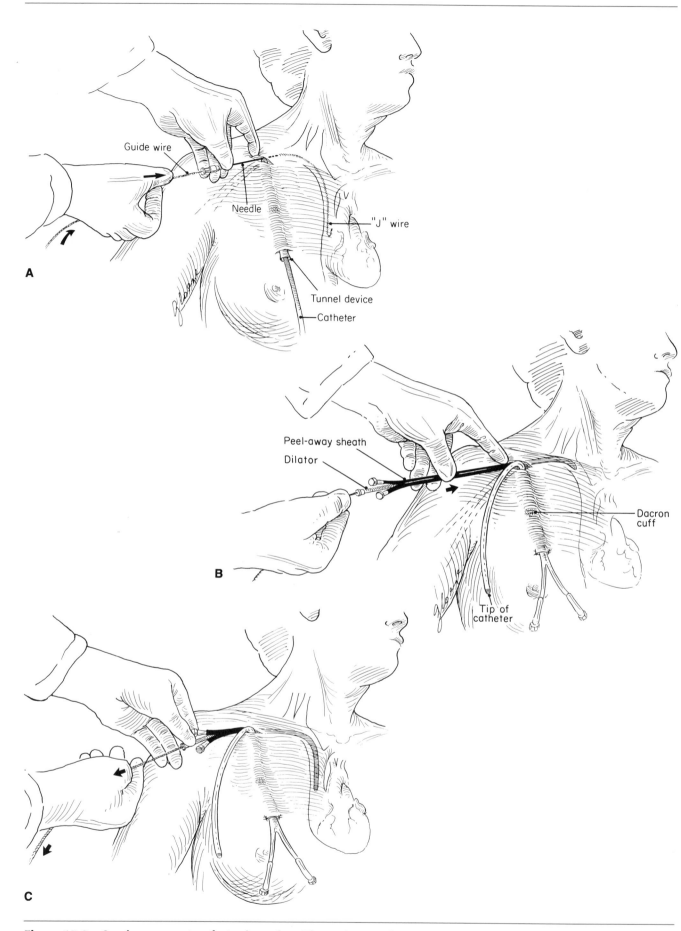

Figure 15.2   Semipermanent catheter insertion. The technique for insertion of the semipermanent (e.g., Hickman) catheter. *A,* A needle is inserted into the right subclavian vein, a guide wire is inserted through the needle, and the needle is withdrawn. *B,* The Cook introducer then is inserted over the guide wire. *C,* After the introducer with its outer sheath is in place in the right subclavian vein, the wire is withdrawn.

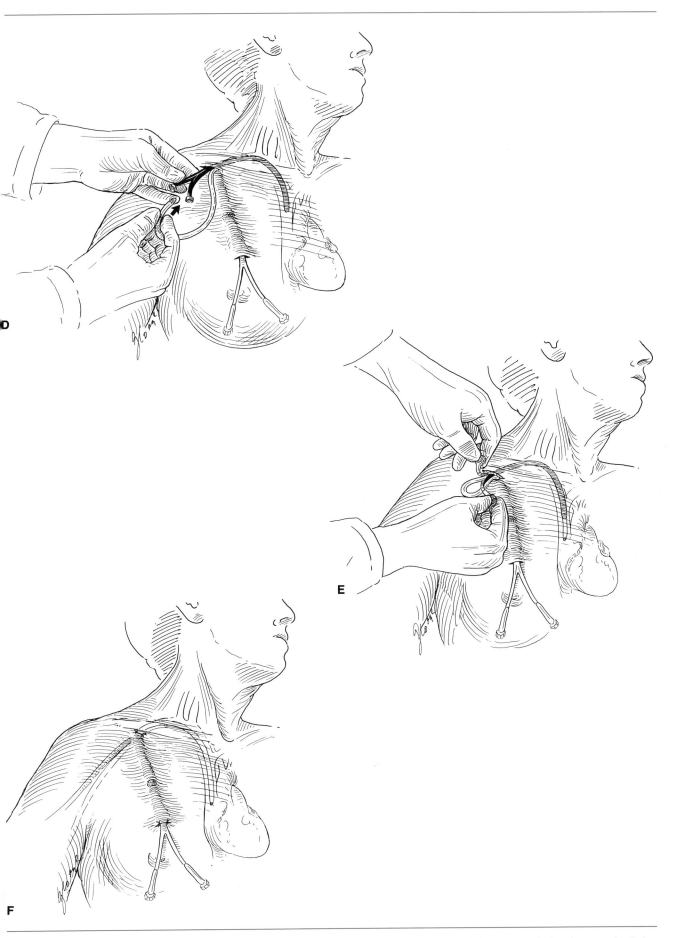

Figure 15.2 continued   *D*, The central catheter of the Cook introducer is withdrawn, and the free end of the semipermanent catheter is inserted through the outer sheath. *E*, The outer sheath of the Cook introducer is peeled away. *F*, The semipermanent catheter is tunneled in the subcutaneous tissue under the skin of the right side of the chest, and the free end is exteriorized.

the semipermanent catheter is threaded through the outer sheath, which remains in the subclavian vein (Fig. 15.2D).

5. After the semipermanent catheter has been inserted, the outer sheath is peeled away, leaving the catheter in place (Fig. 15.2E).

6. The proximal end of the semipermanent catheter is tunneled under the skin of the anterior chest wall and exteriorized through a stab incision in the skin as illustrated (Figure 15.2F).

7. An intravenous line is connected to the catheter's adapter, and fluid is run into the line to establish its patency. The catheter is sutured into place.

Peritoneal Catheters

Peritoneal catheters are used in gynecologic oncology for the instillation of intraperitoneal chemotherapy. A commonly used catheter is the Tenckhoff peritoneal dialysis catheter. This dialysis catheter is designed to minimize the risk of infection, even though it is left in place many months (3). Alternatively, a Hickman venous access catheter can be used.

The catheter is implanted into the peritoneal cavity lateral to the midline laparotomy incision (Fig. 15.3). The catheter is tunneled in the subcutaneous tissue and brought out through a stab incision lateral to the fascial incision. The tip of the catheter in the peritoneal cavity is directed toward the pelvic cul-de-sac.

An alternative peritoneal access catheter is the Port-A-Cath, which is a completely implantable device. The implantable port is attached directly to a peritoneal access

Figure 15.3   Tenckhoff peritoneal catheter. The placement of the Tenckhoff catheter into the peritoneal cavity is illustrated.

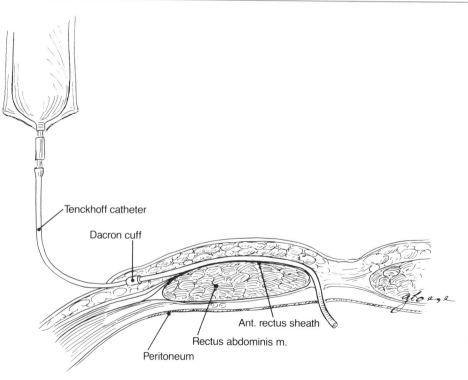

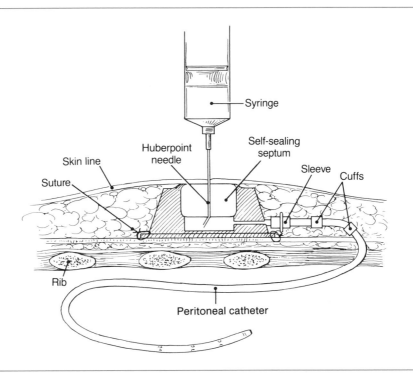

Figure 15.4   Port-a-Cath peritoneal catheter. The totally implantable peritoneal access catheter is tunneled through the subcutaneous tissues into the peritoneal cavity.

Tenckhoff or Hickman catheter. The port is inserted into the subcutaneous tissue and positioned in the left or right lower quadrant of the anterior abdomen for ready access (Fig. 15.4). The port is entered percutaneously with a 21-gauge needle.

The most common problem associated with the catheters is blockage, and there is no effective way to prevent some deposition of fibrin around the catheter. Occasionally, this produces a "ball valve" effect; i.e., fluid will flow in but will not flow out. Minor infections can be treated with antibiotics, and low-grade peritonitis can be treated by the instillation of antibiotics directly via the catheter. For persistent and severe infections, the peritoneal catheter may require removal.

Incisions

Particularly important in the operative plan for any patient is the determination of the type of incision to be made. The surgeon should have a general philosophy and *modus operandi* when planning the surgical procedure. There are certain incisions that are more appropriate in patients who are undergoing surgery for cancer rather than for benign conditions. In addition, special guidelines for the closure of incisions should be followed.

Vertical Incisions

Abdominal incisions used in the gynecologic oncology patient are most commonly vertical. Transverse incisions are also appropriate in certain circumstances. The indications and techniques for these incisions and their modifications are discussed.

Patients with suspected malignancies of the ovary or fallopian tube are best explored through a vertical abdominal incision. With a vertical incision, the patient's disease can be staged properly. Also, this approach permits the removal of any upper abdominal metastases, which cannot always be appreciated preoperatively. The most likely site of resectable upper abdominal disease is the omentum. For an omentectomy, access to the region of the splenic and hepatic flexures is required.

A vertical incision is also necessary in patients being explored for intestinal obstruction or fistulas. The performance of a para-aortic lymphadenectomy is facilitated by a vertical incision. Patients being explored for recurrent malignancies or for possible pelvic exenteration also require a vertical abdominal incision.

The most commonly used vertical incision is in the midline. This incision has the advantage of being easy to perform; it can be accomplished quickly, because the midline is the least vascular area of the abdominal wall, and the smallest depth of tissue must be divided. The principal blood supply to the anterior abdominal wall is from the inferior epigastric vessels, which are located laterally in the rectus sheath posterior to the rectus abdominis muscles, and these vessels are avoided by the midline incision.

The principal problem associated with the midline incision is that it has the highest rate of wound dehiscence when compared with all other incisions. The wound disruption rate is about 0.1–0.65% (4–6), although this rate may be higher in patients with cancer, particularly those with ascites and malnutrition. Dehiscence rates as high as 2–3% have been reported in obese, diabetic patients with cancer (4). The majority of wound dehiscences are associated with wound infection or poor closure technique.

Transverse Incisions

In patients with a probable benign condition who are undergoing abdominal exploration for the first time, a lower transverse abdominal incision is frequently employed. The advantage of this incision is that it is more cosmetic, is generally less painful, and is associated with fewer incisional hernias. The disadvantage is the relative problem of upper abdominal exposure and the more frequent occurrence of wound hematomas.

If exposure to the upper abdomen is required, the surgeon has several choices. The incision can be modified by division of the rectus abdominis muscles in a transverse direction at the level of the incision (i.e., *a Maylard incision*) or the rectus abdominis muscles may be detached from the symphysis pubis (i.e., *the Cherney incision*). After division or mobilization of the rectus muscles, the inferior epigastric vessels are ligated bilaterally and, if necessary, the incision is further extended laterally by incising (with the diathermy) the "strap" muscles of the anterior abdominal wall. The conversion of the incision to a Maylard or a Cherney incision always provides considerably more exposure in the pelvis and low para-aortic area.

If better access to the upper abdomen is required, the incision can be modified further by extending the incision cephalad to form a "**J**", a reverse "**J**", or a "hockey stick" incision. In general, any of these techniques is preferable to the making of a second incision, i.e., a midline incision coincident with the transverse incision, a so-called "**T**" incision. The principal difficulty with the latter approach is the weakness of the incision at the point of intersection of the two incisions.

528

In patients undergoing radical hysterectomy and pelvic lymphadenectomy for early-stage cervical cancer, a lower abdominal transverse incision is acceptable.

Incisional Closure

Of primary importance is the technique of incisional closure (4–6). The closure can be accomplished by closing the peritoneum, fascia, subcutaneous tissue, and skin individually, or a bulk closure can be performed that incorporates the peritoneum and the fascia together. This bulk closure or internal retention suture, the "Smead-Jones" closure, is the strongest closure technique (6). Mass closure with a continuous, single strand of polyglyconate monofilament absorbable suture (Maxon) has been shown to be an effective, safe alternative to the use of interrupted sutures, even in vertical midline incisions (7).

Internal Retention Suture

The Smead-Jones, or internal retention, technique uses interrupted sutures that are placed as illustrated in Figure 15.5. The sutures are placed in a far-far, near-near distribution, which is a modified figure-of-eight. The first suture is placed through the anterior fascia, rectus muscle, posterior fascia, and peritoneum and the second through the anterior fascial layer only. The key is to place the sutures at least 1.5–2.0 cm from the fascial edge and not more than 1 cm apart (6). The disruption rate of midline incisions with this technique was only 0.1% in one

Figure 15.5   Internal retention abdominal closure. The "Smead Jones" far-far, near-near closure.

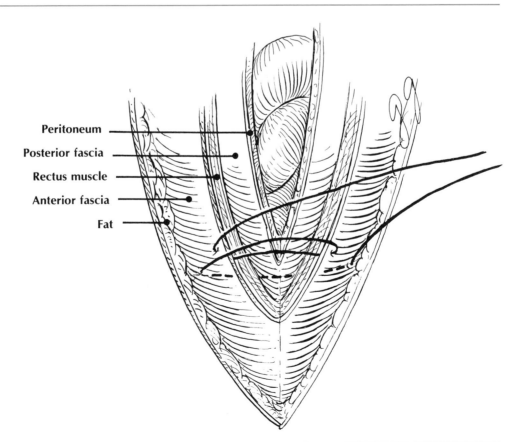

Peritoneum

Posterior fascia

Rectus muscle

Anterior fascia

Fat

series of patients undergoing operations for cancer (4), compared with 0.4% for a closure by the traditional layer-by-layer technique.

Suture Material

The choice of suture should be dictated by the circumstances (8, 9). If there is evidence of significant infection, as with an abscess or an intestinal injury, a monofilament, nonabsorbable suture is most appropriate. The most frequently used substances are nylon sutures, such as Prolene.

For most circumstances, an absorbable synthetic suture offers the best combination of strength, durability, and ease of use. Most frequently either a monofilament polyglyconate suture (Maxon) or a braided, polyglycolic acid suture, such as Vicryl or Dexon, is used. A grade 0 or 1 suture is necessary to provide a suitably strong closure. The tissue reactivity of these synthetic materials is less than that of chromic catgut (9). Nonabsorbable polyfilament materials such as cotton and silk are not used for incisional closure because of the higher potential for "stitch abscess" formation.

External Retention Suture

Retention sutures that are external can be used to prevent evisceration in patients who are at high risk of this potentially catastrophic occurrence. The routine use of internal retention sutures has reduced the need for the external retention sutures. However, in patients who are morbidly obese, patients who have a major wound infection, and patients whose incisions have eviscerated in the past, the addition of external retention sutures may be indicated. These sutures are placed in a manner similar to internal retention sutures, i.e., far-far, near-near, with the far sutures also placed through the skin so that the retention sutures are knotted externally. The preferable suture material for this closure is nylon. The external retention sutures are inserted through a rubber "bolster" that helps to protect the skin from injury from the suture. Sutures are placed at approximately 2–3 cm intervals, and interrupted fascial sutures are placed between them.

Skin Closure

Primary Closure   Skin closure of vertical incisions in cancer patients generally should be interrupted, either with nylon or metal skin clips. Subcuticular closures are not appropriate in most circumstances for vertical incisions, but they are quite cosmetic and acceptable for small transverse incisions where the risk of wound infection is low.

Secondary Closure   A delayed or secondary skin closure is useful in patients whose incisions are infected, e.g., after the drainage of an intra-abdominal abscess or repair of an intestinal fistula. This is achieved by placement of interrupted mattress sutures in the skin, which are not tied, so that the skin remains unapproximated. Thus the skin can be closed later, usually after 3–4 days, when the infection is under control.

Intestinal Operations

Preoperative Intestinal Preparation

If bowel resection is planned or contemplated, a thorough mechanical and antibiotic "bowel preparation" should be undertaken preoperatively. If the intestine is prepared properly, the segment is well vascularized, and there is no sepsis, prior irradiation, or evidence of tumor at the site of anastomosis, colonic reanastomosis can be accomplished without leakage in 98% of the cases (10). More proximal resection of the small intestine can be performed without a bowel preparation, because this portion of the intestine does not contain bacteria.

An effective protocol for bowel preparation is presented in Table 15.1. In a prospective, randomized, double-blind study, serious complications, mostly infection, associated with colonic resection were reduced from 43% in the unprepared group to 9% in the prepared patients (11). The use of magnesium citrate has been replaced by Go-Lytely, which is better tolerated by most patients.

Before laparotomy for small intestinal obstruction caused by ovarian cancer, it is useful to insert a long gastrointestinal tube (e.g., a Cantor tube) at least 48 hours preoperatively (7). The advantage, in an abdomen where multiple adhesions are present, is that the tube can decompress the bowel, help localize the site of obstruction, and differentiate between proximal and distal loops of small bowel. The long tube is particularly useful in patients who have been previously irradiated or who are undergoing exploration for an intestinal fistula. The injection of a radiocontrast through the tube may help to identify the site of obstruction, although multiple obstructions are common in patients with disseminated ovarian cancer.

Minor Intestinal Operations	The most common intestinal operations are lysis of adhesions, repair of an enterotomy, and creation of an intestinal stoma.

Repair of Enterotomy	Intestinal enterotomy is a common inadvertent occurrence in abdominal surgery, and it can occur in the most experienced hands. Factors that predispose to serosal and mucosal injury include extensive adhesions, intra-abdominal carcinomatosis, radiation therapy, chemotherapy, prior abdominal surgery, and peritonitis.

An enterotomy usually does not cause any problems, provided it is identified and repaired. Any defect should be repaired when it occurs or marked with a long stitch so that it will not be overlooked later. At the completion of any intra-abdominal exploration necessitating significant lysis of adhesions, the surgeon must "run the bowel," carefully inspecting it to exclude either a serosal injury or an enterotomy.

Table 15.1   Bowel Preparation

Preoperative day 2 (at home)
   Clear-liquid diet
   Tap water enema at night (optional)

Preoperative day 1 (admit to hospital)
   Clear-liquid diet
   2 liters Go-Lytely (polyethylene glycon) at 8 AM
   Oral neomycin, 1 g every 4 hours for 3 doses (4, 8, 12 PM.)
   Oral erythromycin base, 1 g every 4 hours for 3 doses
   Tap water enemas until no solid stool at night
   Commence IV fluids at 8 PM to correct fluid and electrolyte imbalance caused by bowel
      cleansing

Operation day
   Neomycin retention enema

531

Serosal defects through which the intestinal mucosa can be seen must be repaired. Less complete defects must be repaired in all patients who have had radiation treatment to the abdomen. When in doubt, the defect should be repaired to minimize the risk of intestinal breakdown, peritonitis, abscess, and fistula.

When there is an enterotomy, the repair should be made with interrupted 3-0 or 4-0 sutures on a gastrointestinal needle, placed at 2 to 3 mm intervals along the defect. The suture material most commonly employed for this purpose is silk, although a suitable alternative is Vicryl or Dexon. **The direction of closure should be perpendicular to the lumen of the bowel to minimize the potential for lumenal stricture** (Fig. 15.6).

Figure 15.6 Closure of an intestinal enterotomy. *A,* The edges of the enterotomy are trimmed. *B,* The enterotomy is closed perpendicular to the lumen in two layers.

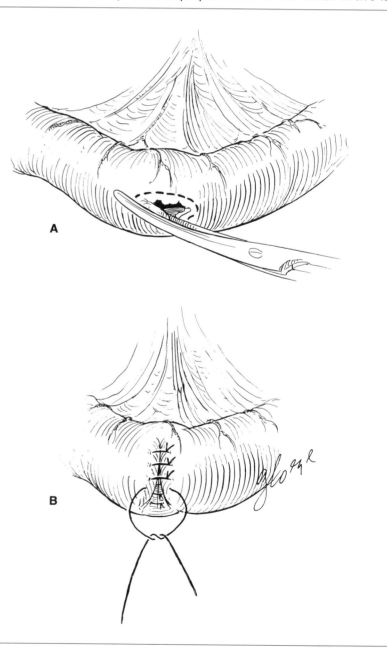

With small defects (i.e., < 5–6 mm), the closure can be accomplished with a single layer of sutures passed through both the serosa and the mucosa. However, it is preferable to close more extensive defects in two layers: an inner full-thickness layer covered with an outer seromuscular layer. Care should be taken to approximate the tissues carefully without cutting through the fragile serosa.

Gastrostomy

A gastrostomy may be necessary in patients with chronic intestinal obstruction, usually from terminal ovarian cancer. It is particularly useful in those who require prolonged intestinal intubation and in whom the underlying intestinal blockage cannot be relieved adequately. This procedure may permit the removal of an uncomfortable nasogastric tube that is irritating to the nasopharynx. The two most common procedures are the Witzel and the Stamm gastrostomies (12).

Stamm Gastrostomy   The simplest technique is the Stamm gastrostomy, in which a small incision is made in the inferior anterior gastric wall. A Foley catheter with a 30 ml balloon is brought into the peritoneal cavity through a separate stab incision in the left upper outer quadrant of the abdomen. Two or three successive pursestring sutures, with 2-0 absorbable suture material, are used to invert the stomach around the tube. Interrupted 2-0 silk sutures are placed in the serosa, and the same material is used to suture the serosa to the peritoneum, approximating the gastric wall to the anterior abdominal wall in an effort to prevent leakage.

Witzel Gastrostomy   The Witzel technique is similar, but the catheter is tunneled within the gastric wall for several centimeters with Lembert sutures of 2-0 silk. This technique results in a serosal tunnel that may further reduce the risk of leakage. The most important step in preventing gastrostomy leakage is approximation of the gastric serosa to the anterior abdominal wall.

Percutaneous Gastrostomy   Another technique for gastrostomy in patients not otherwise undergoing laparotomy is the percutaneous placement of a catheter into the stomach. This method involves the initial passage of a gastroscope. The site for catheter insertion is illuminated by a fiberoptic light source through the gastroscope, and the catheter is introduced into the stomach percutaneously.

Baker Tube Placement

The Baker tube is an 18F tube, which is 270 cm long and has attached to the tip a 5 ml bag that can be filled with saline solution (13). The tube is placed at the time of a laparotomy; it is placed by means of a jejunotomy and advanced through the bowel by milking of the balloon through the lumen until it has passed through the site(s) of chronic obstruction or intestinal damage. The proximal end of the tube is exteriorized through a stab incision in the anterior abdominal wall and connected to a drainage container. It splints the bowel into a position of function, thereby minimizing the likelihood of recurrent obstruction.

The placement of a Baker tube is particularly useful in patients who have had abdominal radiation therapy and have developed a chronic obstruction of the small bowel.

Cecostomy

The performance of a cecostomy may be useful in the occasional patient who has an obstruction of the colon and a grossly dilated cecum and in whom a simple

533

palliative measure to relieve the obstruction is indicated. A more definitive procedure for relief of the obstruction may be appropriate when the patient's condition is more stable.

The cecostomy is performed by placement of a Foley catheter into the dilated portion of the cecum. The tube is sutured into place by the technique employed for a Stamm gastrostomy. The tube is exteriorized through a stab incision in the right lower quadrant of the abdomen and attached to gravity drainage.

Colostomy

Colostomies may be temporary or permanent. A temporary colostomy may be indicated for "protection" of a colonic reanastomosis in patients who have had prior radiation therapy or to palliate severe radiation proctitis and bleeding. It is indicated also in patients who have a large bowel fistula (e.g., rectovaginal fistula) to allow the inflammation to subside prior to definitive repair. A permanent colostomy is indicated in patients who have an irreparable fistula or a colonic obstruction from a pelvic tumor that cannot be resected. Permanent colostomy is also indicated in patients undergoing total pelvic exenteration, unless the distal rectum can be preserved and the colon reanastomosed, and in those who require anoproctectomy because of advanced vulvar cancer.

The site of the colostomy should be selected so that the stomal appliance and bag can be applied to the skin of the anterior abdominal wall without difficulty. The best site is approximately midway between the umbilicus and the anterior iliac crest. The most distal site possible should be employed in the large intestine. After selection of the stomal site, a circular skin incision is made to accommodate two fingers. The subcutaneous tissue is removed and the fascia of the rectus sheath is incised similarly (Fig. 15.7). The end of the colon is brought through the stoma and sutured to fascia with interrupted 2-0 silk, and the stoma is everted to the skin to form a "rosebud" with the use of interrupted 2-0 or 3-0 absorbable braided suture.

Temporary

For patients who require temporary diversion, a transverse or sigmoid colostomy is usually created. The most distal portion of the colon should be used to allow the most formed stool possible. A *loop* colostomy is usually created: a loop of the colon is brought out through an appropriately placed separate incision in the abdominal wall. The loop is maintained by suturing it to the fascia beneath it. It can be reinforced with a rod of glass or plastic passed through a hole in the mesentery. The stoma can be opened immediately by means of an incision along the taenia coli in the longitudinal direction. Alternatively, the loop may be "matured" 1 to 2 days later to minimize the risk of sepsis if the bowel is unprepared.

The colon can be brought out as an *end* colostomy, which requires transection of the colon. This can be readily accomplished by means of a gastrointestinal anastomosis (GIA) stapler, which closes and transects the colon simultaneously. The distal end is sutured to the fascia, and the proximal end is brought out as the colostomy. If the distal colon must also be diverted (because of distal obstruction), either a *double-barrel* or a *loop* colostomy can be created.

Permanent

A permanent colostomy is an end or terminal colostomy, performed as far distally as possible to allow the maximum amount of fluid reabsorption. The distal loop

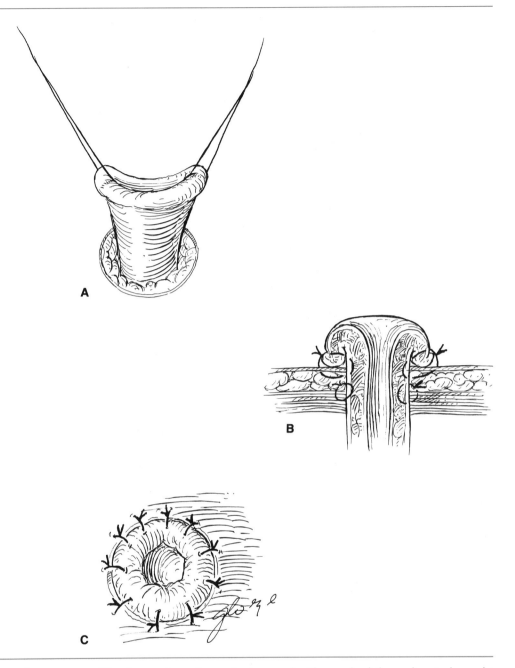

Figure 15.7 The formation of a colostomy. *A*, The end of the colon is brought through the abdominal wall; *B*, it is sutured to the fascia and skin; *C*, the "rosebud" stoma is formed.

of the transected colon may be oversewn to create a *Hartman's pouch* if there is no distal obstruction. In patients in whom there is complete distal obstruction, a mucous fistula should be created.

Enterostomy

If the colon is surgically inaccessible because of extensive carcinomatosis or radiation-induced adhesions, it may become necessary to palliate the bowel obstruction by the creation of a small intestinal stoma. Because the small-bowel contents are loose and irritating compared with colonic contents, an ileostomy or a jejunostomy should be undertaken only when absolutely necessary.

Intestinal Resection and Reanastomosis

After a segment of bowel, along with its wedge-shaped section of mesentery, has been resected, a reanastomosis may be performed. The most commonly used technique for reanastomosis is the *end-to-end* anastomosis, which is performed as either an open two-layered closure or a closed one-layered anastomosis. A *side-to-side* anastomosis may be useful to increase the size of the lumen at the site of anastomosis. Increasingly, the use of surgical stapling devices has permitted more rapid performance of the reanastomosis, which is particularly useful when more than one resection is being carried out or when the duration of the procedure is of major concern.

Hand-Sewn Anastomosis

End-to-End Enteroenterostomy

When the reanastomosis is to be hand sewn, the proximal and distal ends are clamped with Bainbridge clamps (Fig. 15.8A), and the posterior interrupted, seromuscular *Lembert* stitches are placed with 3-0 silk or polyglycolic acid sutures (Vicryl) (Fig. 15.8B). The clamps are removed, the devitalized ends are trimmed, and an inner continuous full-thickness layer of 3-0 chromic catgut or Vicryl is placed to complete the posterior portion of the anastomosis. After the corner is reached, the needle is brought through the wall to the outside, and the continuous layer is completed anteriorly with a *Connell* stitch (outside-in, inside-out) to complete the inner layer (Fig. 15.8C). The anterior seromuscular layer is then placed with interrupted 3-0 silk or Vicryl sutures (Fig. 15.8D). The defect in the intestinal mesentery is repaired.

A single-layered closed technique is occasionally used for colonic reanastomosis in obstructed, unprepared bowel in an effort to minimize peritoneal contamination. In these circumstances, however, the use of the surgical staplers is now recommended (12).

Side-to-Side Enteroenterostomy

The side-to-side anastomosis is particularly useful in patients who are undergoing intestinal bypass rather than resection to palliate bowel obstruction, e.g., in patients with unresectable or recurrent tumor. The loops of intestine are aligned side-to-side, and linen-shod clamps are applied to prevent spillage of intestinal contents. A posterior row of 3-0 silk or Vicryl is placed with interrupted Lembert sutures, and the lumina are created. An inner layer of continuous, full-thickness 3-0 chromic catgut or Vicryl sutures is placed and continued anteriorly to complete the layer with a Connell stitch. The anastomosis is completed by placement of an anterior seromuscular layer with the use of interrupted 3-0 silk or Vicryl sutures.

Intestinal Staplers

The principal advantage of the gastrointestinal staplers is the speed with which they can be employed. There is no increase in the complication rate with the use of staplers as compared with hand-sewn anastomoses (14). The staplers are especially useful in facilitating reanastomosis after low resection of the rectosigmoid colon, because a hand-sewn anastomosis is technically difficult when performed deep in the pelvis. A disadvantage of the staplers is their increased cost, and staplers are difficult to use when the intestinal tissues are very edematous.

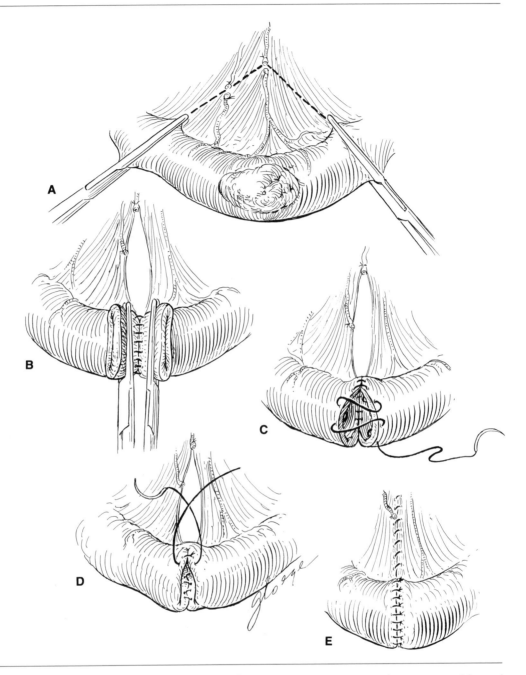

Figure 15.8   Hand-sewn end-to-end enteroenterostomy. *A*, The tumor and bowel are resected along with the mesentery. *B*, The posterior seromuscular layer is sutured. *C*, The Connell stitch is placed. *D*, The anterior seromuscular layer is placed. *E*, The completed anastomosis.

Types of Stapling Devices

The staplers are available in either reusable metal devices or in single-use disposable devices (Fig. 15.9A–C).

Thoracoabdominal (TA) Stapler The thoracoabdominal stapler comes in several sizes, the TA-30, TA-55, TA-60, and TA-90, corresponding to the length, in millimeters, of the row of staples. Individual staples are either 3.5 or 4.8 mm long. The TA closes the lumen in an everting fashion. A TA device is available

537

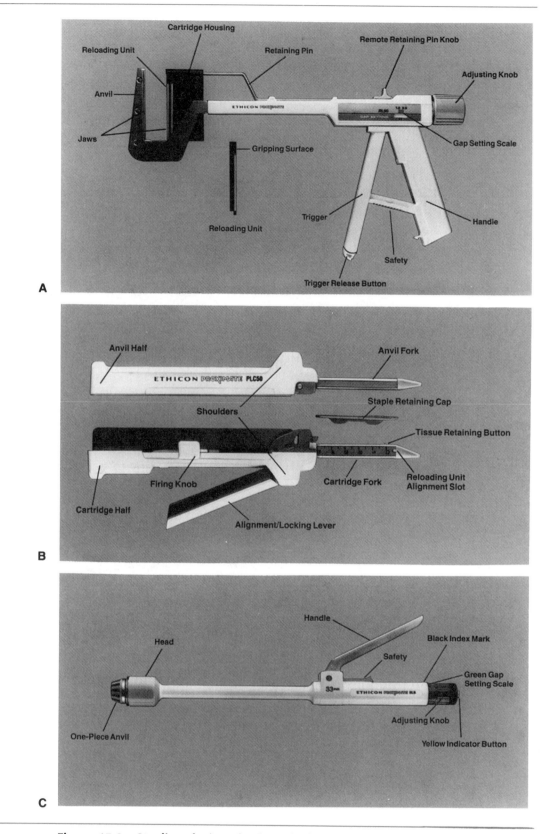

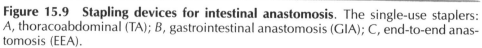

Figure 15.9 Stapling devices for intestinal anastomosis. The single-use staplers: *A*, thoracoabdominal (TA); *B*, gastrointestinal anastomosis (GIA); *C*, end-to-end anastomosis (EEA).

with a reticulating end, called a "Roticulator-55," that can be adjusted for placement into narrow areas (e.g., the deep pelvis).

Gastrointestinal Anastomosis (GIA) Stapler   The GIA device places two double rows of staples and then cuts the tissue between the two rows.

End-to-End Anastomosis (EEA) Stapler   The EEA stapler is used primarily to approximate two ends of the colon, especially to facilitate the reanastomosis of the lower colon after pelvic exenteration or resection of pelvic disease in patients with ovarian cancer. The stapler places a double row of staples, approximates the two ends of the intestine, and cuts the devitalized tissue inside the staple line. It is available in diameters of 21, 25, 28, 31, and 35 mm, and a metal sizing device is used to measure the diameter of the intestinal lumen (7).

Intraluminal (ILS) Stapler   The ILS stapler is a disposable EEA stapler that has a detachable anvil. This removable feature can facilitate the placement of the anvil into a portion of one intestine that is difficult to mobilize. The anvil can be reattached to the rod of the ILS device after it has been placed in the anastomosis.

Stapling Technique

Functional End-to-End Enteroenterostomy Anastomosis   This operation is illustrated in Figure 15.10. The GIA stapler is used to staple and divide each end of the bowel segment to be resected. The antimesenteric borders of the bowel loops are approximated, and the corners are resected. A fork of the GIA device is inserted into each bowel lumen, and after alignment the stapler is fired. The defect where the stapler was introduced then is closed with a TA stapler.

Side-to-Side Enteroenterostomy Anastomosis   When a bypass enteroenterostomy is performed, the two loops of bowel to be anastomosed side to side are aligned, an enterotomy is created in each loop, and a fork of the GIA stapler is slid into each lumen, fired, and removed. This creates the lumen between the two bowel segments, and the enterotomy that is left when the instrument is withdrawn is then approximated with a TA stapler.

Low Colonic End-to-End Anastomosis   A low colonic resection is performed by isolating and removing the portion of the rectosigmoid colon involved with disease. The EEA stapler is inserted through the anus and advanced to the site of the anastomosis. The instrument is opened to allow the anvil to accommodate the proximal colon, which is mobilized and tied over the distal end of the EEA. The distal colon is likewise tied over the EEA with a pursestring suture (Fig. 15.11). The EEA is then closed, approximating the two ends of the colon, and the instrument is fired and removed. A reinforcing layer of interrupted 3-0 silk or Vicryl Lembert sutures is placed anteriorly. The anastomosis is palpated to confirm that it is intact. Also, the pelvis can be filled with saline solution, and air can be insufflated through the rectum to search for bubbles, which would indicate a defect in the anastomosis (14).

An alternative end-to-side (functional end-to-end) low colonic anastomosis can be performed with the use of one of the newer disposable stapling devices, which has a removable distal one-piece anvil, the *intraluminal stapler*. This end-to-side technique is performed by detaching the anvil, which is inserted in the proximal

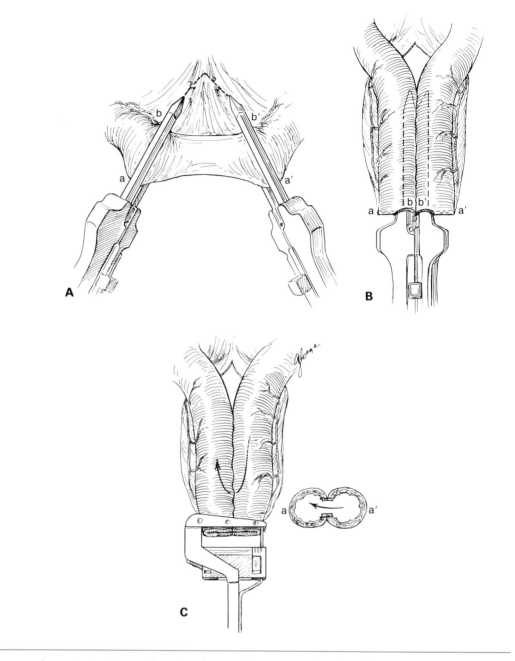

Figure 15.10 Functional end-to-end anastomosis using the stapling technique. *A,* The GIA is used to resect the intestine. *B,* The sides of the transected intestine are placed side to side, and each antemesenteric corner is incised to create two holes into which the two forks of a second GIA are placed. The GIA stapler is fired to create the new intestinal lumen. *C,* The TA stapler is placed over the end and "fired" to close the remaining defect. Note the cross section at a-a'.

colon segment. The center rod of the open EEA instrument without the anvil is inserted through an opening in the bowel or through the anus. Then the rod is inserted through or near the staple line. In the other segment of bowel, a pursestring suture is placed and the free anvil is inserted within the lumen of the bowel within the pursestring suture. The anvil is then screwed onto the rod, the device is closed, and the anastomosis is created.

An alternative side-to-side technique (functional end-to-end) anastomosis of the rectosigmoid colon can be used when the portion of removed bowel is proximal enough to permit this operation (i.e., 10–15 cm of preserved rectum). The GIA instrument is used to perform the colorectal anastomosis. After the segment of colon to be resected is mobilized, the proximal colon to be reanastomosed is closed with either the GIA or the TA-55 instrument. A stab wound is made in the antimesenteric border of the colon about 5 cm proximal to the staple line closure. A corresponding stab wound is made in the left anterolateral wall of the rectum at the proximal point of the planned site of anastomosis. The proximal

Figure 15.11   Low colonic end-to-end anastomosis using the EEA stapler. *A,* After resection of the rectosigmoid colon, the distal end of the descending colon is mobilized and a pursestring suture is placed by hand or with a special instrument (illustrated). A pursestring suture is also placed around the rectal stump. The open end of the EEA stapler is inserted through the anus and the rectal pursestring is tied around the instrument. The end of the descending colon is placed over the end of the EEA and the second pursestring is tied. *B,* The EEA device is closed and "fired."

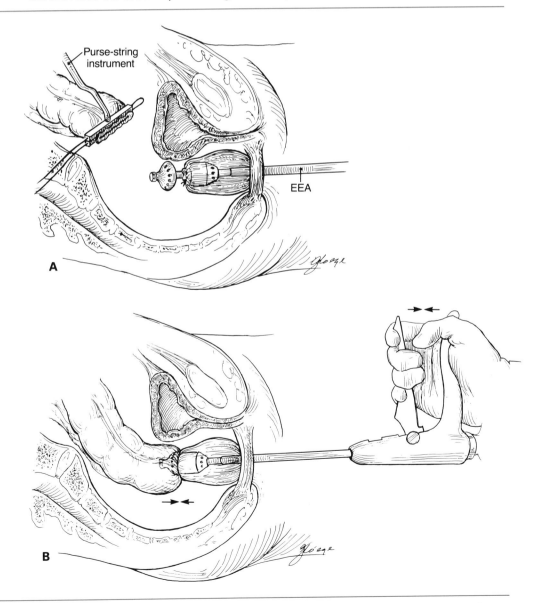

colon is placed into the retrorectal space, side to side along the rectum, the GIA device is placed into the proximal and distal segments, and the instrument is closed and fired. The remaining single defect is closed with either a hand-sewn, double layer of 3-0 sutures or the rotating TA-55 device (Roticulator-55).

Postoperative Care

After resection of the small bowel, a nasogastric tube is usually placed for about 48 hours to reduce the volume of intestinal secretions that must pass through the site of anastomosis. In patients who have received pelvic or abdominal irradiation, the upper intestinal tract should remain intubated until bowel function has returned, as signified by the passage of flatus and stool. Typically, patients who have undergone small bowel resection must be maintained without oral intake for about 5 days, whereas those who have undergone colon resection require about 7 days without oral intake. The diet is advanced gradually as the patient tolerates it. In patients who have undergone colonic resection and reanastomosis, enemas and cathartics should be avoided (15).

Intravenous fluids must be continued while the patient is receiving nothing by mouth. In patients whose recovery is likely to be prolonged beyond 7 days, such as those who have previously received whole-abdominal irradiation, consideration should be given to the use of parenteral nutrition, as discussed in Chapter 18. In such patients, a gastrostomy tube may be useful to avoid prolonged nasogastric intubation.

Urinary Tract Operations

The preoperative evaluation of the urinary tract is important in patients with gynecologic malignancies, because of the frequent involvement of the urinary organs, especially the bladder and the distal ureters (16–20). Renal function and ureteric patency must be assessed preoperatively.

Cystoscopy

Cystoscopy should be performed as part of the staging for cervical and vaginal cancers unless the disease has been diagnosed early (16). Cystoscopy is also indicated in patients with a lower urinary tract fistula or unexplained hematuria. Cystoscopic examination may demonstrate external compression of the bladder by a tumor, bullous edema produced by the blockage of lymphatic vessels from adjacent tumor growth, or mucosal involvement with tumor. When a mucosal lesion is seen, a biopsy can confirm the diagnosis.

Technique Cystoscopy is performed with the patient in the dorsal lithotomy position. After preparation and draping of the area, the cystoscopic obturator and sheath are inserted into the urethra and carefully advanced into the bladder, after which the obturator is removed. The cystoscope is inserted into the sheath. About 250–400 ml of normal saline solution is instilled into the bladder to permit a thorough inspection of the entire mucosa.

Cystostomy

A suprapubic cystostomy catheter is useful in patients who require prolonged bladder drainage. This catheter is particularly useful in patients undergoing radical hysterectomy for cervical cancer or extensive resection of pelvic tumor, because of the temporary disruption of bladder innervation that occurs with these dissections. The suprapubic catheter is easier for the patient to manage than a trans-

542

urethral Foley catheter, and the rate of bladder infection is lower (18, 19). The other convenient aspect of this catheter is that it can facilitate trials of voiding. The patient can clamp the catheter for a specified interval, void, and then unclamp to check for residual urine. When the residual urine is less than 75–100 ml, the catheter can be removed.

Technique The catheter used is an 18F Silastic Foley catheter with a 5–10 ml balloon. This catheter is well tolerated by patients, produces minimal local tissue irritation, and is of sufficient caliber that blockage of the catheter lumen is not a major problem. The placement of a suprapubic catheter involves the following steps:

1. The catheter is inserted through a stab incision in the skin, subcutaneous tissue, and fascia, and a small hole is made in the dome of the bladder.

2. The tip of the catheter is inserted into the bladder, and a seromuscular pursestring suture is placed around the defect with 3-0 Vicryl or chromic catgut.

3. A second reinforcing layer consisting of either 2-0 absorbable braided Vicryl or chromic catgut suture is placed in the bladder.

4. With the Foley balloon distended, the catheter is pulled up so that the bladder is applied snugly to the anterior abdominal wall.

5. The catheter can be attached to a urinary drainage bag, and it can also be attached to a smaller "leg bag," which is more portable and therefore easier for the patient to manage after discharge from the hospital.

Ureteral Obstruction

Ureteral obstruction is the most common urinary complication in patients with gynecologic malignancies. This problem is seen particularly in patients with cervical or vaginal cancer, either at the time of diagnosis or with recurrent disease. It may result from direct tumor extension into the bladder or distal ureters or from compression by lymph node metastases. In patients with intra-abdominal carcinomatosis, most often from ovarian cancer, extensive pelvic tumor may cause significant progressive ureteral obstruction. The most frequent site of lower urinary tract obstruction in gynecologic patients is the ureteral-vesical junction (16).

Postoperative obstruction is usually incomplete and results from edema, possible infection, and partial devascularization of the distal ureter. However, the obstruction may be complete, and when it is, it most often results from inadvertent suture ligature of the distal ureter when the surgeon is attempting to ligate the blood vessels of the cardinal ligament (18). Chronic obstruction can result from stenosis after pelvic irradiation, particularly if pelvic surgery is also performed.

In patients who have a partial ureteral obstruction, the passage of a retrograde stent at the time of cystoscopy might bypass the site of blockage. The retrograde stent used is a 7F to 9F flexible, double "J" retrograde ureteral stent; it is inserted with the aid of a stent-placement apparatus that has an elevator attachment to the cystoscope. Great care must be taken, as this procedure has the risk of ureteral perforation. When the stent does not pass readily, the performance of a percutaneous nephrostomy is preferable.

543

In patients in whom complete ureteral obstruction is suspected (i.e., because of a rising serum creatinine level or the development of an acute unilateral pyelonephritis), an intravenous pyelogram (IVP) should be performed if the serum creatinine value is less than 2.0 mg; an ultrasonogram should be obtained if the level is higher. In patients with complete ureteral obstruction the problem must be corrected immediately, either by temporary urinary diversion by means of a percutaneous nephrostomy or by reexploration and repair of the ureter. Repair may be by either reanastomosis or reimplantation.

Mild degrees of hydroureter are managed by bladder drainage alone in most patients, as these problems are usually temporary and resolve gradually as the edema subsides. Infection should be treated with appropriate antibiotics.

In patients undergoing radical hysterectomy and bilateral pelvic lymphadenectomy, postoperative ureteral damage from devascularization can be decreased by minimizing the collection of fluid in the retroperitoneal space with prophylactic placement of drains (e.g., Jackson-Pratt drains) (17).

Retrograde Pyelography

If an excretory urogram cannot be performed (e.g., because of dye sensitivity) or if the study is inconclusive, retrograde pyelography may be necessary. This procedure is potentially morbid and should be performed only if the information to be gained is critical to the decision regarding diversion of the affected kidney (19). Contrast injected beyond a high-grade obstruction can produce pyelonephritis and sepsis and may require urgent drainage through a percutaneous nephrostomy. The attempted passage of a retrograde ureteral catheter or stent may be useful for diagnosis, and it will stent the ureter if the obstruction has not resulted from a misplaced suture ligature.

Percutaneous Nephrostomy

In patients with an obstructed ureter that cannot be decompressed by means of a retrograde ureteral stent, a percutaneous nephrostomy tube can be placed under fluoroscopic guidance (20). This procedure is relatively easy to perform, and the tube can be changed or replaced as necessary. In addition, an antegrade ureteral catheter or stent can occasionally be passed through a nephrostomy to remove the percutaneous stent in patients in whom a retrograde catheter cannot be passed.

Ureteral Reanastomosis (Ureteroureterostomy)

When the ureter has been transected or damaged beyond repair, it will have to be revised and reanastomosed or reimplanted into the urinary bladder. If the ureteral injury is above the level of the pelvic brim, a simple reanastomosis is the procedure of choice. The two ends of the ureters are trimmed at a 45-degree angle. A double "J" ureteral stent is passed into the distal ureter with one "memory" end inserted into the bladder. The proximal end of the ureter is placed over the stent and sutured to its distal counterpart (21). Interrupted 4-0 absorbable chromic or Vicryl sutures are placed at close intervals in a circumferential fashion (Fig. 15.12). After several weeks, the absence of leakage can be established by means of an IVP, and the stent can be removed through a cystoscope.

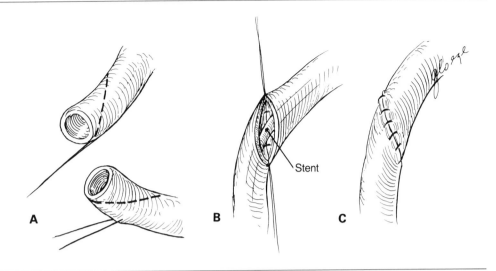

Figure 15.12   Ureteroureterostomy. *A,* The two ends of the ureters are cut diagonally. *B,* A ureteral stent is inserted into the proximal and distal ureter, and interrupted full-thickness sutures are placed. *C,* The completed anastomosis.

Ureteroneocystostomy

The reimplantation of the distal ureter into the bladder is known as the Leadbetter procedure, or ureteroneocystostomy. This operation is preferred for the ureter that has been disrupted distal to the pelvic brim, as long as the bladder can be sufficiently mobilized on the side of reimplantation (22–23). Integral to successful ureteral reimplantation is the creation of a submucosal tunnel (Fig. 15.13). The tunnel minimizes the risk of vesicoureteral reflux and chronic, recurrent pyelonephritis (23).

The technique is as follows:

1. The distal ureter is prepared by careful resection of any devitalized tissue while the maximum length is preserved.

2. The bladder base is mobilized, and the dome of the bladder is affixed laterally to the psoas muscle by means of a lateral cystopexy, a "psoas hitch." This permits stabilization of the bladder as well as extension of the bladder toward the end of the resected ureter, and it is especially important if the ureter is somewhat foreshortened.

3. A cystotomy incision is made, and the tunnel is initiated by injection of the submucosal plane with saline solution to raise the mucosa. The mucosa is incised and a tonsil forceps is inserted submucosally for a length of 1–1.5 cm to the site where the serosa is to be incised. An incision in the serosa is made over the pointed tip of the clamp to create an opening to the tunnel that passes through the muscularis and mucosa of the bladder wall.

4. The ureter is gently pulled through the submucosal tunnel, and mucosa-to-mucosa stitches are placed with interrupted 4-0 chromic suture ma-

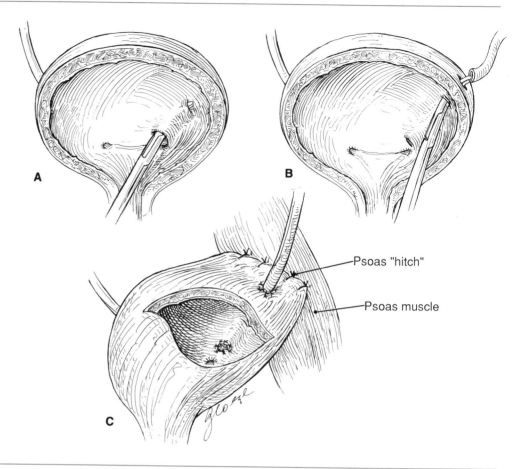

Psoas "hitch"

Psoas muscle

Figure 15.13   Ureteroneocystostomy. *A,* A submucosal tunnel is created. *B,* The ureter is brought into the bladder. *C,* The ureter is passed through the tunnel and sutured to the bladder serosa and mucosa. The serosa of the bladder is sutured to the psoas muscle to stabilize the anastomosis.

terial. A ureteric stent, preferably a soft plastic double "J," is passed up the ureter into the renal calyx, and the other end is placed in the bladder lumen. The site of entrance of the ureter is sutured to the bladder serosa with 4-0 chromic catgut or Vicryl.

5. A suprapubic cystostomy is performed, and the cystostomy is closed with two layers of interrupted 2-0 absorbable suture. The retroperitoneum is drained with a Jackson-Pratt drain. The ureteral stent is left in place 10–14 days and then removed through a cystoscope.

Transureteroureterostomy (TUU)

Another procedure that can be useful in the carefully selected patient is the TUU. When the distal ureter must be resected on one side, and the proximal ureter is too short to permit ureteroneocystostomy, it is possible to implant the distal end of the resected ureter into the contralateral side (24). The distal end of the partially resected ureter is tunneled under the mesentery of the sigmoid colon and approximated, end to side, into the recipient ureter. A ureteral stent is used to protect the anastomosis and is left in place for at least 14 days.

Permanent Urinary Diversion

Permanent urinary diversion must be performed after cystectomy or in patients who have an irreparable fistula of the lower urinary tract. Lower urinary tract fistulas can result from progressive tumor growth or from radical pelvic surgery and/or pelvic irradiation. The most common fistula is the ureterovaginal one.

Urinary Conduit

The most frequently employed techniques for urinary diversion are the creation of an *ileal conduit* (the "Bricker procedure") (25), the creation of a *transverse colon conduit* (26), and the creation of a "continent" urinary conduit (e.g., the Koch, Miami, or Indiana pouch) (27–29). The ileal conduit has been the most widely used means of permanent urinary diversion, and it is suitable for most patients. A segment of transverse colon can be used if the ileum has been extensively injured (e.g., by radiation therapy). The transverse colon is usually away from the irradiated field, and thus its vascularity is not compromised.

More recently, the *continent urinary conduit* has been developed; this may be helpful for gynecologic oncology patients who require exenterative surgery. The continent ileal conduit (or "Koch pouch") requires a longer portion of the ileum (up to 100 cm), a longer operative time (4–6 hours), and the technical skills for creation of the continent conduit (27). Therefore the procedure may be unsuitable in many patients. The operation has the advantage of creating a conduit for which the patient need not wear an appliance, and the urine can be drained by self-catheterization. The continent stoma is created by intussusception of the small intestine so that it forms a stenotic distal lumen.

Another approach to the continent conduit involves the use of the *continent colon conduit*. In this operation, the intestine from the terminal ileum to the midportion of the transverse colon, including the entire ascending colon, the cecum, and the terminal ileum are used to create a urinary reservoir. The colon reservoir (the Indiana or Miami pouch) can be suitable for gynecologic oncology patients, especially those undergoing an exenteration (28, 29). The Indiana and Miami pouches are technically somewhat easier to perform than the Koch pouch; however, the type of continent conduit created is generally determined by the training and preference of the surgeon.

Technique   The technique for the creation of an ileal conduit involves the isolation of a segment of ileum at a site where the intestine appears healthy and nonirradiated. This is typically about 30–40 cm proximal to the ileocecal junction. The conduit requires a segment of ileum measuring approximately 20 cm and its associated mesentery (24). After isolation of the segment, the ileum is reanastomosed (Fig. 15.14). The ureters are implanted into the closed proximal end of the ileal segment, and double "J" ureteric stents are placed into both ureters. A No. 8 pediatric feeding tube made of soft flexible plastic can also be employed for the ureteric stent, as it is relatively atraumatic. The "butt" end of the conduit is sutured to the area of the sacral promontory.

The distal end of the conduit is brought through the anterior abdominal wall of the right lower quadrant, approximately midway between the umbilicus and the anterior superior iliac crest. The ureteral stents should be left in place for about 10 days.

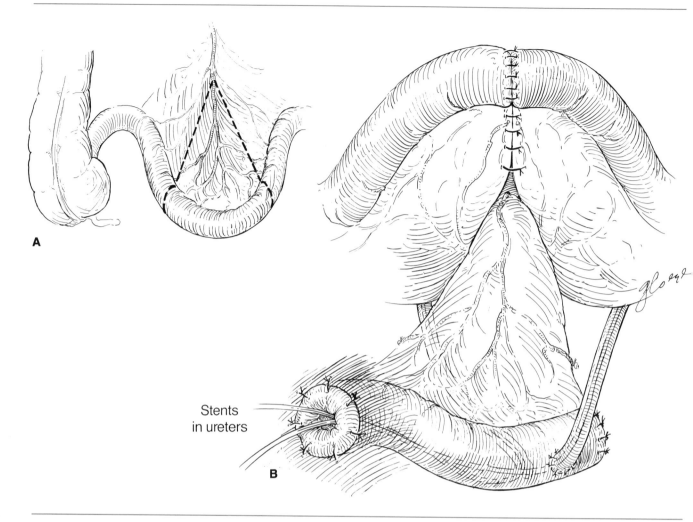

Stents
in ureters

Figure 15.14   Ileal urinary conduit. *A,* A segment of nonirradiated ileum is used for the conduit. *B,* The ileum is reanastomosed, and the ureters are sewn into the "butt" end of the conduit. Note that ureters are stented individually.

When a transverse-colon conduit is selected, the technique is essentially the same. Care must be taken in both techniques to ensure that the vascularity of the intestinal mesentery is not interrupted. The mesentery of the reanastomosed bowel must be reapproximated to prevent herniation of intestinal loops through the defect.

The technique for creation of a Koch pouch has been well described (27). The technique for creation of the Miami pouch (29) involves resection of the intestine from the last 10–15 cm of ileum to the midportion of the transverse colon. The colon is opened along the antimesenteric border through the teniae coli (Fig. 15.15A). The ileum is used to create the continence mechanism (Fig. 15.15B). The ileal-cecal valve serves as the principal portion of the mechanism; the terminal ileum is narrowed, and several pursestring sutures are placed near the valve to reinforce the continence portion of the conduit (Fig. 15.15C). The ascending colon is sutured or stapled to the transverse colon to create a pouch. An ileo-transverse anastomosis is performed to reconstitute the intestine (Fig. 15.15D).

Skin Ureterostomy

In rare instances, a terminally ill patient undergoing exploratory surgery will have a bladder fistula. In such circumstances, one ureter can be ligated, and a skin

Figure 15.15   Colon continent urinary conduit—the "Miami" pouch. *A,* The segment of distal ileum and ascending and transverse colon is isolated, and the segment is opened on its antimesenteric border along the teniae coli; *B,* the ureters are reimplanted into the mesenteric side of the ascending colon and a continence mechanism is created with pursestring sutures and a double staple line is performed with a GIA stapler; *C,* the conduit is closed and the ileal stoma is created; and *D,* the intestines are reconstituted with an ileal-transverse colon anastomosis.

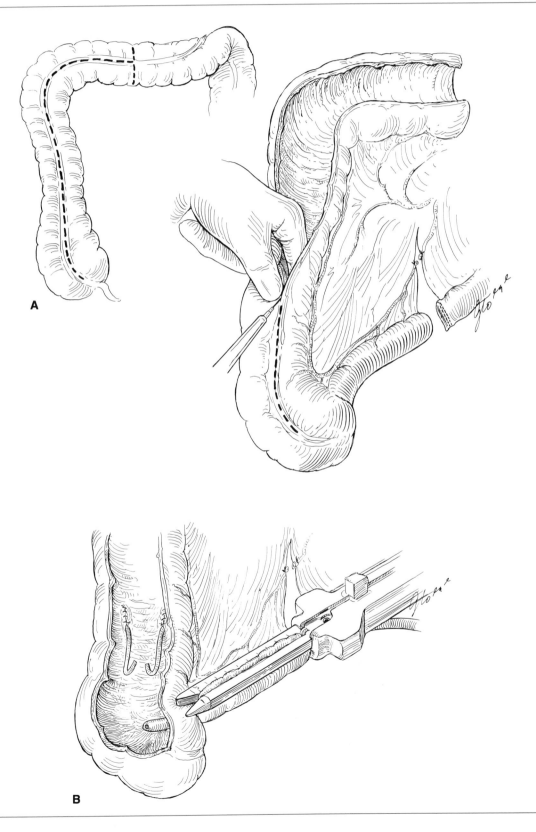

Continued

549

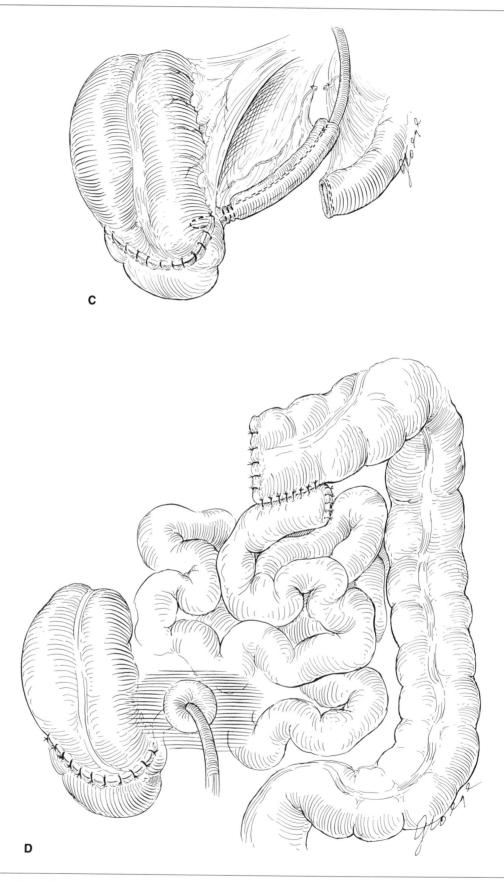

C

D

Figure 15.15 continued

ureterostomy can be created with the other ureter. The ureter is mobilized from its attachments and brought laterally through the retroperitoneal space to the lateral and anterior abdominal wall. The ureter is tunneled through the fascia and brought out through a stab incision in the skin, where it is affixed to create a small stoma (19).

Reconstructive Operations

Reconstructive operations, particularly pelvic floor reconstruction and creation of a neovagina, are important in patients who are undergoing extensive extirpative procedures, such as pelvic exenteration. Vaginal reconstruction helps to provide support to the pelvic floor, thereby reducing the prospect of perineal herniation. By helping to fill the pelvis, vaginal reconstruction also decreases the incidence of enteroperineal fistulas. Pelvic floor reconstruction should be performed in all patients undergoing a pelvic exenteration, and vaginal reconstruction should be performed simultaneously in most patients. The surgeon must be well acquainted with the types of graft that can be employed in the performance of these reconstructive operations and the techniques necessary to accomplish them (30).

Grafts

Grafts used for reconstructive operations in the pelvis are either skin grafts, which can be full or partial (split) thickness, or myocutaneous grafts, which are composed of the full thickness of the skin, its contiguous subcutaneous tissues, and a portion of a closely associated muscle. The most frequently used myocutaneous pedicle grafts contain muscle segments from the gracilis muscle of the inner thigh, the bulbocavernosus muscle of the vulva, the tensor fascia lata muscle of the lateral thigh, or the rectus abdominis muscle.

Skin Grafts

Skin grafts must be harvested under sterile conditions (30). The donor site most frequently used to obtain a split-thickness skin graft is either the anterior and medial thigh or the buttock. Although the thigh may be more readily accessible to the surgeon, the buttock donor site has cosmetic advantages; however, this latter site may be more uncomfortable in the postoperative recovery period. The selection of the donor site should be made preoperatively after discussion with the patient.

A dermatome is used to harvest the skin graft. Several different types of dermatome are available, including the Brown air-powered, electrically driven dermatome and the Padgett hand-driven dermatome. The surgeon should select the instrument with which he or she has the greatest facility, as an equally good graft can be harvested with either one. The technique for obtaining the skin graft is as follows:

1. The graft width and thickness can be determined by adjusting the settings of the dermatome. A split-thickness graft can be obtained by setting the thickness between 14 and 16 one-thousandths of an inch. Full-thickness grafts are 20–24 one-thousandths of an inch.

2. When using the dermatome, the surgeon must apply firm, steady pressure in order to harvest a graft of uniform thickness. To minimize friction,

mineral oil is applied to the skin over which the dermatome is to be passed.

3. The skin to be taken is stretched and flattened by the surgical assistant with the use of a tongue depressor. A second assistant picks up the leading edge of the graft as it is being harvested.

4. The harvested graft is kept moist in saline solution while the recipient site is being prepared.

5. The graft may be "pie crusted" by making small incisions in the surface. This technique maximizes the dimension of the graft while permitting the escape of fluid that might otherwise accumulate between the graft and the recipient site. However, extensive pie crusting may result in contracture when the graft is used to create a neovagina.

Pedicle Grafts

The purpose of the pedicle graft is to provide a substantial amount of tissue along with its blood supply either to repair an anatomic defect or to create a new structure, such as a neovagina (30–34). The pedicle graft can be either a full-thickness skin and subcutaneous tissue graft, as is used frequently for closure of a vulvar defect, e.g., a "Z-plasty" (a "rhomboid flap"), or a myocutaneous graft, e.g., a gracilis.

Before harvesting a pedicle graft, the surgeon should carefully outline the incisions on the skin with a marker pen. During the mobilization of the myocutaneous pedicle, the surgeon must carefully isolate and preserve the neurovascular bundle that supplies the muscle.

Vaginal Reconstruction

Vaginal reconstruction in the gynecologic oncology patient is performed either to revise or replace a vagina that has stenosed as a result of prior vaginal surgery and/or radiation or to create a neovagina when the vagina has been removed (31).

Split-Thickness Graft

When the vagina is fibrotic after irradiation, the scarred vaginal tissue first must be resected before placement of the split-thickness skin graft (32). The skin graft is placed over a vaginal stent that is then inserted into the space created by resection of the old, scarred vagina (Fig. 15.16A). The Heyer-Schulte stent is the vaginal stent preferred for this purpose, because it is inflatable, can be easily removed and replaced by the patient, and has its own drainage tube (Fig. 15.16B).

Split-thickness skin grafts can also be used in patients undergoing exenteration, but this approach is less satisfactory than the use of myocutaneous pedicle grafts, as discussed below. When an anterior exenteration is performed, or when a portion of the rectosigmoid colon is resected but primarily reanastomosed, a neovagina can be created with the use of skin grafts. The omentum is mobilized by ligating and dividing the short gastric vessels along the greater curvature of the stomach, preserving the left gastroepiploic pedicle (Fig. 15.17A). The omentum is then placed into the pelvis and sutured to the rectosigmoid posteriorly and laterally to create a pocket for the neovagina. Split-thickness skin graft(s) are harvested, sewn over a vaginal stent, and inserted into the newly created pelvic space (Fig. 15.17B).

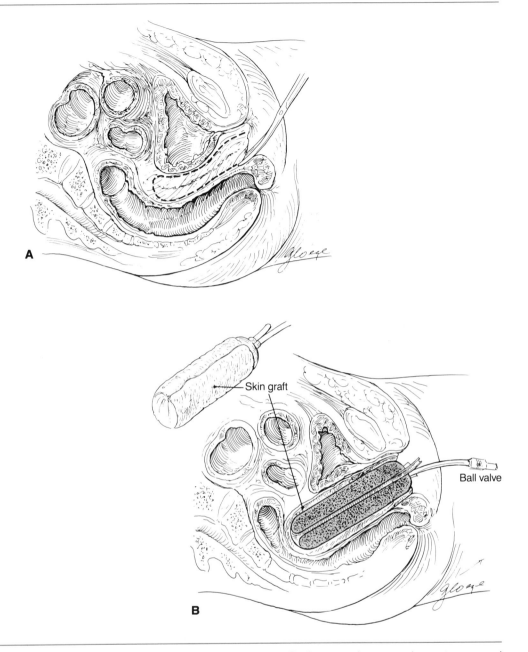

Figure 15.16   Creation of neovagina after radiation. *A*, The vaginal scar is resected in preparation for vaginal reconstruction with split-thickness skin grafts. *B*, A Heyer-Schulte vaginal stent has the skin graft placed around it, and this is inserted into the pelvic space to create a neovagina.

Myocutaneous Gracilis Grafts	Bilateral myocutaneous gracilis pedicle grafts can be used to construct a neovagina. In addition, the grafts provide excellent support for the pelvic viscera (31). The myocutaneous gracilis graft is harvested (Fig. 15.18A) from the inner aspect of the thigh. A line is drawn from the pubic tubercle to the medial epicondyle, and this delineates the anterior margin of the graft. The graft should be about 6 cm wide and about 12 cm long. A skin bridge is preserved between the vulva and the pedicle. The myocutaneous pedicle graft is mobilized by transecting the gracilis muscle distally in continuity with the skin and subcutaneous tissue

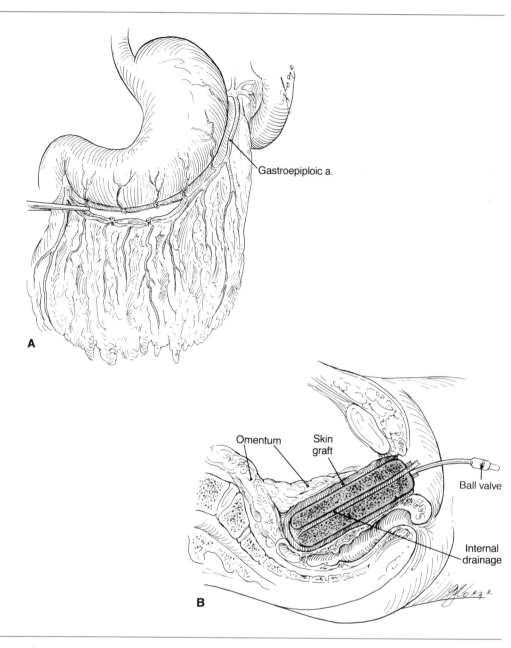

Figure 15.17 Mobilization of the omentum. *A,* This is accomplished by ligating and dividing the right gastroepiploic artery and the short gastric arteries along the greater curvature of the stomach. *B,* The omentum is used to create a "pocket" for the placement of a split-thickness skin graft.

(Fig. 15.18B). The vascular pedicle is proximal, and it must be carefully identified and preserved.

The pedicle is "harvested," brought under the skin bridge of the vulva, and exteriorized through the introitus (Fig. 15.18C). The two grafts are sutured together to create a hollow neovagina (Fig. 15.18D, E). The entire neovagina is placed into the pelvis by posterior and upward rotation and sutured to the introitus (Fig. 15.18F). The apex is sutured to the symphysis pubis and/or the anterior sacrum. At the completion of the procedure, an omental pedicle is brought down over the graft to reconstruct the pelvic floor (Fig. 15.18G).

Bulbocavernosus Pedicle Grafts

The bulbocavernosus myocutaneous pedicle graft has been used for repair of radiation-induced rectovaginal fistulas (Martius procedure), but the procedure has been adopted for the creation of a neovagina (33, 34). The procedure is performed by making an incision over the labium majus, isolating the bulbocavernosus muscle superiorly and anteriorly, and mobilizing it on a posterior vulvar pedicle. The graft is tunneled under a skin bridge at the posterior introitus and sutured to the pedicle of the other side.

Figure 15.18   The gracilis myocutaneous graft. (Reproduced with permission from the American College of Obstetricians and Gynecologists, Berek JS, et al: Vaginal reconstruction performed simultaneously with pelvic exenteration. *Obstet Gynecol* 63:318, 1984.)

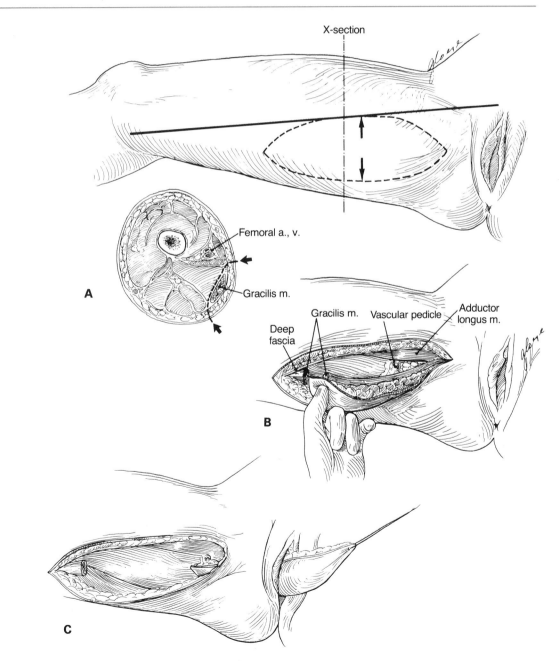

Continued

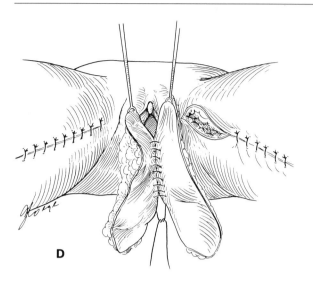

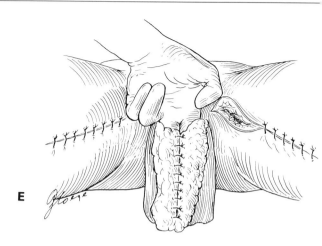

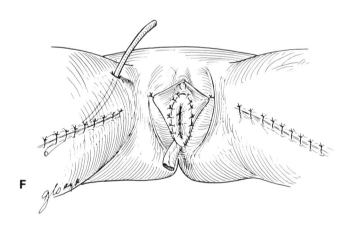

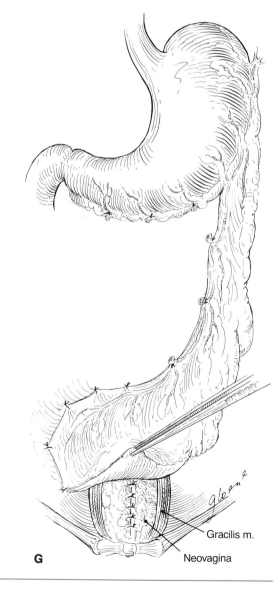

Gracilis m.

Neovagina

Figure 15.18 continued

Colon Segment

Some authors have preferred to use a segment of colon to create a neovagina (32, 35). This technique has had mixed success in the past, but a new approach using a portion of the ascending colon may be an improvement over earlier procedures (35).

Vulvar Reconstruction

Whenever feasible, the vulva should be closed primarily after radical vulvectomy. With radical local excision or a separate incision approach for the groin dissection, primary closure of the vulvar skin can be accomplished in almost all patients.

Rhomboid Pedicle Graft

If there is any tension on the skin edges, the skin can be mobilized by means of a "Z-plasty" using the adjacent skin and subcutaneous tissue. This is called a "rhomboid flap" (36). The technique (Fig. 15.19) involves the repositioning of a rhomboid flap of full-thickness skin and subcutaneous tissue. Use of these pedicle grafts will usually allow for the primary closure of vulvar defects after radical vulvar surgery, but if necessary a split-thickness skin graft can be used. Myocutaneous pedicle grafts, such as a unilateral gracilis graft, can also be used to cover a large vulvar defect.

Tensor Fascia Lata Pedicle Graft

The tensor fascia lata pedicle graft, harvested from the lateral aspect of the thigh, can be useful in covering large defects of the lower abdomen, groin, and anterior vulva. The flap is particularly useful in patients who require extensive resection of large groin recurrences or large, fixed groin nodes.

Figure 15.19   *A,* **The "rhomboid flap"** is used to close a posterior vulvar defect. *B,* The pedicle grafts are bilateral "Z-plasties" that are sutured together in the midline.

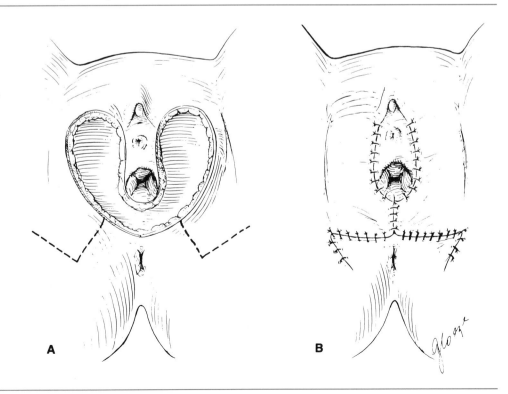

A   B

The graft is obtained by harvesting a myocutaneous pedicle from its proximal origin at the anterosuperior aspect of the iliac bone to its distal insertion on the lateral condyle of the tibia (35). The length of the proposed flaps is determined by measuring the distance from the muscle's vascular supply, located 6–8 cm distal to the anterior superior iliac spine, to the most inferior or distal point of the recipient site (e.g., the posterior vulva). The blood supply is from the lateral circumflex femoral artery located deep to the fascia lata between the rectus femoris and the vastus lateralis. The posterior border of the graft is defined as a line from the greater trochanter of the hip down to the knee, and the distal border is located about 5 cm proximal to the knee. The width of the flap is determined by the width of the defect to be covered, but typically it is 6–8 cm with a length of up to 40 cm.

The pedicle graft is harvested after the defect has been created in order to permit a more accurate measurement of the flap. The flap is first incised distally, and care is taken to avoid injury to the proximal blood supply. Once the flaps are elevated, they are rotated into place and sutured from their most distal point to the proximal. The donor site is closed primarily.

Vulvovaginoplasty

Although the preferred methods for vulvar and vaginal reconstruction are outlined above, there is occasionally a need to perform a vulvovaginoplasty, the so-called "William's procedure." This procedure (37) involves the incision of a horseshoe-shaped flap on the vulva to create a marsupialized pouch that can be used as a neovagina. This operation has the advantage of being relatively simple to perform, and it does not require pelvic dissection. It has the disadvantage of being less anatomically suitable for vaginal intercourse, but its direction can improve with regular use. It may be helpful in a patient who has undergone a pelvic exenteration without vaginal reconstruction.

Pelvic Floor Reconstruction

At the completion of a pelvic exenteration, the pelvic floor must be reconstructed. Probably the most effective procedure is to perform an omental pedicle graft (provided there is sufficient omentum) and to use myocutaneous pedicle grafts whenever possible to reconstruct the vagina. In patients in whom this is not possible, alternatives include the use of a variety of graft materials, either natural or synthetic. A natural material that has been used is dura mater, but this is often unavailable. All areas that can be directly peritonealized should be carefully covered with peritoneal pedicle grafts. Synthetic grafts using Marlex have been associated with a high incidence ($> 20\%$) of infectious morbidity and are therefore much less desirable. However, if a pedicle graft is not feasible, the synthetic material Gore-Tex may be the best alternative.

References

1. **Gajewski JL, Champlin RE:** Vascular access. In Haskell CM (ed): *Cancer Treatment,* ed 3. Philadelphia, WB Saunders, 1990, pp 866–869.

2. **Raaf JH:** Results from use of 826 vascular access devices in cancer patients. *Cancer* 55:1312, 1985.

3. **Hacker NF, Berek JS, Pretorius GR, et al:** Intraperitoneal cisplatin as salvage therapy in residual ovarian cancer. *Obstet Gynecol* 70:759, 1987.

4. **Baggish MS, Lee WK:** Abdominal wound disruption. *Obstet Gynecol* 46:530, 1975.

5. **Helmkamp BF:** Abdominal wound dehiscence. *Am J Obstet Gynecol* 128:803, 1979.

6. **Malt RA:** Abdominal incisions, sutures and sacrilege. *N Engl J Med* 297:722, 1977.

7. **Gallup DG, Nolan TE, Smith RP:** Primary mass closure of midline incisions with a continuous polyglyconate monofilament absorbable suture. *Obstet Gynecol* 76:872, 1990.

8. **Irvin TT, Koffman CG, Duthie HL:** Layer closure of laparotomy wounds with absorbable and non-absorbable suture materials. *Br J Surg* 63:793, 1976.

9. **Murray DG, Blaisdell W:** Use of synthetic absorbable sutures for abdominal and chest wound closure. *Arch Surg* 113:477, 1978.

10. **Schrock TR, Deveney CW, Dunphy JE:** Factors contributing to leakage of colonic anastomosis. *Ann Surg* 177:513, 1973.

11. **Clarke JS, London RE, Bertlett JG:** Preoperative oral antibiotics reduce septic complications of colon operations. *Ann Surg* 186:251, 1977.

12. **Hacker NF, Berek JS, Lagasse LD:** Gastrointestinal operations in gynecologic oncology. In Knapp RC, Berkowitz RS (eds): *Gynecologic Oncology*, ed 2. New York, McGraw-Hill, 1993, pp 361–375.

13. **Baker JW:** Stitchless plication for recurring obstruction of the small bowel. *Am J Surg* 116:316, 1968.

14. **Chassin JL:** *Operative Strategy in General Surgery*, vol 1. New York, Springer-Verlag, 1980.

15. **Berek JS, Hacker NF, Lagasse LD:** Rectosigmoid colostomy and reanastomosis to facilitate resection of primary and recurrent gynecologic cancer. *Obstet Gynecol* 64:715, 1984.

16. **Richie JP, Withers G, Ehrlich RM:** Ureteral obstruction secondary to metastatic tumors. *Surg Gynecol Obstet* 148:355, 1979.

17. **Buchsbaum HJ, Schmidt JD:** *Gynecologic and Obstetric Urology*. Philadelphia, WB Saunders, 1978.

18. **Mattingly RF, Borkowf HI:** Acute operative injury to the lower urinary tract. *Clin Obstet Gynecol* 5:123, 1978.

19. **Kearney GP:** Urinary tract involvement in gynecologic oncology. In Knapp RC, Berkowitz RS (eds): *Gynecologic Oncology*. New York, Macmillan, 1986, pp 447–469.

20. **Dudley BS, Gershenson DM, Kavanauh JJ, et al:** Percutaneous nephrostomy catheter in gynecologic malignancy: M.D. Anderson Hospital experience. *Gynecol Oncol* 24:273, 1986.

21. **Finney RP:** Experience with a new double-J ureteral catheter stent. *J Urol* 120:678, 1978.

22. **Prout GR, Koontz WW:** Partial vesical immobilization: an important adjunct in ureteroneocystostomy. *J Urol* 115:136, 1976.

23. **Mattingly RW:** Operative injuries of the ureters. In Mattingly RW (ed): *Telinde's Operative Gynecology*. Philadelphia, JB Lippincott, 1977, pp 291–307.

24. **Hendren WH, Henske TW:** Transureteroureterostomy: experience with 75 cases. *J Urol* 123:826, 1980.

25. **Bricker EM:** Bladder substitution after pelvic evisceration. *Surg Clin North Am* 30:1511, 1950.

26. **Schmidt JD, Buchsbaum HJ, Jacoby EC:** Transverse colon conduit for supravesical urinary tract diversion. *Urology* 8:542, 1976.

27. **Skinner DG, Boyd SD, Lieskovsky G:** Clinical experience with the Kock continent ileal reservoir for urinary diversion. *J Urol* 132:1101, 1984.

28. **Rowland RG, Mitchell ME, Bihrle R, et al:** Indiana continent urinary reservoir. *J Urol* 137:1136, 1987.

29. **Penalver MA, Bejany DE, Averette HE, et al:** Continent urinary diversion in gynecologic oncology. *Gynecol Oncol* 34:274, 1989.

30. **Berek JS, Hacker NF, Lagasse LD:** Reconstructive pelvic surgery. In Knapp RC, Berkowitz RS (eds): *Gynecologic Oncology*, ed 2. New York, McGraw-Hill, 1993, pp 420–431.

31. **Berek JS, Hacker NF, Lagasse LD:** Vaginal reconstruction performed simultaneously with pelvic exenteration. *Obstet Gynecol* 63:318, 1984.

32. **Berek JS, Hacker NF, Lagasse LD, Smith ML:** Delayed vaginal reconstruction in the fibrotic pelvis following radiation or previous reconstruction. *Obstet Gynecol* 61:743, 1983.

33. **Hatch KD:** Construction of a neovagina after exenteration using the vulvobulbocavernosus myocutaneous graft. *Obstet Gynecol* 63:110, 1984.

34. **White AJ, Buchsbaum HJ, Blyth JF, Lifshitz S:** Use of the bulbocavernosus muscle (Martius procedure) for repair of radiation-induced rectovaginal fistulas. *Obstet Gynecol* 60:114, 1982.

35. **Chafe W, Fowler WC, Walton LA, Currie JL:** Radical vulvectomy with use of tensor fascia lata myocutaneous flap. *Am J Obstet Gynecol* 145:207, 1983.

36. **Barnhill DR, Hoskins WJ, Metz P:** Use of the rhomboid flap after partial vulvectomy. *Obstet Gynecol* 62:440, 1983.

37. **Day TG, Stanhope R:** Vulvovaginoplasty in gynecologic oncology. *Obstet Gynecol* 50:361, 1977.

16 Preoperative Evaluation, Medical Management and Critical Care

Samuel A. Skootsky
John A. Glaspy

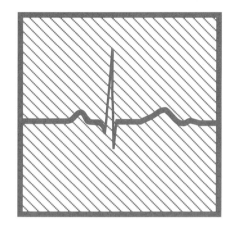

The high incidence of medical problems in gynecologic oncology patients at the time of presentation, coupled with the stresses of aggressive surgical and chemotherapeutic management, necessitates careful monitoring of the patients' medical status. The early identification, evaluation, and management of emerging medical problems are essential, especially in the perioperative period. Comprehensive preoperative evaluation is critical. Those problems most frequently encountered in patients with gynecologic cancers are discussed.

Preoperative Evaluation

The cornerstone of critical care is the anticipation of specific problems. Careful monitoring of patients at risk in the perioperative period minimizes morbidity and mortality.

Cardiovascular

Surgery can represent a major cardiovascular stress because of depression in myocardial contractility, changes in sympathetic tone induced by general anesthetic agents, and rapid changes in intravascular volume due to blood loss and "third spacing" of fluids. The magnitude of cardiovascular stress depends on the nature of the operation, its duration, and whether or not it is elective or emergent (1–3).

Cardiovascular Risk Factors

Goldman et al. (4) identified cardiac risk factors (Table 16.1) by studying 1001 patients over 40 years old who underwent noncardiac surgery. The points assigned to each factor represent the coefficients from the statistical test used. A larger number represents a factor with greater influence over the risk of cardiac complication or death. **A recent myocardial infarction or signs of congestive heart**

561

Table 16.1   Risk Factors for Postoperative Cardiac Complications

Original Multifactorial Index	Points	Modified Multifactorial Index	Points
History		Coronary artery disease	
Myocardial infarction within 6 months	10	MI within 6 months	10
Age > 70	5	MI after > 6 months	5
		CCS angina class III	10
Physical examination		CCS angina class IV	20
S_3 or jugular venous distention	11		
Important aortic stenosis	3	Alveolar pulmonary edema	
		Within 6 months	10
Electrocardiogram		Ever	5
Rhythm other than sinus or sinus plus APBs on last preop. ECG	7	Valvular disease	
		Suspected critical aortic stenosis	20
More than five PVBs/min preop.	7	Electrocardiogram: rhythm other than sinus or sinus plus APBs on last preop. ECG	5
Poor medical status*	3		
		More than 5 PVBs/min preop.	5
Intraperitoneal, intrathoracic, or aortic surgery	3		
		Poor medical status*	5
Emergency operation	4		
		Age > 70	5
		Emergency operation	10
Total points	**53**	**Total points**	**125**

Reproduced, with permission, from Detsky AS, Abrams HB, McLaughlin JR, et al: Predicting cardiac complications in patients undergoing non-cardiac surgery. *J Gen Intern Med* 1:212, 1986.

Abbreviations: APB, atrial premature beat; CCC, Canadian Cardiovascular Society; ECG, electrocardiogram; MI, myocardial infarction; PVB, premature ventricular beats.

*PO_2: < 60 mm Hg; PCO_2 > 50 mm Hg; K < 3.0 mEq/L; HCO_3 < 20 mEq/L; BUN > 50 mg/dl; creatinine > 3 mg/dl; abnormal SGOT; signs of chronic liver disease; bedridden from noncardiac cause.

failure (S_3 or jugular venous distention) had the greatest influence. In the setting of vascular surgery, angina, diabetes, and a Q wave on an electrocardiogram have been proposed as additional clinical risk factors (5). Three studies have attempted to validate the original index (6–8). One of these studies proposed a modified risk factor scale (Table 16.1) (8). This modified risk factor scale is somewhat more clinically useful and includes unstable anginal syndromes, remote myocardial infarction, and pulmonary edema. With use of the assigned points, three score classes were identified, and they represent increasing cardiac risk (Tables 16.2 and 16.3).

In general, an increasing point score is associated with increased risk. Each point class of the modified risk factor scale is associated with a likelihood ratio (Table 16.3). The likelihood ratio is the relative risk of cardiac complications in that point class, compared with the average risk of all patients being rated. Thus the likelihood ratios provide information on the risk of a given patient compared with all patients.

In using these data to predict postoperative cardiac complications, one must take into account that some surgical procedures have more inherent cardiac risk than others (9).

The overall cardiac complication rate varies among institutions, patient populations, and types of surgery. For comparison, the average cardiac complication rate was 11% in a study of patients undergoing abdominal aortic surgery (3), but 3.1% and 5.8% in a study of patients undergoing various noncardiac procedures (4,7). **The overall cardiac complication rate for gynecologic oncology operations is probably similar to that for general surgical operations, about 5%.**

The nomogram in Figure 16.1 can be used to determine the preoperative risk. By means of a straight edge, the estimate of the average cardiac complication rate of gynecologic oncology surgery is used as the left anchor. With the edge set through the patient's point score or likelihood ratio (from the modified index), the estimated postoperative complication rate is defined on the right. Ideally, the estimate of the average cardiac complication rate for gynecologic oncology surgery would be based on data from the local institution where the surgery is performed, rather than on national averages. The cardiac complication rate from one series of general surgery patients in the format of percentages rather than likelihood ratios is presented in Table 16.2.

The details of the calculations are not as important as the concept that important patient risk factors have been identified and that they appear to be valid. However, there are limitations in the predictive value of these indexes. The cardiac risk index may not be valid in the evaluation of critically ill or unstable patients, inasmuch as the data were derived from patients who were clinically stable. Also, the cardiac risk index does not take into account the interventions of the anesthesiologist or internist. Although not proven by specific studies, most clinicians believe that appropriate interventions do lessen the risk of postoperative complications.

In a practical sense, the preoperative evaluation of any patient should include questioning for the factors listed in the cardiac risk indexes, because these have been validated and shown to be related to the majority of cardiac risk. Once

Table 16.2 Cardiac Risk Index: Relationship to Perioperative Cardiac Complications

Class (N)	Point Total	None or Only Minor Complications (N = 943)	Life-Threatening Complications* (N = 39)	Cardiac Deaths (N = 19)
I 537	0–5	532 (99%)	4 (0.7%)	1 (0.2%)
II 316	6–12	295 (93%)	16 (5%)	5 (2%)
III 130	13–25	112 (86%)	15 (11%)	3 (2%)
IV 18	> 26	4 (22%)	4 (22%)	10 (56%)

Reproduced, with permission, from Goldman L, Caldera DL, Nussbaum SR, et al.: Multifactorial index of cardiac risk in noncardiac surgical procedures. *N Engl J Med* 297:845, 1977.
*Documented intraoperative or postoperative myocardial infarction, pulmonary edema, or ventricular tachycardia without progression to cardiac death.

Table 16.3 Relative Risk Using Modified Cardiac Risk Factors*

Class (points)	Major Surgery†	Minor Surgery†	All Surgery†
I (0–15)	0.42	0.39	0.43
II (15–30)	3.58	2.75	3.38
III (> 30)	14.93	12.20	10.60

Adapted, with permission, from Detsky AS, Abrams HB, McLaughlin JR et al.: Predicting cardiac complications in patients undergoing non-cardiac surgery. *J Gen Intern Med* 1:212, 1986.
*Derived from a series of patients in whom the overall cardiac complication rate (myocardial infarction, pulmonary edema, ventricular tachycardia or fibrillation requiring treatment, cardiac death) was 10 percent.
†Relative risk of a patient within one point class relative to all patients. The use of these data to predict the rate of postoperative cardiac complications requires the use of a nomogram.

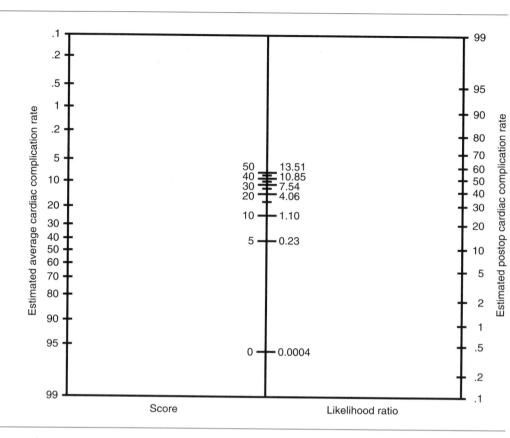

Figure 16.1   Nomogram for predicting postoperative cardiac complications. (Reproduced, with permission, from Detsky AS, Abrams HB, McLaughlin JR, et al: Predicting cardiac complications in patients undergoing non-cardiac surgery. *J Gen Intern Med* 1:212, 1986.)

identified, patients can be stratified (Table 16.2 or 16.3). **In general, patients within the lowest point classifications (Class I in either the Goldman or Detsky schemes) can proceed with surgery. Patients in higher point classes would likely benefit from further evaluation. The surgeon should be wary when patients are in high point classes or have two or more of the following:**

1. Age over 70 years

2. History of ventricular ectopic activity requiring therapy

3. Diabetes requiring other than dietary therapy

4. History of angina, especially if therapy is required

5. Q wave on preoperative electrocardiogram

These factors have been shown to identify a subset of patients at high risk of complications from vascular surgery (5). Although the relevance of these data to gynecologic oncology surgery patients is unknown, these factors probably do identify patients more likely to have significant cardiac disease worthy of evaluation. An algorithm for the evaluation of cardiovascular status is presented in Figure 16.2.

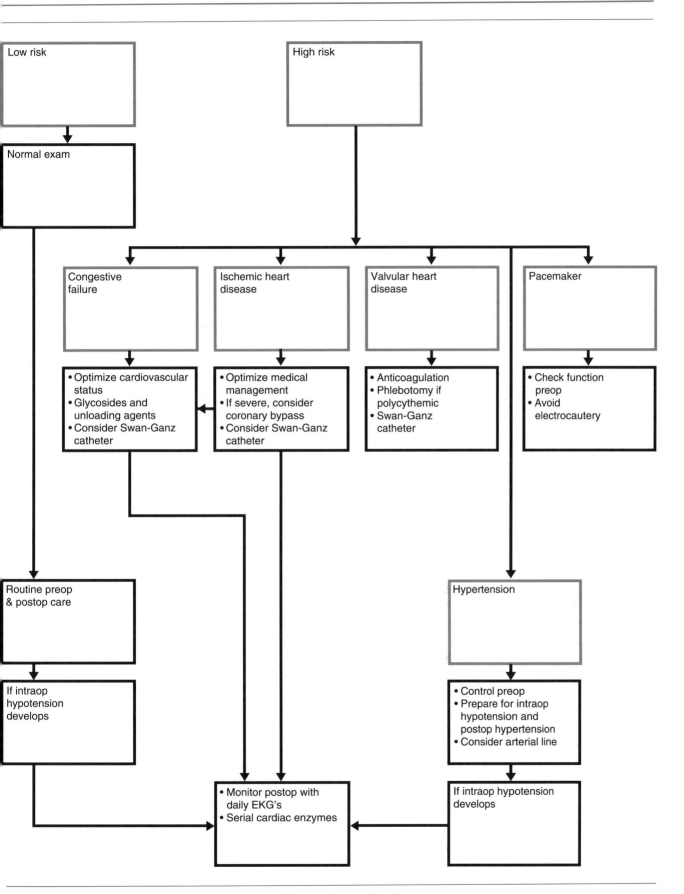

Figure 16.2   Cardiovascular evaluation.

Myocardial Infarction

Postoperative myocardial infarction can be expected in 0.2% of patients undergoing surgery with general anesthesia (3, 10, 11). In the review by Goldman et al. (12), preoperative patient characteristics predictive of postoperative or intraoperative myocardial infarction included:

1. Age over 70 years

2. Pulmonary edema

3. More than five premature contractions per minute documented any time preoperatively

4. A grade II/IV or louder mitral regurgitation murmur

5. Tortuous or calcified aorta on chest radiograph

The risks of postoperative myocardial infarction and of cardiac death increase when surgery is performed after a recent myocardial infarction, especially if the interval between infarction and surgery is less than 6 months. In one study, the risk of myocardial infarction after anesthesia and general surgery was 27% if patients were operated on within 3 months of a previous infarction, 11% if the surgery was delayed 3 to 6 months, and 5% if surgery was delayed more than 6 months (1). There is evidence that this increased risk is decreased substantially by previous coronary artery bypass surgery (12–14).

Postoperative myocardial infarction can be painless in one-third to one-half of the patients (1, 12). **The risk of infarction peaks on the third postoperative day and remains high on the fifth postoperative day** (3). Hence, it is prudent to identify patients at risk of postoperative myocardial infarction and to monitor them with daily electrocardiograms. In especially high-risk patients, serial cardiac enzyme levels should be determined, even in the absence of chest pain.

Because the risk of perioperative myocardial infarction is increased in patients who are subjected to intraoperative hypotension (1, 15), measures must be taken to maintain high-risk patients in a normotensive state during surgery. If intraoperative hypotension (defined as a decrease in systolic blood pressure of 33–50% or more for at least 10 minutes) occurs, the patient should be considered at high risk of postoperative infarction and monitored appropriately. Such reductions in blood pressure during surgery should be rare with modern anesthetic management.

Theoretically, β-blockers would be expected to facilitate the development of intraoperative hypotension because of the additive myocardial depression of these medications with general anesthesia. However, it has been demonstrated that patients tolerate general anesthesia in the presence of continued β-blocker treatment (16) and that abrupt discontinuation of β-blocker medication is associated with a dangerous rebound syndrome (i.e., acute hypertension and angina), with the incidence of the syndrome peaking at 4 to 7 days after discontinuation of the drug (17).

Congestive Heart Failure

Patients with moderate or severe congestive heart failure should be treated preoperatively with appropriate medications to optimize their cardiovascular status. In severe cases, particularly in patients with jugular venous distention, a third heart sound, or valvular heart disease, preoperative placement of a *pulmonary artery (Swan-Ganz) catheter* should be considered to allow cardiac function to be optimized and also to aid in the intraoperative management of fluids and cardiac medications.

Heart Block

Third-Degree Heart Block   Patients who do not have permanent pacemakers and who have third-degree heart block at the time of presentation are at substantial risk of cardiopulmonary arrest during surgery. Typically, they are unable to mount an appropriate pulse response to the vasodilatation and decreased myocardial contractibility induced by general anesthesia or to the volume depletion induced by surgical blood loss. Patients with complete heart block should not be subjected to general surgery without appropriate medical consultation, and strong consideration should be given to preoperative placement of a pacemaker.

Bifascicular Block   In patients with lower degrees of heart block, specifically *bifascicular block (right heart block with left axis deviation)*, the risk of development of a higher degree of ventricular block during surgery is not significantly increased, provided there is no history of previous third-degree heart block or syncope. Such patients rarely require insertion of a temporary pacemaker (12, 18). Patients with bifascicular block who have a history of third-degree heart block should be managed for complete heart block with preoperative cardiology evaluation and pacemaker insertion.

A new bifascicular block developing in the setting of acute myocardial infarction carries a high risk of progression to complete heart block. If this problem occurs postoperatively, the patient should be considered at significant risk for the development of complete atrial-ventricular block. Such patients require a cardiology consultation and insertion of a temporary pacemaker (19).

Patients with permanently implanted pacemakers should have a preoperative cardiology evaluation to allow examination of all pacemaker functions. This precaution will ensure that backup demand pacemaker failure will not be uncovered unexpectedly with the vagotonic stimuli associated with general anesthesia in abdominal surgery (20).

Pacemakers can sense the electromagnetic impulses created by electrocautery, especially when the electrocautery plate is close to the pacemaker unit. It is prudent to place the indifferent electrocautery electrode as far as possible from the chest and to use electrocautery sparingly. An added precaution is introduced if a magnet is available in the operating room to rapidly convert a pacemaker from the demand to a fixed pacing mode if the need arises (21).

Hypertension

The significance of hypertension in patients undergoing surgery remains controversial. This controversy stems from the difficulty in sorting out the risk of hypertension *per se* from the risk of hypertension in the setting of hypertensive or atherosclerotic heart disease.

A large prospective study suggests that uncomplicated mild to moderate hypertension, regardless of treatment status, does not seem to impose an added risk of postoperative cardiac or renal complications (12, 22). However, the presence of hypertension may be of consequence because such patients frequently demonstrate marked intraoperative blood pressure lability and postoperative hypertensive episodes. Blood pressure lability and postoperative hypertension is more frequently associated with major vascular surgery and should be less of a problem with other surgery.

Patients with hypertensive and atherosclerotic heart disease may be at greater risk than those with uncomplicated hypertension. Two studies suggest that postoperative myocardial infarction may be more frequent in patients with hypertension who have underlying heart disease (1, 15). In these patients, postoperative myocardial infarction was related to thoracic and upper abdominal procedures, anesthesia time > 3–4 hours, and significant intraoperative hypotension. As is the case with cardiac complications, the type of surgery is important in understanding the risk of hypertension. Hypotension remains a concern, especially if spinal anesthesia is used.

Hypertensive management begins with identification and then with the development of a plan for control. The patient's blood pressure should be controlled preoperatively as well as possible (23). In general, all antihypertensive medications should be given on the morning of surgery. The question of whether or not chronic diuretics should be given has not been settled but most clinicians do not give them. Although diuretic use is associated with volume depletion and hypokalemia, the importance of correcting mild degrees of diuretic-induced hypokalemia in the absence of significant heart disease is somewhat controversial (24). Repletion should never be rapid and is safest by the oral route or by adjustment of medication.

In the postoperative period, many patients, especially the elderly, will need less antihypertensive medication because of the salutary effects of bed rest and relative sodium restriction. It is wise to reinstate drugs stepwise, beginning with the most active and ending with the diuretic. Patients whose only antihypertensive drug is a thiazide diuretic are best observed in the immediate postoperative period. Certain drugs, such as propranolol and clonidine, have well-recognized abrupt withdrawal syndromes, which can lead to acute myocardial ischemia (especially propranolol), hypertension (especially clonidine), or both. These drugs should be given orally on the morning of surgery and reinstated as soon as possible postoperatively. The use of transdermal clonidine for those patients who are stabilized on clonidine is useful in some cases, but not routinely. Patients who need antihypertensive therapy in the immediate preoperative period should not be treated with diuretics (because of the associated hypovolemia and hypokalemia).

Perioperative hypertensive episodes will occur in about 25% of hypertensive patients. Perioperative hypertension is most common during laryngoscopy and induction (primarily because of sympathetic stimulation) and immediately postoperatively, often in the recovery room. The most important pretreatment consideration is to determine the cause (Table 16.4). In many patients postoperative hypertension will be due to or exacerbated by pain, anxiety, or emergence from anesthesia. Adequacy of ventilation and stable cardiac status should be verified by examination, arterial blood gases, and electrocardiogram. Unrelieved bladder distention can cause hypertension.

Recently, the calcium channel blocker nifedipine has been proposed for treatment of postoperative hypertensive episodes when given by the sublingual route (25), but this can lead to reflex tachycardia and myocardial ischemia. Intravenous short-acting β-blockers and vasodilators (e.g., hydralazine) are often used in the re-

Table 16.4   Causes of Perioperative Hypertension

Cause	Recognition
Chronic hypertension	History, medication review
Laryngoscopy and intubation	Situation
Inadequate anesthesia	Situation
Inadequate ventilation	Arterial blood gas
Pain or anxiety	Patient examination and interview
Bladder distention	Bladder palpation
Emergence from anesthesia	Situation
Excessive fluid administration	OR records, patient examination
Postoperative fluid mobilization	Situation, patient examination
Acute cardiac events (e.g., congestive heart failure)	Patient examination, ECG, chest radiograph
Pheochromocytoma (rare—can be occult)	Unusual clinical responses
Malignant hyperthermia	Unusual clinical responses, fever

covery room and can be considered. Patients with pain and anxiety are best treated with narcotic analgesics. No one agent is best for all situations. It is important for the surgeon to remember that many hypertensive episodes will resolve spontaneously (26).

Pulmonary

General anesthesia and abdominal surgery can compromise respiratory function in all patients. In those with preexisting lung disease, this added stress can precipitate potentially fatal pulmonary complications. Pathophysiologic processes associated with surgery include (27–32):

1. A decrease in lung volume, including vital capacity

2. A decrease in functional residual capacity

3. Shallow, rapid respiration with decreased sighing and atelectasis

4. An alteration in ventilation and perfusion relationships, with a decrease in arterial oxygen saturation

5. A decreased clearance of bacteria because of decreased coughing and impaired ciliary function

These impairments in normal lung function can persist into the second postoperative week and are related to pain, analgesic medications, the supine position, and tight abdominal bandages (33). Postoperative pulmonary complications can occur in up to 70% of high-risk patients undergoing upper abdominal surgery. These include pneumonia and deterioration of arterial blood gases secondary to atelectasis and altered pulmonary physiology (34).

Pulmonary Risk Factors

The study of pulmonary risk factors lacks the multivariate approach that has been applied to the study of cardiac risk. However, sufficient data exist to identify a

569

number of clinical factors associated with perioperative pulmonary complications (35, 36). These are:

1. the anatomic site of surgery (upper abdominal and thoracic surgery having the most complications)

2. smoking cigarettes

3. chronic obstructive lung disease (including asthma)

4. hypercapnia

5. obesity

6. prolonged anesthesia time

7. normal aging (although the effect is less certain)

Abdominal surgery is associated with significant risk of pulmonary complications. Postoperatively, vital capacity (VC) is reduced by 50–60% and functional residual capacity (FRC) is reduced by 20–30%. Approximately one-third of these changes may be related to supine positioning. In one recent study of patients undergoing upper abdominal surgery without any prophylactic measures (38), 48% had postoperative pulmonary complications. This complication rate was reduced considerably by any of several prophylactic measures but was still approximately 20% in the treatment groups. The mechanisms responsible for the high rate of pulmonary complications after upper abdominal surgery have been a subject of great interest. Studies have emphasized that diaphragmatic dysfunction secondary to reduced phrenic nerve output may be an important factor (34).

Current smokers with a history of smoking cigarettes for more than 20 pack-years, or more than one pack a day, appear to have an increased rate of postoperative pulmonary complications. To ameliorate this risk, patients undergoing major oncologic surgery need to stop smoking for at least 8 weeks before the surgery (39).

Patients with chronic obstructive lung disease are at increased risk of postoperative complications. In this group of patients, an increased risk has been associated with:

1. forced vital capacity (FVC) < 70% of predicted

2. a forced expiratory volume (FEV1 %) < 70% of predicted

3. a maximum voluntary ventilation (MVV) < 50% of predicted

4. hypercapnia

However, a recent review concluded that most of the studies on which these cutoff values are based have serious methodologic flaws (40). There is agreement that patients with chronic lung disease, as a group, do have more postoperative pulmonary complications. Among patients with chronic obstructive lung disease, however, the predictive value of abnormal spirometry to identify the subgroup at risk of postoperative complications is poor (41). To the extent that obtaining screening spirometry helps to identify all patients with underlying lung disease who can then receive appropriate preventive measures, a benefit should accrue. For example, a program of preoperative and postoperative treatment that includes smoking cessation, antibiotics, bronchodilation, and chest physiotherapy has been shown to reduce complications significantly (42). Early ambulation is also important.

Normal aging has traditionally been considered a risk factor for pulmonary complications. Physiologic changes associated with normal aging include a reduction in vital capacity, mild hypoxemia, and possible loss of protective airway reflexes (2). However, there is literature to suggest that, when controlled for co-morbidity and pulmonary function (43), age *per se* may not confer independent risk.

Obesity, even if mild, appears to be associated with an increased risk of postoperative atelectasis (44). The obese have a reduced functional residual capacity (FRC) and a reduced effective residual volume (ERV). The reduced ERV frequently results in normal tidal breathing below the closing volume (the lung volume at which airways are believed to undergo closure) and produces a widening of the A–a gradient and hypoxemia. More significant complications, such as pneumonia, are associated with patient weight over 115 kg (45). Postoperative hypoxemia may be more severe or prolonged (46). Even modest weight loss (e.g., 5–10 kg) may reduce the rate of complications (47).

Anesthesia time > 3–4 hours has been reported as a pulmonary risk (1), **even when the site of surgery is considered** (12). For upper abdominal incisions, some older data are conflicting (48).

In practical terms, the preoperative pulmonary evaluation should first be directed at identifying the clinical risk factors (42, 50–53).

1. Patients with chronic pulmonary disease should be free of acute infection (e.g., bronchitis) and should be treated preoperatively with antibiotics if necessary.

2. Smoking cessation should be encouraged, ideally 8 weeks preoperatively.

3. Weight loss is useful and should be encouraged, but it is difficult to accomplish, takes time, and usually is not practical, given the urgency of oncologic surgery.

4. Although screening spirometry does not substitute for history taking and examination, candidates for screening include those patients with symptoms suggestive of pulmonary disease, heavy smokers, those with a productive cough, and the morbidly obese.

5. Patients with abnormal spirometry should have blood gas determinations.

6. Elderly patients who have no symptoms probably do not need screening spirometry before extrafascial hysterectomy, although mild hypoxemia and propensity to atelectasis should be assumed.

7. Patient education is important and should emphasize familiarization with the management plans, especially such respiratory maneuvers as incentive spirometry.

8. Incentive spirometry, because it is inexpensive, effective, and without complications, should be ordered for all patients with risk factors, including the elderly who are otherwise free of symptoms.

In the preoperative and postoperative management of high-risk patients intermittent positive pressure breathing (IPPB) is not superior to the simple use of incentive spirometry, and it may increase the risk of complications (50).

A summary of guidelines to reduce pulmonary complications is presented in Table 16.5. Patients with asthma deserve special comment. **Asthmatic patients are at increased risk of postoperative complications but can do well with proper preparation and postoperative care (49).** The major problems involve exacerbations of asthma, especially as a result of endotracheal intubation or in the immediate postoperative period, and proper steroid coverage is essential if adrenal suppression is suspected. The basic preoperative goal is absence of wheezing on examination, which usually corresponds to the patient's best physical status and pulmonary function. Achievement of this goal may require adjustment of oral or inhaled steroids, inhaled beta agonist, and/or oral theophylline. Modern ambulatory therapy for patients with chronic asthma emphasizes the use of inhaled steroids to suppress bronchial hyperresponsiveness and beta agonists for the symptomatic relief of acute exacerbations.

Stable asthmatic patients who take steroids should receive their usual inhaled dose, or their oral dose should be given intravenously the morning of surgery. Beta agonist inhalational therapy (e.g., albuterol, 2.5 mg/3 ml of normal saline solution or with the patient's own metered-dose inhaler) is also indicated. In the recovery room, exacerbations should be treated initially with beta agonist inhalational therapy. If wheezing persists, intravenous steroids in modest doses (e.g., prednisone 30–60 mg every 6–8 hours) may be added. Patients with adrenal

---

Table 16.5   Measures to Reduce Pulmonary Complications

Preoperative
Identification of patients at risk
Consider screening spirometry for those with risk factors
Patient education to assure optimal pre- and postoperative compliance and performance
Cessation of smoking
Instruction in incentive spirometry
Bronchodilation (e.g., beta agonist via inhaler)
Antibiotics for bronchitis
Control of secretions
Weight reduction

Intraoperative
Avoidance of prolonged anesthesia
Avoidance of aspiration
Maintenance of bronchodilation
Intermittent hyperinflation

Postoperative
Continuation of preoperative measures, especially encouragement of incentive spirometry
Early ambulation
Pain control
Attention to the effects of analgesia on respiration

Adapted, with permission, from Tisi GM: Preoperative evaluation of pulmonary function. *Am Rev Respir Dis* 119:293, 1979.

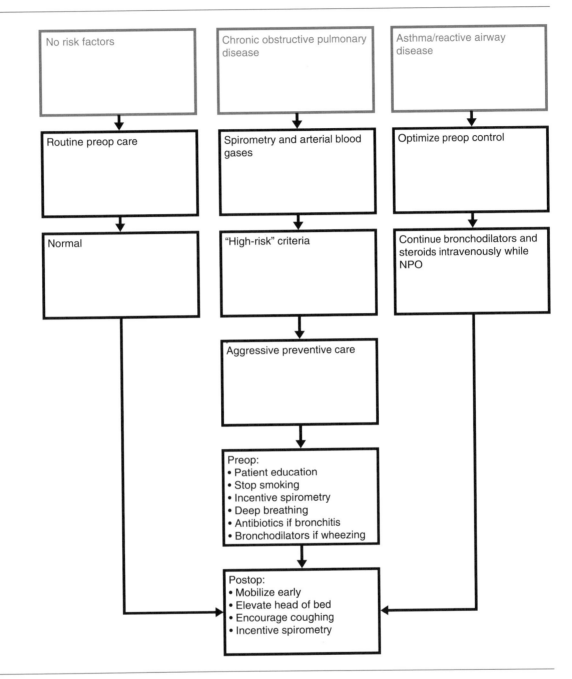

Figure 16.3   Pulmonary evaluation and postoperative care.

suppression will need appropriate coverage (see section concerning corticosteroids). Postoperative beta agonist therapy should be continued for all patients.

An algorithm for the perioperative management of patients with lung disease is presented in Figure 16.3.

Diabetes Mellitus   Diabetes mellitus affects approximately 5% of the adult population in the United States of America. It is now believed that type I diabetes is an autoimmune disease. Persons with type I diabetes have a near total lack of insulin and will develop ketoacidosis if insulin is withheld. They are usually, but not always, young. Persons with type II diabetes are not insulin deficient and thus are not prone to ketoacidosis. The problem in type II diabetes is usually one of relative insulin resistance. Type II diabetics are usually older and overweight. Both groups may develop the complications listed in Table 16.6. It is important to remember that many elderly patients have mild type II diabetes of recent onset related to obesity, are well controlled with diet or oral hypoglycemic drugs, have few overt complications, but may have occult atherosclerotic vascular disease.

The management of diabetes begins with some understanding of the factors that influence perioperative glucose metabolism (54–56). Insulin is the principal glucose-lowering hormone; cortisol, glucagon, growth hormone, and catecholamine are the principal glucose-raising hormones. In the preoperative period, stress and the "dawn" phenomenon may elevate blood glucose. The "dawn" phenomenon is early morning hyperglycemia resulting from nocturnal surges of growth hormone. Intraoperatively, cortisol and growth hormone levels rise. In this period there is hyperglycemia in diabetics and nondiabetics alike. This is caused by glycogenolysis, inhibition of glucose uptake, and decreased insulin release. Postoperatively, in nondiabetics, the hyperglycemia is brought under control by increased endogenous insulin release over a period of 4–6 hours. Diabetics may need additional exogenous insulin.

In addition to these hormonal factors, several other factors are important in modulating the blood glucose level in the perioperative period. Inactivity, stress, and intravenous glucose infusions will tend to raise blood glucose. Decreased caloric intake and semistarvation will tend to lower blood glucose. Because the net effect of these factors is sometimes difficult to anticipate, an important rule is to frequently monitor blood glucose levels.

The goal of management is a blood glucose value of not more than 180–240 mg/dl. This level is chosen because severe glucosuria (and risk of dehydration) is prevented. Furthermore, experimental studies suggest that glucose levels > 240 mg/dl may impair the phagocytic function of leukocytes (57). Finally, experimental studies suggest that hypoinsulinemia may impair wound healing.

The management of the diabetic patient who takes insulin is presented in Table 16.7. It is important to reduce the total daily dose of insulin because caloric intake on the day of surgery will be reduced (58) (hence the recommendation

Table 16.6 Complications of Diabetes	
Complication	*Importance*
Cataracts	Decreased vision
Retinopathy	Decreased vision
Nephropathy	Nephrotic syndrome, hyperkalemia, metabolic acidosis, reduced glomerular filtration rate
Peripheral neuropathy	Decreased peripheral nociception, susceptibility to infection
Autonomic neuropathy	Orthostatic hypotension, gastropathy (delayed gastric emptying, diarrhea), uropathy (urinary retention, overflow incontinence, infection), cardiorespiratory arrest
Coronary artery disease	Silent ischemia, myocardial infarction
Vascular disease	Peripheral arterial insufficiency, coronary artery disease, stroke

Table 16.7   Details of Perioperative Insulin Management for Well-Controlled Patients Taking Insulin

Preoperative

1. Plan for surgery early in the day

2. Measure early AM glucose
(use sliding-scale insulin for glucose > 200–250 mg/dl)

3. Use one-third of NPH (or equivalent) insulin subcutaneously

4. Start D5W at 125 ml/hour

Intraoperative

5. Measure intraoperative glucose frequently (e.g., every 2 hours) and make adjustments

Postoperative

6. Measure recovery room glucose
(use sliding-scale insulin for glucose > 200–250 mg/dl)

7. Measure postoperative glucose every 6 hours
(use sliding-scale insulin for glucose > 250 mg/dl)

8. Use regular insulin according to sliding scale as needed

9. Use one-third of NPH 8–12 hours after AM dose

10. Continue regimen until patient begins to eat (usually next morning)

11. Return to previous regimen incrementally beginning in AM if eating

that one-third of the normal daily dose be given on the morning of surgery and another similar dose 8–12 hours after the first). If control of diabetes is known to be poor, one-half the normal daily dose can be given (unless the reason for the poor control is too much insulin). The need for additional insulin immediately after surgery is anticipated by measurement of glucose level in the recovery room. Care must be taken to restart the normal daily dose while the patient is hospitalized. Hypoglycemia may result if caloric intake is reduced because of discomfort or missed meals. The importance of postoperative blood glucose monitoring every 6 hours (or before each meal if the patient is eating) cannot be overemphasized. This allows the physician to make appropriate adjustments in therapy.

Details of the management of the diabetic who is taking an oral hypoglycemic are presented in Table 16.8. Patients with very well controlled diabetes who take oral agents are at risk of hypoglycemia if an oral hypoglycemic agent is given while the caloric intake is reduced. This is why the oral agent should be withheld on the day of surgery. Oral agents with a long duration of action should be withheld longer (see Table 16.9). As is the case with patients who are taking insulin, care must be taken to restart the normal daily dose while the patient is hospitalized, because the usual dose of oral agent given in the setting of reduced caloric intake may lead to hypoglycemia. This management plan relates to patients whom the surgeon plans to send postoperatively to a general hospital ward.

If a patient is critically ill postoperatively, it is difficult to anticipate the insulin needs resulting from stress and varying caloric loads. Some poorly controlled patients may require urgent or emergency surgery. In these situations, continuous infusion of insulin by pump is probably worthwhile. The patient should be adequately hydrated (dehydration by itself will potentiate hyperglycemia in diabetics secondary to alterations in renal clearance of glucose) and given 5 units of insulin

Table 16.8   Details of Perioperative Diabetes Management for Well-Controlled Patients Taking Oral Hypoglycemics

Preoperative

1. Plan for surgery early in the day

2. Hold oral hypoglycemic on day of surgery;
   long-acting drugs (e.g., chlorpropamide) should be held for 48 hours

3. Measure early AM glucose
   (use sliding-scale insulin for glucose > 200–250 mg/dl)

Intraoperative

5. Measure intraoperative glucose frequently (e.g., every 2 hours).

Postoperative

6. Measure recovery room glucose
   (use sliding-scale insulin for glucose > 200–250 mg/dl)

7. Measure postoperative glucose every 6 hours
   (use sliding-scale insulin for glucose > 200–250 mg/dl)

8. Return to previous regimen incrementally in AM if eating

Table 16.9   Characteristics of Sulfonylureas

Agent	Dose Range (mg)	Duration (hr)	Metabolism
Tolbutamide	500–3000	6–12	Liver
Chlorpropamide	100–500	60	Liver/renal
Acetohexamide	250–1500	12–24	Liver
Tolazamide	100–1000	10–18	Liver
Glyburide	2.5–30	10–30	Liver
Glipizide	5.0–40	18–30	Liver

by intravenous bolus. Regular insulin at 1–5 units per hour should be infused. At blood glucose levels below 250 mg/ml, 5% or 10% glucose in water should be infused to protect against hypoglycemia. Intravenous insulin requires constant monitoring.

Thyroid Disorders

Hypothyroidism is common and may go undetected in patients being prepared for surgery (59). Symptoms include cold intolerance, recent or progressive constipation, hoarseness, fatigability, and changes in cognition. Signs include associated goiter, skin dryness, and a delayed relaxation phase of peripheral reflexes (best demonstrated in the Achilles tendon). Recent studies have suggested that unrecognized mild to moderate hypothyroidism is clinically important, but fears of hyponatremia, prolonged respirator dependency, hypothermia, delayed recovery from anesthesia, or death are probably unwarranted (60, 61). One retrospective study suggested that such patients will have more intraoperative hypotension, postoperative ileus, and confusion and that infection will be less often accompanied by fever.

For patients who are suspected preoperatively of being hypothyroid, thyroid hormone levels should be measured. Hypothyroid patients should be treated with replacement hormone and rendered euthyroid before surgery. In urgent situations, patients who are not myxedematous should be given 1 or 2 days of oral replacement before surgery, with careful postoperative follow-up.

Hyperthyroidism can be a dramatic illness, with tachycardia, fever, and exophthalmos associated with goiter. Other common symptoms and signs include frequent weight loss, fatigue, diarrhea, heat intolerance, tremor, hyperreflexia, and muscle weakness. Hyperthyroidism may be occult in older patients. Unexplained tachycardia, weight loss, arrhythmias, or fever may be the only clinical indicators. With proper preparation (62), hyperthyroid patients undergoing thyroidal surgery do well. However, there are scant data concerning the problems of the hyperthyroid patient undergoing nonthyroidal surgery such as radical hysterectomy. Exacerbation of the illness into a "thyroid storm" is the usual concern. Because of this, when any patient is suspected preoperatively of being hyperthyroid, thyroid hormone levels should be measured. If the diagnosis is confirmed, elective surgery should be delayed until treatment has produced a euthyroid state. In the postoperative period, thyroid hormone levels should be measured when any patient has persistent unexplained tachycardia, fever, or tachyarrhythmias.

Corticosteroids

Patients currently taking corticosteroids or those who have taken them in the recent past should be evaluated for the need of supplemental corticosteroid coverage. In general, patients taking less than the equivalent of 7.5 mg prednisone daily or 40 mg of prednisone on alternate days (63) should not have adrenal suppression. This assumes that a short-acting steroid (e.g., prednisone) is given as a single dose on the morning of surgery. **The amount of steroid needed to cause adrenal suppression is the equivalent of 40 mg of prednisone or more daily for 1 to 2 weeks, or more than 7.5 mg of prednisone daily administered chronically. The recovery from adrenal suppression can take up to nine months** (64). The details of recovery after short courses of high-dose steroid therapy have not been well studied.

Patients who have taken high doses of corticosteroids for more than 1 or 2 weeks within 9 months of surgery are candidates for supplemental steroid coverage. The symptoms of adrenal insufficiency in the postoperative patient can be nonspecific and include fever, nausea, ileus, weakness, and anorexia (65). Because of this, most clinicians err on the side of treatment, as major complications associated with brief steroid coverage are rare.

A suggested regimen of corticosteroid coverage for elective surgery consists of 100 mg of hydrocortisone succinate intravenously on call to the operating room and then the same dose repeated every 8 hours for 24 hours. Assuming that the patient is recovering from surgery uneventfully, the dose is reduced by 50% each day, and then the patient is placed back on her usual steroid dose on the fourth postoperative day.

There are some patients (e.g., those with diabetes) in whom it is important to avoid the unnecessary use of steroids. In these patients, a normal ACTH stimulation test can be used to predict an adequate, but not necessarily normal, response to surgical stress (66). The procedure is to give 250 μg of ACTH intravenously or intramuscularly. The cortisol level is measured immediately before and 30–60 minutes after injection. A normal response is an increase of 12–20 μg/ml.

577

Preoperative Testing

The question of how much preoperative laboratory testing is warranted has been the subject of considerable interest and debate (67–72). The data from these studies confirm that, unless clinical indicators are present, preoperative tests will likely be either normal, falsely positive, or truly positive with no relevance to clinical outcome (70, 71). These studies assume that an "asymptomatic patient" has been identified (i.e., an appropriate negative history and examination are actually obtained). It is recognized that abnormalities do occur in symptom-free patients, but often these are either false-positives or true positives that have no impact on surgical or anesthetic management. The latter case is especially true if age is used as a basis for test ordering.

Preoperative testing *per se* should be directed at uncovering abnormalities that have an impact on surgical or anesthetic management. However, general screening in a population of preoperative patients may often reveal abnormalities that reflect underlying medical conditions worthy of evaluation, although these abnormalities will not always affect surgical or anesthetic management.

Because the prevalence of test abnormalities does increase with age (Table 16.10), age itself is commonly used as a parameter for test ordering. In the older age groups undergoing surgery, many of the traditional preoperative tests can be justified (73). Younger patients generally need few of these tests. Patients with widespread cancer, with or without prior therapy, can have associated coagulation abnormalities; therefore screening for coagulation disturbances is worthwhile. Rappaport (74) argues that in the presence of a negative history, the partial thromboplastin time and platelet count constitute adequate coagulation screening for major surgical procedures. Studies have usually concluded that unexpected coagulation results are rare when the history and physical examination findings are negative (74–76).

Critical Care

Hypertension

Postoperative hypertension, especially severe hypertension lasting longer than 1 hour, is best managed by:

1. Aggressive pain management, usually with narcotics

2. Elimination of hypercarbia via proper ventilatory settings on the respirator

3. Emergence excitement control (i.e., the reduction of sensory stimulation as patients emerge from anesthesia)

4. Intravenous infusion of a vasodilator medication such as nitroprusside, titrated to a diastolic blood pressure of 90 mm Hg

Hypotension and Shock

Shock is defined as a clinical syndrome in which the patient shows signs of decreased perfusion of vital organs, including alterations in mental status with somnolence, and oliguria with an output of < 25 ml/hr. In general, patients with shock evidence a substantial decrease in blood pressure of 50–60 mm Hg, but no absolute value is used to define shock.

578

Table 16.10   Example of the Increase in Prevalence of Preoperative Test Abnormalities by Age; Common Preoperative Laboratory Testing for Anesthesia and Surgery

Test	Indication
Chest radiograph	Age > 60 or clinical history
Electrocardiogram	Age > 40 or clinical history
Creatinine	Age > 40 or clinical history
Glucose	Age > 40 or clinical history
Hematocrit	All females
Complete urinalysis	Clinical history
Electrolytes	Clinical history
Prothrombin time	Anticoagulation or clinical history
Partial thromboplastin time	Anticoagulation or clinical history
Platelet count	Anticoagulation or clinical history

Adapted from Kaplan EB, Sheiner LB, Boeckmann AJ, et al: The usefulness of preoperative laboratory screening. *JAMA* 253:3576, 1985.

The therapeutic approach to these patients is facilitated by a functional classification of shock states. An algorithm for management of the hypotensive patient is presented in Figure 16.4. Each class of shock has its own pathophysiology and requires special acute management. Four varieties of shock have been proposed (77):

1. *Hypovolemic shock*—secondary to bleeding or other fluid losses (e.g., nasogastric suction and diarrhea).

2. *Distributive shock*—secondary to increased venous pooling (e.g., early septic shock, peritonitis, anaphylaxis, and neurogenic shock).

3. *Cardiogenic shock*—secondary to decreased myocardial contractibility and function.

4. *Obstructive shock*—hypoperfusion states secondary to mechanical obstruction (e.g., cardiac tamponade, massive pulmonary embolism, and thrombosed prosthetic valves).

In the perioperative management of patients with gynecologic malignancy, the most common causes of shock are:

1. Hemorrhage (hypovolemia)

2. Sepsis

3. Postoperative myocardial infarction

4. Pulmonary embolus

Hemorrhagic Shock

Adequate volume resuscitation must take place as quickly as possible, because volume repletion with crystalloid or colloid solutions is at least as important as

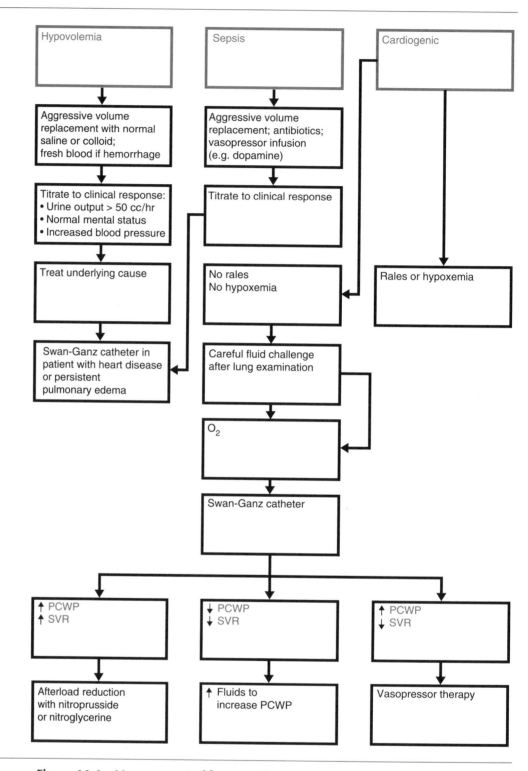

Figure 16.4   Management of hypotension.

the replacement of red cell losses (78). Sufficient volume replacement is more important than the preparation employed, and normal saline solution and Ringer's lactate appear to be equivalent crystalloid preparations (79).

Colloid Versus Crystalloid   There is considerable difference of opinion regarding the relative merits of crystalloid versus colloid solutions in primary resuscitation therapy. Theoretically, aggressive volume replacement with crystalloid solutions risks lowering capillary oncotic pressure and would favor the passage of fluid into the lungs. Because it has been demonstrated that administered radiolabeled albumin leaks into the interstitial spaces, colloid resuscitation would risk increasing pulmonary interstitial oncotic pressure. Several clinical trials have compared crystalloid with colloid fluid management (80–83); these trials have generated contradictory results, and there are no compelling data to support the superiority of either agent in the treatment of hypovolemic shock and in the prevention of postresuscitation pulmonary problems. On a volume basis, approximately half as much colloid solution is required for resuscitation as compared with crystalloid preparations. Colloid therapy has the advantage of efficiency, as it is initially distributed primarily in the intravascular space. Crystalloids have the advantage of ready availability and low cost. **Adequate volume replacement titrated to improvement in blood pressure and urine output and restoration of filling pressures, if they are being monitored, are more important than the preparation used.**

Massive hemorrhage is best treated with fresh red cells rather than with red cells that have been stored for longer than 1 week, as the fresh product is more efficient at oxygen delivery.

Septic Shock

Septic shock has a complex pathophysiology involving:

1. The release of vasoactive kinins with vasodilatation

2. Activation of complement causing increased vascular permeability

3. Activation of the intrinsic clotting cascade with disseminated intravascular coagulation

4. Induction of a fibrinolytic state with bleeding

In the early stages, septic shock is best understood as a form of distributive shock. In the later stages, these patients show evidence of myocardial depression from ischemia associated with hypotension, acidosis, and possibly myocardial depressant factors produced by the infecting organisms. In this phase, septic shock becomes more complicated and can show a mixed picture of distributive and cardiogenic shock.

The treatment of patients with septic shock involves:

1. Aggressive fluid replacement

2. Treatment with vasopressor and inotropic agents

3. Appropriate coverage with broad-spectrum antibiotics

4. Removal of the source of infection (e.g., abscess or infected indwelling venous catheters)

Controversial and unproven aspects of the therapy of septic shock include the use of corticosteroids (84, 85), antiserum to the lipid A portion of gram-negative bacterial endotoxin (86), and naloxone (87).

Cardiogenic Shock

In its pure form, cardiogenic shock presents a complicated problem, and therapy is aimed at optimizing cardiac output. It is important to note that cardiogenic shock can complicate septic shock or hemorrhagic shock; especially in patients with baseline cardiovascular disease.

Appropriate management of cardiogenic shock requires invasive monitoring. Patients with presumed cardiogenic shock who do not have evidence of pulmonary edema on physical examination can be managed initially with careful volume repletion guided by frequent lung examinations. This is a temporizing measure, and further management of these patients—including adjustment of preload with fluids, diuretics, or nitrates and adjustment of afterload with vasopressors or vasodilators—requires invasive monitoring.

Swan-Ganz Catheter The Swan-Ganz catheter is also referred to as a flow-directed, balloon-tipped pulmonary artery catheter. Placement of the Swan-Ganz catheter allows measurement of the *pulmonary capillary wedge pressure (PCWP)*. Because there is an unobstructed column of blood from the pulmonary capillaries to the pulmonary vein and left atrium, **the PCWP is an excellent measure of left atrial pressure and hence a measure of** *left ventricular end-diastolic pressure* **(LVEDP) or "*preload*."** With thermodilution catheters currently available, cardiac output (CO) can be measured reliably. This information, coupled with the mean systemic arterial pressure (MAP), allows calculation of the systemic vascular resistance (SVR) by the following formula:

$$\text{SVR} = \frac{(\text{MAP} - \text{PCWP})}{\text{CO}} \times 80$$

where SVR is measured in dynes/second/cm^{-5}. A normal SVR is approximately 1170 dynes/second/cm^{-5}.

Swan-Ganz catheterization is indicated in any acutely ill patient with underlying heart disease in whom volume management will be necessary. Placement of these catheters should not delay aggressive volume repletion when this is appropriate. In general, catheter insertion is not immediately indicated in the hypotensive patient without rales or hypoxemia.

The Swan-Ganz catheter can be placed either percutaneously or via a surgical cutdown in the antecubital vein, internal jugular vein, subclavian vein, or femoral vein. After catheter lumina have been flushed with heparinized saline solution and transducers and monitoring equipment have been properly prepared, the catheter is advanced in the appropriate vein with the balloon tip deflated until respiratory variations appear on the oscilloscope, confirming the presence of the catheter tip in the thorax. The balloon is inflated with approximately 1 ml of air, and the catheter is advanced until a right ventricular pressure tracing appears on the oscilloscope. Then the catheter is advanced farther until a pulmonary artery tracing is seen and the amplitude of the pressure tracing decreases abruptly. The presence of an atrial pressure waveform with "a" and "v" waves confirms a pulmonary artery wedge position. Before the catheter is sutured into place, the balloon is deflated and the presence of a clear pulmonary arterial waveform is confirmed. A radiograph of the chest should be obtained to confirm placement, to exclude a pneumothorax, and to exclude looping of the catheter in the right ventricle. In patients with cardiomegaly or in whom difficulties are encountered in obtaining adequate pressure tracings, fluoroscopic guidance should be used for placement.

Respiratory Failure

Respiratory failure can be defined as a failure of the respiratory system to accomplish the exchange of oxygen and carbon dioxide between ambient air and red blood cells in amounts required to meet the body's metabolic needs. It can result from diseases involving the central nervous system, the phrenic nerves, the muscles of respiration, the airways, or the terminal gas-exchange units.

The most common causes of respiratory failure in oncology patients are:

1. Nervous system depression secondary to sedative or analgesic medications

2. Bronchospasm

3. Pneumonia

4. Pulmonary edema

5. Lymphangitic spread of cancer

Patients with respiratory failure will initially have abnormal mental status, agitation, somnolence, and disorientation; physical findings include tachycardia, hypertension, and occasionally cyanosis and sweating.

Initial Evaluation

The diagnosis of respiratory failure is based on the demonstration of hypoxemia with an arterial blood gas (ABG) analysis. Hypercapnia, especially in a patient with previously normal blood gases, should also be interpreted as respiratory failure. Careful serial blood gas sampling may be necessary to confirm the diagnosis of early respiratory insufficiency. It is important to obtain a baseline arterial blood gas analysis preoperatively in patients at risk of postoperative respiratory problems.

Interpretation of serial blood gas analyses is simplified by use of the *alveolar-arterial oxygen gradient*, which is a reliable index of the progression of intrinsic lung disease and gas exchange independent of inspired oxygen concentrations. Assuming a normal body temperature and analysis at sea level, alveolar oxygen tension ($P_{AL}O_2$) is expressed by the following equation:

$$P_{AL}O_2 = (F_IO_2 \times 760 \text{ mm Hg}) - (P_aCO_2 \times 1.2)$$

F_IO_2 = the fraction of inspired air which is oxygen (at sea level on room air, approximately 0.21); $PaCO_2$ = the measured arterial tension of carbon dioxide. **The alveolar-arterial oxygen gradient is the pulmonary alveolar oxygen tension minus the measured arterial oxygen tension ($P_{AL}O_2 - P_aO_2$).** The alveolar-arterial oxygen gradient will not be increased by hypoventilation or by changes in inspired oxygen concentrations; hence, increases in this gradient document true deterioration in gas exchange.

Mechanical Ventilation

Indications for mechanical ventilation include:

1. Patients with acute respiratory acidosis (patients who chronically retain CO_2 often do not require intubation).

583

2. Patients with symptomatic and progressive hypoxemia that is not responsive to oxygen supplementation.

3. Patients with a presumptive diagnosis of adult respiratory distress syndrome.

Patients who require mechanical ventilation initially require endotracheal intubation. In the comatose patient, with an absent or markedly diminished gag reflex, intubation is accomplished most easily via the oral approach with a traditional laryngoscope. Patients who have a diminished mental status and some gag reflex may require sedation with a short-acting barbituate (e.g., Brevital) or an opiate (e.g., intravenous morphine sulfate). Patients who are awake and alert may require sedation, but they can often be intubated directly via the nasotracheal approach.

Volume-Cycled Positive-Pressure Ventilator The majority of patients who require mechanical ventilation can be managed on a volume-cycled, positive-pressure ventilator. Ventilator settings are dictated by the results of serial arterial blood gas analyses. Initial ventilator settings should be:

1. Tidal volume: 10 ml/kg body weight.

2. Respiratory rate: 14 breaths/minute with frequent high-volume sighs to prevent atelectasis. The rate should be adjusted and based on the measured P_{CO_2} levels.

3. Inspired F_IO_2: This is dictated by the level required to achieve acceptable arterial oxygen tensions. In patients in whom severe hypoxemia is the reason for ventilator support, the inspired F_IO_2 initially should be 80–100%.

Most ventilators allow a choice of two modes, *intermittent mechanical ventilation* (IMV) or *assist control* (A/C). Patients who have spontaneous respiratory efforts can be placed on the assist control mode, in which the ventilator provides assistance to any inspiration initiated by the patient and additional uninitiated inspirations as necessary, so that a total number of breaths designated in the set backup rate is assured. IMV provides a set number of assisted ventilations, but it does not provide assistance to additional breaths taken by the patient. IMV is therefore useful in patients who hyperventilate and in weaning patients from ventilator support.

In all patients undergoing mechanical ventilation, especially those who have prolonged ventilator support at high ventilatory pressures, there is a risk of barotrauma in the form of a pneumothorax or mediastinal and subcutaneous emphysema. If required ventilatory pressures rise abruptly, suggesting an abrupt decrease in lung compliance, or if arterial blood gases deteriorate abruptly, pneumothorax should be suspected. Patients with hyperresonant lung fields, a tracheal shift, or the unilateral absence of breath sounds require immediate chest tube placement. An algorithm for the management of respiratory failure is presented in Figure 16.5.

Adult Respiratory Distress Syndrome (ARDS)

One pattern of severe respiratory failure that deserves special mention is the adult respiratory distress syndrome, which is characterized by:

584

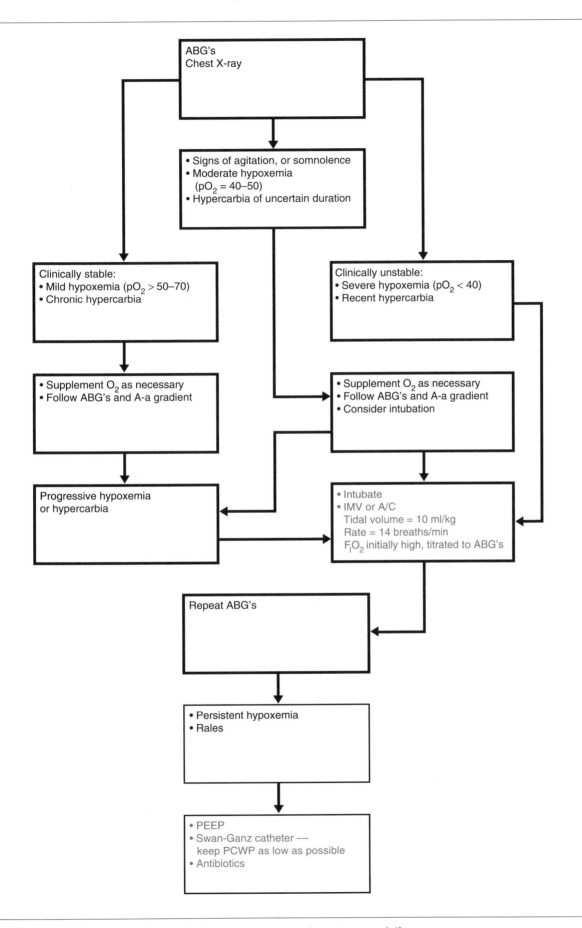

Figure 16.5 Management of respiratory failure.

1. Severe hypoxemia that is not fully corrected by high inspired oxygen concentrations

2. Markedly decreased lung compliance requiring high mechanical ventilatory pressures

3. Diffuse fluffy, interstitial pulmonary infiltrates

4. Rales in the presence of normal or decreased pulmonary capillary wedge pressures, implying increased pulmonary capillary permeability

In gynecologic oncology patients, ARDS can occur as a result of a variety of lung injuries, the most common of which are:

1. Prolonged hypotension ("shock lung")

2. Aspiration pneumonia

3. Septicemia

4. Pulmonary embolism

5. Disseminated intravascular coagulation

In any patient with a known precipitating factor, ARDS must be presumed when progressive hypoxemia develops and requires mechanical ventilatory support and when severe hypoxemia persists despite a high inspired oxygen concentration. These patients have rales despite presumably normal or measured normal left atrial pressure.

Patients with ARDS frequently respond to positive end-expiratory pressure (PEEP) and those suspected of having this syndrome should be given a therapeutic trial of PEEP. If their oxygenation improves, the PEEP can be adjusted as tolerated by the blood pressure. The PEEP must be decreased if hypotension occurs. The inspired oxygen concentration should be maintained at the minimum level to prevent oxygen toxicity. Other adjuncts to management include Swan-Ganz catheter placement to optimize fluid management, diuretics to minimize filling pressures as tolerated by blood pressure, and antibiotics. Treatment of the underlying cause (e.g., infection or pulmonary embolism) is essential. Despite aggressive care, this syndrome is frequently fatal.

Renal Insufficiency

Patients with gynecologic cancer can have renal insufficiency resulting from preexisting unrelated conditions, ureteral obstruction by the malignancy, or nephrotoxic chemotherapeutic agents. Surgery can be performed on patients with severe renal failure who require hemodialysis with less than 5% mortality (88, 89), although morbidity can exceed 50% (90). Patients with previously undiagnosed renal disease should be evaluated and, if possible, the underlying cause should be treated before definitive surgical management of the gynecologic tumor.

Depending on the patient's presentation, work-up might include renal ultrasonography, retrograde pyelography, and renal biopsy. In patients whose renal insufficiency cannot be fully corrected before surgery, the risks of surgery include bleeding due to platelet dysfunction associated with azotemia, volume overload,

586

hyperkalemia, metabolic acidosis, and infection. In the subgroup of patients with nephrotic syndrome, additional risks include hypotension secondary to relative hypovolemia and thrombosis, presumably secondary to antithrombin III deficiency. In the group of patients with untreatable renal insufficiency of mild or moderate severity who do not require hemodialysis (creatinine clearance > 20 ml/min), management includes the avoidance of intravenous contrast agents during imaging procedures, adjustment of drug dosages and administration schedules appropriate for the level of renal insufficiency, careful attention to volume status and electrolyte balance, and avoidance of intraoperative hypotension. Detailed reviews of drug therapy in renal insufficiency are available (91).

Oliguria

The most frequently encountered acute renal problem in critical care medicine is oliguria, which can be defined as a urine output of < 400 ml/day. Although the differential diagnosis of oliguria is extensive and includes intrinsic renal diseases as well as postrenal obstruction, a prerenal disorder first must be excluded in the oliguric patient.

In the gynecologic oncology patient, the most common prerenal cause of oliguria is volume depletion, although congestive heart failure and severe liver disease can cause an identical renal picture. The physical examination should exclude orthostatic blood pressure changes, evidence of liver disease, a palpable bladder, and an elevated postvoid residual urine volume as determined by bladder catheterization.

Laboratory evaluation of the oliguric patient should include determinations of urinary and serum electrolytes, osmolality, and creatinine levels. Urinary electrolytes are uninterpretable in a patient who has been receiving diuretics. *Prerenal azotemia* tends to be associated with the following:

1. High urine osmolality

2. Low urinary sodium

3. High urine-to-plasma creatinine ratio

The best parameter for distinguishing prerenal from renal causes of oliguria is the *fractional excretion of filtered sodium*, which can be calculated as follows:

Fractional excretion of filtered sodium

$$= \frac{\text{Urine sodium} \times \text{Plasma creatinine}}{\text{Plasma sodium} \times \text{Urine creatinine}} \times 100$$

Prerenal azotemia is associated with a fractional excretion of sodium of < 1%, whereas acute obstructive uropathy, as well as acute renal failure, are associated with levels of > 2% (92).

Patients with a history or physical examination suggestive of volume depletion or urinary indices consistent with prerenal azotemia should be treated with fluid administration and frequent examination for evidence of volume overload. Table 16.11 presents a summary of urinary diagnostic indices in patients with various forms of renal impairment.

587

Table 16.11   Urinary Diagnostic Indices*

	Prenal Azotemia	Acute Oliguric Renal Failure	Acute Nonoliguric Renal Failure	Acute Obstructive Uropathy	Acute Glomerulonephritis
Urine osmolality, mosm/kg H_2O	518 ± 35	369 ± 20	343 ± 17	393 ± 39	385 ± 61
Urine sodium, mEq/liter	18 ± 3	68 ± 5	50 ± 5	69 ± 10	22 ± 6
Urine/plasma urea nitrogen	18 ± 7	3 ± .5	7 ± 1	8 ± 4	11 ± 4
Urine/plasma creatinine	45 ± 6	17 ± 2	17 ± 2	16 ± 4	43 ± 7
Fractional excretion of filtered sodium	.4 ± .1	7 ± 1.4	3 ± .5	6 ± 2	.6 ± .2

Reproduced and adapted, with permission, from Miller TR, Anderson RJ, Linas SC, et al: Urinary diagnostic indices in acute renal failure: a prospective study. *Ann Intern Med* 89:47, 1978.
*Values are expressed as mean ± 1 SEM.

Azotemia

Azotemia means that the patient has an elevated serum creatinine value. The initial evaluation of the patient with a rising creatinine level is identical to that of the patient with oliguria; a history and laboratory evaluation are obtained to exclude volume depletion and postrenal obstruction.

In addition to severe volume depletion and ureteral or bladder outlet obstruction, the most common causes of a rising serum creatinine level in the gynecologic oncology patient include:

1. Hypotension

2. Transfusion reactions

3. Contrast dye–induced renal insufficiency (particularly in volume-depleted patients or diabetics)

4. Drug toxicity (e.g., secondary to cisplatin or antibiotics)

5. Hypercalcemia

6. Disseminated intravascular coagulation

If prerenal or postrenal causes of a rising creatinine level cannot be established, examination of the urinary sediment may suggest the underlying cause. Red blood cell casts in the sediment are diagnostic of glomerulonephritis, whereas renal tubular casts and varying degrees of pyuria and hematuria are quite suggestive of acute tubular necrosis. The demonstration of eosinophils in the urine with Wright's stain is diagnostic of interstitial nephritis induced by drugs.

Management of patients with an acutely rising serum creatinine includes (Fig. 16.6):

1. Discontinuation of any nephrotoxic medications

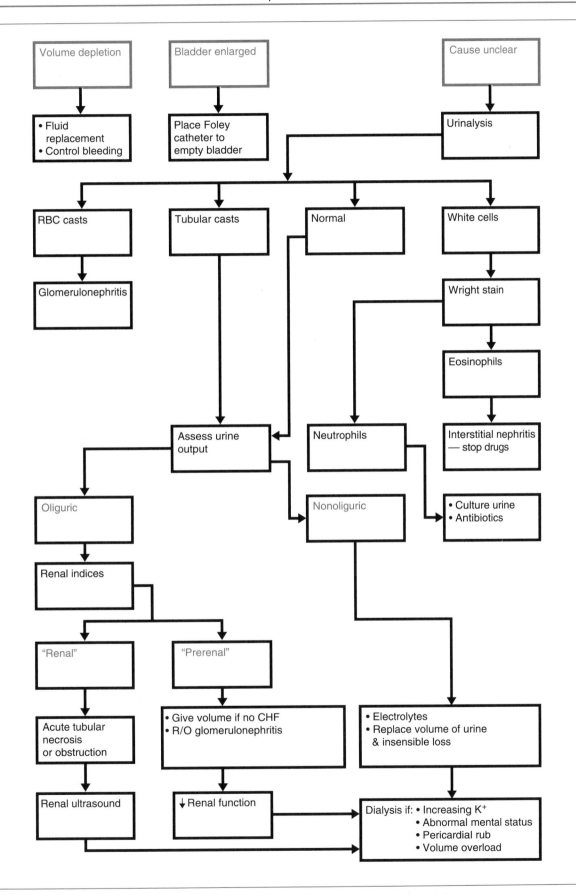

Figure 16.6   Management of a rising serum creatinine.

2. Assurance of adequate hydration with careful attention to volume status to avoid volume overload

3. Careful attention to serum electrolytes, especially avoiding hyperkalemia and hypocalcemia

4. Antibiotics, if disseminated intravascular coagulation is noted or if infection is a possible cause of the initial renal decompensation

Patients with rising serum creatinine levels who also have oliguria can be managed with a therapeutic trial of furosemide (Lasix) or mannitol in an attempt to convert oliguric to nonoliguric renal insufficiency. As a practical matter, these efforts often do not work.

Hemodialysis is indicated in the presence of:

1. Volume overload

2. Hyperkalemia that cannot be controlled with potassium-binding therapy

3. An alteration in mental status

4. A pericardial friction rub

In general, the development of acute renal failure in the postoperative patient indicates serious underlying renal disease and is associated with at least a 50% mortality.

Unusual Causes of Acute Renal Failure

Tumor lysis syndrome is a serious systemic disorder that arises when a large tumor is subjected to chemotherapy, which causes the rapid death of large numbers of tumor cells. The release of intracellular phosphates and urates causes oliguric renal failure, which compounds the tendency toward hyperkalemia induced by release of intracellular potassium. Although this syndrome is seen primarily in the treatment of lymphomas, it should be considered in the differential diagnosis of hyperphosphatemic renal failure in any patient receiving chemotherapy for a tumor that is likely to respond dramatically. When recognized, this syndrome is an indication for urgent hemodialysis.

Thrombotic Thrombocytopenic Purpura (TTP) is a rare disorder that can occur as a paraneoplastic syndrome. This rare and fulminant disease is characterized by:

1. Renal insufficiency

2. Altered mental status

3. Intravascular microangiopathic hemolysis evidenced by schistocytes on the peripheral blood smear

4. Fever

5. Thrombocytopenia

590

TTP is treated by emergency administration of fresh frozen plasma and by plasmapheresis.

Acid-Base Disorders

Disorders of acid-base status are common in critical care medicine, and accurate interpretation of these disorders is important for successful patient management. For an exhaustive review of acid-base disorders, the reader is referred to the excellent summary by Narins and Emmett (93).

Metabolic Acidosis

The most common acid-base disturbance that confronts the physician caring for acutely ill patients is metabolic acidosis. **Metabolic acidosis is defined as a decrease in serum bicarbonate level and occurs as a primary disorder or as a compensation for a respiratory disturbance.**

The first step in evaluating a patient with metabolic acidosis is to measure serum electrolytes and calculate the *anion gap*. A formula for the anion gap is:

$$\text{Anion gap} = [NA^+ + K^+] - [Cl^- + HCO_3^-]$$

With this formula, a normal anion gap is 10–14 mEq/liter. The causes of metabolic acidosis with elevated and normal anion gaps are presented in Table 16.12.

The second step in evaluating patients with metabolic acidosis is assessment of the adequacy of the patient's ventilatory response. The normal response to a process that primarily decreases serum bicarbonate is hyperventilation, which partially corrects the impact of the decreased bicarbonate on pH. The expected ventilatory response to a decrease in bicarbonate can be calculated by the following equation (94):

$$\text{Expected } P_{CO_2} = 1.5 \text{ (measured } HCO_3^-) \pm 2$$

Patients who have metabolic acidosis and whose measured P_{CO_2} levels fall below those expected on the basis of this equation, should be suspected of having a second disturbance, i.e., a primary respiratory alkalosis. In patients with a P_{CO_2} higher than this expected level, primary respiratory acidosis should be suspected of complicating their metabolic disturbance.

The treatment of metabolic acidosis depends on its severity. In the vast majority of cases, identification and treatment of the underlying cause is the only direct therapy necessary. In patients who have profound disturbances and bicarbonate

Table 16.12   Causes of Metabolic Acidosis

Elevated Anion Gap	Normal Anion Gap	Normal-Hyperkalemic Acidosis
A. Renal failure	A. Renal tubular acidosis	A. Early renal failure
B. Ketoacidosis	B. Diarrhea	B. Hydronephrosis
C. Lactic acidosis	C. Posthypocapnic acidosis	C. Addition of HCl
	D. Carbonic anhydrase inhibitors	D. Sulfur toxicity
	E. Ureteral diversions	

levels < 10 and/or pH levels < 7.2, especially if there is associated hypotension or if the underlying disease is expected to worsen, bicarbonate therapy should be considered. **Bicarbonate therapy should be undertaken with caution, as there is a theoretic risk of causing a transient worsening of the cerebrospinal fluid pH level or of inducing fluid overload and "rebound" metabolic alkalosis.**

Metabolic Alkalosis

Metabolic alkalosis is less frequently encountered. In the seriously ill patient who requires ventilatory support and develops a metabolic alkalosis (which may or may not be related to previous respiratory acidosis), metabolic alkalosis can decrease ventilatory drive and make weaning from the ventilator more difficult.

Metabolic alkalosis is best evaluated by recalling that intravascular volume depletion results in increased renal absorption of sodium. Initially, this sodium is accompanied by chloride. However, when urinary chloride levels have become quite low, sodium is accompanied by the negative anion, bicarbonate. Hence, any state associated with avid sodium resorption can result in metabolic alkalosis. A classification of disorders associated with metabolic alkalosis that may be encountered in gynecologic oncology patients is shown in Table 16.13.

In patients who have not received diuretics, a urinary chloride determination will divide patients into two groups:

1. Very low urinary chloride levels: These patients have sodium chloride–responsive metabolic alkalosis and can be treated with the administration of normal saline solution.

Table 16.13 Differential Diagnosis of Metabolic Alkalosis in Gynecologic Oncology Patients

A. *Sodium chloride–responsive* (urine chloride < 10 mmoles/liter)

1. Gastrointestinal disorders
   Vomiting
   Gastric drainage
   Chloride diarrhea

2. Diuretic therapy

3. Correction of chronic hypercapnia

B. *Sodium chloride–resistant* (urine chloride > 20 mmoles/liter)

1. Profound potassium depletion

C. *Unclassified*

1. Alkali administration

2. Milk-alkali syndrome

3. Massive blood or plasma transfusion

4. Nonparathyroid hypercalcemia

5. Glucose ingestion after starvation

6. Large doses of carbenicillin or penicillin

Reproduced and adapted, with permission, from Schrier RW (ed): *Renal and Electrolyte Disorders*, ed 2. Boston, Little Brown, 1980, p 146.

2. Higher urinary chloride levels: These patients will not respond to sodium chloride and must be managed with treatment of their underlying disease.

Fluid and Electrolyte Disorders	Management of water and electrolyte therapy is an important component in the care of the patient who is not able to take nourishment or hydration orally. In the average adult who is taking fluids orally, the average daily loss of water is approximately 3 liters (2 liters as urine and 1 liter as insensible losses from perspiration, respiration, and feces). The condition of critically ill patients may be complicated by additional ongoing losses, frequent derangements in renal function, increased insensible loss, and disturbances in free water metabolism induced by the underlying disease. Successful management of these patients requires frequent monitoring of volume status and serum electrolytes. Predictable losses of fluids and electrolytes must be replaced, particularly those from nasogastric suctioning and the increased insensible losses associated with fever and diarrhea (95).
General Rules	**1.** In a patient with no preexisting renal disease and no disorder of water or electrolyte metabolism, a reasonable maintenance fluid regimen is 3 liters daily of a half-normal saline solution with 20 mEq of potassium chloride added to each liter. **2.** In the presence of significant renal impairment (glomerular filtration rate < 25 ml per minute), potassium therapy should not be given routinely, replacement being based on serial determinations of serum potassium. **3.** In patients suspected of having a defect in free water excretion, because of either hyponatremia at the time of presentation or the presence of such predisposing causes as ascites, edematous disorders, or pulmonary or brain metastases, it is prudent to decrease the free water content of the initial maintenance intravenous fluids. This can be done by alternating normal saline and half-normal saline solutions or by decreasing the total volume administered by one-half and administering normal saline solution only. This latter approach will deliver equivalent quantities of sodium chloride without the accompanying free water. **4.** Gastric fluid is composed of hypotonic saline solution (one-quarter to one-half normal saline), with 5–10 mEq/liter of potassium. In addition to maintenance replacement, patients undergoing nasogastric suction should have replacement milliliter for milliliter, with appropriately constituted intravenous fluids.
Hyponatremia	The most common disorder occurring in critically ill patients is hyponatremia. Serum sodium concentration is independent of total body sodium content, and increases and decreases in sodium concentration reflect changes in total body water. Hyponatremic disorders are best approached with the classification scheme presented by Berl et al. (96). In this scheme, three classes of hyponatremia are recognized:

1. *Hyponatremia associated with a diminished total body sodium content and hence extracellular volume depletion:* In these patients, hyponatremia arises as the body sacrifices osmotic homeostasis to defend the higher-priority volume status, blocking free water excretion by increasing antidiuretic hormone (ADH) secretion. All forms of intravascular volume depletion in patients with normal renal function predispose to this form of hyponatremia, especially when losses have been replaced with hypotonic fluids. The urinary sodium level will be quite low, and signs of volume depletion are frequently present.

2. *Hyponatremia with normal or slightly expanded extracellular volumes:* This is seen in patients with the syndrome of inappropriate ADH secretion and patients with hypothyroidism. Urinary sodium levels reflect free water and sodium intake and can be high or low.

3. *Hyponatremia with increased total body sodium and increased extracellular volume:* The hallmark of these disorders is edema, and urinary sodium levels are low, consistent with intravascular volume depletion. Patients with this category of hyponatremia generally have nephrosis, ascites, or congestive heart failure.

The treatment of hyponatremia is tailored to its pathophysiology:

1. Patients with diminished extracellular volumes are managed with repletion of normal saline solution volume.

2. Patients with normal or increased extracellular volume can be managed initially with free water restriction.

3. Patients with inappropriate ADH syndrome who do not respond to free water restriction and who have symptomatic hyponatremia may have a therapeutic trial of demeclocycline, which induces a nephrogenic diabetes insipidus.

4. Patients without extracellular volume depletion may be managed acutely with furosemide (Lasix) to induce a hypotonic diuresis; urine output is replaced, milliliter for milliliter, with normal saline solution.

Therapy with hypertonic saline solution is rarely necessary, and it should be reserved for patients with profound hyponatremia, particularly those with seizures and neurologic sequelae. An algorithm detailing the approach to the patient with hyponatremia is presented in Figure 16.7.

Hypokalemia

Disturbances in serum potassium concentration are common and important because of the pivotal role played by this ion in maintaining transmembrane potentials in the heart. Because 98% of total-body potassium is intracellular, small changes in serum potassium concentration may reflect very large excesses or deficits in total-body potassium content. For instance, a decrease in plasma potassium concentration to 3 mEq/liter reflects a 100–200 mEq deficit in total-body potassium content; a decrease to 2 mEq/liter reflects a total-body deficit of 300–500 mEq of potassium.

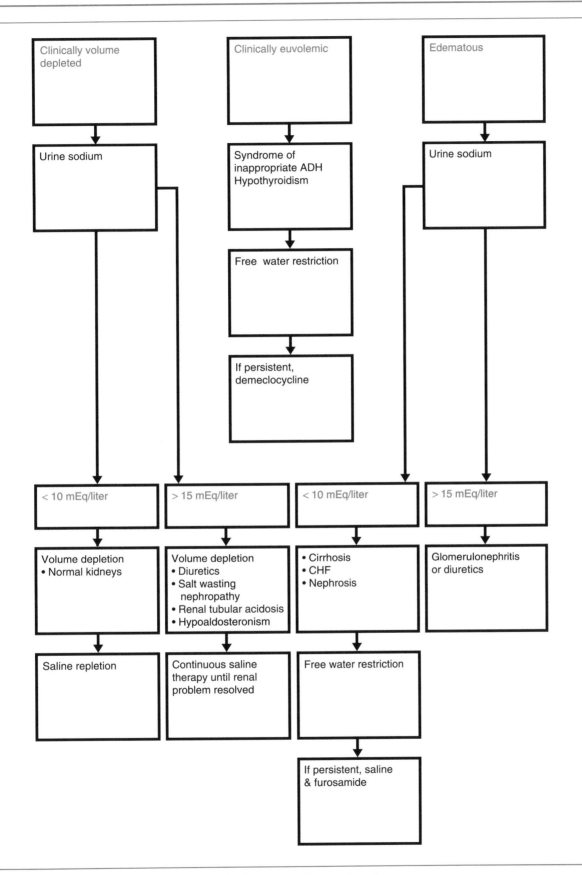

Figure 16.7   Evaluation of hyponatremia.

Changes in hydrogen ion concentration can have an impact on the distribution of potassium between the intracellular and extracellular space. In acidemic patients, there is a shift in potassium from intracellular to extracellular sites. **In a patient who is both acidemic and hypokalemic, plasma potassium concentration will not be appropriately diminished, and total-body potassium deficit will be underestimated.**

Possible causes of hypokalemia include:

1. Fictitiously low levels due to the presence of alkalosis

2. Decreased dietary potassium

3. Insufficient maintenance replacement in a patient with nasogastric suctioning or a gastrointestinal fistula

4. Laxative abuse

5. Diarrhea

6. Diuretic therapy

Patients who are hypokalemic can present with weakness, ileus mimicking intestinal obstruction, and tetany. An electrocardiogram will reveal flattened T waves and the presence of U waves. Hyperglycemia occasionally occurs because of diminished insulin secretion. Left untreated, chronic hypokalemia can result in renal tubular disorders with concentrating defects, phosphaturia, and azotemia.

The treatment of hypokalemia involves reversal of the underlying cause and repletion of the potassium deficit. **Because a rapid increase in serum potassium can result in fatal myocardial depression, potassium should be replaced slowly to allow equilibration across membranes. In general, patients should not receive more than 10 mEq/hour intravenously.** In patients who are treated with a "potassium-sparing" diuretic concomitant with the diagnosis of hypokalemia, potassium levels must be followed carefully during potassium replacement to avoid hyperkalemia. Patients undergoing potassium therapy in the presence of renal failure have a diminished capacity to excrete potassium, and therefore added caution is necessary.

Hyperkalemia

Common causes of an elevated serum potassium concentration include:

1. Increased serum potassium concentration without an increase in total-body potassium content, due to redistribution associated with acidosis (particularly common in diabetic ketoacidosis)

2. Renal insufficiency

3. Adrenal insufficiency

4. Cellular breakdown due to hemolysis or rhabdomyolysis

Occasionally, a high measured serum potassium concentration results from hemolysis of the drawn blood sample prior to laboratory determinations.

596

Although patients with true hyperkalemia may have weakness, the majority of patients with hyperkalemia, even with dangerous levels, have no signs or symptoms. In moderate hyperkalemia, an electrocardiogram will reveal peaked T waves; as the potassium concentration rises above 6 mEq/liter, prolongation of the PR interval, widening of the QRS complex, and loss of P waves occur. As hyperkalemia progresses, the electrocardiogram comes to resemble a sine wave, which is evidence of impending cardiac arrest.

The initial approach to hyperkalemia is to identify and remove the precipitating cause and to assess rapidly any cardiographic changes. In patients with mild hyperkalemia (serum K^+ < 6 mEq/liter) and minimal electrocardiographic changes, treatment of the underlying cause and careful monitoring of serum potassium levels and electrocardiographic changes may be the only therapy necessary. **In patients with potassium levels > 6.5 mEq/liter and electrocardiographic changes of QRS widening, rapid steps should be taken to decrease serum potassium levels with the use of potassium exchange resins and a loop diuretic such as Lasix. If there is associated renal insufficiency, arrangements for dialysis are indicated.** In patients with prolonged QRS intervals approaching the sine wave configuration, or in patients who are hypotensive, emergency treatment includes:

1. Calcium gluconate to reverse the adverse effects of hyperkalemia on the cellular membrane potential

2. Intravenous glucose and insulin (50 ml of 50% glucose solution and one unit of intravenous regular insulin for each 10 g of glucose)

3. Sodium bicarbonate

The latter two facilitate the movement of potassium into cells.

Hypercalcemia

The most common cause of hypercalcemia in hospitalized patients is malignancy (97). There are several mechanisms for the development of hypercalcemia associated with malignancy; in gynecologic oncology patients, the most common mechanism is increased osteoclastic bone resorption without direct bone involvement by tumor. This is occasionally seen in patients with ovarian carcinoma. It is presumed to arise from secretion by the tumor of parathyroid hormone-like substances, prostaglandins, or other humoral factors. When a patient with cancer presents with hypercalcemia, the possibility of primary hyperparathyroidism should be considered, especially if the patient has a cancer that is not traditionally associated with hypercalcemia.

The clinical presentation of hypercalcemia includes lethargy, confusion, psychiatric disturbances, polyuria and polydipsia, constipation, nausea, and occasionally abdominal pain. Some patients have band keratopathy and hypertension. Laboratory findings include electrocardiographic abnormalities, such as prolonged PR and shortened QT intervals, and occasional elevations in serum amylase and creatinine levels.

The acute management of hypercalcemia includes:

1. Hydration with normal saline solution

2. Administration of a loop diuretic (e.g., Lasix) to increase urinary calcium excretion

In severe cases, hydration together with the administration of corticosteroids and oral phosphates to acutely lower serum calcium may be necessary. Subsequently, specific treatment to relieve the underlying cause of hypercalcemia (e.g., treatment of the tumor, parathyroidectomy) is appropriate. In patients in whom the underlying cause of hypercalcemia cannot be eliminated, a therapeutic trial of diphosphonates, prostaglandin inhibitors, or *calcitonin* can be used. In patients with malignancy that is resistant to treatment and causing hypercalcemia, weekly administration of *mithramycin* with careful monitoring of the platelet count may be the only effective management.

Blood Replacement

Red Blood Cells

Red blood cells can be transfused in the form of *whole blood*, which contains red cells as well as platelets and plasma, or *packed red blood cells*, which are red cell concentrates that are prepared by removal of most platelets and all but approximately 100 ml of plasma from a unit of whole blood. In addition, red cells can be washed to remove leukocytes and contaminating plasma proteins for transfusion to selected patients who have had febrile reactions to them.

With the possible exception of the patient who is suffering massive exsanguination, there is little advantage to transfusion of whole blood, and, as a practical rule, packed red blood cells should be used when red cell therapy is indicated. The indications for transfusion of red blood cells include:

1. A decreasing hematocrit value in a patient who, because of bone marrow failure, is unlikely to begin producing red blood cells in the near future.

2. Anemia in a patient with such symptoms as shortness of breath or chest pain. In general, patients will have no symptoms if hemoglobin levels are above 10 g/dl.

Risks of red cell therapy include transfusion hepatitis and acquired immunodeficiency syndrome, as well as acute hemolytic reactions.

Acute Hemolytic Transfusion Reaction   This reaction is life-threatening because of associated hypotension, disseminated intravascular coagulation, and renal failure. It is manifested by fever, chest pain, back pain, hypotension, and red urine. When a patient undergoing a red cell transfusion develops any sign or symptom suggestive of a hemolytic transfusion reaction, the transfusion should be stopped immediately and the remaining aliquot of blood sent to the blood bank, along with a sample of the patient's blood for culture and repeat cross-matching. A screening for disseminated intravascular coagulation, a urinalysis for hemoglobin, and a blood sample for bilirubin also should be obtained. In patients with symptoms of a hemolytic transfusion reaction who, on analysis, show no evidence of hemolysis, a hypersensitivity reaction to transfused leukocytes or plasma proteins contaminating the red cells should be suspected. The incidence of hemolytic transfusion reactions can be minimized by careful attention to clerical information, assuring that the patient is receiving blood cross-matched to her blood sample, and careful cross-matching in the blood bank.

Platelets

Platelet concentrates are prepared by removal of platelets from whole blood fractions. Platelets can be stored for 5 days at 22°C, and each 50 ml platelet unit contains approximately 6×10^{10} platelets.

Platelet transfusions are indicated in patients with:

1. Platelet counts $< 50,000/\text{ml}^3$ who show evidence of bleeding

2. Platelets counts $< 10,000/\text{ml}^3$ as prophylaxis against acute bleeding

Each unit of platelets should be expected to raise the platelet count approximately $5000-10,000/\text{ml}^3$. In general, prophylactic platelet transfusions are indicated only in patients whose platelet count is expected to recover in the future, as platelets express HLA antigens and hence induce antibodies in the recipient. After prolonged platelet therapy, most patients will become resistant to platelet transfusions, presumably because of immune destruction of all transfused platelets.

Plasma Fractions

Several plasma fractions are available for transfusion.

Fresh Frozen Plasma   All coagulation factors (including at least 50% of factors V and VIII present in the original unit of blood) are contained in fresh frozen plasma, and it is an adequate source of all coagulation factors for the treatment of mild coagulation factor deficiencies.

Cryoprecipitate   Cryoprecipitate is produced by freezing of plasma, followed by thawing, and produces a precipitate rich in factor VIII and in fibrinogen. This cryoprecipitate fraction contains approximately 250 mg of fibrinogen per unit and 80 clotting units of factor VIII. When used in the treatment of hemophilic patients, factor VIII level will rise by approximately 2% for each cryoprecipitate unit transfused in the average adult patient.

Factor VIII and Factor IX Concentrates   Factor VIII concentrate for the treatment of classic hemophilia and factor IX concentrate for the treatment of hemophilia B are available. Although the factor VIII product contains only factor VIII, factor IX concentrate also contains factors II, VII, and X in high concentrations, in addition to containing 500 clotting units of factor IX. Factor IX concentrate has been associated with thrombosis and disseminated intravascular coagulation in patients with liver disease, and this preparation is contraindicated in such patients.

Clotting Disorders

Massive Blood Transfusion

Several problems occur in patients who require massive transfusion, including the following:

1. Replacement with red cell preparations alone can cause *dilutional thrombocytopenia* and a *"washout" of protein clotting factors*. The net result is an increased risk of generalized microvascular bleeding (98). This has led to the recommendation that platelets, and occasionally fresh frozen plasma, be administered with every 6–12 units of red cell products

in patients undergoing massive transfusions. However, a randomized clinical trial of prophylactic platelet transfusions and fresh frozen plasma administration in this setting failed to show benefit from routine use of these supplements (99). A prudent approach to massive transfusion would be to follow carefully the patient's platelet count and clotting parameters. If abnormalities are noted, appropriate supplements of clotting factors or platelets should be administered, provided disseminated intravascular coagulation has been excluded.

2. Several events take place during the storage of red blood cells: decreased oxygen affinity, increased osmotic fragility, decreased deformability, and decreased viability. Most important of these "storage lesions" is the decreased oxygen affinity. In a patient who has had massive transfusions and whose blood contains essentially only transfused blood, there is a theoretic problem with oxygen delivery by the transfused blood (100). **Although randomized clinical trials are lacking, a prudent approach would be to opt for the use of fresh blood or blood that has been stored for less than 1 week in patients undergoing transfusions of more than 10 units of red blood cells.**

3. Widespread bleeding from mucous membranes, sites of blood drawing, or intravenous catheter sites is usually secondary to disseminated intravascular coagulation or "washout coagulopathy" associated with massive transfusions. Washout coagulopathy will resolve when transfusion therapy is diminished; in the presence of bleeding, it can be treated with replacement of appropriate factors.

Disseminated Intravascular Coagulation (DIC)

DIC is a syndrome that complicates the course of a variety of disease states and is characterized by the pathologic activation of the coagulation cascade and the fibrinolytic system. In gynecologic oncology patients, it is usually seen in association with the following conditions:

1. Malignancy *per se*, especially mucin-producing adenocarcinomas

2. Sepsis

3. Acute vasculitis

4. Acute and chronic liver disease

5. Hemolytic transfusion reactions

In its acute form, DIC appears rapidly in the critically ill patient and is manifested by bleeding from multiple sites, including venipunctures, surgical wounds, gingiva, gastrointestinal tract, and skin. Purpura and hemorrhagic bullae may occur (101). Thrombosis is uncommon. Mortality rates exceed 80%.

Direct demonstration of DIC would require demonstration of intravascular fibrin deposition. The laboratory diagnosis of DIC depends on indirect evidence of circulating thrombin and plasmin activity (102). Useful laboratory tests can be divided into screening and confirmatory tests (103). Screening tests include:

1. *Platelet count*, which is decreased in 90% of cases.

2. *Prothrombin time*, which is significantly prolonged in 90% of cases.

3. *Fibrinogen*, which is < 150 mg in 70% of cases.

If results of all three of the above tests are found to be abnormal in the absence of severe liver disease, this triad is diagnostic of DIC. If one or two screening tests are positive, confirmatory plasma tests are required. These include:

4. *Fibrin degradation products*, which are > 5 mg/ml in 95% of patients with DIC but are also positive in many postoperative patients. Plasma levels > 40 mg/ml are quite specific for DIC.

5. *Protamine sulfate*, which screens for the presence of circulating fibrin monomers and is very sensitive for diagnosing DIC but somewhat non-specific.

6. *Factor VIII assay*, which will be decreased in DIC but not in liver disease.

The therapy of DIC is controversial. Because the majority of patients with acute DIC die of their underlying disease, the primary treatment is aimed at controlling the underlying cause. Treatment should include:

1. Empiric antibiotic therapy, even in patients who are not febrile and in whom another cause of DIC can be found

2. Treatment of other conditions adversely affecting coagulation, such as vitamin K deficiency

3. Replacement with appropriate hemostatic factors in patients with active bleeding

4. Consideration of some of the controversial options, such as anticoagulation, factor replacement, epsilon aminocaproic acid with heparin, and antiplatelet drugs

The diagnosis of DIC is not *ipso facto* an indication that the disorder should be treated aggressively. Treatment decisions must be based on the individual clinical situation. Heparin is of clear benefit only in patients with thrombotic or thromboembolic complications.

Chronic DIC   Chronic DIC follows a variable clinical course in a patient who is chronically ill over a period of months, with thrombotic complications much more common than bleeding complications. This problem is seen occasionally in gynecologic oncology patients, because chronic DIC is frequently associated with adenocarcinomas (particularly those containing mucin), as well as in patients with cirrhosis or vascular abnormalities.

Symptoms are significantly relieved in 60% of the patients treated with heparin (104) but may recrudesce on discontinuation of the heparin therapy. Warfarin is not as effective as heparin. Hence, in patients with thrombotic complications from underlying adenocarcinomas, long-term heparin therapy is frequently necessary (105). This may include self-injection of heparin at home.

Thromboembolic Disease Prophylaxis

Patients undergoing oncologic surgery are at substantial risk of thromboembolic disease. Patients can be stratified according to clinical history as follows (106):

High risk — History of recent pulmonary embolism, extensive surgery for cancer, or orthopedic procedures of the lower limbs

Moderate risk — > 40 years of age undergoing general surgery with < 30 minutes of anesthesia. Other risk factors important.

Low risk — < 40 years of age or those > 40 years of age and < 30 minutes of anesthesia. Other risk factors possibly important.

These groupings are associated with the following rates of thrombosis and embolism without treatment:

	Calf	Proximal	Fatal pulmonary embolus
High risk	40–80	10–20	1–5
Moderate risk	10–40	2–10	0.1–0.7
Low risk	< 10	< 1	< 0.01

Table 16.14 lists patient-related factors that predispose to thromboembolic disease. Any patient undergoing surgery with one or more of these risk factors would be at a higher level of risk. Inherited disorders typically become manifest in younger patients, but for the older patient attention to the acquired factors is more important.

Some form of thromboembolic prophylaxis should be considered for every patient undergoing surgery. Several methods of prophylaxis have been studied. These

---

Table 16.14   Factors Related to Increased Risk of Thromboembolic Disease

Inherited disorders

Antithrombin III deficiency
Protein C deficiency
Protein S deficiency
Dysfibrinogenemia
Disorders of plasminogen and plasminogen activation

Acquired disorders

"Lupus anticoagulant"
Anticardiolipin antibody
Nephrotic syndrome
Paroxysmal nocturnal hemoglobinopathy
Cancer
Stasis (e.g., congestive heart failure)
Age > 70
Estrogen therapy
Sepsis
Bed rest
Stroke
Polycythemia rubra vera
Inflammatory bowel disease
Obesity
Prior thromboembolism

Adapted, with permission, from NIH Consensus Conference: Prevention of venous thrombosis and pulmonary embolism. *JAMA* 256:744–749, 1986.

include low-dose heparin, warfarin starting preoperatively or postoperatively (used in orthopedic surgery), adjusted-dose heparin, dextran, and external pneumatic compression (106).

A recent meta-analysis, which combined the results of several trials, suggested that low-dose heparin may be effective in many types of surgery (107). The use of low-dose heparin will reduce postoperative deep venous thrombosis by approximately 50%. Gynecologic oncology surgery is associated with a particularly high rate of thromboembolism, and prior studies of low-dose heparin begun in standard fashion postoperatively showed it not to be effective. Recently, low-dose heparin (5000 units) started preoperatively (every 8 hours for at least two doses) and then continued every 8 hours postoperatively has been shown to be effective for prophylaxis (108, 109). Many clinicians also use external pneumatic compression, which is equally effective. The two may be used together for added protection.

Low-dose heparin and external pneumatic calf compression are approximately equally cost-effective.

Screening for Hemostatic Defects

In a hemostatic history, the most important information involves the results of prior hemostatic stress and the family history. The patient should be asked about the need for prior transfusions. Minor surgical procedures should not have required transfusion. A history of postoperative bleeding 2 or 3 days postoperatively also should be suspect. Most patients have had tooth extractions. Bleeding should not last more than 24 hours and should not start again after stopping. A familial history of bleeding or suspected bleeding should be investigated. Large ecchymoses, especially if they are of recent onset, should be evaluated initially with a platelet count. It should be remembered that many older patients have senile purpura, a benign condition that is not associated with a hemostatic defect.

Von Willebrand's disease is the most common inherited disorder of hemostasis, occurring in as many as 1 in 800 persons. The template bleeding time can be used to screen for the most common form of Von Willebrand's disease (type I).

Deep Venous Thrombosis

Clinical signs of deep venous thrombosis are notoriously unreliable and are present in only 50% of the cases. Because of this, laboratory confirmation of a diagnosis of deep venous thrombosis is essential. *Contrast venography* remains the reference standard for the diagnosis of deep vein thrombosis (DVT). However, its use is limited because of its invasive nature and side effects. Recently, *impedance plethysmography (IPG)* and *compression B-mode ultrasonography*, two noninvasive methods, have been developed. IPG was developed first, and initial studies reported that IPG had a sensitivity of about 95% for proximal DVT. However, IPG is insensitive for calf DVT. Subsequent studies showed that up to 25% of patients with symptoms and with proven DVT who initially had a normal IPG examination developed abnormal examination findings during serial testing. This is probably related to the fact that IPG is not very sensitive for nonocclusive thrombi. A recent report cautioned against overreliance on this method (110). Real-time compression ultrasonography has been shown to have a sensitivity of 97% (range 83–100%) and a specificity of 97% (range 86%–100%) (111). Although ultrasonography is much better than IPG for detection of nonocclusive thrombi, it also is insensitive in the detection of calf DVT. Thus, patients with symptoms in whom initial ultrasonographic examinations are negative should have repeat studies. Although compression ultrasonography appears to be superior to IPG, clinical management trials with ultrasound are lacking.

Once documented, deep venous thrombosis requires treatment to decrease the risk of pulmonary thromboembolism. Patients who do not have an overriding contraindication to anticoagulation should be treated immediately with heparin, 5000 units by intravenous bolus, followed by continuous heparin infusion of 10–15 units/kg/hr. The rate of heparin infusion customarily is adjusted to achieve an *activated partial thromboplastin time* (aPTT) approximately two to three times that of the control value. It is important to wait at least 6 hours after the initial heparin bolus before obtaining the first aPTT, as levels obtained earlier invariably will be above the final steady-state level. After 2–3 days of full heparinization, patients should be placed on a regimen of oral warfarin. The heparin is continued for 7–10 days until the effect of the warfarin has been documented by a pro-thrombin time (PT) that is 1.5 to 2.5 times the control value. The optimal duration of oral anticoagulation for deep venous thrombosis remains controversial, but in general these medications are continued for 3–6 months.

Pulmonary Embolism

Pulmonary embolism is a frequent and life-threatening complication of the peri-operative state. Presenting symptoms can include pleuritic chest pain, shortness of breath, cough with or without hemoptysis, and in the case of massive pulmonary embolism, sudden syncope or death (112). On physical examination, tachypnea, tachycardia, cyanosis, hypotension, signs of right-sided congestive heart failure, and a pleural friction rub are sometimes found. Laboratory findings can be helpful. Arterial blood gas sampling can reveal hypoxemia, associated with a widened alveolar-arterial gradient. Although frequently normal, chest radiography can reveal a focal area of oligemia or a pleural effusion representing evidence of pulmonary infarction. With massive pulmonary emboli, the electrocardiogram can reveal right axis deviation, with the classic pattern including an S wave in lead I, a significant Q wave in lead III, and T wave inversion in lead III (113). Although the constellation of a high-risk patient with classic symptoms and characteristic physical and laboratory findings may lead to a high index of suspicion, the differential diagnosis will include myocardial infarction, dissecting aortic aneurysm, and pneumonia. Documentation of pulmonary embolism is critical.

In patients with a normal chest radiograph, the initial diagnostic test is usually a radioisotopic *ventilation-perfusion scan*. If the initial perfusion phase is entirely normal, there is less than a 1% chance that the patient has a pulmonary embolus, and further tests are not usually necessary. In patients with perfusion abnormalities, ventilation scans are obtained. If an area of perfusion defect is not matched by a ventilation defect, the scan can be interpreted by experts as highly suggestive of pulmonary embolus, and further diagnostic endeavors are not necessary. In the remaining patients, including those with matching ventilation and perfusion defects, *pulmonary angiography* is necessary. This is the definitive diagnostic test for pulmonary embolism. There is a small risk of severe complications from pulmonary angiography, including death from cardiac arrest (113) due to acute arterial spasm in patients with severe preexisting pulmonary hypertension.

If the pulmonary embolus is less than 1 week old, thrombolytic therapy with urokinase or streptokinase should be considered. In general, thrombolytic therapy has not been shown to decrease mortality in patients with pulmonary embolism, but these agents may be useful in improving long-term pulmonary function and in decreasing the incidence of chronic pulmonary hypertension in patients with large, hemodynamically significant emboli. Contraindications to the use of thrombolytic agents include major surgery within the last 10 days, a history of gastrointestinal bleeding, hypertension, left atrial thrombosis, age over 75 years, pregnancy, diabetic retinopathy, and bacterial endocarditis (114). Patients who are not candidates for thrombolytic therapy should be treated with heparin, followed by warfarin anticoagulation for 6 months.

Infections

In general, infections in patients with gynecologic malignancies should be managed as in all septic patients, i.e., with antibiotics chosen initially on the basis of the presumed infecting organism and changed if necessary when the results of culture and sensitivity testing are available. Some clinical settings deserve specific discussion.

Fever in the Neutropenic Patient

When the absolute granulocyte count falls below 1000/mm^3, the incidence of severe infection rises, and infected patients frequently decompensate rapidly. Hence, it has become a maxim of oncologic care that febrile neutropenic patients should be treated immediately with broad-spectrum intravenous antibiotics, despite the absence of focal signs of infection or of a positive culture result. Frequently encountered pathogens in the neutropenic patient include *Staphylococcus aureus*, and gram-negative enteric organisms such as *Escherichia coli*, *Klebsiella*, and *Pseudomonas aeruginosa*. Less frequently encountered are fungal infections.

Whereas many acceptable combinations of antibiotics can achieve the goal of covering the most likely pathogens, an acceptable initial approach is to give the patient a broad-spectrum semisynthetic penicillin with some activity against *Pseudomonas*, combined with either an aminoglycoside or a third-generation cephalosporin. Meticulous daily follow-up and adjustment of antibiotic coverage is more important than the precise initial combination chosen. Before initiation of antibiotic therapy, blood cultures and urinalysis should be obtained. The patient should be placed in reverse isolation, a low-bacterial diet should be started, and therapy with nonabsorbable bowel-sterilizing antibiotics, such as neomycin tablets, should be initiated.

Although there is some evidence that granulocyte transfusions facilitate clinical improvement in granulocytopenic patients with documented gram-negative infections (115, 116), there has been no consistent demonstration of improvement in survival in these patients, presumably because of inadequate doses of granulocytes delivered in trials to date (117). **The prophylactic transfusion of granulocytes in neutropenic patients without infection has not led to improved survival.** Complications of granulocyte transfusions have included febrile reactions, the transmission of cytomegalovirus, leukoagglutinin reactions in the lungs producing transient respiratory insufficiency, and transmission of graft-versus-host disease. At present, granulocyte transfusions for neutropenic fever, especially during its initial recognition and treatment, cannot be recommended.

Growth Factor Rescue of Febrile Neutropenia Another approach to the management of patients with febrile neutropenia is administration of granulocyte-colony stimulating factor (G-CSF). In a pilot study by Metcalf and Morstyn (118), 12 patients with lymphoid malignancies or solid tumors with febrile neutropenia after chemotherapy were treated with daily intravenous or subcutaneous injections of G-CSF (20–60 μg/kg/day). Compared with a group of historical controls, there appeared to be a 4-day shortening of the duration of neutropenia in the patients receiving G-CSF ($p < 0.007$). A double-blind, placebo-controlled trial is now in progress in such patients, in which half receive G-CSF and the other half receive a placebo in addition to a standard empiric antibiotic combination (tobramycin and piperacillin) to determine whether the duration of the febrile episodes is shortened and the outcome is improved. In the future, it may be appropriate to treat the febrile episode with both G-CSF and antibiotics while full-dose chemotherapy is continued, rather than making a dose reduction.

Fungemia

Fungemia is a life-threatening postoperative complication of surgery and severe medical illness. The typical patient at risk is receiving multiple antibiotics and hyperalimentation and has intravenous access lines and a Foley catheter (119, 120). Additional important risk factors are cancer, chemotherapy, corticosteroids, and hyperglycemia. The clinical presentation of disseminated disease is identical to that of gram-negative sepsis. These patients may have signs of local fungal disease, such as oral thrush. The principal organism found will be *Candida* species, usually *C. albicans*. Reported mortality is 40–50%. Because this organism is associated with retinal lesions, a funduscopic examination is mandatory if fungemia is suspected. The characteristic skin lesions of disseminated disease are 0.5–1.0 cm erythematous papulonodules on the extremities and trunk that tend to become hemorrhagic, especially if the patient has thrombocytopenia. These lesions may resemble ecthyma gangrenosum, a necrotic skin lesion associated with disseminated *Pseudomonas aeruginosa*. The treatment of choice for severe disseminated disease is amphotericin B. Clinical studies are currently under way to determine the role of fluconazole and other oral antifungal agents in the prophylaxis of patients at risk of fungemia.

Prophylaxis

Endocarditis In general, patients with structural cardiac valvular abnormalities, either congenital or acquired, should be treated with prophylactic antibiotics while undergoing procedures that are likely to result in transient bacteremia. Although the need for endocarditis prophylaxis in patients with mitral valve prolapse is controversial, it is reasonable to administer prophylactic antibiotics to patients in whom mitral regurgitation accompanies the mitral valve prolapse. **In gynecologic oncology, operations in which there is a possibility of bowel or vaginal incisions should be considered procedures appropriate for endocarditis prophylaxis.** Assuming normal renal function and no penicillin allergy, appropriate prophylaxis would include intravenous aqueous penicillin G, 1.0 million units, and gentamicin, 1.5 mg/kg, given 1 hour before surgery and then every 8 hours for two additional doses. Intravenous ampicillin, 1 g, can be substituted for the penicillin. In patients who are allergic to penicillin, 1 g intravenous vancomycin can be substituted.

Perioperative Although prophylactic antibiotics for the prevention of wound infection are controversial, it is reasonable to administer 1 gm cefotetan intravenously or intramuscularly just before surgery and then every 6 hours for two additional doses in patients undergoing extensive gynecologic oncology surgery. A recent study demonstrated that **preoperative antibiotics must be given within 2 hours of surgery to be effective** (121). In addition, if incision of the colon or rectum is anticipated, bowel preparation with neomycin and erythromycin base, coupled with mechanical cleansing of the bowel on the day before surgery, is prudent, as discussed in Chapter 15.

References

1. **Steen PA, Tinker JH, Tarhan S:** Myocardial infarction after anesthesia and surgery. *JAMA* 239:2566, 1978.

2. **Skinner JF, Pearce ML:** Surgical risk in the cardiac patient. *J Chron Dis* 17:57, 1964.

3. **Tarhan S, Moffitt RA, Taylor WF, Giulian ER:** Myocardial infarction after general anesthesia. *JAMA* 220:1451, 1972.

4. **Goldman L, Caldera DL, Nussbaum SR, et al:** Multifactorial index of cardiac risk in noncardiac surgical procedures. *N Engl J Med* 297:845, 1977.

5. **Eagle KA, Coley CM, Newall BA, et al:** Combining clinical and thallium data optimizes preoperative assessment of cardiac risk before major vascular surgery. *Ann Intern Med* 110:859, 1989.

6. **Jeffrey CC, Kunsman J, Cullen DJ, Brewster DC:** A prospective evaluation of cardiac risk index. *Anesthesiology* 58:462, 1983.

7. **Zeldin RA, Math B:** Assessing cardiac risk in patients who undergo noncardiac surgical procedures. *Can J Surg* 27:402, 1984.

8. **Detsky AS, Abrams HB, McLaughlin JR, et al:** Predicting cardiac complications in patients undergoing non-cardiac surgery. *J Gen Intern Med* 1:212, 1986.

9. **Lette J, Walters D, Lassonde J, et al:** Multivariate clinical models and quantitative dipyridamole-thallium imaging to predict cardiac morbidity and death after vascular reconstruction. *J Vasc Surg* 14:160, 1991.

10. **Mauncy FM, Ebert PA, Sabistan DC:** Postoperative myocardial infarction: a study of predisposing factors, diagnosis, and mortality in high-risk group of surgical patients. *Ann Surg* 172:497, 1970.

11. **Plumlee JE, Boettner RB:** Myocardial infarction during and following anesthesia and operation. *South Med J* 65:886, 1972.

12. **Goldman L, Caldera DL, Southwick FS, et al:** Cardiac risk factors and complications in non-cardiac surgery. *Medicine* 57:357, 1978.

13. **Mahar LJ, Steen PA, Tinker JH, et al:** Preoperative myocardial infarction in patients with coronary artery disease with and without aorta-coronary bypass grafts. *J Thorac Cardiovasc Surg* 76:533, 1978.

14. **McCollum CH, Garcia-Rinald R, Graham JM, DeBakay ME:** Myocardial revascularization prior to subsequent major surgery in patients with coronary artery disease. *Surgery* 81:302, 1977.

15. **Mauncy FM, Ebert PA, Sabistan DC:** Postoperative myocardial infarction: a study of predisposing factors, diagnosis and mortality in a high risk group of surgical patients. *Ann Surg* 172:497, 1970.

16. **Caralps JM, Mulet J, Wienke HN, et al:** Results of coronary artery surgery in patients receiving propranolol. *J Thorac Cardiovasc Surg* 67:526, 1974.

17. **Goldman L:** Noncardiac surgery in patients receiving propranolol: case reports and a recommended approach. *Arch Intern Med* 141:193, 1981.

18. **Pastore JO, Yurchak PM, Janis KM, et al:** The risk of advanced branch block in surgical patients with right bundle branch block and left axis deviation. *Circulation* 57:677, 1978.

19. **Rooney SM, Goldiner PL, Muss E:** Relationship of right bundle branch block and left axis deviation to complete heart block during general anesthesia. *Anesthesiology* 44:64, 1976.

20. **Pulroth MC, Hultgren HN:** The cardiac patient and general surgery. *JAMA* 232:1279, 1975.

21. **Simon AB:** Perioperative management of the pacemaker patient. *Anesthesiology* 46:127, 1977.

22. **Goldman L, Caldera DL:** Risks of general anesthesia and elective surgery in the hypertensive patient. *Anesthesiology* 50:285, 1979.

23. **Prys-Roberts C, Meloche R, Foex P:** Studies of anesthesia in relation to hypertension. I. Cardiovascular responses of treated and untreated patients. *Br J Anaesth* 43:122, 1971.

24. **Vitez TS, Soper LE, Wong KC, Soper P:** Chronic hypokalemia and intraoperative dysrhythmias. *Anesthesiology* 63:130, 1986.

25. **Adler AG, Leahy JJ, Cressman MD:** Management of perioperative hypertension using sublingual nifedipine: experience in elderly patients undergoing eye surgery. *Arch Intern Med* 146:1927, 1986.

26. **Gal TJ, Cooperman L:** Hypertension in the immediate postoperative period. *Br J Anaesth* 47:70, 1975.

27. **Anscombe AR, Buxton R St J:** Effect of abdominal operations on total lung capacity and its subdivisions. *Br Med J* 2:84, 1958.

28. **Diament ML, Palmer KNV:** Postoperative changes in gas tensions of arterial blood and in ventilatory function. *Lancet* 2:180, 1966.

29. **Egbert LD, Bendixen HH:** Effect of morphine on breathing patterns: a possible factor in atelectasis. *JAMA* 188:485, 1964.

30. **George J, Hornum I, Mellengard K:** The mechanism of hypoxemia after laparotomy. *Thorax* 22:382, 1966.

31. **Ross BB, Gramiak RA, Rahn H:** Physical dynamics of the cough mechanism. *J Appl Physiol* 8:264, 1955.

32. **Kilburn KH:** A hypothesis for pulmonary clearance and its implications. *Am Rev Respir Dis* 98:449, 1968.

33. **Tisi GM:** Preoperative evaluation of pulmonary function: validity, indications, benefits. *Am Rev Respir Dis* 119:293, 1979.

34. **Stein M, Koota GM, Simon M, Frank HA:** Pulmonary evaluation of surgical patients. *JAMA* 181:103, 1962.

35. **Jackson CV:** Preoperative pulmonary complications. *Arch Intern Med* 148:2120, 1988.

36. **Tisi GM:** Preoperative evaluation of pulmonary function. *Am Rev Resp Dis* 119:293, 1979.

37. **Churchill ED, McNeil D:** The reduction in vital capacity following operation. *Surg Gyn Obstet* 44:483, 1927.

38. **Celli BR, Rodriguez KS, Snider GL:** A controlled trial of intermittent positive pressure breathing, incentive spirometry, and deep breathing exercises in preventing pulmonary complications after abdominal surgery. *Am Rev Resp Dis* 130:12, 1984.

39. **Warner MA, Divertie MB, Tinker JH:** Preoperative cessation of smoking and pulmonary complications in coronary artery bypass patients. *Anesthesiology* 60:380, 1984.

40. **Lawrence VA, Page CP, Harris MD:** Preoperative spirometry before abdominal operations: a critical appraisal of its predictive value. *Arch Intern Med* 149:280, 1989.

41. **Gracey DR, Divertie MB, Didlier EP:** Preoperative pulmonary preparation of patients with chronic obstructive pulmonary disease: a prospective study. *Chest* 76:123, 1979.

42. **Stein M, Cassara EL:** Preoperative pulmonary evaluation and therapy for surgery patients. *JAMA* 211:787, 1970.

43. **Mohr DN, Jett JR:** Preoperative evaluation of pulmonary risk factors. *J Gen Intern Med* 3:277, 1988.

608

44. **Latimer RG, Dickman M, Day WC, et al:** Ventilatory patterns and pulmonary complications after upper abdominal surgery determined by preoperative and postoperative computerized spirometry and blood gas analysis. *Am J Surg* 122:622, 1971.

45. **Garibaldi RA, Britt MR, Coleman ML, et al:** Risk factors for preoperative pneumonia. *Am J Med* 70:677, 1981.

46. **Vaughn RW, Engelhart RC, Wise L:** Postoperative hypoxemia in obese patients. *Ann Surg* 180:877, 1974.

47. **Gould AB Jr:** Effect of obesity on respiratory complications following general anesthesia. *Anesth Analg* 41:448, 1962.

48. **Wightman JAK:** A prospective survey of the incidence of postoperative pulmonary complications. *Br J Surg* 55:85, 1968.

49. **Oh SH, Patterson R:** Surgery and corticosteroid dependent asthmatics. *J Allergy Clin Immunol* 53:345, 1974.

50. **Dahi S, Gold MI:** Comparison of two methods of postoperative respiratory care. *Chest* 73:592, 1978.

51. **Bartlett RH, Gazzaniga AB, Geraghty TR:** Respiratory maneuvers to prevent postoperative pulmonary complications: a critical review. *JAMA* 224:1017, 1973.

52. **Egbert LD, Batlet GG, Welch CE, Bartlett KM:** Reduction of postoperative pain by encouragement and instruction of patients. *N Engl J Med* 270:835, 1964.

53. **Ward RJ, Danzinger F, Bonica JJ, et al:** An evaluation of postoperative respiratory maneuvers. *Surg Gynecol Obstet* 123:51, 1966.

54. **Goldberg NJ, Wingert TD, Levin SR, et al:** Insulin therapy in the diabetic surgical patient: metabolic and hormone response to low dose insulin infusion. *Diabetes Care* 4:279, 1981.

55. **Taitelman U, Reece EA, Bessman AN:** Insulin in the management of the diabetic surgical patient: continuous intravenous infusion vs subcutaneous administration. *JAMA* 237:658, 1977.

56. **Schwartz SS, Horwitz DL, Zehfus B, et al:** Use of a glucose controlled insulin infusion system (artificial beta cell) to control diabetes during surgery. *Diabetologia* 16:157, 1979.

57. **McMurray JF:** Wound healing with diabetes mellitus: better glucose control for better wound healing in diabetics. *Surg Clin North Am* 64:769, 1984.

58. **Steinke J:** Management of diabetes mellitus and surgery. *N Engl J Med* 282:1472, 1970.

59. **Drucker DJ, Burrow GN:** Cardiovascular surgery in the hypothyroid patient. *Arch Intern Med* 1585, 1985.

60. **Ladenson PW, Levin AA, Ridgway ED, Daniels GH:** Complications of surgery in hypothyroid patients. *Am J Med* 77:261, 1984.

61. **Weinberg AD, Brennan MD, Gorman CA, et al:** Outcome of anesthesia and surgery in hypothyroid patients. *Arch Intern Med* 143:893, 1983.

62. **Lennquist S, Jortso E, Andberg B, Smeds S:** Beta-blockers compared with antithyroidal drugs as preoperative treatment in hyperthyroidism: drug tolerance, complications, and postoperative thyroid function. *Surgery* 98:1141, 1985.

63. **Ackerman GL, Nolan CM:** Adrenocortical responsiveness after alternate day corticosteroid therapy. *N Engl J Med* 278:405, 1968.

64. **Axelrod L:** Glucocorticoid therapy. *Medicine* 55:39, 1976.

65. **Steer M, Fromm D:** Recognition of adrenal insufficiency in the postoperative patient. *Am J Surg* 139:443, 1980.

66. **Kehlet H, Binder C:** Value of an ACTH test in assessing hypothalamic-pituitary-adrenocortical function in glucocorticoid-treated patients. *Br Med J* 2:147, 1973.

67. **Shapiro MF, Greenfield S:** The complete blood count and leukocyte differential count: an approach to their rational application. *Ann Intern Med* 106:65, 1987.

68. **Tape TG, Mushlin AI:** The utility of routine chest radiographs. *Ann Intern Med* 104:663, 1986.

69. **Goldberger AL, O'Konski M:** Utility of the routine electrocardiogram before surgery and on general hospital admission. *Ann Intern Med* 105:552, 1986.

70. **Kaplan EB, Sheiner LB, Boeckmann AJ, et al:** The usefulness of preoperative laboratory screening. *JAMA* 253:3576, 1985.

71. **Blery C, Charpak Y, Szatan M, et al:** Evaluation of a protocol for selective ordering of preoperative tests. *Lancet* 1(8473):139, 1986.

72. **Rohrer MJ, Michelotti MC, Nahrwold DL:** A prospective evaluation of the efficacy of preoperative coagulation testing. *Ann Surg* 208:554, 1988.

73. **Roizen MF, Kaplan EB, Schreider BD, et al:** The relative role of the history and physical examination, and laboratory testing in preoperative evaluation for outpatient surgery: the "Starling" curve of preoperative laboratory testing. *Anesth Clin North Am* 5:15, 1987.

74. **Rappaport SI, ed:** *Introduction to Hematology,* ed 2. Philadelphia, JB Lippincott, 1987, pp 470–482.

75. **Suchman AL, Griner PF:** Diagnostic uses of the activated partial thromboplastin time and prothrombin time. *Ann Intern Med* 104:810, 1986.

76. **Suchman AL, Mushlin AI:** How well does the activated partial thromboplastin time predict postoperative hemorrhage? *JAMA* 256:750, 1986.

77. **Weil MH, Shubin H, Carlson R:** Treatment of circulatory shock: use of sympathomimetic and related vasoactive agents. *JAMA* 231:1280, 1975.

78. **Shoemaker WC:** Comparison of the relative effectiveness of whole blood transfusions and various types of fluid therapy in resuscitation. *Crit Care Med* 4:71, 1976.

79. **Lowery BD, Cloutier CT, Carcy LC:** Electrolyte solutions in resuscitation in human hemorrhagic shock. *Surg Gynecol Obstet* 133:273, 1971.

80. **Lowe RJ, Moss GS, Jilak J, Levine HD:** Crystalloid vs colloid in the etiology of pulmonary failure after trauma: a randomized trial in man. *Surgery* 81:676, 1977.

81. **Weil MH, Henning RS, Puri VK:** Colloid oncotic pressure: clinical significance. *Crit Care Med* 7:113, 1979.

82. **Skillman JS, Restall DS, Salzman EW:** Randomized trial of albumin vs electrolyte solutions during abdominal aortic operations. *Surgery* 78:291, 1975.

83. **Jelenko C III, Williams JB, Wheeler MC, et al:** Studies in shock and resuscitation. I. Uses of a hypertonic, albumin-containing, fluid demand regimen (HALFD) in resuscitation. *Crit Care Med* 7:157, 1979.

84. **Weitzman S, Berger S:** Clinical trial design in studies of corticosteroids for bacterial infections. *Ann Intern Med* 81:36, 1974.

85. **Schumer W:** Steroids in the treatment of clinical septic shock. *Ann Surg* 184:333, 1976.

86. **Zieglon EG, McCutchan JA, Braude AI:** Clinical trial of core glycolipid antibody in gram-negative bacteremia. *Trans Assoc Am Phys* 91:253, 1978.

87. **Faden AI, Holadzy JW:** Opiate antagonists: a role in the treatment of hypovolemic shock. *Science* 205:317, 1979.

88. **Hampas CL, Bailey GL, Hager EB, et al:** Major surgery in patients on maintenance hemodialysis. *Am J Surg* 115:747, 1968.

89. **Hata M, Remmers AR Jr., Lindley JD, et al:** Surgical management of the dialysis patient. *Ann Surg* 178:134, 1973.

90. **Brenowitz JB, Williams CD, Edwards WS:** Major surgery in patients with chronic renal failure. *Am J Surg* 134:765, 1977.

91. **Bennett WM, Singer I, Galpor T, et al:** Guidelines for drug therapy in renal failure. *Ann Intern Med* 86:754, 1977.

92. **Miller TR, Anderson RJ, Linas SC, et al:** Urinary diagnostic indices in acute renal failure: a prospective study. *Ann Intern Med* 89:47, 1978.

93. **Narins RG, Emmett M:** Simple and mixed acid-base disorders: a practical approach. *Medicine* 59:161, 1980.

94. **Albert MD, Dell RB, Winters RW:** Quantitative displacement of acid-base equilibrium in metabolic acidosis. *Ann Intern Med* 66:312, 1967.

95. **Schrier RW (ed):** *Renal and Electrolyte Disorders*, ed 2. Boston, Little Brown, 1980.

96. **Berl T, Anderson RJ, McDonald KM, et al:** Clinical disorders of water metabolism. *Kidney Int* 10:117, 1976.

97. **Mundy GR, Ibbotson KJ, D'Souza SM, et al:** The hypercalcemia of cancer: clinical implications and pathogenic mechanisms. *N Engl J Med* 310:1718, 1984.

98. **Counts RB, Haisch C, Simon TL, et al:** Hemostasis in massively transfused trauma patients. *Ann Surg* 190:91, 1979.

99. **Reed RL, Ciavarella D, Heimbach DM, et al:** Prophylactic platelet administration during massive transfusion. *Ann Surg* 203:40, 1986.

100. **Collins JA:** Problems associated with the massive transfusion of stored blood. *Surgery* 75:274, 1974.

101. **Mant MJ, Kong EG:** Severe acute disseminated intravascular coagulation: a reappraisal of its pathophysiology, clinical significance, and therapy based on 47 patients. *Am J Med* 67:557, 1979.

102. **Ockelford PA, Carter CJ:** Disseminated intravascular coagulation: the application and utility of diagnostic tests. *Semin Thromb Hemostas* 8:198, 1982.

103. **Colman RW, Robboy SJ, Minna JD:** Disseminated intravascular coagulation: a reappraisal. *Ann Rev Med* 30:359, 1979.

104. **Feinstein DI:** Diagnosis and management of disseminated intravascular coagulation: the role of heparin therapy. *Blood* 60:284, 1982.

105. **Sack GH, Levin J, Bell WR:** Trousseau's syndrome and other manifestations of chronic disseminated coagulopathy in patients with neoplasms: clinical, pathophysiologic and therapeutic features. *Medicine* 56:1, 1978.

106. **Hull RD, Raskob GE, Hirsh J:** Prophylaxis of venous thromboembolism: an overview. *Chest* 89:374S, 1986.

107. **Collins R, Scrimgeour A, Yusuf S, Peto R:** Reduction in fatal pulmonary embolism and venous thrombosis by perioperative administration of subcutaneous heparin. *N Engl J Med* 318:1162, 1988.

108. **Clark-Pearson DL, De Long E, Synan LS, et al:** A controlled trial of two low-dose heparin regimens for the prevention of postoperative deep-vein thrombosis. *Obstet Gynecol* 75:684, 1990.

109. **Clark-Pearson DL, Olt G:** Thromboembolism in patients with gynecologic tumors: risk factors, natural history, and prophylaxis. *Oncology* 3:39, 1989.

110. **Anderson DR, Lensing AWA, Wells PS, et al:** Limitations of impedance plethysmography in the diagnosis of clinically suspected deep-vein thrombosis. *Ann Intern Med* 118:25, 1993.

111. **Buller HR, Lensing AWA, Hirsh J, ten Cate JW:** Deep vein thrombosis: new noninvasive diagnostic test. *Thromb Haemost* 66:133, 1991.

112. **Bell WR, Simon TL, DeMets DL:** The clinical features of submassive and massive pulmonary emboli. *Am J Med* 62:355, 1977.

113. **Mosser K:** Diagnostic approaches to pulmonary embolism. *J Respir Dis* 2:78, 1981.

114. **Thrombolytic therapy in thrombosis:** A National Institutes of Health consensus development conference. *Ann Intern Med* 93:141, 1980.

115. **Alavai JB, Root RK, Djerassi I, et al:** A randomized clinical trial of granulocyte transfusions for infection in acute leukemia. *N Engl J Med* 296:706, 1977.

116. **Herzig RH, Herzig GP, Graw RG, et al:** Successful granulocyte transfusion therapy for gram-negative septicemia: a prospectively randomized controlled study. *N Engl J Med* 296:701, 1977.

117. **Higby DH, Burnett D:** Granulocyte transfusions: Current status. *Blood* 55:2, 1980.

118. **Metcalf D, Morstyn G:** Colony-stimulating factors: general biology. In DeVita VT, Hellman S, Rosenberg SA (eds): *Biologic Therapy of Cancer.* Philadelphia, JB Lippincott, 1991, p 436.

119. **Wey SB, Mori M, Pfaller MA, et al:** Risk factors for hospital-acquired candedemia. *Arch Intern Med* 149:2349, 1989.

120. **Faser VJ, Jones M, Dunkel J, et al:** Candidemia in a tertiary care hospital: epidemiology, risk factors, and predictors of mortality. *Clin Infect Dis* 15:414, 1992.

121. **Classen DC, Evans RS, Pestotnik RL, Burke JP:** The timing of prophylactic administration of antibiotics and the risk of surgical wound infection. *N Engl J Med* 326:281, 1992.

Hormone Therapy

Peter E. Schwartz
Frederick Naftolin

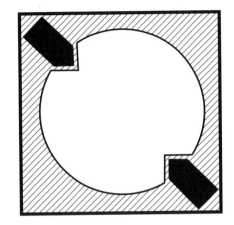

Gynecologic cancers arise in steroid-dependent tissues and thus may be subject to control by these hormones. An understanding of the mechanism of action of these hormones permits the development of a rationale for their use in these neoplasms. The relative ease of administration and low toxicity of hormone therapies make them potentially useful in selected patients with gynecologic cancer.

Hormone Receptors

The discovery of the estrogen receptor (ER) was an important advance in the understanding of the biology of tumors that arise in hormonally sensitive tissues. New technology, including the development of radiospectrometers and the synthesis of a radioactive estradiol with specific activity sufficient to enable detection of the ER protein, has permitted the development of a receptor assay that can be used as a clinical tool (1). When the radioactive estradiol probe was synthesized, the technology became available to measure the quantity and activity of steroid hormone receptors in cancer patients and to correlate these findings with hormone treatment and patient outcome (2).

The presence of cellular ER has been well established in breast cancer (3). Studies have confirmed a good correlation between ER content and the response of breast cancer patients to endocrine ablative therapy. Subsequently, the presence of receptors in other tissues, including normal endometrium, hyperplastic endometrium, endometrial carcinoma, and carcinoma of the ovary, has been established (4-8).

Mechanism of Action

The criteria established for the hormone's recognition of its receptor protein include (2):

613

1. *High receptor binding affinity*: The hormone and the nuclear receptor have a particular biochemical affinity for one another in preference to other nuclear proteins.

2. *Finite binding capacity*: The hormone binds to receptors that permit only a finite quantity of hormone to interact with the nucleus of the cell.

3. *Hormonal specificity*: A specific hormone has a receptor with which it primarily and specifically interacts.

4. *Tissue specificity*: Those tissues that specifically contain a particular hormonal receptor react to the hormone after binding preferentially to the hormone.

5. *Correlation between exhibition of the hormone and biologic response*: The initiation of cellular activity, especially protein synthesis, as a result of the hormone interaction with the receptor.

Estrogen Receptors

The biochemical events that allow estrogen to bind to its receptor and induce growth are summarized in Fig. 17.1 (9). Estrogen is a very small molecule (molecular weight approximately 300 daltons), which allows it to enter readily into any cell.

Figure 17.1 1, Estrogen. 2, Entry of estrogen into cell. 3, Entry of estrogen into nucleus. 4, Binding of estrogen with ER. 5, Binding of estrogen—ER complex to chromatin. 6, Transcription resulting in increased RNA. 7, Translation resulting in increased protein synthesis. 8, Replenishment of ER.

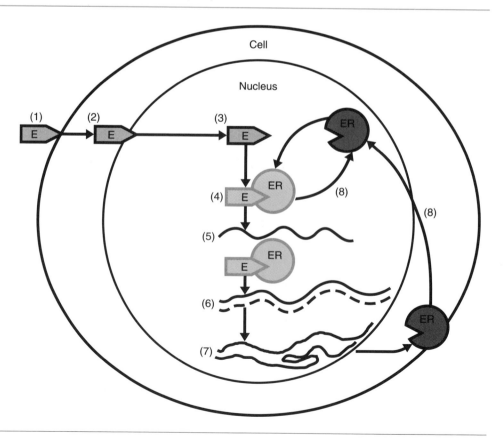

Estrogen–ER Complex

For estrogen to have its effect in the cell, it first must bind to (or ligand) its receptor (ER). The ER is a soluble macromolecule that until recently was thought to be present in the cytoplasm until it binds with estrogen. It is clear that the ER is produced in the cytoplasm. However, it appears that the association of unbound ER with the cytoplasm is an artifact of the *in vitro* technique, and immunohistochemical investigations suggest that most of the unbound receptors reside in the nucleus (10).

Complex–Chromosome Binding

Once the estrogen–ER complex is formed within the nucleus, it binds to one of two sites on the chromosomes:

1. *Acceptor sites*, which are specific complexes of chromosomal proteins (believed to be *nonhistone proteins*) that the ER complex recognizes and binds with a very high affinity.

2. *Nonacceptor sites*, which are secondary sites on chromatin where the ER complex can bind with a lower affinity.

Nonacceptor sites are present in much larger numbers than acceptor sites and are thought to maximize the estrogen binding within the nucleus.

Activation of Synthesis

Once the estrogen–ER complex binds the acceptor sites, gene sites become available for transcription by RNA polymerase. This event results in:

1. Elevated cellular RNA

2. Protein synthesis through translation of the message by ribosomes

This process leads to hypertrophy and hyperplasia of specific target organs. The nuclear binding of estrogen-occupied ER complexes also results in the replenishment of ER. The mechanism may be either synthesis of new receptor molecules or reutilization of the same receptor (11).

Progestin Receptors

Among estrogen-dependent tissues, progestin receptors (PR) are also induced after estrogen binding to its receptor.

Progestins also bind to receptor molecules, which are thought to reside in the nucleus of progestin-sensitive cells. The binding of the progestin to its receptor results in a complex that binds to acceptor sites on DNA, resulting in progestin-mediated responses.

The progestin responses are often antiestrogenic and reduce the synthesis of both ER and PR.

Receptor Methods

The most commonly used methods for determination of ER and PR are the *dextran-coated charcoal analysis* (DCCA) and the *sucrose density gradient anal-*

615

ysis (SDGA). These methods have been generally comparable in their accuracy, but most institutions employ the DCCA method because it is simpler and less costly. The DCCA method involves the use of charcoal, which binds and absorbs radioactive (tritiated) unbound or "free" hormone, leaving the radiolabeled hormone bound to its receptor to be measured. New techniques, particularly the use of a *monoclonal antibody* directed toward the ER and PR proteins, are currently being studied (12, 13). Although these immunohistochemical techniques are still investigational, they appear to be very sensitive and may be useful in localizing ER to specific cells, in detecting ER in tumors that are falsely negative by biochemical assays, and retrospectively evaluating paraffin-embedded tissue.

Growth Factors

Growth factors may act as estrogen-induced "second messengers" in the estrogen-responsive growth of human cancer. *In vitro* data suggest that the interaction of estrogen with its receptor results in the synthesis of *growth factor proteins*, including *a) insulin-like growth factor* and *b) transforming growth factor* alpha, which binds to the *epidermal growth factor* receptor (11). Further study is necessary to establish the significance of these growth factors.

Androgen Receptors

The presence of androgen receptors (AR) in specimens of epithelial ovarian cancer is now well recognized. Friberg el al. (14) originally described their presence in 8 of 10 (80%) samples assayed. Overall, detectable AR levels have been identified in 243 of 342 (71%) epithelial ovarian cancers assayed (14–21), and the presence of measurable levels of AR do not appear to be directly related to the histologic type of the cancer. Although estrogen and progestin assays have been reported more frequently in the literature (22), measurable levels of AR are identified in a higher percentage of epithelial ovarian cancers.

Luteinizing Hormone (hLH) and Follicle-Stimulating Hormone (hFSH) Receptors

Epithelial ovarian cancer most often occurs in perimenopausal and postmenopausal women, suggesting that changes in the hormonal milieu may account at least in part for the occurrence of these tumors. Nakano et al. (23) analyzed benign and malignant epithelial neoplasms and were able to establish the presence of hLH binding sites in one of three mucinous cystadenomas. No hLH binding sites could be found in two mucinous, seven serous, or two clear cell carcinomas. Similarly, the same investigators found hFSH binding sites in two of three mucinous and one of two serous cystadenomas but were unable to identify hFSH binding sites in any of the malignant epithelial tumors they studied.

Breast Cancer

The value of oophorectomy in the management of disseminated breast cancer has been established since 1896 (24). Since then, various hormonal manipulations, including ablative surgery or the addition of such hormones as estrogen, androgen, or progestin, have been used with varying degrees of success for the management of metastatic breast cancer. Recently, some form of medical ablative treatment based on receptor status, has been used to block the biologic effect of estrogen by blocking formation of the ligand (e.g., aminoglutethemide), inhibiting the enzyme aromatase (25), or competing for estrogen receptor sites (tamoxifen) (26). Tamoxifen has been used both therapeutically and prophylactically for breast cancer (26). Some patients have developed endometrial cancer while taking tamoxifen, and our own studies indicate a high incidence of poorly differentiated tumors in such cases. Overall, about 30% of patients with disseminated disease will respond to some form of hormonal manipulation (27), and thus far there seems to be no clear "best approach," the choice of agent being determined by the patient's tolerance of the drug.

Receptors

ER and PR should be measured on every biopsy specimen of breast cancer. The tumor must be handled properly because ER and PR are labile and temperature-sensitive. On removal of the tissue, fat should be trimmed from the tumor, and the pathologist should obtain a frozen section confirming the malignant nature of the tissue. The tumor should be frozen in liquid nitrogen until the assay can be done. If tissue must be sent to an outside laboratory, it should be sent frozen in dry ice. Approximately 0.75–1.0 g of tissue is required for an ER and PR assay. Tumor can be obtained from either the primary tumor or a metastasis because a high correlation exists between receptor status of the primary and metastatic breast lesions (28).

Relationship to Outcome

The quantity of ER present in breast cancer specimens is related directly to the endocrine response of the patient (29–37). Patients with a tumor that contains low or undetectable levels of ER infrequently respond to endocrine therapy, whereas those with a tumor that contains elevated levels of ER frequently respond. An increasing response rate with increasing levels of ER has been established. Hormonal manipulation is the treatment of choice for metastatic breast cancer in patients with ER-positive tumors, because such manipulation has fewer side effects and a longer duration of response than cytotoxic chemotherapy.

About one-third of premenopausal and two-thirds of postmenopausal women have ER-positive tumors. In such cases, determination of ER and PR levels is extremely valuable in predicting the response of patients to endocrine manipulation. Of patients with ER- or PR-positive tumors, 80% will improve with hormone therapy, whereas 55% of patients with ER-positive/PR-negative tumors will respond. It has been proposed that "ER-negative/PR-positive" tumor status results from the presence of a truncated ER that can carry out certain ER actions, such as PR induction (38), even though it has minimal estrogen binding. In any case, patients with ER-negative tumors have a 10% chance of responding to hormonal manipulation and probably should be started on chemotherapy with or without adjuvant hormonal therapy.

Treatment

Surgical ablative therapy (i.e., removal of ovaries and adrenal glands) in the routine management of hormonally sensitive breast cancer has become less frequent since the introduction of tamoxifen. The latter is an "antiestrogen," or estrogen "agonist-antagonist," with primarily antagonist qualities. Tamoxifen is an oral preparation that is well tolerated and can be used in combination with standard radiation or chemotherapeutic regimens (34). Short-term side effects are usually limited to warm flashes and occasional nausea.

Mouridsen et al. (35) reported 1650 high-risk patients with breast cancer selected at random to receive radiation therapy or radiation therapy plus 1 year of tamoxifen after total mastectomy and axillary lymph node sampling. Patients were designated

617

"high-risk" if positive lymph nodes were found, the tumor was 5 cm in diameter, or invasion of the skin or fascia was present. Patients with distant metastases were excluded. Overall recurrence-free survival at 6 years was 39% in the radiation group and 48% in the radiation-plus-tamoxifen group. Although the overall improvement was not statistically significant, four subgroups of patients were found to benefit from tamoxifen:

1. Patients < 69 years of age

2. Patients with ≥ 4 positive axillary nodes

3. Patients with grade 1-2 tumors (low-grade)

4. Patients with high ER-positive levels (> 100 fmole/mg)

The lack of significant side effects with tamoxifen and the uncertainty about beneficial effects of adjuvant chemotherapy for postmenopausal women led Cummings et al. (36) to design a double-blind trial comparing tamoxifen given for 2 years postoperatively with a placebo for women over the age of 65 years with Stage II breast cancer. There were 170 women eligible for the trial. With a median follow-up of 55 months, the overall disease-free survival at 4 years was 73% for those treated with tamoxifen and 52% for those treated with placebo. In this study, patients who particularly benefited from tamoxifen were similar to those identified in the earlier study, i.e., patients with 4–10 positive axillary lymph nodes and ER-positive cancers measuring less than 3 cm in diameter. **The conclusion of the National Institutes of Health consensus panel for breast cancer was that tamoxifen should now be regarded as standard therapy for postmenopausal patients with positive axillary lymph nodes and positive hormone receptor status, because tamoxifen significantly improves disease-free survival** (37). A summary of the role of hormonal therapy in combination with chemotherapy is presented in Chapter 14.

Summary

A prototype flow chart for the use of hormonal therapy has evolved primarily from the vast experience with breast cancer (Fig. 17.2). This plan is now applied to patients with endometrial and ovarian cancers as discussed below.

Endometrial Cancer

Progestin therapy for endometrial cancer was well established even before the biochemical identification of ER and PR (39). A differential sensitivity to progestin therapy has been recognized, and many factors have been identified as being important in this sensitivity (40).

The correlates of response to progestin therapy include:

1. The extent and location of metastases

2. Recurrence within prior radiation therapy fields

3. The degree of histologic differentiation

4. The interval between primary treatment and diagnosis of recurrence

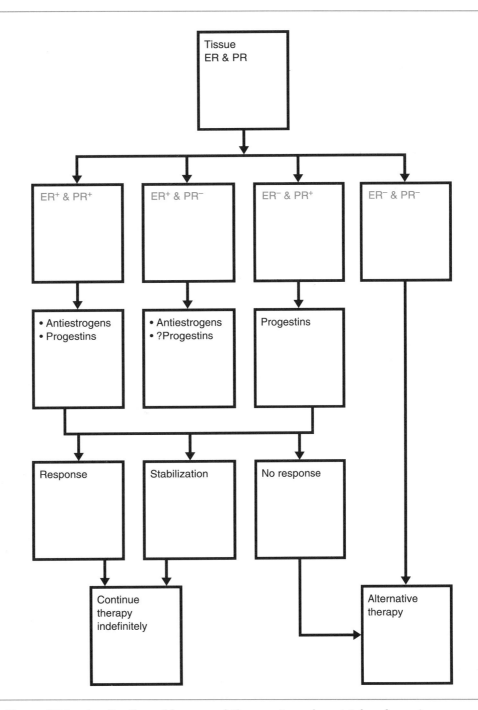

Figure 17.2   Application of hormonal therapy in endometrial and ovarian cancer based on tissue levels of ER and PR.

5. The age of the patient

6. The type and dose of progestin therapy

7. The duration of progestin therapy

Several mechanisms for the progestin effect, including immunologic mechanisms, alterations in the endogenous hormonal status of the patient, and a direct anties-

619

trogen effect at the cellular level, have been postulated (40). The identification of the ER and PR proteins has permitted a more precise approach to the hormonal management of endometrial cancer; i.e., ER- and PR-poor endometrial cancers are more likely to respond to cytotoxic chemotherapy than endometrial cancers with higher receptor levels (41).

Progestin Receptors

There is a close correlation between PR levels in endometrial cancer and 17β-hydroxysteroid dehydrogenase (17β-HSD) activity, the enzyme that converts highly biologically active estradiol to the less active estrone. 17β-HSD activity can be induced in well-differentiated endometrial cancers exposed to progestins and is induced in normal endometrium after ovulation.

Tissue Processing

Estimation of ER and PR content of endometrial cancers is usually based on endometrial samples obtained by dilatation and curettage (42–47). The difficulty with this approach is that the curettings may contain normal endometrium as well as endometrial cancer. Even in the postmenopausal patient, normal endometrial tissue has measurable levels of ER and PR.

A second important factor that may influence hormonal receptor analysis is the time elapsed between obtaining of the tissue and analysis of the specimen. Delaying the analysis may cause loss of receptor protein. Most reports of ER and PR have been determined on stored tissue, so these data may be inaccurate.

Tumor Grade

Most investigators have documented that the ER and PR content of endometrial cancers correlates with the differentiation of the tumor (Table 17.1).

Whereas about four-fifths of well-differentiated lesions contain receptors, only about three-tenths of poorly differentiated lesions contain significant ER and PR levels. Also, early-stage cancers tend to be well differentiated, whereas advanced-stage cancers tend to be poorly differentiated.

One study of 82 patients with previously untreated endometrial cancer (46) reported a direct correlation between receptor content and histologic grade. The

Table 17.1 Endometrial Cancer: Grade versus Receptor Content

Tumor Grade	E_2R/PrR Positive (DCCA >7 FM) (%)	E_2R/PrR Positive (SDGA >3 FM 8S) (%)
1	20/24 (83)	17/24 (71)
2	14/24 (58)	11/24 (46)
3	5/16 (31)	5/16 (31)
Recurrence	5/14 (36)	5/14 (36)

Reproduced, with permission, from Creasman WT, McCarty KS Sr, Barton TK, McCarty KS Jr: Clinical correlates of estrogen- and progesterone-binding proteins in human endometrial adenocarcinoma. *Obstet Gynecol* 55:363, 1980.
DCCA = Dextran-coated charcoal analysis.
SDGA = Sucrose density gradient analysis.

mean level of PR was 265 fmole/mg cytosol protein for grade 1 lesions, 150 fmole/mg for grade 2, and 40 fmole/mg for grade 3. The quantity of ER was 87 fmole/mg cytosol protein for grade 1 lesions, 35 fmole/mg for grade 2 lesions, and 35 fmole/mg for grade 3 lesions. Each grade 1 or 2 cancer had detectable levels of PR, and most had detectable levels of ER. Grade 3 cancers frequently had no significant levels of PR or ER. Cancer specimens from 52 of 82 patients were available for both PR and ER assessment: 25 of the 52 (48%) were ER-positive/PR-positive, 16 (31%) were ER-negative/PR-positive, 11 (21%) were ER-negative/PR-negative, and none were ER-positive/PR-negative.

Reference Values

Patients are typically considered to have an ER-rich cancer if the content of receptor is > 30 fmole/mg and a PR-rich tumor if the receptor content is > 20 fmole/mg, but these values are based on breast data rather than on endometrial cancer data. In fact, from a review of the literature, it is unclear what the limits should be for considering endometrial cancers to be receptor-rich or receptor-poor (42–47). Studies vary between values of 7–50 fmole/mg for PR positivity. For grade 2 cancers, the limits can make a significant difference in terms of receptor status. If lower reference values are used (42, 46), tumors are twice as likely to be considered rich in ER and PR.

Depth of Invasion

An inverse correlation between depth of invasion and receptor content of endometrial cancers has been reported (41, 48). Kauppila et al. (48) showed that when Stage I endometrial cancers have infiltrated deeper into the myometrium, their ER and PR levels are lower. Mean PR levels of 390 fmole/mg were found when there was no superficial myometrial invasion. With deep invasion, however, the mean PR content was 61 fmole/mg. Similarly, ER levels decreased from a mean of 145 to a mean of 32 fmole/mg as tumors were found to have more deeply invaded the myometrium.

Progestin Therapy

Progestin therapy has been employed for the treatment of advanced endometrial cancer, and responses have been documented. The likelihood of a response correlates with the differentiation of the tumor (Table 17.2). In fact, primary tumors are more likely to be well differentiated than tissue from metastatic lesions, which are more likely to be poorly differentiated. Therefore, correlation of the PR level with response depends on the source of the tissue that is evaluated. For metastatic disease, it is not clear whether the PR level of the primary tumor can be used to determine a patient's likely response to hormone therapy. As seen in Table 17.3, responses to progestin therapy have been reported frequently. In the series by Martin et al. (44), 13 patients had an objective response, but only two patients with vaginal apex recurrences had complete disappearance of their tumors. These patients regularly had stabilization of disease as their "objective response" to progestin therapy.

A report by Ehrlich et al. (46) supports the use of progestin therapy based on the PR content of the cancer. With a reference level for PR positivity of 50 fmole/mg, seven of eight patients (88%) with PR-positive tumors responded to hormonal therapy, compared with only 1 of 16 PR-negative patients (6%). **These data indicate that very high levels of PR are predictive of response.**

Table 17.2   Endometrial Cancer: Response to Progestins versus Tumor Grade

Grade	Objective Response (%)
1	30/58 (51.7)
3	7/45 (15.5)
Total	37/103 (35.9)

Reproduced, with permission, from Kohorn E, et al.: Progesterone therapy in metastatic endometrial cancer. *Gynecol Oncol* 4:398, 1976.

Table 17.3   Endometrial Adenocarcinoma: Relationship Between Response to Progestins and PR Content

Author	Responders		Nonresponders	
	PR+	PR−	PR+	PR−
Creasman et al. (42)	4	0	1	8
Martin et al. (44)	13	1	0	6
Benraad et al. (45)	6	2	1	5
Ehrlich et al. (46)	7	1	1	15
Schwartz & Naftolin	1	0	7	4
Total	31 (89%)	4 (11%)	9 (19%)	38 (81%)

At Yale University, 41 patients with endometrial cancer were treated with oral medroxyprogesterone acetate (Provera); 27 had recurrent disease, and 12 had advanced primary disease. Only one patient (2%) had a complete response, and two patients (5%) had partial responses. The patient with the complete response had a Stage II, grade 1 cancer and had developed lung metastases, which responded dramatically to progestin therapy. Her disease recurred 2½ years later and resulted in her death. The two partial responses occurred in patients whose tumors had elevated PR levels. Four patients with elevated PR levels had stable disease, and three had progressive disease. Stabilization of disease averaged 12 months in previously untreated patients with no clinically detectable cancer but averaged only 6.6 months in patients with clinically detectable disease. Stabilization averaged 10.3 months for recurrent disease that was not clinically detectable and 6.6 months when recurrent disease was clinically evident. Overall, the progression-free interval with progestins was 11.4 months for patients with no clinical evidence of disease.

Antiestrogen Therapy

Tamoxifen should to be effective in the management of endometrial cancer. It decreases the levels of ER, making the cell less responsive to estrogen stimulation. However, tamoxifen also stimulates the synthesis of PR, a phenomenon observed in patients whose initial levels of PR were undetectable but became measurable after tamoxifen treatment (49).

For reasons that are poorly understood, most patients treated with tamoxifen alone for recurrent endometrial cancer do not have an objective response to the therapy (49). In our experience, only one of eight patients had a partial response that lasted 4 months. Two additional patients had stabilization of disease for 5 and 6 months, respectively. These three patients had ER-positive tumors, but three of five patients who did not respond to tamoxifen also had ER-positive tumors.

Summary

Currently available data suggest the following conclusions regarding steroid receptors and endometrial cancer:

1. PR levels correlate with histologic grade, myometrial invasion, and stage of disease.

2. Response to progestin therapy can be predicted by histologic grade.

3. Patients with a histologically well-differentiated advanced or recurrent endometrial cancer should initially be given a trial of progestin therapy.

4. Patients with a histologically poorly differentiated advanced or recurrent endometrial cancer are best treated with cytotoxic chemotherapy.

5. There is a lack of uniformity in defining assay levels for receptor-rich and receptor-poor endometrial cancer.

6. Tamoxifen alone or in sequential administration with progestins may stabilize advanced or recurrent endometrial cancer, but will rarely provide long-term benefit.

7. The role of steroid receptor determinations in the routine management of endometrial cancer has yet to be established.

Ovarian Cancer

Ovarian cancer has emerged as the *bete noir* of gynecologic cancer because of the difficulty of early diagnosis. The poor survival of patients treated with combination chemotherapy has given impetus to clinical investigation of hormonal therapy in the management of these tumors, and the past decade has witnessed the identification of ER and PR in epithelial cancers of the ovary. In 1978 Schwartz et al. (50) presented the first series of epithelial ovarian cancers to be studied specifically for the presence of estrogen-binding macromolecules. Subsequent experience with 30 previously untreated epithelial ovarian cancers confirmed the presence of ER in 16.

Heterogeneity of ER content in primary ovarian cancer samples and metastases has been documented (51). Consistent levels of ER can be demonstrated in the primary tumor, but metastases and primary tumors differ in ER content. Primary cancers rich in receptors may have receptor-poor metastases, and occasionally receptor-poor primary tumors may have receptor-rich metastases.

Receptors and Histology

A report of 113 primary epithelial ovarian cancers correlated multiple histologic parameters (histologic type, grade, necrosis, fibrosis, lymphocyte infiltration, mitotic rate, tumor giant cells, psammoma bodies, stroma) with the ER and PR content of the tumors (51). The significant finding was that very poorly differentiated (grade 4) cancers had a greater likelihood of ER positivity than lower-grade cancers, 61% and 22%, respectively. Among grade 3 tumors, those containing abundant mitoses were more often ER-positive than those containing fewer mitoses. PR content correlated universally with the presence of lymphocytic infiltration; i.e., PR was more often positive in tumors with minimal lymphocytic infiltration.

With the exception of a small group of grade 3 or 4 tumors, ER content of epithelial ovarian cancers was independent of all histologic features studied. Similarly, with the exception of lymphocytic infiltration, PR content was also independent of these histologic parameters.

Recurrent Ovarian Cancer

Progestin Therapy

Because traditional chemotherapy for ovarian epithelial cancer has not been successful, wide-ranging strategies of hormonal therapy have been used. Progestin therapy has been used for the past 30 years in the treatment of epithelial ovarian cancers (52–58) (Table 17.4). Early reports tended to be vague in distinguishing objective tumor responses from subjective responses.

Delalutin

There are three reports (52–54) on the use of Delalutin (17 hydroxyprogesterone in oil) for the treatment of advanced and recurrent epithelial ovarian cancer. Five objective responses were observed in 39 patients (13%), with a response duration of 3 to 6 months. No toxicity was reported. Subjectively, an increased sense of well-being was noted by many patients.

Provera

The progestational agent most commonly used for the management of advanced or recurrent ovarian cancer is Provera (medroxyprogesterone acetate), an agent that has been administered in both oral and intramuscular forms. Oral Provera has produced only three objective responses among 87 patients treated, but no toxicity has been reported (55–58).

Results of intramuscularly (IM) administered Provera in oil (Depo-Provera) have been no more encouraging. Three reports of IM administration of Provera to a

Table 17.4 Progestin Therapy in Advanced and Recurrent Ovarian Cancer

Progestin	Author	Year	Patients Treated	Patients Responding	Response (%)
Delalutin (IM)	Varga and Henriksen (53)	1964	6	1	16
	Ward (54)	1972	23	3	13
	Jolles (65)	1983	10	1	10
Provera (PO)	Kaufman (55)	1966	11	1	9
	Malkasian et al. (56)	1977	19	1	5
	Mangioni et al. (57)	1981	30	0	0
	Aabo et al. (58)	1982	27	1	4
Provera (IM)	Slayton et al. (59)	1981	19	0	0
	Mangioni et al. (57)	1981	33	5	15
	Tropé et al. (60)	1982	25	1	4
Megace (PO)	Geisler (63)	1985	31	10	32
	Ahlgren (64)	1985	26	1	4
	Schwartz	1987	12	0	0
Total			**272**	**25**	**9**

Delalutin: 17-α-Hydroxyprogesterone caproate.
Provera: Medroxyprogesterone acetate.
Megace: Megestrol acetate.

total of 77 patients demonstrated objective responses in only six patients (8%) (57, 59, 60). The more recent series used more objective response criteria than the earlier series with Delalutin. The toxicity of IM Provera included hypertension associated with fluid retention in one patient. Oral Provera (200 mg four times daily) in combination with cytotoxic chemotherapy (mitomycin and vinblastine) has been reported in the treatment of recurrent epithelial ovarian cancer (61), and none of 13 patients had an objective response. **Provera seems ineffective in the treatment of ovarian cancer.**

Megace

Geisler (62, 63) used high-dose oral megestrol acetate (Megace), 800 mg daily for 1 month and then 400 mg daily thereafter, in the management of advanced or recurrent ovarian cancer. Ten of 31 patients (32%) had an objective remission. Six patients had a complete response lasting 5–36 months (mean = 16.5), and four patients had a partial response with a progression-free interval ranging from 4–10 months. Toxicity was not reported; nor were PR values. Ahlgren et al. (64) reported their experience with the same dosage of Megace in 26 patients who had failed prior cytotoxic chemotherapy. Only one partial response lasting 4 months was observed. We have treated 12 such patients with high-dose megestrol acetate, and no objective responses have been seen. **We do not recommend Megace for the treatment of ovarian cancer.**

Combination Estrogen and Progestin Therapy

Recognition of the need for hormones to bind to their receptors in target tissues in order to evoke a hormone-induced response resulted in a study combining estrogen and progestins as second-line therapy in a series of patients in whom cisplatin combination chemotherapy had failed (65). Sixty-five patients received oral ethinyl estradiol, 0.1 mg daily, for 25 days of a 30-day cycle and oral Provera, 100 mg daily, on days 8 through 25, followed by no therapy on days 26 through 30. The cycle was then repeated. Nine patients (14%) had objective responses. One patient had a cerebrovascular accident during her first course of hormonal therapy. One patient who had a partial response was the only one who discontinued therapy because of severe nausea. We do not consider this sufficient evidence to recommend treatment with estrogens and progestins in ovarian cancer.

Antiestrogen Therapy

Tamoxifen Therapy

The identification of the ER led to establishment of treatment programs designed to determine the role of the estrogen agonist-antagonist tamoxifen in the management of epithelial ovarian cancers. In our series (66), 13 patients with advanced or recurrent epithelial ovarian cancer were treated with oral tamoxifen. Most patients had previously undergone unsuccessful chemotherapy or radiation therapy and had ER determinations of their tumors before treatment. Patients initially received tamoxifen 10 mg twice daily, and in those who did not respond the dose was doubled every 4 weeks to a maximum daily dose of 320 mg. No complete response was observed, but one patient had a partial response that lasted 2 months and in four patients the disease was stabilized for 11 to 30 weeks. Eight patients had no response to tamoxifen, but five of those eight had a partial small-bowel obstruction and may not have absorbed the tamoxifen. These five patients died within 9 weeks of treatment, and the three other patients who did not respond died within 24 weeks.

Each patient who showed stabilization of disease on the tamoxifen regimen had a cancer rich in ER (23–169 fmole/mg). However, ER-rich tumors were also present in the group that failed to respond. There were no differences in the two groups of patients with respect to histologic type, grade of tumor, or time from initial diagnosis to initiation of tamoxifen therapy.

Eight subsequent reports have shown an objective response rate for tamoxifen therapy varying from 0–27.6% (Table 17.5) (67–73). The most significant experience was that of Hatch et al., (73) who reported 10 complete responses (9.5%) and 8 partial responses (7.6%) among a group of 105 women with refractory ovarian cancer who were treated with tamoxifen. The clinical value of tamoxifen in the management of epithelial ovarian cancer awaits further study.

Primary Ovarian Cancer

Progestin Therapy

Berqvist et al. (74) administered IM Provera to four patients with advanced, previously untreated ovarian cancer, and they observed objective responses in three patients. Each of three patients with mucinous carcinomas responded to progestin therapy, but in the fourth patient, a Stage IV serous carcinoma rapidly progressed during therapy (Table 17.6).

The well-documented observation that endometrial cancer may respond to progestin therapy led Rendina et al. (75) to study a series of 41 patients with endometrioid ovarian cancers given high-dose IM Provera as primary therapy (Table 17.6). Of the 31 patients with advanced cancer, 26 had well-differentiated tumors. Thirty patients had Stage III disease, and one had Stage IV disease. Estrogen receptors were present in 81.3% of the primary tumors, and progesterone receptors were present in 72.1%. ER and PR content appeared to correlate with the histologic grade. Only 14% of the well-differentiated cancers were receptor-negative. Seventeen of 30 patients had an objective response; three had a complete response, and 14 had a partial response. In eight patients the disease was stable, and in six patients the disease progressed. Ten patients with Stage III disease

Table 17.5 Tamoxifen Therapy in Refractory Ovarian Cancer

Study	Year	No. of Patients	Response Complete (CR)	Response Partial (PR)	Stable	CR + PR%
Schwartz et al. (66)	1982	13	0	1	4	7.7%
Pagel et al. (67)	1983	29	1	7	12	27.6%
Hamerlynck et al. (68)	1985	18	0	1	2	5.6%
Shirley et al. (69)	1985	23	0	0	19	0
Slevin et al. (70)	1986	22	0	0	1	0
Weiner et al. (71)	1987	37	1	2	6	8.1%
Osborne et al. (72)	1988	53	0	1	5	1.9%
Hatch et al. (73)	1991	105	10	8	40	17.1%
Total		**300**	**12**	**20**	**89**	**10.7%**

CR = Complete response; PR = partial response.

Table 17.6   Progestin Therapy as Primary Treatment in Ovarian Cancer

Progestin	Author	Year	Patients Treated	Patients Responding	Response (%)
Provera (IM)	Berqvist et al. (74)	1984	4	3	75
	Rendina et al. (75)	1982	31*	17	58
Depostat (IM)	Timothy (76)	1982	15	3	20
Total			**50**	**23**	**46**

Depostat: Gestronol hexanoate.
Provera: Medroxyprogesterone acetate.
*All patients had endometrioid ovarian carcinoma.

were alive after 3 years. For the entire series, complete and partial responses to progestin therapy were observed only in that group of patients whose cancers contained ER or both ER and PR. Six of eight patients with steroid receptor-poor tumors demonstrated progressive disease, and the remaining two had stable disease. **The results of this study clearly support the concept that endometrioid ovarian cancers, like endometrial cancers, are hormonally sensitive tumors, and responses to progestin therapy may be correlated with the steroid receptor content of the primary cancer.**

Timothy (76) reported 15 patients with epithelial ovarian cancer who received IM Depostat as primary therapy (Table 17.6). Seven patients with Stage III or IV disease had progression-free intervals of 9 to 48 months. Two patients had complete responses that lasted 9 and 18 months, respectively, and one had a partial response that allowed easy surgical excision; she survived 48 months. In addition, all eight patients with Stage I–II disease remained free of disease 6–72 months after diagnosis. Patients reported an increased sense of well-being despite advanced disease. These results are consistent with those of others cited above and strongly suggest that progestins might be used as first-line therapy for patients with epithelial ovarian cancer. However, data on ER and PR content are not consistently available in these reports, and a method of identifying patients who might benefit from progestin therapy remains to be established.

Estrogen Therapy

There is a paucity of literature on the role of estrogen therapy in the management of advanced epithelial ovarian cancer. Long and Evans (77) reported 14 patients with advanced metastatic ovarian cancer who were given oral diethylstilbestrol (DES) at high doses of 15–30 mg per day. Five of the patients were lost to follow-up. Two of the nine evaluable patients had an objective response for more than 1 year after the initiation of therapy. One patient had a papillary adenocarcinoma with generalized metastases, and the other had myxomatous peritonei. Three patients noted an increased sense of well-being similar to that experienced with progestin therapy. In at least one patient the disease was thought to have been aggravated by DES therapy. Possibly, the DES suppresses gonadotropin, and this may result in the observed therapeutic effects. A summary of hormonal medications is shown in Table 17.7.

Hormonal and Cytotoxic Chemotherapy

Tamoxifen

At Yale University School of Medicine, a prospective randomized trial employing tamoxifen in combination with cytotoxic chemotherapy was initiated in patients

627

Table 17.7   Hormones and Hormonal Antagonists

Drug	Route of Administration	Common Treatment Schedules	Common Toxicities	Common Cancers Treated
Estrogens				
Diethylstilbesterol	Oral	15 mg daily	Gynecomastia, nausea and vomiting, fluid retention, changes in libido, hypercalcemia, endometrial carcinoma	Postmenopausal breast
Progestins				
Hydroxyprogesterone caproate (Delalutin)	IM	1 g twice weekly	Fluid retention, epithelial changes in the genital tract, nausea, sterile abscesses from injections	Endometrium, ovary, breast
Medroxyprogesterone acetate (Provera)	IM	300 mg weekly		
	Oral	150 mg daily		
Megesterol acetate (Megace)	Oral	160–320 mg daily		
Androgens				
Testosterone propionate (Oreton proprionate)	IM	50–200 mg twice weekly	Virilization in females, change in libido, fluid retention, cholestatic jaundice, hypercalcemia	Breast
Fluoxymesterone (Halotestin)	Oral	10–40 mg daily		
Corticosteroids				
Prednisone	Oral	40–210 mg daily	Fluid retention hypertension, diabetes mellitus, gastric irritation, potassium loss, psychosis	Breast, neurologic symptoms from metastatic disease, hypercalcemia
Dexamethasone (Decadron)	Oral	0.5–4 mg daily		
Hormone Antagonists				
Tamoxifen	Oral	20 mg daily	Myelosuppression, retinitis	Breast, ovary
Gonadotropin-Releasing Hormone Analogues				
Leuprolide (Lupron)	SQ	1 mg daily	Fluid retention	Ovary
D-TRP-6-LHRH (Decapeptyl)	IM	3 mg monthly (sustained release)	Vaginal dryness	

with Stage III or IV ovarian cancer after determination of receptor status (78). Patients were randomly selected to receive intravenous Adriamycin and cisplatin every 4 weeks, to a maximum of 18 treatments, with or without oral tamoxifen, 10 mg twice daily throughout the treatment. Of 100 patients treated, 51 received cytotoxic chemotherapy alone and 49 received tamoxifen in combination with cytotoxic chemotherapy. Survival was no different in patients who received the combination of tamoxifen and cytotoxic chemotherapy than in those who received cytotoxic chemotherapy alone.

Progestin

Kahanpaa et al. (79) reported 10 patients with advanced ovarian cancer (five primary, five recurrent) who received Provera (1 g IM weekly) and combination chemotherapy with cisplatin, Adriamycin, and Cytoxan. This group of patients was compared with 10 patients who received chemotherapy only. No objective responses were observed in patients who received combined progestin and chemotherapy, but two complete responses and one partial response were documented in those who received only the chemotherapy. The authors noted that the patients had unfavorable therapeutic and prognostic factors and that no ER or PR levels were available.

Radiolabeled Estrogen Therapy

The identification of ER proteins in approximately 50% of epithelial ovarian cancers and the synthesis of a gamma-emitting estrogen ($16\alpha^{125}$I-iodoestradiol) that binds with high affinity to the ER led us to initiate a study to determine whether the compound might be useful in imaging ER-rich cancers and might subsequently have a therapeutic role in ovarian cancer (80). In 11 patients with epithelial ovarian cancer who were undergoing surgery, 0.3 mCi of $16\alpha^{125}$I-iodoestradiol was injected, and at specific times after administration portions of the cancer, control tissues (muscle, fat), and blood were removed and counted in a scintillation counter. There was a strong correlation between ER concentration in the cancer specimens and the amount of nuclear radioactivity but no correlation between the radioactivity in the tumor and that in the muscle or fat. A substantial proportion (approximately 30%) of the radioactivity was present in the cell nucleus, consistent with a steroid receptor–mediated process. Whereas rapid liver metabolism of this compound precludes its use for the routine imaging of ER-rich cancers, the synthesis of analogues that are protected from inactivation may lead to compounds that will be of diagnostic and therapeutic value for ER-rich ovarian cancers.

Androgen Therapy

The presence of androgen receptors (AR) has supported research in androgen therapy (14–21). Kaufman (55) treated advanced refractory ovarian cancers with unspecified androgens but was unable to demonstrate a beneficial effect. Recently, Kavanagh et al. (81) treated 16 women who had refractory ovarian cancer with fluoxymesterone (*Halotestin*). Unfortunately, no objective responses were observed.

Gonadotropin-Releasing Hormone Analogue Therapy

In three reported studies (82–84) gonadotropin-releasing analogues have been used in the treatment of refractory ovarian cancer (Table 17.8). Parmar et al. (82) used D-Trp-6-luteinizing hormone (*Decapeptyl*) in 39 women with refractory ovarian cancer and demonstrated partial remissions in 6 patients (15%). Kavanagh et al. (83) and Bruckner et al. (84) each used leuprolide acetate (*Lupron*) to treat patients who had refractory ovarian cancer, and 7 of 28 (25%) demonstrated objective responses. Responses occurred most often in women who had well-differentiated tumors. This may be a promising avenue for treatment, but further studies will be required.

Hormone Replacement Therapy After Cancer

Postmenopausal hormone therapy for women who have been treated for potentially hormonally dependent cancers is controversial. However, there are limited data to justify either withholding or administration of estrogen therapy. Although most authors agree with the use of hormone replacement therapy in patients with a history of treated invasive squamous carcinomas of the cervix, vulva, and vagina, there exists little consensus on the recommendation for the use of such therapy in those with a previous diagnosis of adenocarcinomas of the endometrium, ovary,

Table 17.8   Gonadotropin-Releasing Hormone Analogues in Refractory Ovarian Cancer Treatment

Study	Year	No. of Patients	Complete (CR)	Partial (PR)	Stable	CR + PR%
			\<Response\>			
Parmar et al. (82) (D-TRP-6 LHRH)	1988	39	0	6	5	15.4%
Kavanagh et al. (83) (Leuprolide)	1989	23	0	4	2	17.2%
Bruckner et al. (84) (Leuprolide)	1989	5	1	2	2	60.0%
Total		67	1	12	9	19.4%

CR = Complete response; PR = partial response.

and breast. Hormone replacement therapy in such high-risk women has yet to be evaluated in prospective randomized trials to determine the benefit of the therapy versus the risk of recurrent disease.

There are now several studies in which women who have previously had endometrial cancer have received hormone replacement therapy. **In general, the series have failed to show that replacement estrogen therapy was deleterious to the health of the women who previously had been treated for endometrial cancer.** However, the women who received treatment in these series had well- or moderately well-differentiated adenocarcinomas that had very little likelihood of recurrence (1–4). Ironically, the women at highest risk of their cancers being stimulated by hormonal therapy (those with well- or moderately well-differentiated endometrial cancers) are the ones who receive the therapy. Women with poorly differentiated cancers who are less likely to have steroid hormones present in their tumor cells have been the ones who have not received hormone replacement therapy. The natural history of well-differentiated adenocarcinomas of the endometrium treated with hysterectomy, with or without additional radiation therapy, is so good that it would appear that hormone replacement therapy does not put the patient at excess risk. In general, we recommend waiting at least 6 months to 1 year from completion of the endometrial cancer treatment before hormone replacement therapy is initiated. The risks as well as the benefits of this treatment should be clearly understood by the patient and her family.

Less information is available regarding the risk/benefit ratio for hormone replacement therapy after a prior diagnosis of epithelial ovarian cancer. Although estrogen and progestin receptor proteins are present in about half of the ovarian cancer specimens measured, it has yet to be established whether these are functional receptors. The minimal information currently available would suggest that the receptors tend not to be functional in epithelial ovarian cancers, with the possible exception of well-differentiated endometrioid adenocarcinomas of the ovary. Eelles et al. (89) have retrospectively reviewed a series of 373 women under the age of 50 who were treated for ovarian cancer; 78 of these patients received hormone replacement therapy. After consideration of other therapy factors (stage of cancer, differentiation of tumor, histology), no significant difference in overall or disease-free survival was noted in the group receiving hormone replacement therapy compared with the group who did not receive hormones. **Therefore one should consider giving replacement estrogen therapy to women who have been castrated as part of their ovarian cancer management.** Nevertheless, multi-institutional trials will be necessary to establish whether there is a beneficial or detrimental effect on the management of such patients.

Hormone replacement therapy after diagnosis of breast cancer is quite controversial, and data regarding the value of such an approach are extremely limited (90–92). Therefore, until such data are available, we do not recommend routine hormone replacement therapy for women with hormone receptor–positive breast cancers.

References

1. **Jensen EV, DeSombre ER, Jungblut PN:** Estrogen receptors in hormone responsive tissues and tumors. In Wissler RE, Dao TL, Wood S (eds): *Endogenous Factors Influencing Host-Tumor Balance*. Chicago, University of Chicago Press, 1967, p 15.

2. **Clark JH, Peck EJ Jr:** Steroid receptor characterization and measurement. In *Female Sex Steroids Receptors and Function*. New York, Springer-Verlag, 1979, pp 4–36.

3. **Jensen EV:** The pattern of hormone-receptor interactions. In Griffiths K, Pierrepoint CG (eds): *Some Aspects of the Etiology and Biochemistry of Prostatic Cancer*. Cardiff, Alpha Omega Alpha, 1970, p 151.

4. **Janne O, Kauppila A, Kontula K, et al:** Female sex steroid receptors in normal, hyperplastic and carcinomatous endometrium: the relationship to serum steroid hormones and gonadotropin and changes during medroxyprogesterone acetate administration. *Int J Cancer* 24:545, 1979.

5. **Martin PM, Rolland PH, Gammerre M, et al:** Estradiol and progesterone receptors in normal and neoplastic endometrium: correlations between receptors, histopathological examinations and clinical responses under progestin therapy. *Int J Cancer* 23:321, 1979.

6. **Benraad RJ, Friberg LG, Koenders AJM, Kullander S:** Do estrogen and progesterone receptors (E_2R and PR) in metastasizing endometrial cancers predict the response to gestagen therapy? *Acta Obstet Gynecol Scand* 59:155, 1980.

7. **Holt JA, Caputo TA, Kelly KM:** Estrogen and progestin binding in cytosols of ovarian adenocarcinomas. *Obstet Gynecol* 53:50, 1979.

8. **Schwartz PE, ViVolsi VA, Hildreth N, et al:** Estrogen receptors in human ovarian epithelial carcinoma. *Obstet Gynecol* 59:229, 1982.

9. **Clark JH, Hardin JW, McCormack SA:** Estrogen receptor binding and the stimulation of normal and abnormal growth. In Witliff JL, DaPunt O (eds): *Steroid Receptors and Hormone Dependent Neoplasia*. New York, Masson Publishing USA, 1980, pp 19–28.

10. **DeSombre ER, Greene GL, King WJ, Jensen EV:** Estrogen receptors, antibodies and hormone dependent cancer. In Gurpide E, Calandra R, Levy C, Soto RJ (eds): *Hormones and Cancer*. New York, Alan R Liss, 1984, pp 1–21.

11. **Dickson RB, McManaway ME, Lippman ME:** Estrogen-induced factors of breast cancer cells partially replace estrogen to promote tumor growth. *Science* 232:1540, 1986.

12. **Carcangiu ML, Chambers JT, Voynick IM, et al:** Immunohistochemical evaluation of estrogen and progesterone receptor content in 183 patients with endometrial carcinoma. Part I. Clinical and histologic correlations. *Am J Clin Pathol* 94:247, 1990.

13. **Chambers JT, Carcangiu ML, Voynick IM, Schwartz PE:** Immunohistochemical evaluation of estrogen and progesterone receptor content, in 183 patients with endometrial carcinoma. Part II. Correlation between biochemical and immunohistochemical methods and survival. *Am J Clin Pathol* 94:255, 1990.

14. **Friberg LG, Kullander S, Persian JP, et al:** On receptors for estrogen (ER) and androgens (DHT) in human endometrial carcinoma and ovarian tumors. *Acta Obstet Gynecol Scand* 57:261, 1978.

15. **Galli MC, Giovanni CDE, Nicolletti G, et al:** The occurrence of multiple steroid hormone receptors in disease-free and neoplastic human ovary. *Cancer* 47:1297, 1981.

16. **Quinn MA, Pearce P, Rome R, et al:** Cytoplasmic steroid receptors in ovarian tumours. *Br J Obstet Gynaecol* 89:754, 1982.

17. **Wurz H, Wassner E, Citoler P, et al:** Multiple cytoplasmic steroid hormone receptors in benign and malignant ovarian tumors and in disease-free ovaries. *Tumor Diagn Ther* 4:15, 1983.

18. **Kuhner R, DeGraff J, Rao BR, et al:** Androgen receptor predominance in human ovarian carcinoma. *J Steroid Biochem* 26:393, 1987.

19. **Kuhner R, Rao R, Poels LG, et al:** Multiple parameter analyses of human ovarian cancer: morphology, immunohistochemistry, steroid hormone receptors and aromatase. *Anticancer Res* 8:281, 1988.

20. **Slotman BJ, Rao BR:** The presence of a hitherto undefined high-capacity androgen binding macromolecule in human ovarian cancer tissue. *J Steroid Biochem* 33:105, 1989.

21. **Rao BR, Slotman BJ, Geldof AA, et al:** Correlation between tumor histology, steroid receptor status, and adenosine deaminase complexing protein immunoreactivity in ovarian cancer. *Int J Gynecol Pathol* 9:47, 1990.

22. **Rao BR, Slotman BJ:** Endocrine factors in common epithelial cancers. *Endocrine Rev* 12:14, 1991.

23. **Nakano R, Kitagama S, Yamoto M, et al:** Localization of gonadotropin binding sites in human ovarian neoplasms. *Am J Obstet Gynecol* 161:905, 1989.

24. **Beatson GT:** On the treatment of inoperable cases of carcinoma of the mammary gland: suggestions for a new method of treatment with illustrative cases. *Lancet* 2:104, 162, 1986.

25. **Brodie AM, Santen RJ:** Aromatase in breast cancer and the role of aminoglutethimide and other aromatase inhibitors. *Crit Rev Oncol Hematol* 5:361, 1986.

26. **Love RR:** Tamoxifen therapy in primary breast cancer: Biology, efficacy, and side effects. *J Clin Oncol* 7:803, 1989.

27. **Jensen EV:** Hormone dependency of breast cancer. *Cancer* 47:2319, 1981.

28. **Sundaram GS, Manimekalai S, Wenk RE, Goldstein PJ:** Estrogen and progesterone receptor assays in human breast cancer: a brief review of the relevant terms, methods and clinical usefulness. *Obstet Gynecol Surv* 39:719, 1984.

29. **Knight WA, Livingston RB, Gregory EJ, McGuire WL:** Estrogen receptor as an independent prognostic factor for early recurrence in breast cancer. *Cancer Res* 37:4669, 1977.

30. **Lippman M, Allegra JC:** Estrogen receptor and endocrine therapy of breast cancer. *N Engl J Med* 299:930, 1978.

31. **Hubay CA, Arafah B, Gordon NH, et al:** Hormone receptors: an update and application. *Surg Clin North Am* 64:1155, 1984.

32. **Giuliano AE:** Breast. In Benson RC (ed): *Current Gynecologic Diagnosis and Treatment*, ed 5. Los Altos, Calif., Lange Medical Publishers, 1985.

33. **Ingle JN, Ahmann DL, Green SJ, et al:** Randomized clinical trial of diethylstilbestrol versus Tamoxifen in postmenopausal women. *N Engl J Med* 304:16, 1981.

34. **Mouridsen HT, Palshof T, Patterson J, Battersby L:** Tamoxifen in advanced breast cancer. *Cancer Treat Rev* 5:131, 1978.

35. **Mouridsen HT, Andersen AP, Brincker H, et al:** Adjuvant tamoxifen in postmenopausal high-risk breast cancer patients: present status of Danish breast cancer cooperative group trials. *Natl Cancer Inst Monogr* 1:115, 1986.

36. **Cummings FJ, Gray R, Davis TE, et al:** Tamoxifen versus placebo: Double-blind adjuvant trial in elderly women with stage II breast cancer. *Natl Cancer Inst Monogr* 1:119, 1986.

37. **Introduction and Conclusions:** National Institutes of Health Consensus Development Panel on Adjuvant Chemotherapy and Endocrine Therapy for Breast Cancer. *Natl Cancer Inst Monogr* 1:1, 1986.

38. **Fuqua SAW, Fitzgerald SD, Chamness GC, et al:** Variant human breast tumor estrogen receptor with constitutive transcriptional activity. *Cancer Res* 51:105, 1992.

39. Gurpide E, Fleming H, Holinka CF: Steroid receptors and responsiveness to hormones in endometrial cancer. In Hollander VP (ed): *Hormonally Responsive Tumors*. Orlando, Academic Press, 1985, pp 69–94.

40. Pollow K, Schmidt-Gollwittzer M, Pollow B: Progesterone- and estradiol-binding proteins from normal human endometrium and endometrial carcinomas: a comparative study. In Witliff JL, Dapunt O (eds): *Steroid Receptors and Hormone-Dependent Neoplasia*. New York, Masson Publishing USA Inc, 1980, pp 69–94.

41. Kauppila A, Janne O, Kausansuu E, Vihko R: Treatment of advanced endometrial adenocarcinoma with a combined cytotoxic therapy: predictive value of cytosol estrogen and progestin receptor levels. *Cancer* 46:2162, 1980.

42. Creasman WT, McCarty KS Sr, Barton TK, McCarty KS Jr: Clinical correlates of estrogen- and progesterone-binding proteins in human endometrial adenocarcinoma. *Obstet Gynecol* 55:363, 1980.

43. Janne O, Kauppila A, Kontula K, et al: Female sex steroid receptors in normal, hyperplastic and carcinomatous endometrium: the relationship to serum steroid hormones and gonadotropins and changes during medroxyprogesterone acetate administration. *Int J Cancer* 24:545, 1979.

44. Martin PM, Rolland PH, Gammerre M, et al: Estradiol and progesterone receptors in normal and neoplastic endometrium: correlations between receptors, histopathological examinations and clinical responses under progestin therapy. *Int J Cancer* 23:321, 1979.

45. Benraad TJ, Friberg LG, Koenders AJM, Kullander S: Do estrogen and progesterone receptors (E_2R and PR) in metastasizing endometrial cancers predict the response to gestagen therapy. *Acta Obstet Gynecol Scand* 59:155, 1980.

46. Ehrlich CE, Young PCM, Cleary RE: Cytoplasmic progesterone and estradiol receptors in normal, hyperplastic, and carcinomatous endometrium: therapeutic implications. *Am J Obstet Gynecol* 141:539, 1981.

47. Neumannova M, Kauppila A, Vihko R: Cytosol and nuclear estrogen and progestin receptors and 17 beta-hydroxy steroid dehydrogenase activity in normal and carcinomatous endometrium. *Obstet Gynecol* 61:181, 1983.

48. Kauppila A, Janne O, Kausansuu E, Vihko R: Cytosol estrogen and progestin receptors in endometrial carcinoma in patients treated with surgery, radiotherapy, and progestin: clinical correlates. *Cancer* 50:2157, 1982.

49. Schwartz PE, MacLusky N, Naftolin F, Eisenfeld A: Tamoxifen-induced increase in cytosol progestin receptor levels in a case of metastatic endometrial cancer. *Gynecol Oncol* 16:41, 1983.

50. Schwartz PE, Eisenfeld A: Steroid receptor proteins in epithelial ovarian cancer. *Proc Felix Rutledge Society,* 1978.

51. Schwartz PE, Merino MJ, Livolsi VA, et al: Histopathologic correlations of estrogen and progestin receptor protein in epithelial ovarian carcinomas. *Obstet Gynecol* 66:428, 1985.

52. Jolles B: Progesterone in the treatment of advanced malignant tumors of breast, ovary and uterus. *Br J Cancer* 16:209, 1962.

53. Varga A, Henriksen E: Effect of 17-alpha-hydroxyprogesterone 17-n-caproate on various pelvic malignancies. *Obstet Gynecol* 23:51, 1964.

54. Ward HWC: Progestogen therapy for ovarian carcinoma. *J Obstet Gynecol Br Commonw* 79:555, 1972.

55. Kaufman RJ: Management of advanced ovarian carcinoma. *Med Clin North Am* 50:845, 1966.

56. Malkasian GD, Decker DG, Jorgensen EO, Edmonson H: Medroxyprogesterone acetate for the treatment of metastatic and recurrent ovarian carcinoma. *Cancer Treat Rep* 61:913, 1977.

57. Mangioni C, Franceschi S, LaVecchia C, D'Incalci M: High-dose medroxyprogesterone acetate (MPA) in advanced epithelial ovarian cancer resistant to first- or second-line chemotherapy. *Gynecol Oncol* 12:314, 1981.

58. Aabo K, Pedersen AG, Hald I, Dombernowsky P: High-dose medroxyprogesterone acetate (MPA) in advanced chemotherapy-resistant ovarian carcinoma: a phase II study. *Cancer Treat Rep* 66:407, 1982.

59. **Slayton RE, Pagano M, Creech RH:** Progestin therapy for advanced ovarian cancer: a phase II Eastern cooperative oncology group trial. *Cancer Treat Rep* 65:895, 1981.

60. **Tropé C, Johnson JE, Sigurdsson K, Simonsen E:** High-dose medroxyprogesterone acetate for the treatment of advanced ovarian carcinoma. *Cancer Treat Rep* 66:1441, 1982.

61. **Ozols RF, Hogan WM, Ostchega Y, Young RC:** MVP (mitomycin, vinblastine, and progesterone): a second-line regimen in ovarian cancer with a high incidence of pulmonary toxicity. *Cancer Treat Rep* 67:721, 1983.

62. **Geisler HE:** Megestrol acetate for the palliation of advanced ovarian carcinoma. *Obstet Gynecol* 61:95, 1983.

63. **Geisler HE:** The use of high-dose megestrol acetate in the treatment of ovarian adenocarcinoma. *Semin Oncol* 12:20, 1985.

64. **Ahlgren JD, Thomas D, Ellison N, et al:** Phase II evaluation of high dose megestrol acetate in advanced refractory ovarian cancer. *Proc Am Soc Clin Oncol* 4:124, 1985.

65. **Jolles CJ, Freedman RS, Jones LA:** Estrogen and progestogen therapy in advanced ovarian cancer: preliminary report. *Gynecol Oncol* 16:352, 1983.

66. **Schwartz PE, Keating F, MacLusky N, et al:** Tamoxifen therapy for advanced ovarian cancer. *Obstet Gynecol* 59:583, 1982.

67. **Pagel J, Rose C, Thorpe S, et al:** Treatment of advanced ovarian carcinoma with tamoxifen: a phase II trial. (abstr) *Proc 2nd Eur Conf Clin Oncol*, 1983.

68. **Hamerlynck JVTH, Vermorken JB, van der Burg MEL, et al:** Tamoxifen therapy in advanced ovarian cancer: a phase II study (abstr). *Proc Am Soc Clin Oncol* 4:115, 1985.

69. **Shirley DR, Kavanagh JJ Jr, Gershenson DM, et al:** Tamoxifen therapy of epithelial ovarian cancer. *Obstet Gynecol* 66:575, 1985.

70. **Slevin ML, Harvey VJ, Osborne RJ, et al:** A phase II study of tamoxifen in ovarian cancer. *Eur J Cancer Clin Oncol* 22:309, 1986.

71. **Weiner SA, Alberts DS, Surwit EA, et al:** Tamoxifen therapy in recurrent epithelial ovarian carcinoma. *Gynecol Oncol* 27:208, 1987.

72. **Osborne RJ, Malik S, Slevin ML, et al:** Tamoxifen in refractory ovarian cancer: the use of a loading dose. *Br J Cancer* 57:115, 1988.

73. **Hatch KD, Beecham JB, Blessing JA, et al:** Responsiveness of patients with advanced ovarian cancer to tamoxifen: a gynecologic oncology group study of second-line therapy in 105 patients. *Cancer* 68:269, 1991.

74. **Berqvist A, Kullander S, Thorell J:** A study of estrogen and progesterone cytosol receptor concentration in benign and malignant ovarian tumors and a review of malignant ovarian tumors treated with medroxyprogesterone acetate. *Acta Obstet Gynecol Scand (Suppl)* 101:75, 1981.

75. **Rendina GM, Donadio C, Giovannini M:** Steroid receptors and progestinic therapy in ovarian endometrioid carcinoma. *Eur J Gynaecol Oncol* 3:241, 1982.

76. **Timothy I:** Progestogen therapy for ovarian carcinoma. *Br J Obstet Gynaecol* 89:561, 1982.

77. **Long RTL, Evans AM:** Diethylstilbestrol as a chemotherapeutic agent for ovarian carcinoma. *Mo Med* 60:1125, 1963.

78. **Schwartz PE, Chambers JT, Kohorn EI, et al:** Tamoxifen in combination with cytotoxic chemotherapy in advanced epithelial ovarian cancer: a prospective randomized trial. *Cancer* 36:1074, 1989.

79. **Kahanpaa KV, Karkkainen J, Nieminen U:** Multi-agent chemotherapy with and without medroxyprogesterone acetate in the treatment of advanced ovarian cancer. *Excerpta Med Int Congr Ser* 611:477, 1982.

80. **Hochberg RB, MacLusky JN, Chambers JT, et al:** Concentration of $[16\alpha^{-125}]$ iodoestradiol in human ovarian tumors in vivo and correlation with estrogen receptor content. *Steroids* 46:775, 1985.

81. **Kavanagh JJ, Wharton JT, Roberts WS:** Androgen therapy in the treatment of refractory epithelial ovarian cancer. *Cancer Treat Rep* 71:537, 1987.

82. **Parmer H, Rustin G, Lightman SL:** Response to D-Trp-6-luteinizing hormone releasing hormone (Decapeptyl) microcapsules in advanced ovarian cancer. *Br Med J* 296:1229, 1988.

83. **Kavanagh JJ, Roberts W, Townsend P, et al:** Leuprolide acetate in the treatment of refractory or persistent epithelial ovarian cancer. *J Clin Oncol* 7:115, 1989.

84. **Bruckner HW, Motwani BT:** Treatment of advanced refractory ovarian carcinoma with gonadotropin-releasing hormone analogue. *Am J Obstet Gynecol* 161:1216, 1989.

85. **Creasman WT, Henderson D, Hinshaw W, Clarke-Pearson DL:** Estrogen replacement therapy in the patient treated for endometrial cancer. *Obstet Gynecol* 76:326, 1986.

86. **Lee RB, Burk TW, Park RC:** Estrogen replacement therapy following treatment for stage I endometrial carcinoma. *Gynecol Oncol* 36:189, 1990.

87. **Baker DP:** Estrogen replacement therapy in patients with previous endometrial carcinoma. *Compr Ther* 16:28, 1990.

88. **Bryant GW:** Administration of estrogen to patients with a previous diagnosis of endometrial adenocarcinoma (letter). *South Med J* 83:725, 1990.

89. **Eelles RA, Tan S, Wiltshaw E, et al:** Hormone replacement therapy and survival after surgery for ovarian cancer. *Br Med J* 302:259, 1991.

90. **Spicer D, Pike MD, Henderson BE:** The question of estrogen replacement therapy in patients with a prior diagnosis of breast cancer. *Oncology* 4:49, 1990.

91. **Theriault RL, Sellin RV:** A clinical dilemma: estrogen replacement therapy in postmenopausal women with a background of primary breast cancer. *Ann Oncol* 2:709, 1991.

92. **Staffa JA, Newschaffer CJ, Jones JK, Miller V:** Progestins and breast cancer: an epidemiological review. *Fertil Steril* 57:473, 1992.

18 Nutritional Therapy

David Heber

The diagnosis and management of the nutritional problems of the gynecologic oncology patient must not be overlooked in the presence of the more pressing medical and surgical concerns. Awareness of the methods for classification of malnutrition and appropriate treatment may improve the patient's ability to undergo definitive oncologic therapy, including surgery, radiation, or chemotherapy, and may improve the patient's quality of life.

Malnutrition

In hospitalized patients on general medical and surgical wards, the prevalence of malnutrition is 30–50% (1–3).

Risk Factors

Predisposing conditions frequently found in malnourished hospitalized patients include:

1. Heart failure

2. Chronic obstructive pulmonary disease

3. Infection

4. Gastrointestinal disorders

5. Psychiatric disorders

6. Renal insufficiency

7. Malignancy

It is typical for undernourished patients to have more than one predisposing condition (3).

637

These patients commonly will have vitamin and mineral deficiencies, particularly iron and vitamins A, D, E, and B_{12}. Decreased stores of these vitamins can be detected in early malnutrition. Because vitamins are stored in small amounts, the provision of only dextrose and water intravenously will lead to their rapid depletion, abnormal enzyme function, and clinical signs of vitamin deficiency.

Normal Body Metabolism

Each day a variety of foods are ingested to provide the energy needed to maintain life. According to the *first law of thermodynamics,* the energy ingested must equal the energy expended or stored in the body at equilibrium. Although the quantity of energy intake and the amount expended and stored in any 24-hour period do not correspond exactly, body weight eventually reflects the balance between energy intake and energy expenditure.

Calorie

The unit of energy exchange is the calorie, which is the amount of heat required to raise the temperature of 1 ml of water 1°C at one atmosphere of pressure.

Dietary Calorie

The dietary calorie equals 1000 calories. Thus 1500 dietary calories are equal to a 1500-kcalorie diet. This notation is used to examine body stores of energy and the quantity of food ingested.

Body Stores

Although the patient ingests a variety of foods, the body breaks them down into monosaccharides, amino acids, fatty acids, and glycerol. These are then redistributed to body stores or metabolized for energy.

The body stores of energy are very different from the composition of the diet (Fig. 18.1). The average diet has from 30–50% fat calories, 40–60% carbohydrate calories, and 15–20% protein calories. The body contains only 1200 carbohydrate calories as stored glycogen in muscle and liver, whereas it contains 130,000–160,000 calories as fat. The body also contains about 54,000 calories as protein in muscle and organs, but only 30–50% of this is available to be burned for energy. Protein is essential to life, and greater than 50% depletion of total body protein is incompatible with life (4).

Metabolism During Starvation

During starvation the body will adapt to spare the vital protein stores. The *carbohydrate stores* of the body are depleted within 3 days of total starvation at rest or more rapidly if the body's energy requirements are elevated by the metabolic effects of certain illnesses. Many organs use glucose in large amounts, obligating the breakdown of 75 g/day of muscle early in starvation (5). If the muscle were to continue to be broken down at this rate, starvation would lead to death in 45–60 days. Over a period of 6 weeks, however, the body adapts from the carbohydrate economy of the fed state to the fat fuel economy of starvation (Fig. 18.2). In this adaptation, peripheral tissues and organs use *ketone bodies,* a breakdown product of fat, in place of glucose. Because the body contains fat equivalent to 160,000 calories, survival can now be extended to 140–160 days. Some muscle breakdown continues, limiting survival, because the brain and the red blood cells continue to require enough glucose to cause the breakdown of 20 g/day of muscle.

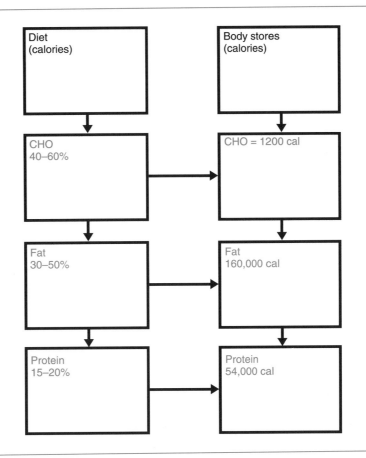

Figure 18.1.   Body stores of energy versus dietary calories.

Clinical Features

Regardless of the metabolic features of malnutrition, weight loss is usually the presenting sign. To detect this sign, it is essential to know the patient's usual weight, as well as her ideal weight for height.

Ideal Body Weight

For the purposes of screening for malnutrition in gynecologic patients, a practical formula to use for determining the ideal body weight is the following:

Ideal weight = 100 lb for 5 ft + 5 lb/inch > 5 ft

For example, a woman whose height is 5 feet 4 inches would have an ideal body weight of 120 pounds. For many common cancers, loss of as little as 6% of usual body weight can have significant prognostic effects on survival (6). It is important to question patients about usual body weight, because some patients can be 70% of ideal body weight all their lives as a result of differences in frame size or habits, such as chronic smoking, which affect body weight.

Weight Loss

Weight loss can result from loss of body fat, body protein, or body water. Each liter of body water lost represents a weight loss of 2.2 pounds, but this weight loss can be corrected rapidly with rehydration. The degree to which losses of

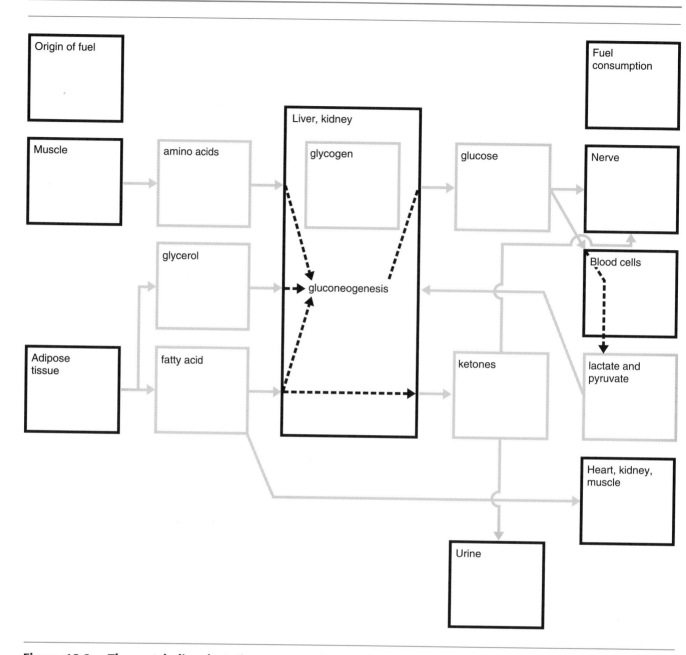

Figure 18.2. The metabolic adaptation to starvation. Redrawn, with permission, from Cahill GF, Owen OE: Some observations on carbohydrate metabolism in man. In Dickens F, Randle PJ, Whelan WJ (eds): *Carbohydrate Metabolism and Its Disorders.* New York, Academic Press, 1968, p 497.)

body protein or body fat dominate the clinical picture is a reflection of the body's ability to adapt to a *fat fuel economy* in the face of inadequate nutrition (7). There are three basic types of malnutrition: kwashiorkor, marasmus, and a combination of the two, cachexia (Fig. 18.3).

Kwashiorkor This form of malnutrition is variously termed protein calorie malnutrition, hypoalbuminemic malnutrition, protein energy malnutrition, or kwashiorkor-like malnutrition of the adult. If malnutrition is rapid and occurs in the face of disease factors that affect nutrition, a rapid depletion of protein stores can occur out of proportion to the loss of body weight. Kwashiorkor refers to a tropical pediatric disease and means "separation from the breast" in the African language of Swahili. Children are removed from their natural mother at 1 year of age and given to the care of an aunt or other adoptive mother. These children are then fed a diet consisting of cassava fruit, which is high in carbohydrates but contains no protein or fat, leading to a rapid depletion of body protein stores with hypoalbuminemia, edema, hypopigmentation, and an enlarged fatty liver.

In hospitalized patients, the major signs of protein depletion are:

1. Decrease in serum albumin to < 3.5 mg/dl

2. Decrease in absolute lymphocyte count to < 1500/mm^3

Figure 18.3   Classification of malnutrition.

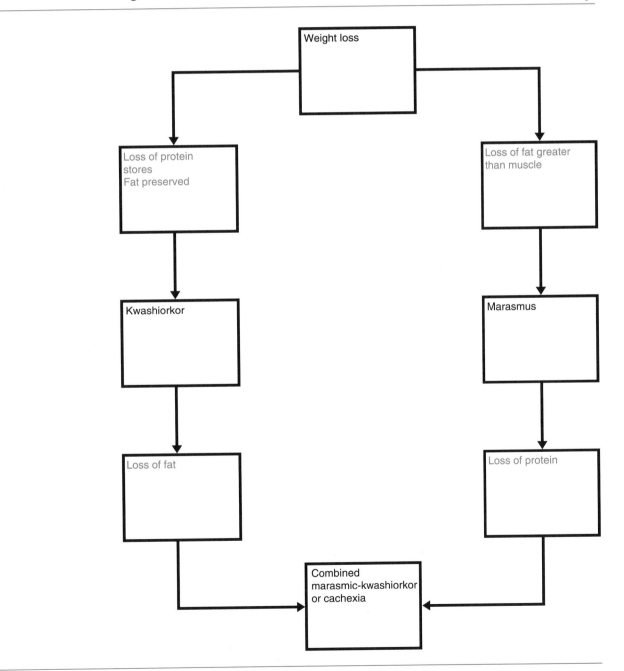

3. Decrease in serum transferrin to < 150 mg/dl

4. Loss of reactivity to common skin test antigens

It is possible for this form of malnutrition to occur in the absence of weight loss if the hypoalbuminemia leads to ascites or edema.

Marasmus   The other major form of malnutrition in adults is called marasmus or chronic inanition. Primary malnutrition resulting from anorexia or dietary inadequacy usually is seen with this form of malnutrition. It is characterized by a depletion of fat stores and the obvious appearance of malnutrition with visible loss of muscle and fat in the arms and legs. Although weight loss is often significant in these thin patients, protein stores can be remarkably preserved. It is not uncommon for the patient to have normal serum albumin and transferrin levels, a normal lymphocyte count, and normal skin test responses.

Cachexia   When the two major forms of malnutrition occur together in patients with advanced malnutrition, the condition is called cachexia. In this advanced condition, there is depletion of body fat stores and body protein stores, which produces visible emaciation with loss of body muscle and fat as well as decreased circulating serum proteins. Cachexia is a life-threatening condition and has also been termed *combined marasmic-kwashiorkor* or mixed-form malnutrition of the adult.

In tropical environments and other areas of endemic starvation, the most common cause of death is simple, uncomplicated pneumococcal pneumonia (7). Although the exact contribution of malnutrition to mortality in hospitalized gynecologic oncology patients is often difficult to quantify, immune impairment and an increased susceptibility to infections, poor wound healing, and cardiorespiratory impairment are all important negative effects of malnutrition on patient survival. These functions relate to the overall status of body proteins in vital organs, circulating cells, and serum.

Diagnosis

Serum levels of circulating proteins can be decreased and reflect impaired function of the liver and other organs, even in the absence of marked depletion of visceral and muscle protein (8). This usually occurs in the setting of excessive metabolic demands caused by specific illnesses that impair the body's ability to conserve protein.

Similarly, protein and fat stores can be depleted markedly while circulating proteins remain in the normal range. This occurs with anorexia and primary malnutrition in otherwise normal adults, in whom a gradual adaptation to starvation occurs.

Anthropometry, in which body stores are estimated by direct measurements, and *biochemical markers* that assess circulating proteins must be used in concert to determine the specific type of malnutrition in any given patient (Table 18.1).

Anthropometric techniques include the measurement of body weight and height in adults. The simple formula presented above is used to calculate the percent of ideal weight for height. From the history it is also possible to obtain the percent of usual weight. The fat stores can be measured by assessing *skin-fold thickness*. The most commonly used skin fold in practice is the triceps. For this measure-

642

Table 18.1   Physical/Biochemical Markers of Malnutrition

	Marasmus	*Kwashiorkor*	*Cachexia*
Albumin	Normal	↓	↓
Transferrin	Normal	↓	↓
WBC	Normal	↓	↓
Skin tests	Normal	Negative	Negative
Body weight	↓	Normal	↓
Body fat	↓	Normal	↓

ment, the patient sits with the right arm hanging freely at the side. For bedridden patients, the right arm is flexed at the shoulder while the forearm crosses the chest (9). The midpoint between the acromion and the olecranon posteriorly over the triceps muscle is marked. The skin and subcutaneous tissue at the midpoint are then pinched and pressure-regulated calipers (10) are applied for 3 seconds before a reading is taken. The calipers are designed to deliver a pressure of 10 g/mm² regardless of the fold thickness and can be used to compare the same patient's progress over time as well as to assess the severity of malnutrition.

Protein Store Assessment   Protein stores can be assessed by assaying a number of circulating proteins, most of which are secreted by the liver (11, 12). Their synthesis and secretion are inhibited rapidly in the presence of protein malnutrition, and they decrease to a variable extent in the circulation according to their metabolic half-lives. The most widely used markers are albumin and transferrin. Each of these proteins has advantages and disadvantages (11).

Albumin   Albumin has a long half-life, and significant decreases may not occur for up to 1 month after the onset of starvation. Albumin may be decreased by rapid loss of serum proteins (e.g., excessive losses from the gastrointestinal tract). Restoration of the serum albumin to normal levels by nutritional means is slow and often lags behind clear improvement in nutritional status by other criteria.

Transferrin   Transferrin is synthesized in the liver and other sites where it can act as a growth-promoting peptide. In the liver, synthesis is modulated by the iron stores in the hepatocytes as well as by the overall protein status. The half-life of the protein is only 8–10 days, and the body pool is only 5 g. The synthetic rate is the major factor determining serum levels, and serum transferrin will increase within 10 to 14 days of nutritional repletion. The problems with the interpretation of transferrin levels are that degradation rates increase during illness, and iron deficiency will falsely elevate the levels.

For these reasons, both transferrin and albumin must be taken into consideration, together with the anthropometric determinations of body weight and triceps skin-fold thickness.

Retinol- and Thyroxine-Binding Proteins   Retinol-binding protein and thyroxine-binding prealbumin also are synthesized in the liver, with half-lives of 10 hours and 2 days, respectively. At present these markers are not widely used clinically. Their levels drop acutely with metabolic stress, and retinol-binding

Table 18.2 Serum Half-Life of Circulating Proteins Decreased in Malnutrition

Protein	Half-life
Albumin	3–4 weeks
Transferrin	1 week
Thyroxine-binding prealbumin	2 days
Retinol-binding protein	10 hours

protein is also filtered and broken down by the kidney. These factors complicate the interpretation of serum levels for diagnosis of malnutrition, but they can be used in a research setting to assess response to nutrition.

The serum half-lives of these circulating proteins are listed in Table 18.2.

Immune Function

The absolute lymphocyte count and delayed cutaneous hypersensitivity responses to skin test antigens are nonspecific markers of impaired immune function in malnourished patients (13) (Fig. 18.4). In areas of endemic starvation, malnourished patients are at increased risk of opportunistic infections in the hospital and ambulatory settings because of the following:

1. Depressed levels of complement components, including C3

2. Reduced amounts of secretory IgA in external body secretions

3. Abnormal T cell function

4. Impairment of nonspecific defenses, including decreased epithelial integrity, decreased mucus production, and decreased cilial motility

The precise nutritional deficiency that leads to decreased immune function remains unknown.

Most patients with protein and caloric malnutrition have multiple deficiencies, and almost any single nutritional deficiency, if severe enough, can affect immune function (14). Correction of malnutrition will improve immune function; this is especially true in the gynecologic oncology patient, whose immune function can be impaired by therapy as well as by the tumor itself.

Absolute Lymphocyte Count The absolute lymphocyte count is calculated by multiplying the percentage of lymphocytes by the total white blood cell count. The absolute lymphocyte count and skin tests are the most widely used immune markers of nutritional status. A normal lymphocyte count is $> 2000/\text{mm}^3$ in patients who are not receiving chemotherapy.

Most circulating lymphocytes are T cells, and involution of the tissues producing T cells occurs early in the course of malnutrition. The delayed-hypersensitivity skin test response reflects three processes:

1. Processing of the antigen by macrophages resulting in the generation of both effector and memory T cells

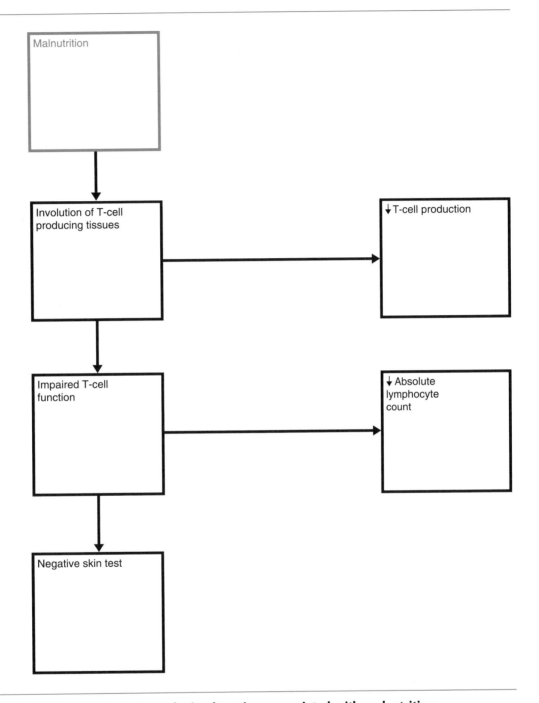

Figure 18.4.   Immunologic alterations associated with malnutrition.

2. Recognition of antigen rechallenge resulting in blast transformation, cellular proliferation, and generation of lymphokine-producing effector cells

3. Production of a local wheal and flare secondary to the actions of lymphokines and chemotactic factors at the skin site

Antigens that are frequently tested include purified protein derivative, streptokinase-streptodornase, mumps, *Candida,* trichophyton, and coccidioidin. The prevalence of nonreactivity to skin test antigens is about 50% in patients whose serum albumin level is < 3.0 g/dl, but it can be as high as 30% in patients whose serum albumin level is > 3.0 g/dl. Other problems with interpretation of skin tests include:

1. Only about 60% of healthy patients respond to most of the antigens, so that failure to respond to one or two antigens may not be predictive.

2. Primary illnesses, including sarcoidosis and lymphoma, as well as immunosuppressive drugs, will produce anergy.

The assessment of malnutrition by means of clinical examination in combination with routinely available laboratory tests will provide an accurate estimation in more than 70% of patients (15). Difficulties with each of these tests have kept the nutritional assessment from becoming part of the routine data base for every hospitalized patient.

Impact of Disease

Many systemic illnesses, including cancer, predispose patients to malnutrition (Fig. 18.5). Although abnormalities of metabolism, digestion, absorption, and utilization of nutrients all contribute to malnutrition in such patients, decreased nutrient intake is still a universal finding in most malnourished patients, with the exception of those with uncomplicated hyperthyroidism.

Anorexia

Decreased appetite, or anorexia, is the major factor contributing to decreased intake in many disease processes. Although anorexia can be a feature of such

Figure 18.5. Impact of disease factors on nutrition.

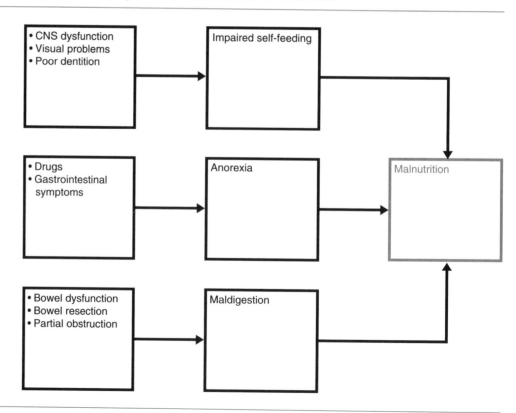

646

Table 18.3   Metabolic Consequences of Cancer

Host Metabolic Abnormality	Consequence
Increased glucose production	Rapid weight loss, muscle breakdown
Increased lipid mobilization	Hypertriglyceridemia, rapid wasting
Insulin resistance	Hyperglycemia, hypertriglyceridemia
Hypoglycemia secondary to tumor humoral factors	Syncope, fatigue
Diarrheal syndromes due to tumor humoral factors	Electrolyte disturbances

diseases as cancer, it can also be a side effect of many drugs. These include antineoplastic drugs, which are most pertinent for the gynecologic oncology patient. A number of commonly used drugs (e.g., anticholinergics, antihistamines, methyldopa, sympathomimetics, clonidine, and tricyclic antidepressants) may cause a dry mouth. The latter can decrease sensation and food palatability.

Another common type of anorexia is a learned aversion to food when it is known to cause adverse physical symptoms. Gastrointestinal diseases, including reflux esophagitis, gastritis, and peptic ulcer, frequently cause dyspepsia. Irritable bowel syndrome, food allergies, lactose intolerance, diverticuli, and biliary disease can cause diarrhea or flatulence. All of these gastrointestinal problems can cause patients to avoid foods altogether or to ingest an unbalanced diet.

Intestinal Dysfunction

Mechanical malfunction of the bowel is a particularly common problem among patients who have undergone abdominal radiation or extensive abdominal surgery. Postoperative or postirradiation adhesions can lead to partial or complete bowel obstruction. In patients with disseminated intra-abdominal malignancy such as ovarian cancer, an *adynamic ileus* or *intestinal pseudo-obstruction* can result in a nonfunctional gastrointestinal tract. Impaired capacity for self-feeding can also markedly decrease food intake.

Metabolic Disturbances

Cancer specifically affects nutrient metabolism. Patients with metastatic and localized cancer have increased rates of whole-body glucose metabolism, whole-body protein breakdown, and insulin resistance (16, 17). Improved nutrition often fails to correct such abnormalities, once severe malnutrition is present, despite continuous parenteral or enteral alimentation with adequate nutrients (17–19). Specific metabolic disturbances and their consequences are presented in Table 18.3.

Nutritional Support

Nutritional support is an adjunct to primary therapy for the gynecologic oncology patient. The aim is to prevent deterioration of nutritional status during planned primary therapy, such as radiation, surgery, and chemotherapy. Early initiation of nutritional support prior to any deterioration of nutritional status is desirable. This goal necessitates early evaluation, the proper choice of nutritional therapy modalities, and an accurate assessment of requirements.

Once a protein deficiency occurs, it is difficult to reverse, inasmuch as less than 5% of the protein will be replaced per day, regardless of the amount of substrate provided. Vitamins and minerals are replaced more easily, but there is no substitute for adequate planning to meet caloric and protein requirements essential for nutritional maintenance of vital functions.

Caloric Requirements

The protein and caloric requirements can be estimated at 1 g/kg/day and 35 kcal/kg/day for healthy adults, respectively. If malnutrition exists or if the patient's metabolism is elevated by infection or other metabolic stresses, then 1.5 g/kg/day of protein and 45 kcal/kg/day should be supplied. More exact formulas are available for pediatric patients and patients at the extremes of height and weight.

Need for Support

There are two key aspects of the patient's nutritional status that affect decisions about nutritional support:

1. The degree of prior malnutrition at the time of assessment

2. The degree of hypermetabolism or metabolic abnormality expected to interfere with nutritional rehabilitation

If the degree of prior malnutrition is minimal and the patient has only mild hypermetabolism after elective surgery, a temporary form of nutritional support can be used. On the other hand, if the patient is going to require excess calories to restore preexisting severe malnutrition, forced intake of calories by an enteral or parenteral route must be used. The following guidelines can be used:

1. If a patient is to be without nutrition for a period of 7 days, some form of nutritional support should be used.

2. If nutritional support is to be continued for more than 2 weeks, a permanent entry port for enteral or parenteral nutritional support should be employed and arrangements made for home enteral or parenteral nutrition.

Method of Support

The choice between *parenteral* and *enteral* therapy should be made on the basis of the availability and functional status of the gastrointestinal tract (Fig. 18.6). If the gastrointestinal tract is functioning normally, the expense and complications of parenteral nutrition argue against its use.

Enteral

If the gastrointestinal tract is atrophied from prior malnutrition, a period of rehabilitation with special formula diets can be used to renourish the patient gradually so that routine formula diets can be used (20). The epithelium of the gastrointestinal (GI) tract will be directly nourished by the infused nutrients in the formula diet bathing these cells, and ultimately a complete formula diet can be used. If the patient is already severely malnourished and hypermetabolic, careful consideration should be given to initiation of concurrent parenteral nutrition to provide calories and protein during the period of nutritional rehabilitation of the GI tract.

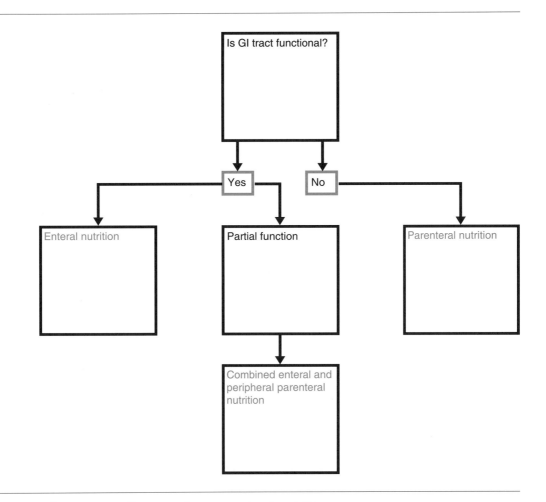

Figure 18.6.   Parenteral versus enteral nutrition.

When fewer calories than those required for total support are provided by the parenteral route, a peripheral vein can be used. The 10% glucose solution will irritate the peripheral veins by causing a chemical phlebitis. This may limit the use of any single peripheral vein to a period of about 10 days. A large central vein is required for the 20–25% glucose solution plus added amino acids required for total parenteral nutrition. In patients receiving chemotherapy, peripheral veins are often sclerosed, and a central venous route for nutrition and medications must be used.

In view of the difficulties inherent in the use of parenteral nutritional support, every effort should be made to use the enteral route whenever possible. A gastrostomy tube or a jejunostomy tube can be easily placed early in the course of management without interfering with the patient's lifestyle. The gastrostomy port can be used at night for enteral support therapy by continuous infusion of isotonic enteral supplements at a rate of ≤ 100 kcal/hour. The next day, the patient can cover the port with a dressing and go through her usual daily activities. This approach is often more acceptable to patients than a nasogastric tube, which is visible and irritating. In some patients, the gastrostomy port has the added advantage that the stomach can be used as a reservoir for bolus feeding, which is more convenient. In cases of abnormal gastric motility, esophageal reflux, or possible aspiration of gastric contents, continuous slow infusion of supplement should be used, or a tube should be passed beyond the pylorus into the jejunum.

Diarrhea is often a complication of enteral feeding and can be dealt with in the following ways:

1. The rate of infusion can be decreased. If the GI tract dysfunction is due to atrophy of the epithelial cells, a gradual increase in infusion rate is often tolerated, starting with an initial rate of 25 ml/hour and increasing by twofold increments every 48 hours.

2. The type of enteral formula can be changed to an isosmolar formula. Many of the high-calorie or high-nitrogen supplements are also hyperosmolar. Changing to an isotonic formula will often decrease intestinal hypermotility.

3. A number of specific medications can be used to decrease intestinal motility. In the presence of partial obstruction, such medications must be used with caution.

4. The level of enteral support can be decreased and temporarily combined with peripheral parenteral alimentation until intestinal motility problems respond to the maneuvers discussed above.

Parenteral

Total parenteral nutrition (TPN) is the provision of all calories in an intravenous solution of dextrose, amino acids, and emulsified lipids. This form of therapy, although appearing more invasive and definitive, confers no special advantage to the malnourished patient with a functional GI tract. In some patients receiving chemotherapy or radiation therapy, mucosal inflammation, nausea, and vomiting impair normal intake. In such patients, TPN may be needed as an adjunct to restore functional status and allow continuation of therapy. Patients with GI fistulas often require avoidance of enteral feeding.

TPN is usually administered through a central venous catheter surgically placed in the subclavian vein, although there are other vessels that can be used when needed, as described in Chapter 16. The patient must be given special training in aseptic handling of the catheter site and use of the infusion equipment required. Many medical centers have special home parenteral nutrition support teams, whereas in other areas private firms provide this service. Potential medical problems for these patients depend to a great extent on the experience of the team providing home parenteral support. It is not uncommon for patients to require hospitalization for blood cultures and other studies to investigate a fever.

Combined Enteral-Parenteral Feeding

Sometimes combined parenteral and enteral nutritional therapy can be used to advantage. For example, parenteral nutrition can be used in postsurgical patients when the GI tract is functional but the total caloric requirement cannot be met by the enteral route.

Evaluation of Response to Nutritional Support

Because the goal of nutritional support is the attainment of an anabolic state or reduction of nitrogen losses, assessment of nitrogen balance is the most useful clinical tool to determine the effectiveness of therapy. **Nitrogen balance is defined as the difference between nitrogen intake and nitrogen excretion.**

One gram of nitrogen is equivalent to 6.25 g of protein. Hence, *nitrogen intake* can be determined by dividing protein intake, as determined from dietary records, by 6.25. *Nitrogen excretion* is defined as the urinary nitrogen excreted per 24 hours plus a fixed estimate of 4.0 g/24 hr for unmeasured nitrogen losses from cellular sloughing into the feces (1 g), losses from the skin (0.2 g), and nonurea nitrogen losses in the urine (2 g) (21). Because nitrogen balance is most usefully applied in a serial fashion in the same patient, the particular constants used to estimate unmeasured excretion are important only for comparison of published results.

At any given level of nitrogen intake, nitrogen balance improves with increased administration of nonprotein calories. The maximum benefit is achieved when the ratio of nonprotein calories to grams of nitrogen is 150:1 (22).

Proteins vary in their biologic value according to their mixture of essential and nonessential amino acids. Albumin has the ideal mixture of amino acids for optimal use of protein and is assigned a biologic value of 100. Casein is close to albumin in its biologic quality whereas meat proteins, such as those found in steak or tuna, have a biologic value of 80. Corns and beans, each with biologic values of 40 or less, can be combined in a protein mixture with a biologic value of 80, because the amino acid mixtures of the two proteins are complementary. **The protein requirement for normal persons is 0.55 gm/kg for protein with a high biologic value, such as milk or albumin, but is 0.8 gm/kg for the mixture of proteins found in the average American diet** (23).

Effect of Nutritional Support on Prognosis   Although it is easy to demonstrate the impact of renutrition on a patient with uncomplicated starvation or an inability to absorb calories because of a loss of intestinal tissue, it is much more difficult to demonstrate the beneficial effect of nutritional support in a patient with a chronic illness such as cancer (24). Often the course of the underlying illness will mask the beneficial effects of nutritional therapy.

In patients with mild disease or elective surgery, malnutrition is relatively well tolerated from a clinical standpoint. In such cases, nutritional rehabilitation usually occurs without any special effort as the underlying medical or surgical condition runs its course. In patients with severe disease, nutrition is often relegated to the secondary list of problems as the progress of the primary illness dictates therapeutic decisions. In both of these instances, however, nutritional therapy may play a beneficial role in either preventing or retarding malnutrition in individual patients (25). On the other hand, an extensive meta-analysis of 53 published studies of parenteral and enteral nutrition showed that survival was improved in 6 studies, unchanged in 43, and worse in 2 (26). The judicious application of nutritional support for gynecologic oncology patients may lead to the prevention of progressive malnutrition as well as an improvement in the quality of life and prognosis.

Complications   Complications can occur after either enteral or parenteral nutrition. Complications of enteral nutrition are either mechanical or metabolic, whereas complications of parenteral nutrition can be mechanical, infectious, or metabolic (27).

Mechanical problems of enteral feeding include aspiration, especially in semi-conscious patients or patients with abnormalities of swallowing. This problem can be minimized by proper placement of the feeding tube and by determination of the volume of the residual gastric contents 8 hours after feeding to eliminate the possibility of gastric outlet obstruction or gastric atony. If these latter problems occur, the feeding tube can be placed into the jejunum. Proper placement should be assured radiologically. Irritation of the oropharynx and the gastric mucosa can occur, especially with the use of larger-bore and less flexible feeding tubes. This problem can be minimized with the use of inert silicone rubber and polyurethane tubes.

Diarrhea is the most common complication associated with tube feeding (28). Carefully increasing the rate of administration will help avoid this problem. Prolonged starvation can lead to gastrointestinal epithelial atrophy and maldigestion, which in turn can result in diarrhea. Diarrhea also can be due to the effects of other medications, colonic infections (e.g., *Clostridium difficile*), or overly rapid administration of hypertonic enteral formulations. Most enteral formulations are free of lactose, so that lactose intolerance is not likely to cause diarrhea.

Dehydration with hypernatremia can be a problem in the elderly, in whom inadequate fluid intake can occur during the administration of a hypertonic enteral formula. When high-carbohydrate enteral formulas are used, *glucosuria* can occur in some patients without a prior history of diabetes.

The complications of parenteral nutrition are often more serious than those associated with enteral nutrition (29). *Pneumothorax* and *subclavian venous thrombosis* are the most common catheter-related complications. Pneumothorax should occur in only about 1–2% of catheter insertions, but this rate is higher when transthoracic puncture is used rather than open surgical placement or when less experienced persons insert the catheter (30). A chest radiograph to confirm proper catheter placement and to exclude a pneumothorax is essential. A pneumothorax will usually resolve spontaneously, but a chest tube may be required in some cases. Thrombosis of the catheter in the central veins has been reported in 5–10% of patients receiving parenteral nutrition, especially with the hypercoagulable states of sepsis or cancer (31). In such patients, the catheter should be flushed with heparin solution (300 units/ml) to prevent this complication. **When thrombosis occurs, the catheter must be removed.** Peripheral venous nutrition must be used while a full course of heparin is given to treat the thrombosis. Infections most commonly occur from skin contaminants, such as gram-positive organisms, but can include fungi and unusual bacteria, especially if acquired during hospitalization. Infected catheters must be removed before the systemic treatment of catheter-related sepsis. In patients committed to lifelong parenteral nutrition, this decision must be made carefully because only eight external sites are available for central venous catheter placement.

Infections **occur in 2–5% of central catheters placed for parenteral nutrition.** When the patient is febrile and a peripheral source of infection is not found within 96 hours, the catheter should be removed and cultured for evidence of catheter-related infection. Infected catheters can be a source of life-threatening phlebitis. Blood-borne infections from sources other than the catheter can be treated with intravenous antibiotics without removal of the catheter, but the patient should be observed carefully because the catheter is a foreign body in the vascular system and can be seeded with bacteria.

In patients treated with broad-spectrum antibiotics, *systemic candidiasis* can occur. The eyegrounds should be examined for the presence of cotton-wool exudates that are pathognomonic of systemic candidiasis, and blood cultures should be sent for special fungal isolation procedures. If present, these infections require treatment with amphotericin, which has significant systemic side effects.

A variety of *metabolic complications* can occur during parenteral nutrition. The most common is overfeeding, which results in excess CO_2 production that can add to respiratory problems in patients with pulmonary disease (32). Hyperglycemia can occur in some as a result of transient insulin resistance or relative insulin deficiency. Both subcutaneous insulin and insulin added to the parenteral solutions can be used to treat this complication (33). Metabolic acidosis, which occurred commonly when potassium and sodium were administered only as chloride salts, is less frequently a problem since acetate buffers have been used in parenteral solutions. Abnormalities of phosphate, potassium, calcium, and magnesium can occur because of excessive or inadequate administration, particularly in the presence of underlying disorders, such as renal failure or gastrointestinal fistulas, which themselves predispose to electrolyte abnormalities (34, 35). Deficiencies of trace minerals such as zinc, copper, and chromium rarely occur, because these are now added routinely to parenteral solutions (36). Azotemia can occur in patients with renal failure or when there is excessive administration of amino acids relative to nonprotein calories, and this is simply treated by reduction of the amino acid load (37). Essential fatty acid deficiency rarely occurs because the use of intravenous lipid emulsions has become so common (38). In most cases, the metabolic complications associated with parenteral nutrition respond to careful fluid and electrolyte management with daily monitoring of input and output.

Multiple Organ Failure Syndrome   Multiple organ failure syndrome can develop in the critically ill patient secondary to a decline in cellular oxygen consumption, leakage of intracellular enzymes, and cell death (39). A cascade of events leads to these terminal events, including at different times hypoperfusion/hypoxia, immunodysfunction, endocrine dysfunction, acute starvation, and metabolic derangement. Early organ failure usually appears from 5 to 7 days after the initial insult but can occur as late as 21 days later.

The nutritional therapy provided to such patients has been called metabolic support to differentiate it from the nutritional support given to more stable patients with chronic anorexia and starvation. In nutritional support, the goals are simply to provide adequate calories and nutrients to restore nutritional deficiencies and to maintain protein synthesis, positive nitrogen balance, and lean body mass (40). Metabolic support of the critically ill patient at risk of multiple organ failure syndrome is directed at partial caloric replacement, sustenance of important cellular and organ metabolism, and the avoidance of overfeeding. Metabolic costs of overfeeding include lipogenesis, gluconeogenesis, and thermogenesis. Excessive infusion rates and choice of the wrong mixture of macronutrients can be harmful in the critically ill patient (41).

A breakdown in the physical and immunologic barriers of the gastrointestinal tract can promote multiple organ failure syndrome. The gastrointestinal tract is particularly susceptible to ischemic and reperfusion injury. Glutamine, a preferred fuel for the gut epithelium, may promote healing of the gastrointestinal tract epithelium after an injury (42). In animal studies, an enteral formula containing glutamine has been shown to improve gastrointestinal mucosal integrity and nitrogen balance (43). Research is under way on utilization of the physiologic properties of specific nutrients to prevent multiple organ failure syndrome. However, the critical therapeutic difference between the multiple organ failure syndrome and chronic malnutrition is the need to avoid overfeeding by providing a hypocaloric protein-sparing nutritional regimen in the former.

Calculation of Requirements

There are many methods of estimating basal energy requirements. The following are guidelines:

1. Obese patients will maintain their body weight when given only 25 kcal/kg actual body weight per day.

2. Lean patients will maintain their weight when given 35 kcal/kg/day.

3. In patients with malnutrition, there is a cost of anabolism that involves the calories necessary for new protein synthesis. For patients with very severe illnesses and in whom malnutrition may be combined with sepsis or trauma to elevate energy requirements, 45 kcal/kg/day may be required.

There are many other formulas for estimating energy requirements that take the patient's height into consideration. Taller patients have a higher resting energy expenditure at the same weight than shorter patients, because they have larger livers and other vital organs. In older persons, metabolic rates tend to fall, in part because of a decrease in lean body mass. Whereas such equations are useful for clinical nutrition research, they are generally unnecessary for clinical management. A more practical set of guidelines is as follows:

Estimation of Total Caloric Requirement

Severity of Illness	Daily Caloric Requirement
Mild	35 kcal/kg
Moderate	40 kcal/kg
Severe	45 kcal/kg

Estimation of Protein Requirement   Once the caloric requirement has been estimated, the protein requirement can be estimated at about 1.0 g/kg of usual or ideal body weight.

Estimation of Nonprotein Calories   One may estimate the nonprotein calorie requirement by initially estimating the amount of nitrogen administered according to the following formula: 1 g nitrogen = 6.25 g protein. By either the parenteral or the enteral route, 150 nonprotein calories must be provided for each gram of nitrogen administered. Therefore, estimation of nonprotein calories can be achieved as follows:

$$\text{Nonprotein calories} = \frac{\text{Protein requirement} \times 150}{6.25}$$

An alternative is simply to subtract the protein calories from the total number of calories.

Determination of Carbohydrate Requirement   It is usual to give about half the total calories as carbohydrates. Most nutritional solutions are already pre-mixed, and the precise formulas available will vary in different hospitals.

Determination of Fat Requirement   The absolute fat requirement for essential fatty acids (i.e., linoleic acid and linolenic acid) is only 4% of the total calories. However, the amount of fat usually administered either enterally or parenterally exceeds this amount. Indeed, the remainder of the calories necessary to fulfill the minimum total caloric requirement after the protein and carbohydrate calories have been calculated can be given as fat. In all cases, the number of calories given as fat will be far less than 60% of the total calories, which is the maximum fat that should be given.

Sample Calculations

Sample calculations for both enteral and parenteral formulations are presented.

Enteral

A 50-year-old woman who weighs 45 kg has a usual body weight of 70 kg and is severely ill with sepsis and postsurgical stress. Her gastrointestinal tract is functional, and enteral formulation must be prescribed. The following steps allow calculation of the specific requirements:

1. The total daily caloric requirement is estimated by multiplying the caloric requirement based on severity (in this case, 45 kcal/kg/day) by the patient's weight (i.e., 45 kg). Therefore, the caloric requirement is 45 kcal/kg × 45 kg = 2025 kcal.

2. The minimum protein requirement is determined by multiplying the ideal body weight by 1.0 g/kg, e.g., in this case 70 kg, and 1.0 g/kg = 70 g. Because protein = 4 kcal/g, the protein caloric need is 280 kcal.

3. The estimation of nonprotein calories is determined by multiplying the protein requirement (70 g) by 150, and this figure is divided by 6.25. Therefore, the minimum nonprotein calories required = $\dfrac{70 \text{ gm} \times 150}{6.25} = 1680$ kcal.

4. The determination of specific carbohydrate and fat needs is empiric; i.e., if about one-half the total caloric need is given in carbohydrates (in this case, 1010 kcal), the remainder of the calories may be given as fat. Therefore, fat calories = 2025 − (1010 + 280) = 735 kcal.

5. An enteral formula that approximates these caloric requirements should be employed. A standard formula containing 1.0 kcal/ml, 15% protein, 34% fat, and 51% carbohydrate, would provide about 150 kcal of protein, 340 kcal of fat, and 510 kcal of carbohydrate for every liter of formula given to the patient. Therefore, this patient's caloric requirements would be met by giving her approximately 2 liters of formula per day.

Parenteral

A 45 kg 70-year-old woman has lost 15 kg as a result of postirradiation changes to the bowel. In view of her poor gastrointestinal function, parenteral alimentation is appropriate. The estimation of her nutritional requirements is as follows:

1. The total daily caloric requirement is estimated by multiplying the caloric requirement based on severity by the patient's weight (i.e., 45 kcal/kg × 45 kg = 2025 kcal).

2. The minimum protein requirement is determined by multiplying the usual body weight (60 kg) by 1.0 g/kg = 60 g. At 4 kcal/g, the protein caloric need is 240 kcal.

3. The nonprotein caloric requirement thus equals about 1785 kcal, which should include about 775 kcal fat and 1010 kcal carbohydrate.

4. A standard TPN formula containing 20% dextrose and 3.5% protein (e.g., Travasol), would provide 680 kcal of dextrose per liter and 35 g (140 kcal) of protein per liter. Therefore, 1.7 liters of this formula would approximate the carbohydrate and protein needs of the patient. The parenteral solution is administered at a rate of 75 ml/hr.

5. A single unit of 10% intravenous (IV) fat emulsion provides 550 kcal/unit. Therefore, the usual amount of fat given would be provided by 1.4 units (or 700 ml). Because fat emulsions are available in single units, it is preferable to give this patient 2 units of fat emulsion per day.

In this typical example, the IV fat emulsion provides needed additional calories, allowing for the more complete utilization of the administered protein. An additional reason to provide fat emulsions parenterally is the need to provide essential fatty acids at a minimum level of 4% of total calories. For example, 4% × 2000 kcal = 80 kcal/day. This requirement can be met by one 550 kcal unit of IV fat emulsion per week. In the absence of any fat administration, essential fatty acid deficiency develops in 4–6 weeks in most persons, once endogenous stores of essential fatty acids are depleted. Because the cost of lipid emulsions has decreased considerably, fat is being used as a parenteral caloric source in amounts exceeding that needed to meet the minimal essential fatty acid requirements, as outlined in the example above.

Standard electrolytes per liter of solution are listed by most pharmacies, and they are designed together with acetate buffers to deliver a nonacid solution with a pH of between 5.3 and 6.8. In special fluid and electrolyte situations, the composition of the solution can be custom designed, but this significantly increases

Table 18.4   Typical Parenteral Nutrition Solutions

Solution	Na+ (mEq/liter)	K+ (mEq/liter)	Mg++ (mEq/liter)	Acetate (mEq/liter)	Cl− (mEq/liter)	Protein (g/liter)	Calories/liter (D 20)*
FreAmine III 3%	35	24.5	5	44	40	29	800
Aminosyn 4.25%	70	66	10	142	98	85	850
Travasol 4.25%	70	60	10	135	70	89	850
Travasol 3.5%	25	15	5	54	25	37	820

*If admixed with a solution of 20% dextrose.

656

the cost of parenteral nutrition. The use of standard fluid and electrolyte solutions with supplements as necessary is preferable. Typical parenteral nutrition solutions are shown in Table 18.4.

Osmolarity and caloric content of the parenteral solution are related to the glucose concentration. For lipid preparations, the osmolarity and caloric content are also related to the percentage of lipid in the solution (Table 18.5).

Recommended vitamins that should be provided on a daily basis in parenteral solutions are listed in Table 18.6. These substances are available in preformulated ampules, and one ampule per day added directly to the parenteral solution will meet all the requirements in most patients. In patients who are especially stressed

Table 18.5 Osmolarity and Caloric Content of Glucose and Lipids in Parenteral Nutritional Solutions

Glucose Concentration (wt/vol)	Osmolarity (mOsmol/liter)	Calories (kcal/dl)
5%	250	17
10%	500	34
20%	1000	68
50%	2500	170
70%	3500	237
Lipid Concentration (wt/vol)		
10%	280	110
20%	340	200

Table 18.6 Guidelines for Daily Adult Parenteral Vitamin Supplementation

Vitamin	Daily Intravenous Dose
A	3300 IU
D	200 IU
E	10 IU
B_1 (thiamin)	3.0 mg
B_2 (riboflavin)	3.6 mg
B_3 (pantothenic acid)	15.0 mg
B_5 (niacin)	40.0 mg
B_6 (pyridoxine)	4.0 mg
B_7 (biotin)	60.0 mg
B_9 (folic acid)	400.0 mg
B_{12} (cobalamin)	5.0 mg
C (ascorbic acid)	100.0 mg
K	5.0 mg/week*

From American Medical Association/Nutrition Advisory Group Guidelines. *J Paren Ent Nutr* 3:258, 1979.
*Parenteral vitamin K supplementation is not included in the official recommendation as some patients are receiving anticoagulants.

(e.g., septic), 500 mg of vitamin C should be given. Patients receiving common medications such as Dilantin may require additional specific vitamin supplements (e.g., vitamin D).

Major mineral requirements are listed in Table 18.7. The daily requirement has a wide range that depends largely on the extent of gastrointestinal and renal losses. In patients with an abnormally high excretion, the losses must be replaced aggressively.

Supplementation with zinc, copper, chromium, and selenium is essential in parenteral nutrition (Table 18.8). *Deficiency states* of these trace elements have been described in patients who have been receiving parenteral nutrition without supplementation. These patients respond to the specific replacement of deficient trace elements.

Manganese has not been clearly established as an essential component of TPN solutions, but it has been included in some recommended regimens. Iodine is not

Table 18.7 Range of Daily Requirements of Major Minerals and Electrolytes in Parenteral Solutions

Electrolyte	Daily Requirement Range
Sodium	50–250 mEq
Potassium	30–200 mEq
Chloride	50–250 mEq
Magnesium	10–30 mEq
Calcium	10–20 mEq
Phosphorus	10–40 mmole

Modified from Alpers DH, Clouse RE, Stenson WF: *Manual of Nutritional Therapeutics.* Boston, Little, Brown & Co., 1983, p. 238.

Table 18.8 Suggested Daily Adult Intravenous Requirements of Essential Trace Elements and Associated Deficiency Syndromes

Trace Element	Requirement	Deficiency Syndrome
Iron	10–18 mg/day	Anemia
Copper*	30 mcg/kg/day	Rare hemolysis
Zinc*	15 mg/day	Blepharitis, conjunctivitis, growth retardation, dermatitis, diarrhea
Selenium*	50–200 mcg/day	Cardiomyopathy
Chromium*	20 mcg/day	Glucose intolerance, hypercholesterolemia, hyperaminoacidemia
Manganese	3–5 mg/day	Dermatitis, hypocholesterolemia, hair color change, decreased hair and nail growth
Iodine	100 mcg/day	Hypothyroidism
Fluoride	1.5–4.0 mg/day	Anemia, growth retardation
Molybdenum†	200–500 mcg/day	Muscle cramps

Adapted from *JAMA* 241:2051, 1979.
*Required in TPN solutions.
†Not absolutely required but included in most formulations.

658

normally supplemented because the transdermal absorption of iodine-containing solutions that are used to clean catheter sites permits the intake of the required amount of iodine.

In the presence of excessive gastrointestinal losses (e.g., small-bowel fistula), additional zinc should be given for replacement. It is recommended that 12.2 mg of additional zinc per liter of small-bowel loss should be given.

In patients who are being given enteral supplementation, 2 liters of formula per day will include all the recommended dietary allowance for vitamins, minerals, and trace elements.

References

1. **Bistrian BR, Blackburn GL, Hallowell E, Heddle R:** Protein status of general surgical patients. *JAMA* 230:858, 1974.

2. **Bistrian BR, Blackburn GL, Vitalle J, et al:** Prevalence of malnutrition in general medical patients. *JAMA* 235:1567, 1971.

3. **Willard MD, Gilsdorf RB, Price RA:** Protein–calorie malnutrition in a community hospital. *JAMA* 243:1720, 1980.

4. **Alpers DH, Clouse RE, Stenson WF:** *Manual of Nutritional Therapeutics.* Boston, Little, Brown & Co., 1983, pp 3–51.

5. **Young VR:** Energy metabolism and requirements in the cancer patient. *Cancer Res* 37:2336, 1977.

6. **Moore FD, Brennan MF:** Surgical inquiry: body composition, protein metabolism and neuroendocrinology. In Ballinger WF, Collins JA, Drucker WR, et al (eds): *Manual of Surgical Nutrition.* Philadelphia, WB Saunders, 1975, pp 169–222.

7. **Cahill GF:** Starvation in man. *N Engl J Med* 282:668, 1970.

8. **Blackburn GL, Bistrian BR, Maini BS:** Nutritional and metabolic assessment of the hospitalized patient. *J Parenter Enter Nutr* 1:11, 1977.

9. **Burgert SL, Anderson CF:** An evaluation of upper arm measurements used in nutritional assessments. *Am J Clin Nutr* 32:2136, 1979.

10. **Jensen TG, Dudrick SJ, Johnston DA:** A comparison of triceps skinfolds and upper arm circumference measurements taken in standard and supine positions. *J Parenter Enter Nutr* 5:519, 1981.

11. **Heymsfield SB, Arteaga C, McManus BS, et al:** Measurement of muscle mass in humans: validity of the 24 hr urinary creatinine method. *Am J Clin Nutr* 37:478, 1983.

12. **Grant JP, Custer DB, Thurlow J:** Current techniques of nutritional assessment. *Surg Clin North Am* 61:437, 1981.

13. **Chandra RK:** Immunocompetence testing and nutritional status. *Diagn Med* 5:53, 1982.

14. **Gross RL, Newberne PM:** Role of nutrition in immunologic function. *Physiol Rev* 60:188, 1980.

15. **Baker JP, Detsky AS, Wolman SL, et al:** Nutritional assessment: a comparison of clinical judgement and objective measurements. *N Engl J Med* 306:969, 1982.

16. **Heber D, Chlebowski RT, Ishibashi DE, et al:** Abnormalities in glucose and protein metabolism in noncachectic lung cancer patients. *Cancer Res* 42:4815, 1982.

17. **Heber D, Byerley MS, Chi J, Grosvenor M, Bergman R:** Pathophysiology of malnutrition in the adult cancer patient. *Cancer* 58:1867, 1986.

18. **Brennan MF:** Total parenteral nutrition in the cancer patient. *N Engl J Med* 305:375, 1981.

19. **Silberman H, Eisenberg D:** Parenteral nutrition: the lipid system. In Silberman H, Eisenberg D (eds): *Parenteral and Enteral Nutrition for the Hospitalized Patient.* East Norwalk, Conn, Appleton-Century-Crofts, 1982, pp 182–190.

20. **Laughlin EH, Dorosin NN, Phillips YY, et al:** Total parenteral nutrition: a guide to therapy in the adult. *J Fam Pract* 5:947, 1977.

21. **Sirba E:** Effect of reduced protein intake on nitrogen loss from the human integument. *Am J Clin Nutr* 20:1158, 1978.

22. **Calloway D, Spector H:** Nitrogen balance as related to caloric and protein intake in active young men. *Am J Clin Nutr* 2:405, 1954.

23. **Recommended Dietary Allowances,** 10th edition, National Academy Press, Washington DC, 1989.

24. **Pillar B, Perry S:** Evaluating total parenteral nutrition: final report and statement of the technology assessment and practice guidelines forum. *Nutrition* 6:313, 1990.

25. **Meguid MM, Mughal MM, Meguid V, Terry JJ:** Risk-benefit analysis of malnutrition and perioperative nutritional support: a review. *Nutr Int* 3:25, 1987.

26. **Koretz RL:** What supports nutritional support? *Digest Dis Sci* 29:577, 1984.

27. **Bethel RA, Jansen RD, Heymsfield SB, Nixon DW, Rudman D:** Nasogastric hyperalimentation through a polyethylene catheter: an alternative to central venous hyperalimentation. *Am J Clin Nutr* 32:1112, 1979.

28. **Voit KAJ, Echave V, Brown RA, Gund FN:** Use of elemental diet during the adaptive stage of short gut syndrome. *Gastroenterology* 65:419, 1973.

29. **Heymsfield SB, Bethel RA, Ansley JD, Nixon DW, Rudman D:** Enteral hyperalimentation: an alternative to central venous hyperalimentation. *Ann Intern Med* 90:63, 1979.

30. **Feliciano DV, Mattox KL, Graham JM:** Major complications of percutaneous subclavian catheters. *Am J Surg* 138:869, 1979.

31. **Ryan A, Abel M, Abbot WM:** Catheter complications in total parenteral nutrition. *New Engl J Med* 290:757, 1974.

32. **Covelli HD, Black JW, Olsen MS, Beekman JF:** Respiratory failure precipitated by high carbohydrate loads. *Ann Intern Med* 95:579, 1981.

33. **Ryan JA:** Complications of total parenteral nutrition. In: Fischer JE (ed): *Total Parenteral Nutrition.* Boston, Little, Brown & Co., 1976, p 55.

34. **Ruberg R, Allen T, Goodman M:** Hypophosphatemia with hypophosphaturia in hyperalimentation. *Surg Forum* 22:87, 1971.

35. **Fleming CR, McGill DB, Hoffman HN, Nelson RA:** Total parenteral nutrition. *Mayo Clin Proc* 51:187, 1976.

36. **Fleming CR, Hodges RE, Hurley LS:** A prospective study of serum copper and zinc levels in patients receiving total parenteral nutrition. *Am J Clin Nutr* 29:70, 1976.

37. **Chen WJ, Ohashi E, Kasai M:** Amino acid metabolism in parenteral nutrition: with special reference to the calorie:nitrogen ratio and the blood urea nitrogen level. *Metabolism* 23:1117, 1974.

38. **Goodgame JT, Lowry SF, Brennan MF:** Essential fatty acid deficiency in total parenteral nutrition:time course of development and suggestions for therapy. *Surgery* 84:271, 1978.

39. **Blackburn GL, Wan JM, Teo TC, et al:** Metabolic support in organ failure. In: Behari DJ, Cerra FB (eds): *New Horizons: Multiple Organ Failure.* Fullerton, California, Society of Critical Care Medicine, 1989, pp. 337–370.

40. **Cerra FB:** Hypermetabolism, organ failure, and metabolic support. *Surgery* 101:1, 1987.

41. **Windmueller HG:** Glutamine utilization by the small intestine. *Adv Enzymol* 53:210, 1982.

42. **Fox AD, Kripke SA, DePaula JA:** Glutamine supplemented diets prolong survival and decrease mortality in experimental enterocolitis. *J Parenter Enter Nutr* 12 (suppl 1): 8S, 1988.

43. **Thomas RJS:** The response of patients with fistulas of the gastrointestinal tract to parenteral nutrition. *Surg Gynecol Obstet* 153:77, 1981.

Psychological Issues

Barbara L. Andersen

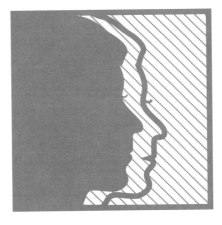

For the majority of women, a diagnosis of gynecologic cancer is a crisis. There follows a period of extreme emotional distress, but this slowly dissipates with recovery. For others, cancer may become a chronic stressor, a way of life, either because the disease is disseminated and can be controlled only with radical treatments or because their coping strategies are not adequate for this life experience. In any case, management of patients with gynecologic malignancies needs to go beyond routine medical care and take into account the psychologic and behavioral aspects of the disease.

A review of the data on psychologic and behavioral issues surrounding gynecologic cancer is presented. In addition, practical information that can be used to conceptualize and deal with a woman's personal response to her disease is summarized. These issues are presented within a disease "time frame," from the appearance of symptoms to recovery or recurrence and death (Fig. 19.1).

Symptoms, Signs, and Delay

Early detection and prompt treatment can reduce the morbidity and mortality associated with most gynecologic cancers. The length of time women tolerate symptoms before consulting a physician is therefore an important factor in outcome. Local and national cancer societies have sought to combat delay through educational campaigns aimed at the general public. For example, "unusual bleeding or discharge," a common symptom of gynecologic cancer, is listed by the American Cancer Society as one of the seven warning signs. Unfortunately, these interventions have yielded limited success in shortening patient delay (1).

Why do women with gynecologic symptoms delay seeking medical attention?
To help answer this question, women who had a diagnosis of primary or recurrent cancer were interviewed before treatment (2). This study and a review of the literature revealed four factors that account for delay in seeking a cancer diagnosis. These factors may be categorized as follows:

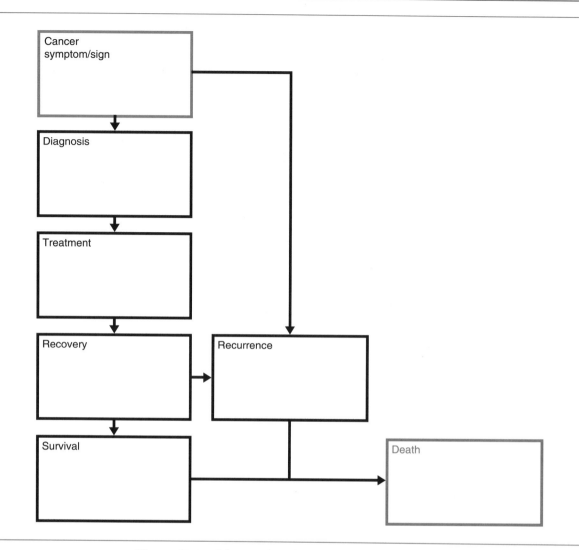

Figure 19.1 Disease time intervals.

1. Symptom characteristics

2. Symptom interpretation

3. Knowledge of cancer

4. Sociodemographic characteristics

Symptom Characteristics Gynecologic symptoms can be nonspecific and easily confused with less consequential conditions. For example, women with ovarian cancer may misinterpret their symptoms as indigestion or recurrence of a previous infection (3), and those with endometrial cancer, particularly perimenopausal women, often believe their abnormal bleeding is an indication of menopause (4).

The site of a symptom can account for delay. Rectal and genital cancers appear to be characterized by greater patient delay than other sites (5), and vulvar malignancies in particular foster lengthy patient and physician delays (6). One explanation for this is the wide availability of nonprescription remedies for symptomatic relief. Patients with symptoms of vulvar cancer often seek a physician's diagnosis only after attempts at self-treatment of those symptoms have failed (7). Likewise, physicians may not suspect carcinoma and may prescribe a regimen of topical treatments (6).

Severity is a characteristic that appears to affect delay—a severe sensation is more likely than a weak or vague sensation to lead a patient to seek treatment early (8). Related to severity is the extent to which a symptom interferes with the activities of the person. Because people may define illness according to their ability to perform physical and social roles (9), disabling symptoms will likely bring a patient to seek medical attention earlier than symptoms that do not interfere with normal activities.

Also related to severity is the existence and extent of pain. Among patients with breast (10) and ovarian cancer (3), the presence of pain as an early symptom has been noted to reduce delay in seeking a diagnosis. Pain with intercourse (dyspareunia) is also influential in a woman's decision to seek a diagnosis of early cervical or endometrial cancer (11).

Symptom Interpretation

Once persons detect a bodily change, they begin to consider explanations and to assess the consequences of the change; i.e., the process of symptom interpretation begins. This process, however, may be subverted. For example, a woman may delay contacting a physician because she is busy caring for a sick husband or child or because a long-awaited vacation has been planned. If such environmental events have negative connotations, attention to bodily events may be increased and reporting of symptoms hastened (12), whereas more positive events may distract the person and lengthen delay.

Women who believe that their symptoms are caused by "normal" life circumstances delay longer in seeking a diagnosis; conversely, women who believe their symptoms are indicative of cancer seek earlier consultation. Not surprisingly, **few women think cancer is the cause of their symptoms. Even patients with recurrent cancer do not consider cancer as an explanation any more rapidly than those who learn of their diagnosis for the first time** (2).

The symptoms of cancer recurrence can be dissimilar to those experienced with the initial episode. For instance, if hysterectomy has been performed, recurrent cervical cancer might be manifest as rectal or back pain, rather than as the vaginal bleeding that signaled the initial disease. A patient then may conclude erroneously that her symptoms do not signal cancer but are caused by hemorrhoids or a strained muscle. Patients with recurrent cancers do seek medical consultation more rapidly.

Failure to regard symptoms as consequential is an important contributor to delayed diagnosis in patients with cancer (13). For example, heavy bleeding, in contrast to light spotting, might prompt a woman to act sooner because of the fear of anemia or lethargy.

Studies of the relationship between delay and emotional responses to symptoms have yielded equivocal results. Denial has been reported to be associated with greater delay (14), although this finding is controversial (15). Discrepant results also abound regarding fear or worry (3). Among gynecologic patients, women who are more anxious tend to believe a physician's care is necessary earlier than women who are less anxious (2).

Knowledge

Lack of general information regarding cancer may increase delay in seeking a diagnosis (16); yet educational campaigns to provide such knowledge appear to have had little impact. In fact, there is no significant relationship between a woman's knowledge of her own cancer (e.g., site, treatment, prognosis) and the length of delay (2). A more important type of knowledge may be past experience with symptoms. Patients whose symptoms are similar to those of a previous illness or condition often interpret their present illness as a recurrence of the familiar and/or less consequential condition.

Sociodemographic Characteristics

In studies of delay, few sociodemographic characteristics exhibit a consistent association (13, 17, 18), although this may be due to the small sample sizes in such studies (usually < 100 cases). Sociodemographic characteristics—age, race, marital status, education, and income—are believed to play a role in delay because of their general importance as mediators for health-promoting and/or health-damaging behaviors (19). These same characteristics also relate to the psychologic, behavioral, and disease outcome after diagnosis.

Age Specifically for gynecologic cancer, there is a consistent increase in the incidence rates from younger to older cohorts, and death rates for the elderly are also increased.

Race White women have a higher incidence of endometrial and ovarian cancer, whereas black women have twice the incidence of cervical cancer (20, 21). Black women have a lower survival rate for both cervical and endometrial cancer (approximately 10% lower for each), whereas there are no differences in survival rates for ovarian cancer.

Marital Status Married persons live longer and have a lower mortality for almost every major cause of death than never married, separated, widowed, or divorced persons. More specifically, population-based studies of adults with cancer indicate that unmarried persons have a decreased overall survival. They present initially with more advanced disease (longer delay), have a higher likelihood of not being treated for cancer, and, after adjustment for both factors, respond less well to treatment (23). There are two possible explanations for this. One is the benefit from the higher socioeconomic status of married persons, and the other is the importance of social support. The significance of the latter has been reliably underscored in large community cohort studies that have controlled for income (24, 25).

Socioeconomic Status There is a relationship between both family income and educational level and age-adjusted cancer incidence and survival. The poor cervical cancer results for black women appear to be due in large part to their socioeconomic status (26). Blacks represent one-third of the poor, one-fourth of the unemployed, but only one-tenth of the population (27). Thus examination of the psychologic responses of various socioeconomic groups necessitates consideration of the circumstances that may arise from a lack of education, unemployment, substandard housing, poor nutrition, risk-promoting lifestyle and behavior, and diminished access to health care (27).

Intervention

Providing information to women on the hallmarks of gynecologic cancer, such as irregular or postmenopausal bleeding, is essential. In addition to noting the symptoms, however, educational campaigns must also emphasize the similarity of the symptoms to other benign conditions that women may experience, such as dysfunctional uterine bleeding or bleeding from postmenopausal atrophy. Finally, women treated for gynecologic cancer need to be alerted to the most common signs of recurrence.

Diagnosis

Cancer patients face difficult circumstances throughout their illness, but the shock of learning the diagnosis is the first, and often the most difficult, experience. The term *existential plight* has been used to describe this period and the emotional turmoil that continues for the immediate months (28).

The emotions and sources of distress may include:

1. *Depression* from life disruption and doubts concerning the future.

2. *Anxiety* anticipating cancer treatment.

3. *Confusion* from dealing with a complex medical environment.

4. *Anger* from the loss of childbearing capacity and the opportunity to choose whether or not to have children.

5. *Guilt* from concerns that previous sexual activity may have "caused" the cancer. The guilt may be mixed with concerns about how future sexual activity will be disrupted after cancer treatment.

In a prevalence study of psychiatric illness among cancer patients, Derogatis et al. (29) estimated that approximately **50% of cancer patients would justify a psychiatric diagnosis and of those, 85% had symptoms of depression and/or anxiety.** Most diagnoses (68%) were classified as an *adjustment disorder*—a maladaptive emotional reaction to a life stressor.

In a similar investigation of 83 women with gynecologic cancer, Evans et al. (30) reported that 23% met appropriate psychiatric criteria for *major depression*, 24% met criteria for *adjustment disorder with depressed mood,* and 14% had other psychiatric diagnoses. In a study of depressive symptomatology, Cain et al. (31) studied 60 newly diagnosed patients with cervical, endometrial, or ovarian malignancies. They classified the depression as severe in 35% of the patients, moderate in 35%, and mild in 30%.

Initial Diagnosis

To clarify the pattern of mood disturbance common to a diagnosis of cancer, we asked women to complete a self-report inventory on the emotions they experienced during their initial evaluation (32). Their responses were compared with those from two matched groups, one with benign gynecologic disease anticipating surgery and the other with no disease (i.e., healthy women).

665

Findings were as follows:

1. Only women with cancer described themselves as significantly depressed.

2. In contrast, high anxiety was reported by both groups with disease, whether benign or malignant.

3. There were no differences in the level of anger between the groups.

4. High levels of confusion were reported only by the cancer patients.

5. There were equivalent levels of fatigue among the disease groups.

Recurrence

Patients with recurrent cancer have an even greater level of distress than women receiving their initial diagnosis. This appears to result from higher levels of depression and anger. In contrast, the levels of anxiety and confusion are comparable to those reported by women receiving their first diagnosis. Thus the worries of a poorer prognosis, the anger about treatment failure, and the anticipatory concerns of beginning further treatment are evidenced.

Intervention

Severe emotional distress consequent to cancer diagnosis and during cancer treatments can be reduced with psychologic efforts. Two studies, both using nonequivalent control group designs, have explored the effectiveness of brief psychologic interventions for gynecologic cancer patients.

Capone et al. (33) provided a crisis-oriented intervention to newly diagnosed women. The structured counseling assisted women to express feelings and fears related to their diagnosis or upcoming treatment, provided information about treatment sequelae, and attempted to enhance self-esteem, femininity, and interpersonal relationships. For sexually active women, an additional sexual therapy component included information on how to reduce anxiety when resuming intercourse. The format involved at least four individual sessions during the surgical hospitalization; the length of each session or total therapy time was not specified. Two psychologists were the therapists. Fifty-six newly diagnosed women (51% were Stage I, 22% Stage II, 15% Stage III, and 12% IV or unstaged) receiving treatment at a university medical center participated; the participation rate was 87%. The sociodemographic characteristics were as follows: mean age was 50 years, 60% had at least a high school education, 64% were married, 79% were white, and 21% were black. A nonequivalent control group was obtained by recruiting previously treated women as they returned for posttreatment follow-up. Standardized outcome measures were used to assess emotional distress and self-concept and were supplemented with self-reports of return to employment and frequency of intercourse. Data were gathered before treatment and at 3, 6, and 12 months after treatment for the intervention women and at the same posttreatment intervals for the comparison women. Analyses indicated no differences between groups or within the intervention group on the measures of emotional distress or self-concept. A trend in the percentage of women returning to work favored the intervention participants (e.g., 50% vs. 25% at 3 months). In contrast, substantial differences were found between the groups in the return to and frequency of intercourse across all posttreatment assessments (e.g., 16% of the intervention group vs. 57% of the control women reported less or no sexual activity at 12 months posttreatment).

The second quasi-experimental investigation was reported by Houts et al. (34) and examined the efficacy of a peer counseling model. The structured intervention included encouragement to maintain interpersonal relationships, to make positive plans for the future, to query the medical staff regarding treatments, side effects, and sexual outcomes, and to maintain normal routines. These interventions were delivered in three telephone contacts (before treatment and at 5 and 10 weeks after treatment), with provision of a booklet and audiotape description of the coping strategies at the pretreatment hospital visit. Two social workers were the peer counselors; subjects were not informed that former cancer patients were also trained as social workers. Thirty-two women with diagnosed gynecologic cancer (stage not specified) participated (14 intervention and 18 control); participation rate was 78%. The sociodemographic characteristics included a mean age of 50 years and at least a high school education in 65%. Fifty-one percent of the women were married. Control subjects were recruited on alternate weeks. A standardized outcome measure assessed emotional distress and an experimenter-derived measure assessed coping strategies. Data were gathered before treatment and at 6 and 12 weeks after treatment. Analysis indicated no differences between the groups at any point in time. **In summary, the quasi-experimental design suggested that interventions for gynecologic cancer patients produced limited gains, except in the area of sexual functioning. The latter finding is consistent with longitudinal descriptive data of gynecologic cancer patients showing low morbidity in the areas of emotional distress, marital adjustment, and social adjustment but moderately severe problems with sexual functioning (32, 54).**

These and other studies involving patients with newly diagnosed cancer (see reference 35 for a review) focus on the trauma of learning that one has a potentially life-threatening illness. **Regarding psychologic support, a crisis intervention or brief therapy model appears to be most appropriate.** This provides a rapid early assessment of the patient's emotional distress and other difficulties, a present-day focus on the problems facing her, limited therapeutic goals, and a therapist who is actively making suggestions for coping and problem management and prompt interventions. Therapeutic components may include *emotional support* and *comfort,* which acknowledges the difficulty of the situation and provides a context for the patient to openly discuss her fears and anxieties about the disease, *information about the disease* and *treatment, behavioral coping strategies* (e.g., role playing difficult discussions with family or the medical staff), *cognitive coping strategies,* (i.e. identifying the patient's troublesome worries and thoughts and providing alternative appraisals of the situation), and *relaxation training* to lower anxiety and/or bodily tension and enhance one's sense of control.

The studies of women with cancer, specifically gynecologic or breast cancer, highlight the need for *focused interventions* for sexual functioning. Briefly, at least three components are essential: *sexuality information* (e.g., male and female sexual anatomy, the sexual response cycle, sexual dysfunctions, and potential sources of difficulty after cancer treatment), *medical interventions* (e.g., hormonal therapy, reconstructive surgery), and *specific sex therapy suggestions*.

Because psychologic interventions may not alleviate all problems, pharmacologic agents may be potentially useful. Unfortunately, they are rarely used. A survey of psychotropic drug prescriptions for cancer patients found that antidepressants, for example, were prescribed for only 1% of these patients. One-third of the prescriptions were written for conditions other than depression (36). This finding

667

is especially surprising in view of the demonstrated effectiveness of pharmacologic agents in controlled trials with psychiatric patients as well as cancer patients. For example, thioridazine (75 mg daily) is superior to placebo in relieving the distress of cancer patients suffering from anxiety or depression (37). In another study, 80% of depressed radiotherapy patients given imipramine showed improvement, compared with 42% of such patients who did not receive the drug (38). More research is needed to determine which agents alleviate distress among specific groups of patients.

Cancer Treatment

It is most important for a woman to receive information about the treatment plan for her disease. Despite efforts to allay concerns and provide accurate information, misconceptions abound, and anxiety will remain high as patients approach surgery, radiotherapy, or chemotherapy.

Patients experiencing high levels of distress have many other difficulties. These include problems understanding and remembering all that they are told. This may include simple information (e.g., what time they are to be admitted) or more complex information (e.g., what organs the surgery will remove and the nature of side effects). There may be difficulty in managing personal affairs (e.g., contacting one's insurance company or arranging for child care during recovery), and difficulty may also be experienced with expected behaviors (e.g., being a "patient" and allowing others to care for one's needs). In addition, most patients are unfamiliar with major medical treatments.

Even for those with previous knowledge, cancer treatment can be qualitatively different. For example, a woman's mother, sister, or a close friend may have related her experiences with hysterectomy. Even if the surgery involved an abdominal rather than a vaginal approach, the preoperative and postoperative experience for the woman with cancer will be notably different from the patient's expectations (e.g., bowel preparation, length of recovery, vaginal shortening, bladder disruption). Thus it is normal for *any* patient to experience cognitive, emotional, and behavioral difficulties, and it is the rare patient who will not require supportive assistance as treatment approaches.

Surgery

Although there have been few investigations of patients' psychologic reactions to cancer surgery, there are numerous descriptive studies of the reactions of relatively healthy persons undergoing surgery for benign conditions (e.g., uterine fibroids). This research has indicated that there is a direct relationship between the magnitude of preoperative and postoperative anxiety; i.e., those patients who are the most anxious before surgery are also the most anxious afterward, albeit less so. In addition, the magnitude of postoperative distress often correlates with behavioral indicants of recovery (e.g., time out of bed, pain reports, days in hospital). Research that has examined emotional distress during recovery has differentiated the outcomes for patients undergoing surgery for benign versus malignant conditions. Gottesman and Lewis (39) noted greater and more lasting crisis feelings and a stronger sense of helplessness among cancer patients for as long as 2 months after discharge from the hospital.

Gynecologic cancer surgery may pose further emotional burdens. Women of childbearing age who are nulliparous or have not yet achieved their desired family size are often distraught and have feelings of loss after hysterectomy. Acceptance of this change may not come for months, and in the interim it may be difficult for the woman to socialize with sisters or female friends who are pregnant or who have young children. Because the age of childbearing among women in the United States has risen in recent years, the likelihood of this situation occurring for women with gynecologic cancer will increase. Radical surgical procedures, such as radical vulvectomy or pelvic exenteration, which produce genital and/or pelvic disfigurement and involve long hospitalization and lengthy recovery, produce depression, feelings of isolation, and significant body concerns (40, 41).

Intervention

Efforts to reduce distress from surgery or to facilitate recovery are typically of a psychotherapeutic or informational nature. **Informational interventions—including detailed descriptions of the procedure, sensations, or side effects to be anticipated—and behavioral coping strategies—e.g., relaxation training or distraction exercises for pain management—have generally proved effective.** In this regard, prepared patients tend to have shorter hospital stays, use fewer medications, and report less severe pain than patients receiving standard hospital care and preoperative nursing information (42, 43). It is hypothesized that this type of preparation reduces stress by helping to build accurate expectations and by enhancing feelings of control and predictability for the patient.

Radiation Therapy

Approximately 60% of women with a diagnosis of gynecologic cancer will receive radiation therapy. Although there are differences in the experiences of patients receiving external radiation therapy and intracavitary radiation, the majority of patients report confusion and negative emotions regarding these treatments. Misinformation is common, with some patients fearing permanent contamination from treatment and others assuming that radiation attacks only "bad" cells, leaving others unaffected. A patient's prior knowledge of radiotherapy may be based on the experiences of a friend or relative, and if their treatment was unsuccessful or difficult, she may enter treatment believing it will be the same for her (44).

External Radiation

The initiation of external therapy brings fears or uneasiness about the size or the safety of treatment machines and distress from being in a radiation therapy department where other cancer patients in obvious ill health are seen. For some women, disrobing and exposing the pelvic area can be a daily embarrassment, and field-marking tattoos are visible reminders of the disease. Such concerns are common early in treatment; in one study, roughly 80% of patients receiving ERT expressed an unwillingness to discuss these concerns with their physicians (45). This occurs because patients may perceive their physicians as too busy, or they may have difficulty devising "intelligent" questions for their physicians.

As the procedures of radiation therapy become more routine, many patients report less emotional distress, but the side effects of fatigue, diarrhea, and anorexia appear by the second week. These side effects complicate living, requiring, for example, activity reductions and dietary modifications. Previously symptom-free patients may begin to feel and think of themselves as "ill," doubting their positive prognosis. Premenopausal women experience hot flushes, a salient and distressing symptom of the loss of their fertility.

At the termination of treatment, these patients might be expected to report a drop in anxiety and fear, similar to the pattern exhibited by relatively healthy persons undergoing surgery. Instead, gynecologic patients (46), as well as other cancer patients (47), report a different pattern of anxiety responses. Women with high pretreatment anxiety are less anxious on the last treatment day than on the first, although they remain the most distressed. Those with moderate levels of pretreatment distress report little diminution in distress by the last treatment, and surprisingly, those with low levels of anxiety at the onset of treatment report significantly greater anxiety on the last treatment day. As expected, physical symptoms of fatigue, abdominal pain, anorexia, diarrhea, and skin irritation are significant for all patients at the conclusion of treatment.

Recovery from the physical and psychologic distress of radiotherapy is not rapid. Nail et al. (48) have documented an incidence of nausea in 5%, anorexia in 15%, diarrhea in 15%, and fatigue in 32% of gynecologic patients treated as long as 3 months previously. In addition, new long-term complications, such as radiation proctitis or fistulas, can emerge. Decreased lubrication and vaginal tenderness also result in significant sexual disruption during recovery, with dyspareunia a problem.

Intracavitary Radiation

In contrast to external-beam radiation, few patients have heard of intracavitary radiation. Worries about lengthy isolation and permanent contamination are common, and women may cope with the impending treatment by diverting their attention to less distressing thoughts (49). During intracavitary radiation, women report significant physical discomfort, even when there has been liberal analgesic medication (50). Gas pains, burning sensations, and lower backache are typical physical complaints, and emotional distress is also pervasive. The visitation restrictions limit contact with one's family and friends, and this may be frightening to a patient if it is perceived as isolation from nurses or physicians. It is not surprising that many women feel irritable and/or upset during treatment.

A second application is received by 50—75% of women. Whereas physicians see their patients as better adjusted during a second treatment, patients do not "get used to" this treatment. In fact, women report feeling more anxious and debilitated after their second treatment than after their first; women with lower levels of anxiety before their first intracavitary treatment experience reported elevated levels of anxiety after their second application (50).

Intervention

The patterns of emotional distress, as well as the patients' descriptions of themselves as anxious, confused, and uncomfortable about expressing such concerns, provide targets for intervention. Patients most vulnerable to distress and most likely to need psychologic assistance during treatment may include (47, 50, 51):

1. Those who exhibit relatively little emotional distress before treatment

2. Those with a history of emotional problems

3. Those with a disease causing chronic discomfort

4. Those who are socially isolated

Several strategies may be useful to address the anxiety-based concerns of the radiotherapy patient. General counseling focused on the patient's problems may

670

be offered. For example, Forrester et al. (52) provided weekly sessions in which women receiving external radiation could discuss any topic, although the majority of sessions were supportive and informational. Improved functioning was found when these patients were compared with those receiving no intervention; intervention patients reported lower levels of emotional distress and less severe side effects.

Other interventions have focused primarily on provision of information. Topics worthy of discussion include simulation, radiation equipment, side effects of radiation, length of recovery, and strategies for managing side effects (e.g., diet modification, skin care, adequate rest). Research on patient preparation suggests that such information needs to be simplified and repeated. Instead of providing all information to patients on one occasion at the start of treatment, an alternative is to repeat portions of it as it becomes more relevant. For example, Israel and Mood (53) provided information about therapeutic procedures early in the treatment, about radiation side effects and their management at the midpoint of treatment, and about emotional issues and the length of recovery toward the end of therapy.

A special category of information for the gynecologic oncology patient is that of vaginal care and sexuality after radiation treatment. *Dyspareunia* is the most frequent complaint, and it appears to be most severe among women receiving both external and internal radiation, although patients receiving only external therapy also report this symptom (54). The magnitude of pain during intercourse appears to decrease during the months after treatment for women who maintain sexual activity.

A regimen of vaginal care is necessary for all patients to reduce pain and maintain, as much as possible, vaginal plasticity. Women who are not sexually active should be supplied with a vaginal dilator of sufficient length and width that, when lubricant is applied, it can be inserted comfortably and held in place. They should be instructed to use their dilator regularly (e.g., two to three times per week for 10–15 minutes). If the frequency of intercourse is low (i.e., less than once a week), women should use a dilator intermittently.

If not contraindicated, topical estrogen cream may promote healing and improve the vaginal epithelium (55). Despite these interventions, pain during intercourse may occur until sufficient healing of the vaginal epithelium has occurred.

Once any type of information has been delivered, patient understanding needs to be assessed inasmuch as many patients become confused or forgetful when too much information is given. One way to assure understanding is to ask the patient to explain in her own words what she has been told, as if she were telling her husband or a close friend. This strategy provides an opportunity for reinforcement of her understanding as well as for correction of misconceptions.

Chemotherapy

Patients' reactions to learning that they need chemotherapy can range from extreme negativity (i.e., feeling angry or depressed), to relief that some kind of treatment is available to them (56). This mix of emotions reflects the distress at having to undergo a difficult treatment, which many patients believe is only for "hopeless" cancers, and they fear that it will not control the disease or prevent a recurrence.

To allay patients' concerns, medical personnel usually spend a session or two providing descriptions of, and written materials about, the effects and side effects of treatment. Yet, as many as 10% of such patients may still report an uncertainty and lack of knowledge when beginning treatment (56). Others may approach chemotherapy optimistically and believe that they will belong to the small subset of persons who will not experience any side effects.

Patients experience a significant and constant level of distress throughout chemotherapy. As treatment occupies more and more of a patient's life, worries become intrusive, and the intense and noxious side effects generate stronger feelings of illness. Women who attempt to control the side effects and fail become more distressed than those who report that they have coped successfully (56).

Anticipatory nausea and vomiting may complicate the course of chemotherapy for approximately 25% of patients. This refers to nausea and/or vomiting prior to the administration of chemotherapy. It is hypothesized that this disturbing situation develops because the stimuli surrounding the administration of chemotherapy (e.g., needles and smell of alcohol) become paired with posttreatment nausea and vomiting. With repeated cycles, the stimuli become conditioned and are able to evoke nausea or vomiting prior to the administration of chemotherapy. Once anticipatory reactions develop, they can become more general (e.g., alcohol-containing substances such as perfume may elicit the response), and they occur progressively earlier (e.g., on entering the hospital, rather than on entering the treatment room).

Factors that place a patient at risk of developing anticipatory nausea and vomiting include (57):

1. Age under 50 years

2. Lengthy infusion of chemotherapy

3. Severe posttreatment nausea or vomiting in the early cycles

4. Extreme anxiety and/or depression

5. Previous susceptibility to motion sickness

Another concomitant of some chemotherapy is confusion, a distressing symptom for the patient and her family. Pharmacologic effects of chemotherapeutic agents account for some cognitive changes (58), and such changes further emphasize the illness and its consequences to the patient.

Intervention

To the extent that posttreatment nausea and vomiting can be controlled or lessened with antinauseants from the start of a regimen, the likelihood of anticipatory problems developing will be reduced. Once anticipatory nausea and vomiting develop, *behavioral interventions* have demonstrated some effectiveness in breaking the chain of responses. These efforts have included (57):

1. Hypnotic or biofeedback-assisted relaxation training

2. Systematic desensitization

3. Instruction in coping strategies

672

Such problems can be reduced or eliminated within limits. Continuous intervention (i.e., relaxation instruction prior to the administration of each chemotherapy) is often necessary (57). "Live" rather than audiotaped relaxation training instruction is more effective.

Recovery

Psychologic

For decades there has been the clinical impression that psychologic and behavioral outcomes after cancer diagnosis and treatment were troubled (e.g., 59–61). **Data now indicate that the majority of patients cope successfully; many former patients report renewed vigor in their approach to life, stronger interpersonal relationships, and a "survivor" adaptation (62, 63).** Recent longitudinal data also confirm this scenario for gynecologic cancer patients.

Andersen et al. (32, 54) compared longitudinal data on the psychologic and sexual outcomes of women with gynecologic cancer (Stage I or II; $N = 47$) with two matched comparison groups, women treated for benign gynecologic disease ($N = 18$) and gynecologically healthy women ($N = 57$). All women were assessed after diagnosis but before treatment and then reassessed 4, 8, and 12 months after treatment. Considerable sexual disruption occurred, but this represented the only major life disruption. The significant emotional distress at diagnosis was transitory and resolved after treatment. There was no evidence of a higher incidence of relationship dissolution or poorer marital adjustment in the cancer patients, but 30% reported that their sexual partners had some difficulty in reaching orgasm (i.e., delayed ejaculation) during the recovery year. There was no evidence of impaired social adjustment. Finally, women treated for gynecologic cancer retained their employment and occupations, although their involvement (e.g., hours worked per week) was significantly reduced during recovery.

Sexuality

Increased national attention has been given to the sexual difficulties of cancer patients (64) and to women with gynecologic cancer in particular (65). **Of women treated for gynecologic disease, 30–90% experience significant sexual disruption,** and much of the variability in this estimate can be accounted for by disease site or treatment. When patients have been queried about sexuality, strategies for alleviating pain during intercourse, or the schedule for resuming sexual activity after treatment, all have indicated that these are important concerns that need to be addressed (40, 41, 66).

Female Sexual Response Cycle and Dysfunction

A conceptual model for understanding sexual response includes the phases of sexual desire, excitement, orgasm, and resolution.

Sexual Desire

Sexual desire is the least understood of all the phases. It has been conceptualized as a drive or motivation for sexual activity, and androgen is hypothesized as the hormonal basis for sexual desire in women. Data in support of the latter point come from a prospective crossover experiment in women with surgically induced menopause (67). Exogenous androgen enhanced the intensity of sexual desire and arousal, but estrogen had no effect.

The term *inhibited sexual desire* characterizes those persons who report that they are generally uninterested in sexual activity. Such an attitude can be manifest by avoidance of sexual contacts, refusal of sexual activity, or infrequent initiation of sexual activity. Inhibited persons report an absence or low frequency of sexual fantasy or other pleasant, arousing sexual thoughts. Persons with sexual desire dysfunction may experience sexual excitement and/or orgasm when engaging in sexual activity; however, disruption in the focus, intensity, or duration of sexual activity is typical, and excitement and/or orgasmic phase dysfunctions commonly occur.

Sexual Excitement

The phase of sexual excitement begins with psychologic or physical stimulation. Physiologic responses that occur during the excitement phase include vaginal engorgement and lubrication. Maximal vasocongestion produces a congested orgasmic platform in the lower one-third of the vaginal barrel.

Dysfunctional responses during the phase of sexual excitement would include insufficient response so that penetration during heterosexual intercourse would be difficult or uncomfortable. Psychologically, a woman may report that she does not feel aroused and/or that her body is not responding. As with desire phase difficulties, subsequent orgasmic disruption could easily result from lowered levels of excitement.

If such disruption occurs after treatment of gynecologic cancer, it is likely to be due to nerve damage or to the structural changes imposed. Women report that their bodies do not feel aroused; concurrently, they report few arousing feelings or thoughts (54). Also, normal excitement responses can be disrupted with treatment side effects. For example, dyspareunia is a common problem after radiation therapy, particularly intracavitary treatment. It is likely that this pain results from the direct trauma to the vaginal epithelium, decreased vascular engorgement, and reduced vaginal lubrication.

Orgasm

Although the specific neurophysiologic mechanism of orgasm is not known, it has been proposed that orgasm is triggered when a plateau of excitement has been reached (68).

Subjectively, a woman's awareness of orgasm typically focuses on pelvic sensations, centered in the clitoris, vagina, and uterus. Orgasm is marked by rhythmic contractions of the uterus, the orgasmic platform, and the rectal sphincter. A woman's awareness of orgasm is reported to be similar, regardless of the manner in which it is achieved (69).

Among cancer patients, the typical difficulty is a dramatic decline in frequency of orgasm or a failure of orgasm to occur. This problem is typically accompanied by the excitement difficulties described above, so that the woman feels she does not become sufficiently aroused to approach the plateau necessary for orgasm.

Resolution

If effective stimulation ends and/or orgasm occurs, the anatomic and physiologic changes that occurred during excitement reverse. The orgasmic platform disappears, the uterus moves back into the true pelvis, and the vagina shortens and narrows. Such bodily responses after orgasm generally are accompanied by subjective feelings of tension release, relaxation, and contentment. If orgasm does not occur, the same physiologic processes are completed at a much slower rate.

Women with excitement or orgasmic dysfunctions typically report discontentment with the resolution period as well, with symptoms of continued pelvic vasocongestion, residual sexual tension, lack of satisfaction, and/or negative affect. Complaints with resolution after unimpaired excitement and orgasm are infrequent; when they occur, they may be prompted by inhibitory affects, such as guilt or marital discord, that are associated with sexual activity generally.

When all previous sexual responses are satisfactory for cancer patients, resolution responses are similar to those of healthy women. When difficulties arise, problematic resolution responses among cancer patients can be quite varied. Those with lowered desire and excitement and/or orgasmic disruption may have sexual tension, disappointment, and concern that their sexual responsiveness has been changed permanently. Those who experience pain during intercourse often have residual discomfort. Such outcomes, not unexpectedly, often lower a woman's interest in sexual activity.

Sexual Outcomes

Extensive data on sexual outcomes for cervical cancer patients are available (see reference 70 for a review). Sexual outcomes have been reported for treatments ranging from cervical conization for *in situ* disease to pelvic exenteration for recurrence. In contrast, patients with endometrial and vulvar cancer have been less well studied. There has been no study of the sexual outcomes for ovarian cancer patients.

Cervix

Preinvasive Lesions   After conization of the cervix, there appears to be no significant decline in the frequency of sexual intercourse or in sexual satisfaction and no concomitant increase in sexual dysfunction (71).

Invasive Lesions   In a prospective pretreatment study of patients with cervical and endometrial cancer, Andersen et al. (11) reported a surprisingly high frequency of major sexual disruption in the months immediately *prior to* diagnosis. This disruption seemed to be related to the appearance of disease symptoms (i.e., fatigue, postcoital bleeding, vaginal discharge, or pain). The difficulties were pervasive and included loss of desire, arousal problems. and orgasmic difficulties. For example, orgasm during intercourse occurred about half as often as usual.

Retrospective studies of posttreatment outcomes report diminished sexuality in up to 78% of patients after radical hysterectomy, 44–79% of patients after radiation therapy, and 33–46% of patients after combined treatment (54, 70). Many oncologists believe that radiotherapy is significantly more disruptive to sexual functioning than surgery. However, prospective research has documented that surgery and radiotherapy produce comparable rates of disruption, with 30–40% of all patients experiencing significant sexual problems (72).

The most comprehensive descriptive study of sexual outcomes in women with gynecologic cancer comes from Andersen et al. (32, 54), who compared women with clinical Stage I or II gynecologic cancer ($N = 47$) with two matched comparison groups, women treated for benign gynecologic disease ($N = 18$) and gynecologically healthy women ($N = 57$). All women were assessed after diagnosis but before treatment and then reassessed 4, 8 and 12 months after treatment. The frequency of intercourse declined for women treated for disease, whether malignant or benign. Considering the sexual response cycle, diminution of sexual excitement was pronounced for women with disease; however, this difficulty was more severe and distressing for the women with cancer, possibly because of significant coital and postcoital pain, premature menopause, and/or treatment side effects. Changes in desire, orgasm, and the resolution phase of the sexual response cycle also occurred. In approximately 30% of the women treated for cancer, a sexual dysfunction was diagnosed. Table 19.1 provides a summary of the rates of sexual dysfunction 12 months after treatment. The nature, early timing, and maintenance of sexual functioning morbidity suggest the instrumental role that cancer and cancer treatments play in these deficits (particularly arousal problems).

Pelvic Exenteration Pelvic exenteration is clearly a radical and disfiguring operation. Not surprisingly, clinical studies have reported the cessation of sexual activity for 70–80% of patients after surgery (41, 73–75). Although vaginal reconstruction offers the possibility that future sexual activity can include intercourse, it is not a panacea. Some women have specific difficulties related to the reconstruction (e.g., the cavity is too large or too small). Others have problems due to hampered healing (e.g., there may be a persistent vaginal discharge). In addition, some women avoid sexual intercourse because of the fear of vaginal bleeding or dyspareunia.

Endometrial Cancer

Limited information is available on sexual functioning after treatment for early-stage endometrial cancer. In the only retrospective study addressing this issue, 25% of the patients treated with surgery and 44% who had both surgery and radiotherapy experienced a decrease in the frequency of sexual activity (76). The majority of women who reported such a change also reported dyspareunia and diminished lubrication. Several women reported diminished arousal, but this factor was not influential in affecting the frequency of intercourse. These findings were replicated with data from the sexual partners. Approximately one-third of the sample reported the end of all sexual activity after treatment.

Vulvar Cancer

Despite the mutilating nature of surgical procedures for vulvar cancer, there has been minimal study of the sexual outcomes for these patients. Carcinoma *in situ* of the vulva is increasing in frequency and occurring at an earlier age (77). The

Table 19.1   Percentage of Sexual Dysfunction Diagnoses by Gynecology Group at 12 Months Posttreatment

Group	Frequency of Sexual Dysfunction at 12 Months Posttreatment			
	Desire	*Excitement*	*Orgasm*	*Dyspareunia*
Cancer	32%	29%	29%	29%
Benign	13%	20%	14%	14%
Healthy	9%	9%	6%	6%

From Andersen BL, Anderson B, deProsse C: Controlled prospective longitudinal study of women with cancer. I. Sexual functioning outcomes. *J Consult Clin Psychol* 57:683, 1989.

original treatment advocated for vulvar carcinoma *in situ* was wide local excision, but until recently many gynecologists removed the entire vulva, arguing that the disease was frequently multicentric. The main nonsurgical approaches for *in situ* disease have included the topical use of chemotherapy or CO_2 laser vaporization. The cosmetic and sexual results are thought to be optimal with these procedures, although confirming data have not yet been obtained. Patient tolerance of 5-FU is low because of intense burning and pruritus (78).

Andersen et al. (66) retrospectively studied sexual outcomes after surgical treatment, vulvectomy versus wide local excision, for patients with *in situ* vulvar disease. A pattern of sexual disruption was found. The *in situ* patients did not report diminished sexual desire despite excitement and orgasmic difficulties. There was a threefold to fourfold increase in sexual dysfunction from pretreatment to posttreatment, and more than 30% of the sample were not sexually active at follow-up. Also, **the type of surgery was significantly correlated with the magnitude of sexual difficulties, with greater sexual problems among those who underwent total vulvectomy rather than wide local excision.**

Radical vulvectomy has been regarded as standard treatment for invasive vulvar cancer, but there are advocates of individualized treatment and less radical surgery (79, 80). Radical vulvectomy causes substantial emotional and sexual disruption (40). Such patients have a limited capacity for sexual arousal but little diminution in sexual desire. As many as 50% stop all sexual activity except "friendly" kissing with their partner. This may result from negative feelings by the woman or her partner about the changed bodily appearance or from the severe dyspareunia that can occur with a surgically narrowed introitus (81, 82).

Intervention

If the sexual problems for women that occur as a result of gynecologic cancer treatment are to be minimized, a significant investment of time, energy, and resources will be necessary. Such an effort must include additional time spent in consultation with patients, development of psychologic interventions or written educational materials, and delivery of services by professionals or well-trained and closely supervised paraprofessionals experienced in the assessment and treatment of difficult medically related sexual problems. Because institutions differ in the services they are able to provide, a system for intervention development will be described.

Preparation

Physicians and nurses need to be informed about the potential sexual outcomes for gynecologic cancer patients that have been detailed here. It is best if this information is part of a broad understanding of normal female sexual function and response. **Patients make few inquiries, despite their concerns, so care providers need to initiate discussion of sexuality topics. When questions do arise, an informed and understanding response will encourage future disclosure of questions and concerns.**

Departments caring for gynecologic cancer patients need to determine how they will provide psychosexual help. For the individual patient, preventive rather than rehabilitative efforts are desirable. This should include the routine provision of sexual information to patients, particularly those at high risk of sexual problems

(83). Longitudinal data indicate that if sexual difficulties are to develop, the majority will be evidenced in the early months of recovery (54); thus information should be provided before and immediately after treatment, with a gradual decrease in the therapeutic efforts across time. Women at greatest risk of problems include those with vulvar or vaginal cancer and those who have had a pelvic exenteration.

In contrast to preventive services, rehabilitative services may be considered for women at less risk (e.g., a 55-year-old radical hysterectomy patient). With such a system, women would usually be seen only after sexual problems had developed. Although they might be more difficult to treat then, the positive benefit of having a readily available treatment program would be important to the patients. Patients returning for follow-up need to be informed of the availability of such a resource.

Assessment

A brief sexual history should be obtained from all patients before treatment. Obtaining a sexual assessment can achieve three goals:

1. It identifies sexuality as an area of importance to the gynecologic cancer patient.

2. It provides the healthy "baseline" data necessary to evaluate any future changes in sexual functioning. Retrospective reports are subject to the patient's recollections of past sexual activity and responses.

3. It provides an informed context for future discussions about sexuality with the medical team.

Even for the older woman or the woman who is not presently sexually active, such information is desirable. **The most important determiner of the frequency of sexual activity for a woman is the presence of a healthy and interested sexual partner, not age** *per se* (84). Women who are not presently sexually active may wish to be so in the future and will need to know how their functioning may be changed.

A pretreatment sexual history is best obtained by questioning the patient directly. Questionnaires can be used to assess such topics as sexual behavior (85, 86) or sexual arousal (87). The following areas can be briefly surveyed during a discussion with a patient:

1. Marital status and availability of current sexual partner(s)

2. Frequency of sexual activities (e.g., intercourse)

3. Presence of female sexual dysfunction (e.g., lack of desire, orgasmic difficulties)

4. Presence of sexual dysfunction in the partner (e.g., premature ejaculation, erectile difficulties)

Treatment

There have been few clinical (88, 89) and empirical (33, 90) reports of sexual intervention for female cancer patients. Two investigations provided brief counseling to gynecologic cancer patients on a variety of topics, such as causes of cancer, relaxation training, diet, exercise, and sexuality (33, 91). Sexual function was significantly less disrupted among counseled patients than among uncounseled controls.

Provision of Information

Information *per se* is an important component of sexual therapy interventions, even for healthy women (92). Patients should be well informed of the potential *direct* effects that the treatments may have on sexuality. Such effects include changed general health (e.g., chronic fatigue), structural changes to the genitals, hormonal changes, and direct interference with the physiologic components of the sexual response cycle. The range of sexual behaviors possible after treatment should be outlined.

Although sexual problems for the majority of gynecologic cancer patients are more difficult to treat than those of healthy persons, such information may prevent problems resulting from ignorance or misconception and may decrease the severity of problems that arise from other factors.

Medical Therapy

Specific medical interventions may enhance sexual functioning for selected patients (see reference 93 for a complete discussion). For example, hormonal medication may be used for menopausal symptoms; after vulvectomy the introitus may be narrowed, and the defect may be surgically correctable; the regular use of a sterile lubricant may be necessary for radiotherapy patients. Despite these efforts, certain sexual activities may remain impossible. For example, surgical modification of the introitus for a patient with vulvar cancer may not be successful, so the woman and her partner will need to reorient themselves to a sexual lifestyle that does not include vaginal intercourse.

Behavioral Therapy

Although the sexual problems of the gynecologic cancer patient are more difficult to treat than those of healthy women, behavioral techniques offer a useful place to begin. They should be conducted by a professional who is trained broadly in sexual therapy and familiar with the specific difficulties of the gynecologic cancer patient.

Desire Problems   In the treatment of desire problems, a careful determination of cause is important. Many women with cancer may experience direct disruption of excitement or orgasm from their treatments, which in turn may lead to loss of sexual desire. Women may report that the body does not respond or they do not feel the bodily sensations of arousal. Because interventions to enhance arousal or orgasm may, unfortunately, be met with limited success, such desire problems may remain and require direct intervention. Desire problems commonly occur in the earliest months of recovery. Therefore a lack of desire may not be a problem but, rather, evidence of a normal, prolonged recuperative process. Several interventions for desire problems can be considered, including:

1. Determining what conditions for sexual activity are more or less appealing and encouraging sexual activity under the most desirable circumstances

2. Increasing the frequency and variety of intimate activities (not only sexual behaviors) that the woman might find pleasurable

679

3. Increasing the frequency and variety of the woman's sexual fantasies during sexual activity and on other occasions

Enhancing Arousal Many desire-phase interventions have been used to enhance arousal, including the use of individual and couple body-touching exercises (i.e., sensate focus). Graduated steps for sexual activity are suggested to the woman or to the couple, with each stage employing more intimate touching and higher levels of arousal. For example, the couple's sensate focus could involve steps that include caressing of hands, arms, and face; caressing the whole body without genitals, breasts, or buttocks; caressing whole body without genital stimulation; caressing the whole body; and, finally, caressing the whole body with focused stimulation. Individual masturbation activities can be designed according to the same principles. Whereas activities such as these are useful to all couples, they are particularly important for women who are unable to resume intercourse. Such graduated activities have several potential benefits:

1. They can reintroduce relaxing and enjoyable sexual activity to a woman or a couple. This is important because many patients come to sexual therapy after many frustrating, discouraging, or unsatisfactory sexual encounters.

2. The activities are not strenuous, which is helpful to the woman who is not fully recovered or who tires easily.

3. The activities do not focus on a particular body part or area, and one objective is to find new, previously unexplored areas or methods of stimulation.

4. Touching of an area affected by treatment can be eliminated or introduced gradually.

Such a strategy can be less anxiety provoking for a woman and her partner. Also, both partners can learn what sensitivity, if any, remains in affected areas. Some areas will have sensations similar to those prior to cancer treatment, whereas others may feel unpleasant to the touch. Some couples may prefer not to explore certain areas. When this is done in the context of sensate focus exercises, other areas remain for touching, and a loving, sexual relationship can prevail, rather than a rejecting or anxiety-provoking one.

Reducing Negative Sexual Reactions Women may react negatively to their changed bodies after radical surgery—such as vulvectomy or pelvic exenteration—although the same reactions can occur for any person with cancer (94). Extreme responses may include disgust, anxiety when looking at the site, and fear of being seen by others. Many healthy women with sexual difficulties or anxieties have similar feelings. For such women, anxiety-reducing techniques, particularly systematic desensitization (95, 96) or individual sensate focus exercises (97, 98), have proved effective. Although such activities may not change a woman's negative body feelings to positive, the feelings may become neutral, or at least nondisruptive, to her sexual activities and overall mood.

Resuming Sexual Intercourse The graduated sexual activities described here provide a relaxing and sensual context in which intercourse can be resumed. Although there is no "correct" intercourse position, there may be positions that are more or less comfortable for the woman recovering from cancer treatment. If the patient tires easily or needs body support, the male superior position is the least strenuous for the woman. In contrast, if a woman is having pain with intercourse, (e.g., after intracavitary radiation), it is important that she have control over the depth of penetration and the rate of thrusting. In this case, the female superior position is often optimal. If this position does not provide relief from pain and a longer period of healing is necessary, it is important that couples be told to wait before resuming intercourse and to engage in other intimate activities if they wish.

During this period, the woman should be using a vaginal dilator regularly. In addition to keeping the vagina "open," the dilator exercises will provide a source of feedback to the woman regarding her degree of persistent vaginal discomfort. This information will help her to decide when it might be most comfortable to resume intercourse.

Orgasmic Dysfunction   Orgasmic dysfunction among women after gynecologic treatment is common. The difficulty is typically acute, with disruption occurring immediately after treatment. It is also pervasive, with the woman who was regularly orgasmic with coital activity before treatment becoming nonorgasmic. With this pattern, it is likely that the difficulty is a result of altered structure or innervation. For some women, orgasm is more difficult to achieve, although it does occur intermittently.

Before beginning a treatment program for orgasmic difficulties, it is important that other reasons for orgasmic difficulties be assessed, including insufficient arousal or dyspareunia. The most successful treatment programs for healthy nonorgasmic women include a series of individual sexuality and masturbation exercises. The early steps of such programs involve body examination, identification of genital anatomy, actual body and genital self-examination to identify pleasurable sensations, and focused genital stimulation. Even though pelvic or genital anatomy after cancer treatment is changed, it is possible that orgasm can still be experienced through other means, because women can experience orgasm without genital stimulation or without specific organs such as the clitoris, once believed critical to the response.

If the woman is motivated to undertake treatment, the exercises are completed with conscientious effort, and orgasm does not occur, the change in orgasmic ability may be long-standing. Even in this case, the exercises may help the woman to take a more active role in her sexuality, give her an improved body concept, and allow her to discover new modes of experiencing sexual pleasure (98, 99).

Resolution Disruption   Sexual dysfunction or difficulty during resolution is seldom noted in healthy women. However, in view of the kinds of sexual difficulties that occur for women with gynecologic cancer, disruption during this phase is common. Sources of difficulty may include residual pain if there has been dyspareunia or continued arousal from lack of orgasm. The most straightforward remedy to such problems is enhanced functioning during earlier phases of the sexual response cycle so that the resolution period is satisfactory. However, for those women with permanent sexual changes, efforts should be made to counteract feelings of discouragement, "letdown," or continued tension that might predominate a woman's view of her sexual functioning during the resolution phase. The woman should be reoriented to focus on the positive aspects of her sexual life,

681

such as the continued ability to engage in sexual activity, the experience of physical closeness and intimacy with her partner, and the sharing of alternative sexual activities with her partner.

New Strategies

Although sexual difficulties for the gynecologic cancer patient may have a different cause, be of greater magnitude, and be more resistant to successful treatment, they do not differ in principle from the sexual problems of many healthy women. The first step in treating these sexual difficulties should be a consideration of medically based interventions. For many women, however, consideration of behaviorally oriented techniques will be necessary. In addition to those discussed here, new strategies undoubtedly will be necessary. For example, biofeedback has had some use in the treatment of sexual dysfunctions and has been important in the area of physical rehabilitation. It has been used with healthy women to enhance sexual arousal (100) and as an aid to masturbation training for patients with secondary orgasmic dysfunction (101). It may have some role, for example, in providing feedback during masturbation treatment of women who have had radical genital surgery. Structural or neural changes may be such that women are not able to perceive the low level of genital sensation generated, and biofeedback may provide the necessary amplification. Techniques will also have to be developed to overcome common and troublesome difficulties such as dyspareunia. At present, however, there are sufficient behaviorally oriented techniques available so that preventive and rehabilitative efforts can begin.

References

1. **Robinson E, Mohilever J, Zidan J, Sapir D:** Delay in the diagnosis of cancer: possible effects on the stage of disease and survival. *Cancer* 54:1454, 1984.

2. **Cacioppo JT, Andersen BL, Turnquist DC, Petty RE:** Psychophysiological comparison processes: interpreting cancer symptoms. In Andersen B (ed): *Women With Cancer: Psychological Perspectives.* New York, Springer-Verlag, 1986, pp 141–171.

3. **Smith E, Anderson B:** The effects of symptoms and delay in seeking diagnosis and stage of disease at diagnosis among women with cancers of the ovary. *Cancer* 56:2727, 1985.

4. **Cochran SD, Hacker NF, Berek JS:** Correlates of delay in seeking treatment for endometrial cancer. *J Psychosom Obstet Gynecol* 5:245, 1986.

5. **Lynch HT, Krush AJ:** Delay: a deterrent to cancer detection. *Arch Environ Health* 17:204, 1968.

6. **Franklin EW:** Malignancy of the vulva. In McGowan L (ed): *Gynecologic Oncology.* New York, Appleton-Century-Crofts, 1978, p 148–168.

7. **Kutner B, Makover H, Oppenheim A:** Delay in the diagnosis and treatment of cancer: a critical analysis of the literature. *J Chron Dis* 7:95, 1958.

8. **Safer MA, Tharps QJ, Jackson TC, Leventhal H:** Determinants of three stages of delay in seeking care at a medical clinic. *Med Care* 17:11, 1979.

9. **Baumann B:** Diversities in conceptions of health and physical fitness. *J Health Soc Behav* 2:39, 1961.

10. **MacArthur C, Smith A:** Delay in breast cancer and the nature of presenting symptoms. *Lancet* 1:601, 1981.

11. **Andersen BL, Lachenbruch PA, Anderson B, deProsse C:** Sexual dysfunction and signs of gynecologic cancer. *Cancer* 57:1880, 1986.

12. **Mechanic D:** Social psychological factors affecting the presentation of bodily complaints. *N Engl J Med* 286:1132, 1972.

13. **Berkanovic E:** Seeking care for cancer relevant symptoms. *J Chron Dis* 35:727, 1982.

14. **Greer S:** Psychological aspects: delay in the treatment of breast cancer. *Proc R Soc Med* 67:470, 1974.

15. **Watson M, Greer S, Blake S, Shrapnell K:** Reaction to a diagnosis of breast cancer: relationship between denial, delay and rates of psychological morbidity. *Cancer* 53:2008, 1984.

16. **Temoshok L, DiClemente RJ, Sweet DM, et al:** Factors related to patient delay in seeking medical attention for cutaneous malignant melanoma. *Cancer* 54:3048, 1984.

17. **Marshall JR, Gregorio DI, Walsh D:** Sex differences in illness behavior: care seeking among cancer patients. *J Health Soc Behav* 23:197, 1982.

18. **Worden JW, Weisman AD:** Psychosocial components of lagtime in cancer diagnosis. *J Psychosom Res* 19:69, 1975.

19. **Matthews KA:** Are sociodemographic variables markers for psychological determinants of health? *Health Psychol* 8:641, 1989.

20. **Bean JA:** Epidemiologic review of cancer in women. In Andersen B (ed): *Cancer in Women: Psychological Perspectives.* New York, Springer-Verlag, 1986, pp 59–92.

21. **American Cancer Society.** (1992). *Cancer Facts and Figures—1992.* New York.

22. **Ortmeyer CF:** Variations in mortality, morbidity, and health care by marital status, In Erhardt LL, Berlin JE (eds): *Mortality and morbidity in the United States.* Cambridge, Mass, Harvard University Press, 1974, pp 159–184.

23. **Goodwin JS, Hunt WC, Key CR, Samet JM:** The effect of marital status on stage, treatment, and survival of cancer patients. *JAMA* 258:3125, 1987.

24. **Berkman LF, Syme SL:** Social networks, host resistance, and mortality: a nine year follow-up study of Alameda County residents. *Am J Epidemiol* 109:186, 1979.

25. **House JS, Robbins C, Metzner HL:** The association of social relationships and activities with mortality: prospective evidence from the Tecumseh community health study. *Am J Epidemiol* 116:123, 1982.

26. **Baquet CR, Horm JW, Gibbs T, Greenwald P:** Socioeconomic factors and cancer incidence among blacks and whites. *J Natl Cancer Inst* 83:551, 1991.

27. **Freeman HP:** Cancer in the socioeconomically disadvantaged. *CA- Cancer J Clin* 39:266, 1989.

28. **Weisman AD, Worden JW:** The existential plight in cancer: significance of the first 100 days. *Int J Psychiatry Med* 7:1, 1976.

29. **Derogatis LR, Morrow GR, Fetting J, et al:** The prevalence of psychiatric disorders among cancer patients. *JAMA* 249:751, 1983.

30. **Evans DW, McCartney CF, Nemeroff CB, et al:** Depression in women treated for gynecological cancer: clinical and neuroendocrine assessment. *Am J Psychiatry* 143:447, 1986.

31. **Cain EN, Kohorn EI, Quinlan DM, et al:** Psychosocial reaction to the diagnosis of gynecologic cancer. *Obstet Gynecol* 62:635, 1983.

32. **Andersen BL, Anderson B, deProsse C:** Controlled prospective longitudinal study of women with cancer. II. Psychological outcomes. *J Consult Clin Psychol* 57:692, 1989.

33. **Capone MA, Good RS, Westie KS, Jacobsen AF:** Psychosocial rehabilitation of gynecologic oncology patients. *Arch Phys Med Rehabil* 61:128, 1980.

34. **Houts PS, Whitney CW, Mortel R, Bartholomew MJ:** Former cancer patients as counselors of newly diagnosed cancer patients. *J Natl Cancer Inst* 76:793, 1986.

35. **Andersen BL:** Psychological interventions for cancer patients to enhance the quality of life. *J Consult Clin Psychol* 60:552, 1992.

36. **Derogatis LR, Meyer JK:** The invested partner in sexual disorders: a profile. *Am J Psychiatry* 136:1545, 1979.

37. **Johnston B:** Relief of mixed anxiety-depression in terminal cancer patients. *NY State J Med* 2315, 1972.

38. **Purohit DR, Navlakha PL, Modi RS, et al:** The role of antidepressants in hospitalized cancer patients. *J Assoc Physicians India* 26:246, 1978.

39. **Gottesman D, Lewis M:** Differences in crisis reactions among cancer and surgery patients. *J Consult Clin Psychol* 50:381, 1982.

40. **Andersen BL, Hacker NF:** Psychosexual adjustment after vulvar surgery. *Obstet Gynecol* 62:457, 1983.

41. **Andersen BL, Hacker NF:** Psychosexual adjustment following pelvic exenteration. *Obstet Gynecol* 61:331, 1983.

42. **Wallace L:** Psychological preparation as a method of reducing the stress of surgery. *J Hum Stress* 10:62, 1984.

43. **Hayward DJ:** *Information: A Prescription Against Pain.* London, Whitefriars Press, 1975.

44. **Peck A, Boland J:** Emotional reactions to radiation treatment. *Cancer* 40:180, 1977.

45. **Mitchell GW, Glicksman AS:** Cancer patients: knowledge and attitudes. *Cancer* 40:61, 1977.

46. **Andersen BL:** Psychological aspects of gynaecological cancer. In Broome AK, Wallace LM (eds): *Psychology and Gynecologic Problems.* London, Tavistock Publications Ltd, 1984, pp 117–141.

47. **Andersen BL, Tewfik HH:** Psychological reactions to radiation therapy: reconsideration of the adaptive aspects of anxiety. *J Pers Soc Psychol* 48:1024, 1985.

48. **Nail LM, King KB, Johnson JE:** Coping with radiation treatment for gynecologic cancer: mood and disruption in usual function. *J Psychosom Obstet Gynaecol* 5:271, 1986.

49. **Karlsson JA, Andersen BL:** Radiation therapy and psychological distress in gynecologic oncology patients: outcomes and recommendations for enhancing adjustment. *J Psychosom Obstet Gynaecol* 5:283, 1986.

50. **Andersen BL, Karlsson JA, Anderson BA, Tewfik HH:** Anxiety and cancer treatment: response to stressful radiotherapy. *Health Psychol* 3:535, 1984.

51. **Mages N, Mendelson G:** Effects of cancer on patients lives: a personalogical approach. In Stone G, Cohen F, Adler N (eds): *Health Psychology.* San Francisco, Jossey Bass, 1980.

52. **Forester B, Kornfeld DS, Fleiss JL:** Psychotherapy during radiotherapy: effects on emotional and physical distress. *Am J Psychiatry* 147:22, 1985.

53. **Israel MJ, Mood DW:** Three media presentations for patients receiving radiation therapy. *Cancer Nurs* 5:57, 1982.

54. **Andersen BL, Anderson B, deProsse C:** Controlled prospective longitudinal study of women with cancer. I. Sexual functioning outcomes. *J Consult Clin Psychol* 57:683, 1989.

55. **Pitkin RM, Van Voorhis LW:** Postirradiation vaginitis: an evaluation of prophylaxis with topical estrogen. *Ther Radiol* 99:417, 1971.

56. **Leventhal H, Easterling D, Coons HL, et al:** Adaptation to chemotherapy treatments. In Andersen BL (ed): *Women With Cancer: Psychological Perspectives.* New York, Springer-Verlag, 1986, pp 172–203.

57. **Carey MP, Burish TG:** Providing relaxation training to cancer chemotherapy patients: a comparison of three methods. *J Consult Clin Psychol* 55:732, 1986.

58. **Silberfarb PM, Philibert D, Levine PM:** Psychosocial aspects of neoplastic disease. II. Affective and cognitive effects of chemotherapy in cancer patients. *Am J Psychiatry* 137:597, 1980.

59. **Bard M, Sutherland AM:** Adaptation to radical mastectomy. *Cancer* 8:656, 1952.

60. **Cohen MM, Wellisch DK:** Living in limbo: psychosocial intervention in families with a cancer patient. *Am J Psychother* 32:560, 1978.

61. **Wortman CB, Dunkel-Schetter C:** Interpersonal relationships and cancer: a theoretical analysis. *J Soc Issues* 35:120, 1979.

62. **Andersen BL (ed):** *Women With Cancer: Psychological Perspectives.* New York, Springer-Verlag, 1986.

63. **Taylor SE:** Adjustment to threatening events: a theory of cognitive adaptation. *Am Psychol* 38:1161, 1983.

64. **Andersen BL:** Sexual functioning morbidity among cancer survivors: present status and future research directions. *Cancer* 55:1835, 1985.

65. **Andersen BL:** Sexual functioning morbidity and the woman with gynecologic cancer: outcomes and directions for prevention. *Cancer* 60:2123, 1987.

66. **Andersen BL, Turnquist D, LaPolla JP, Turner D:** Sexual functioning after treatment of *in situ* vulvar cancer: preliminary report. *Obstet Gynecol* 71:15, 1988.

67. **Sherwin BB, Gelfand MM, Brender W:** Androgen enhances sexual motivation in females: a prospective, crossover study of sex steroid administration in the surgical menopause. *Psychosom Med* 47:339, 1985.

68. **Masters WH, Johnson VE:** *Human Sexual Response.* Boston, Little, Brown & Co., 1966.

69. **Newcomb MD, Bentler PM:** Dimensions of subjective female orgasmic responsiveness. *J Pers Soc Psychol* 44:862, 1983.

70. **Andersen BL, van der Does J, Anderson B:** Sexual outcomes following gynecologic cancer. In Coppelson M, Morrow P, Tattersall M (eds): *Gynecologic Oncology, 2nd ed.* Edinburgh, Churchill Livingstone, 1992, pp 1481–1497.

71. **Kilkku P, Gronroos M, Dunnonen R:** Sexual function after conization of the uterine cervix. *Gynecol Oncol* 14:209, 1982.

72. **Vincent CE, Vincent B, Greiss FC, Linton EB:** Some marital-sexual concomitants of carcinoma of the cervix. *South Med J* 68:552, 1975.

73. **Brown RS, Haddox V, Posada A, Rubio A:** Social and psychological adjustment following pelvic exenteration. *Am J Obstet Gyencol* 114:162, 1972.

74. **Dempsey GM, Buchsbaum HJ, Morrison J:** Psychosocial adjustment to pelvic exenteration. *Gynecol Oncol* 3:325, 1975.

75. **Vera MI:** Quality of life following pelvic exenteration. *Gynecol Oncol* 12:355, 1981.

76. **Cochran SD, Hacker NF, Wellisch DK, Berek JS:** Sexual functioning after treatment for endometrial cancer. *J Psychosoc Oncol* 5:47, 1987.

77. **Buscema J, Woodruff JD, Parmley TH, Genadry R:** Carcinoma in situ of the vulva. *Obstet Gynecol* 55:225, 1980.

78. **Lifshitz S, Roberts JA:** Treatment of carcinoma in situ of the vulva with topical 5-fluorouracil. *Obstet Gynecol* 56:242, 1980.

79. **DiSaia PJ, Creasman WT, Rich WM:** An alternate approach to early cancer of the vulva. *Am J Obstet Gynecol* 133:825, 1979.

80. **Hacker NF, van der Velden J:** Conservative management of early vulvar cancer. *Cancer* 71(Suppl 4): 1673, 1993.

81. **Moth I, Andreasson B, Jensen SB, Bock JE:** Sexual function and somatopsychic reactions after vulvectomy. *Dan Med Bull* 30:27, 1983.

82. **Tamburini M, Filiberti A, Ventafridda V, DePalo G:** Quality of life and psychological state after radical vulvectomy. *J Psychosom Obstet Gynaecol* 5:263, 1986.

83. **Andersen BL:** Predicting sexual and psychological morbidity and improving quality of life for women with gynecologic cancer. *Cancer* 71(Suppl 4): 1678, 1993.

84. **Bachmann, GA, Leiblum SR, Kemmann E, et al:** Sexual expression and its determinants in the postmenopausal woman. *Maturitas* 6:19, 1984.

85. **Derogatis LR, Melisaratos N:** The DSFI: a multidimensional measure of sexual functioning. *J Sex Marital Ther* 5:244, 1979.

86. **Andersen BL, Broffitt B:** Is there a reliable and valid measure of sexual behavior? *Arch Sexual Behav* 17:509, 1988.

87. **Andersen BL, Broffitt B, Karlsson JA, Turnquist DC:** A psychometric analysis of the Sexual Arousability Index. *J Consult Clin Psychol* 57:123, 1989.

88. **Lamont JA, DePetrillo AD, Sargeant EJ:** Psychosexual rehabilitation and exenterative surgery. *Gynecol Oncol* 6:236, 1978.

89. **Witkin MH:** Psychosexual counseling of the mastectomy patient. *J Sex Marital Ther* 4:20, 1978.

90. **Christensen DN:** Postmastectomy couple counseling: an outcome study of a structured treatment protocol. *J Sex Marital Ther* 9:266, 1983.

91. **Cain EN, Kohorn EL, Quinlan DM, et al:** Psychosocial benefits of a cancer support group. *Cancer* 57:183, 1986.

92. **Kilmann PR, Mills KH, Bella B, et al:** The effects of sex education on women with secondary orgasmic dysfunction. *J Sex Marital Ther* 9:79, 1983.

93. **Berek JS, Andersen BL:** Sexual rehabilitation: surgical and psychological approaches. In Hoskins WJ, Perez CA, Young RC (eds): *Gynecologic Oncology: Principles and Practice*. Philadelphia, JB Lippincott, 1992, pp 401–416.

94. **Steinberg MD, Juliano MA, Wise L:** Psychological outcome of lumpectomy versus mastectomy in the treatment of breast cancer. *Am J Psychiatry* 142:34, 1985.

95. **Jones W, Park P:** Treatment of single partner sexual dysfunction by systematic desensitization. *Obstet Gynecol* 39:411, 1972.

96. **Lazarus A:** The treatment of chronic frigidity by systematic desensitization. *J Nerv Ment Dis* 136:272, 1963.

97. **LoPiccolo J, Lobitz WC:** The role of masturbation in the treatment of orgasmic dysfunction. *Arch Sex Behav* 2:163, 1972.

98. **Wallace DH, Barbach LG:** Preorgasmic group treatment. *J Sex Marital Ther* 1:146, 1974.

99. **Cotten-Huston AL, Wheeler KA:** Preorgasmic group treatment: assertiveness, marital adjustment, and sexual function in women. *J Sex Marital Ther* 9:296, 1983.

100. **Cerny JA:** Biofeedback and the voluntary control of sexual arousal in women. *Behav Ther* 9:847, 1978.

101. **Reisinger JJ:** Effects of erotic stimulation and masturbatory training upon situational orgasmic dysfunction. *J Sex Marital Ther* 4:177, 1978.

20 Palliative Care and Pain Management

J. Norelle Lickiss

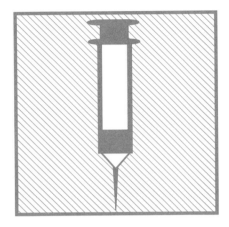

Palliative care is active treatment that is carefully focused to serve the real needs of the patient and her family, with emphasis on facilitating comfort, autonomy, dignity, and personal rehabilitation and development, in the midst of serious, usually life-threatening circumstances. It is not a cessation of treatment, and it is not focused on dying; nor is it a marginated activity removed from mainstream cancer care. **Palliative care is directed toward allowing the patient to live until she dies with an attitude of realistic expectations and in a context of well-grounded hope in what will not fail, not false hope in what must inevitably fail. It should be concurrent with good antitumor treatment and not seen as commencing when all antitumor treatment has failed.**

The World Health Organization, in a recent statement, offers a definition embodying these elements (1):

Palliative care is the active total care of patients whose disease is not responsive to curative treatment. Control of pain, of other symptoms, and of psychological, social and spiritual problems are paramount. The goal of palliative care is achievement of the best possible quality of life for patients and their families. Many aspects of palliative care are also applicable earlier in the course of the illness, in conjunction with anticancer treatment. Palliative care:

- *affirms life and regards dying as a normal process;*
- *neither hastens nor postpones death;*
- *provides relief from pain and other distressing symptoms;*
- *integrates the psychological and spiritual aspects of patient care;*
- *offers a support system to help patients live as actively as possible until death;*
- *offers a support system to help the family during the patient's illness and in their own bereavement.*

687

Radiotherapy, chemotherapy and surgery have a place in palliative care, provided that the symptomatic benefits of treatment clearly outweigh the disadvantages. Investigative procedures are kept to a minimum.

In the last 50 years, there have been significant advances in gynecologic cancer care, especially since recognition of the subspecialty field of gynecologic oncology in the early 1970s. Patients with gynecologic cancer still get distressing symptoms, however, and a significant proportion of patients continue to have progressive or relapsing disease. Gynecologic cancer is a potent cause of chronic as well as acute morbidity.

In general, effective antidisease therapy offers the best chance of good symptom relief if the patient is a "responder," but the quality of life of a "nonresponder" to chemotherapy may be worse than that of an untreated patient. Many gynecologic oncologists will not have expertise in palliative care therapeutics that is comparable to that in surgery, chemotherapy, and radiation therapy. All four disciplines, together with good primary care and psychologic and pastoral support, are essential, especially in that phase of treatment where the goal is restoration and maintenance of good-quality life for as long as possible. Gynecologic oncologists need to have access to clinical colleagues with expertise in contemporary palliative therapeutics throughout the course of a patient's treatment, so that good symptom management not based on antidisease strategies can be achieved. Just as the last movement of a symphony is a crucial section of the work, so the last phase of life is crucial in the completion of a human life. It is the responsibility of the medical and nursing professions to facilitate maximum autonomy and quality of life for each woman "walking her last mile" or "creating the last section of her symphony." Such concepts are not sentimental but realistic, and the attitude of the physician to the last phase of life and to death may color clinical judgment.

When the patient's condition is clearly deteriorating, and a plateau in therapy has been reached with a high price being paid for very small gains, a revision of management is essential, preferably with involvement of a palliative care physician. It is crucial for the bond between the patient and her primary care physician, the gynecologic oncologist, to be strengthened at this time. One of the skills required of the palliative care practitioner is to be nonintrusive wherever possible. Indeed, the patient's own primary care physician becomes central, assisted when needed by specialist palliative medical and nursing staff, preferably those already known to the patient. **Continuity of as many professional relationships as possible is beneficial, and as the patient moves from a chronic phase into a deteriorating late phase, a total change of personnel is undesirable.**

Every effort is needed to ensure that care is simple, gentle, inexpensive, and efficient. It is inappropriate to resort to intravenous techniques if oral or percutaneous techniques have not been adequately explored. Careful research has established the efficiency of such techniques for control of pain and other symptoms.

The organization of palliative care services varies from place to place, but there is a genuine right to good-quality management of symptoms. Equity of access for all patients should be one of the objectives. The most efficient strategies should be used, and good management of symptoms should become the norm so that uncontrolled pain and other symptoms are rare. While there is more to quality of life than relief of symptoms, this is at least a basic prerequisite.

Practical Aspects of Palliative Care

The care of a woman with advanced gynecologic malignancy involves several components: diagnosis, delineation of therapeutic possibilities, implementation of treatment, and evaluation of outcome. A further diagnostic and therapeutic effort may be necessary if new problems develop with the passage of time. The concept of the *patient as subject* must be understood: the patient as a person with capacities to perceive, know, understand, love and receive love, and establish priorities within a specific geographic and cultural context, and within a network of personal relationships.

It is essential initially to make a *comprehensive diagnosis,* which includes listening to the patient's experience with her cancer. It is crucial to give her the opportunity to tell her experience of the prediagnostic period and the circumstances of diagnosis (listening especially for delay), of initial treatment, and of treatment difficulties, including failure (especially with respect to trials to which she gave her consent). Her current hierarchy of problems must be ascertained, together with her current hopes, plans, and expectations for herself and for her significant others. Her perception of her care system should also be sought—its problems, limitations, and capacity. A comprehensive diagnosis involves at least:

1. Ascertainment of the patient's symptoms and other problems, in her order of priority

2. Clarification of the nature and the extent of the neoplastic process, with careful consideration of other pathology that may be contributing to the present problems

3. Delineation of the personal and social contexts within which the patient is living and from which she may draw support

4. Elucidation of her personal objectives at this time

The pursuit of an adequate diagnosis may involve not only interaction with the patient but also, if the patient gives consent, interaction with family members and friends. The woman herself should give consent to the transfer of information to her husband in all but exceptional circumstances. In seeking information from family members or friends, the patient's privacy must be safeguarded; the more powerless the patient, the more onerous is the charge.

On the basis of a comprehensive diagnosis, with or without further investigations to elucidate the mechanisms of troublesome symptoms, it is normally possible to *delineate the therapeutic possibilities.* If the symptoms are not adequately ascertained, the mechanisms are not adequately understood, and the patient's priorities are not appreciated, then therapeutic endeavors are likely to be ineffective.

Palliative care is concerned with the facilitation of freedom, and the choice among therapeutic options should reflect this. In general, the least restrictive alternative involving the least dependence on medical facilities and the least use of the patient's time, resources, and personal energy should be selected. Careful consideration of other relevant antitumor measures (surgery, radiotherapy, or chemotherapy) is mandatory, because control of the neoplastic process usually offers the best chance of alleviating symptoms. Decision-

making in this area requires genuine clinical wisdom, going far beyond the consideration of known statistics with respect to specific outcomes.

Decisions concerning treatment should normally involve the patient, who should be adequately informed about the foreseeable advantages and disadvantages of the various options. Although the patient should share in decision making in so far as she wishes, her physician should, on the whole, clearly indicate the course of action he or she favors and ultimately take the responsibility for an intervention. This is not necessarily true for an omission, if the patient clearly prefers not to have an advised intervention. The burden of decision making is considerable, and ways of reaching decisions vary according to social, cultural, economic, and medical contexts. However, the physician has the duty to bear a part of the burden so that a distressing outcome should not engender guilt in the patient and her family. This being said, the physician should not compromise his or her better judgment or conscience in the face of patient or family pressure. **There are no circumstances that justify a physician's declaring to a patient or her family that "there is nothing more that can be done."**

Evaluation of palliative interventions is best performed by the informed patient, although the observations of the medical and nursing staff are also important. Monitoring in some form is essential, because time, often the patient's most precious possession, should not be wasted by ineffective intervention if further treatment options are available or modifications are possible. The more restricted the life expectancy, the more grave is the misuse of time. Formal outcome measures based on subjective criteria should ideally be introduced into routine clinical practice.

Mention needs to be made of the *art of prognostication,* because this matter will inevitably arise. While there are various factors that allow a gynecologic oncologist to give a particular patient a probability figure for survival, in the case of the individual patient, the outcome is fairly uncertain and it is cruel indeed for a clinician to be too specific about the likely duration of survival. In the face of a question concerning prognosis, there is a strong case for responding by offering some time boundaries within which death may eventually occur. Such boundaries are useful for thinking and planning and certainly reinforce the fact that, as in the case of all mortals, time is finite and the "horizon is in view." They do not give a patient or her family an agonizing date around which to focus; nor do they suggest that what is still quite uncertain can be predicted precisely. The completion of life is too serious a matter to be diverted by such a false focus.

The clinical process also involves the clear *recognition that a patient is in fact dying,* when this is obviously the case. There are many indicators of this phase, and these are well known to clinicians, nurses, and family members. There may be a change in the tempo of the disease, a manifest change in the function of the critical organs with no possibility for reversibility, or a rapid deterioration in strength or physical performance in the absence of reversible factors, such as gross anemia, septicemia, hypercalcemia, or drug interactions. What is medically possible at this stage, such as treatment of septicemia or hypercalcemia, may not necessarily be medically wise.

There are other psychologic signs that a patient is actually dying. An experienced clinician will note the gradual withdrawal of the patient from interest in the wider world, from interest in personal friends, and even the gradual loosening of bonds

690

with those very close. In some patients, this "cutting of the moorings" is very obvious; intrapersonal activity may be very intense and may be expressed only to a few trusted persons. The patient herself may clearly articulate her awareness that she is now close to death, or she may choose not to speak of it. The essence of clinical response is to respect the mystery of the individual.

Symptoms and Their Relief

Symptoms are subjective, even though the person with severe symptoms may have objective manifestations, such as vomiting. A patient in severe pain may or may not show signs of distress. Her behavior will be influenced by cultural and environmental factors, as well as by personal and interpersonal relationships. A patient suffering unrelieved pain may show no facial changes, nor complain to medical or nursing staff; yet she may admit to a trusted confidant that the pain is almost unbearable. **Accurate assessment of symptoms requires skill, patience, active listening, and unconditional regard for the patient. The patient is always right about symptoms because of their intrinsic subjectivity.**

Symptoms vary in their significance. Certain symptoms (e.g., vaginal bleeding) may cause much emotional distress, while other symptoms that are more serious in their physiologic consequences (e.g., severe constipation) may not evoke the same fear. It is important to give the patient a chance to express her fears and to offer some simple explanation for the symptom, as this will at least reduce her anxiety. Whatever the cause, symptom relief is essential and usually possible with relatively simple measures.

Symptoms may arise from the tumor itself, from the treatment, and/or from unrelated causes. In gynecologic cancer, symptoms tend to cluster, and some major symptom complexes can be delineated. Each of these can logically be dealt with on the basis of rational palliative therapeutics:

1. Pelvic mass symptoms, from pressure and infiltration effects on the bladder, rectum, pelvic blood vessels, ureters, lymphatics, or nerves

2. Abdominal mass symptoms, from compression and dysfunction of the stomach, small bowel, and large bowel

3. Perineal symptoms, including referred pain to the perineum or pain and discomfort from ulceration, particularly with urination and defecation

4. Pulmonary symptoms, including dyspnea or debilitating coughing

5. Radiation- and chemotherapy-induced symptoms, including emesis, pain, neuropathy, weakness, and diarrhea

Symptoms may well precede signs or radiologic evidence of spread of disease. This is particularly true in the case of lumbosacral plexopathy. Magnetic resonance imaging or a computed tomography scan may demonstrate a lesion suspected on the basis of symptoms. Waiting for hard signs may be disastrous in certain circumstances, such as the early diagnosis of remediable spinal cord compression. Feinstein (2) pointed out the prognostic significance of symptoms at the time of diagnosis of certain tumors, and symptoms are also of value in pointing to potential complications. There is now a considerable literature concerning the understanding and therapy of major symptoms in cancer (3–6); attention will be given here to common matters and practical points.

Pain Management

Pain has been defined by the International Association for the Study of Pain as "an unpleasant sensory and emotional experience associated with actual or potential tissue damage or described in terms of such damage." Pain is a subjective phenomenon, an experience. It is not surprising, therefore, that there are difficulties both in measuring pain and in pain management. Because of its subjective nature, the patient is always correct in her appraisal of the severity of the pain.

The advances of the last decade in pain management should be readily available to all patients with advanced gynecologic cancer. Improvements have been based on a more adequate understanding of pain physiology and classification, as well as on precise research with respect to drug management (7–9). Conolly (10) recently stated, "What is needed now is not a stunning new understanding of pain pharmacology, but the consistent and rational application of what is already known." Cancer pain assessment and treatment guidelines have recently been developed by the American Society of Clinical Oncology (11).

Cautious optimism is justified, and many approaches to pain management have been published. The following simple schema may provide some guidelines in the face of the complexity of recent research and practice. Pain management may be considered as having four steps.

Step One—Reduce the Noxious Stimulus at the Periphery

This step demands an adequate understanding of the mechanisms of the pain stimulus in the individual patient, on the basis of a carefully focused history, physical examination, and, if necessary, other investigations. A precise history, including the mode of onset, characteristics, distribution, aggravating factors, trends over time, and response to therapeutic endeavors, provides the fundamental guide to the likely mechanism (or mechanisms). Pain caused by treatment (e.g., radiotherapy) requires as close attention as that resulting directly from tumor. Pain in gynecologic cancer may be due to soft tissue infiltration, bone involvement, neural involvement, muscle spasm (e.g., psoas spasm), infection within or near tumor masses, or to intestinal colic. Therapeutic approaches vary according to the mechanism that is operative.

Consideration should be given to specific therapeutic measures (e.g., radiotherapy, chemotherapy, antibiotics, regional neural blockade, or occasionally surgical approaches), whether or not peripherally acting analgesic drugs are being used.

Bone metastases frequently cause inflammatory changes with release of prostaglandins that may sensitize the tissues to other noxious stimuli. When the pain is clearly arising from bone metastases and has the characteristics of bone pain, the use of drugs that interfere in some way with prostaglandin synthesis, e.g., *nonsteroidal anti-inflammatory drugs (NSAIDS)*, is logical. These drugs should be avoided or used with caution in patients who have a history of peptic ulceration, excessive alcohol consumption, bleeding diatheses, or known idiosyncratic reactions to *aspirin* or related drugs. Where the use of *NSAIDS* is precluded, *acetaminophen* is useful, although the mechanism of action of this drug is obscure. It may have central effects as well as some peripheral action. While *acetaminophen* is fairly well tolerated and safe, it should be used in reduced dosage in patients with extensive liver damage, especially alcoholic cirrhosis.

Peripherally acting drugs such as *acetaminophen* and *NSAIDS* are also useful for pain arising in nonosseous sites and for postoperative pain. They should rarely be omitted from drug analgesic regimens, even in moribund patients. Rectal preparations may prove useful as an adjunct to rectal *morphine* in patients who are unable to take oral drugs.

Muscle spasm requires muscle relaxants such as diazepam, as well as gentle massage. Psoas spasm is not infrequent in gynecologic cancer. It should be suspected if there is difficulty with full extension of the hip in a patient with retroperitoneal disease.

Step Two—Raise the Pain Threshold

The concept of threshold is useful, and it is clear that the threshold for pain perception is varied by many factors. **The threshold for pain may well be raised significantly by comfort, care, concern, diversion, and various forms of relaxation, and lowered by depression, anxiety, loneliness, and isolation.** A wide range of strategies exists to facilitate coping with pain, and simple nontherapeutic measures should be tried initially. The diagnosis of anguish as a component of pain in an individual patient is difficult and may not be clear until an empiric approach to pain therapy has been initiated.

Occasionally, anxiety and depression are so clearly pathologic that the patient is impeded in her attempts to relate to her loved ones and to come to terms with her disease. In such circumstances, a formal psychiatric consultation may be of assistance and anxiolytics or antidepressants may prove helpful. In general, threshold issues, including extreme anguish, feelings of futility, loss of sense of meaning, personal guilt, and other forms of spiritual pain require a different approach, with help from skilled counsellors, pastors, and, above all, those persons who are so close to the patient that admission into the private space of suffering is welcome.

Step Three—Reduce Pain Perception by the Careful and Precise Use of Opioid Drugs

There is abundant literature on opioid use, with a range of opioids available (7–12). In practice, weak opioids such as *codeine* or *dextraproxyphene*, or stronger opioids, typically *morphine*, are combined with peripherally acting drugs such as *acetaminophen* or *aspirin*, with due regard to the contraindications. **It is now widely recognized that opioids should be given regularly, at precisely determined doses and at fixed intervals in accordance with the half-life of the drug concerned, rather than haphazardly in response to a severe pain stimulus.**

1. The most commonly used *morphine* preparation, *morphine sulfate* solution, is best given every 4 hours, with a double dose (or one and one-half times the standard dose in the frail) at bedtime and a break of approximately 8 hours overnight to permit sleep for both patient and carers. Many find the following schedule to be useful: 6 AM, 10 AM, 2 PM, 6 PM, and 10 PM.

2. A reasonable starting dose of oral *morphine* in a patient not already on an opioid drug would be 5–10 mg in a patient of average size or 3–5 mg in the frail or elderly patient, with repetition of the original dose in 1–2 hours if there has been no relief of pain.

3. Over the next 24–48 hours, dose finding is undertaken by prescription of regular doses given every 4 hours together with the provision of one or two "break-through" doses equal to the standard dose. The correct dose may range from 2 mg to over 100 mg every 4 hours, but the majority of patients will need less than 50 mg every 4 hours.

4. Occasionally, the oral route cannot be used, and calibration can then be undertaken by the subcutaneous route with doses one-third to one-half the oral dose.

If significant drowsiness or other *morphine* toxicity occurs after the first 24 hours without relief of pain, the *morphine* level is probably above the therapeutic range for that patient. Other causes of drowsiness should be excluded, such as sedating drugs or hypercalcemia, but the *morphine* dose should not be raised further. In such circumstances, the pain therapy usually requires another approach. Some types of pain are relatively unresponsive to opioids. These include pain caused by bone metastases, nerve irritation, or extreme muscle spasm.

Controlled-release *morphine* tablets (such as *MS Contin*) represent a significant advance in convenience of administration, with the proviso that dose finding should be initially undertaken with use of *morphine sulfate* solution. Once the correct dose has been determined, the total 24-hour dose can be given in two fractions (every 12 hours) or occasionally in three fractions (every 8 hours). It is essential that the tablets not be crushed. Controlled release *morphine* should not be used in patients with uncontrolled or unstable pain or in patients with extensive upper abdominal disease that is likely to interfere with drug absorption or normal gastric motility. Aqueous *morphine* or subcutaneous *morphine* is a wiser choice in such circumstances.

The efficacy of the regular dosing approach to *morphine* administration may be dependent on the contribution of an active metabolite (*morphine 6-glucuronide*), which is a more powerful analgesic than *morphine*. Hepatic impairment, if severe, interferes with *morphine* metabolism to glucuronides. Renal impairment, even if only moderate, interferes with excretion of these metabolites, and in both of these circumstances dose reduction is essential.

Whether an opioid is effective usually is not dependent on the route of administration but, rather, on the cause of the pain. The oral route is usually available for opioids, but the rectal route is a useful alternative in some patients (e.g., patients with vomiting). If parenteral drugs are essential, the subcutaneous route is satisfactory, either with intermittent injections through an indwelling butterfly needle every 4 hours or with a continuous infusion via a battery-driven syringe driver. There is usually no need for the intramuscular route, and intravenous pulses give short-lived analgesia. In general, a parenteral dose of one-half or one-third of the oral dose appears equianalgesic. If oral or subcutaneous morphine is efficacious but the side effects are troublesome, the epidural route is occasionally advantageous. **The intravenous route can be hazardous, one risk being the development of acute tolerance, which may not always be overcome by the**

**addition of further *morphine* (13). Cessation of the infusion ₐ
of appropriate subcutaneous doses every 4 hours is often he**

Simultaneously it is important to review other aspects of mana
the possible need for *NSAIDS*, or drugs relevant to neuropath
offers no advantage over *morphine* except higher solubility, and it
as a pro-drug, as its efficacy depends on metabolism to *morphiₙ*

Morphine (if correctly used) does not hasten death or lead to
vast majority of cases, but some physicians continue to harbor
about its use. When *morphine* is to be commenced, counseling
essary, and three issues should be stressed to counteract widely

1. The use of *morphine* with careful dose-finding and monₜ
   in the vast majority of patients, lead to addiction (al
   dependence occurs).

2. The introduction of *morphine* does not mean that the pₐ
   dying but, rather, that *morphine* is the most appropriₐ
   time. It is the type of pain and its severity, not the p
   patient, that dictate whether an opioid should be introd

3. Patients and their families may need to be reassured that
   of *morphine* will not mean that there will be no adₑ
   available at a later stage in the illness when the situatioₙ

Tolerance to *morphine* may be a major clinical problem if the ₗ
introduced and calibrated correctly. When the drug is used corr
requirements during the course of an illness usually signify an
noxious stimulus, rather than a reduction in the effectiveness of

Although *morphine* is currently the most useful opioid, other str
occasionally preferable. Availability varies, but gynecologic onₑ
become familiar with a narrow range of opioids, e.g., *morphi*
codeine and other relevant drugs (Table 20.1).

Oxycodone (available as tablets, suspension, and suppositories) iₛ
equianalgesic with *morphine*, being most often used in a dose of
4 to 6 hours. Some patients tolerate *oxycodone* better than *morph*
dose, and vice versa.

Meperidine (pethidine) is of very little value in palliative care.
the drug is clearly neurotoxic and can add much to the distress of
If a patient is already receiving *meperidine* subcutaneously or
and does not show evidence of neurotoxicity, conversion to *m*
achieved with approximately 10% of the *meperidine* dose as sub
phine or 30% of the *meperidine* dose as oral *morphine* every 4 hₒ
calibration of the *morphine* dose may proceed as usual.

Methadone is occasionally useful, but its long half-life is somet
tageous, and its sedative action outlasts its analgesic activity, m
difficult to use. Transdermal preparations of such opioids as *Fentₑ*
to be very convenient if used correctly. Such opioids as *codeine*, ₑ
with *aspirin* or *acetaminophen* or *dextrapropoxyphene*, are usefuₗ

695

Table 20.1 Equivalency of Various Narcotic Analgesics to 10 mg of Intramuscular Morphine

Drug	Route	Dose (mg)	Duration (hr)	Plasma (T ½)	Comments
Morphine	IM PO	10 30–60	4–6	2–3.5	Also available in a slow-release form and as rectal suppositories
Codeine	IM PO	130 200	4–6	3	Metabolized to morphine
Oxycodone	IM PO	15 30	3–4	—	Often, 5 mg combined with ASA and acet-aminophen
Levorphanol	IM PO	2 4	4–6	12–16	May accumulate and result in delayed toxicities
Hydromorphone	IM PO	1.5 7.5	4–5	2–3	Available up to 10 mg/ml for injection and as rectal suppositories
Oxymorphone	IM PR	1 10	4–6	2–3	No oral preparation
Meperidine	IM PO	75 300	2–3	3–4	Toxic metabolite causes CNS excitation; avoid in renal failure
Methadone	IM PO	10 20	4–6	15–30	May accumulate and result in delayed toxicities
Fentanyl	IV Patch	0.1 0.5	0.5–1 72	3–12	Transdermal delivery requires days to reach steady state

Reproduced, with permission, from Grossman SA: Is pain undertreated in cancer patients? *Advances Oncol* 9:11, 1993.
T ½, half-life; IM, intramuscular; PO, oral; ASA, acetylsalicylic acid (aspirin); PR, rectally; CNS, central nervous system.

but these opioids should not be combined with *morphine*. Care should be taken to use only one opioid at a time; a combination of two opioids is unwise, unnecessary, and hazardous. A change from one opioid to another, however, is frequently justified; usually this involves a change from another opioid to *morphine*.

The side effects of opioid drugs are in large part avoidable by precise prescribing. Predictable side effects such as constipation can usually be prevented with concomitant use of a laxative that combines softening and stimulant properties. Care should be taken to avoid laxatives that increase the bulk of the stool in patients liable to bowel obstruction. Nausea is uncommon unless the patient is very anxious, inadequately counseled, or already constipated. It can also occur if *morphine* is introduced in such a manner that serum levels rise rapidly.

In addition to anxiety or preexisting constipation, *morphine* induced nausea may have several mechanisms including gastric stasis, stimulation of the chemosensitive-trigger zone (CTZ) and, rarely, stimulation of the vestibular centers. *Metaclopramide*, 10–20 mg every 6 hours (orally or subcutaneously), and *haloperidol*, 1.5–3 mg at night (orally or subcutaneously), are useful antinauseants, the former

having action on both the gastrointestinal center and the CTZ, the latter being specific for the CTZ. Routine prescription of antinauseant drugs is not necessary for patients who are receiving *morphine* but may be advisable if factors known to increase the likelihood of nausea are present. *Haloperidol* would usually be the wiser choice under such circumstances.

If fecal impaction has occurred as a result of opioids given without a laxative, pelvic and abdominal pain may occur and nausea may be made more likely. Such patients are in preventable misery, and the diagnosis should always be suspected in a patient with diarrhea, nausea, abdominal distention, abdominal pain, or, in the case of an elderly patient, confusion.

Step Four—Recognize Neuropathic Pain and Treat Correctly

Neuropathic pain may be due to irritation or destruction of peripheral nerves. It may be neuralgic or may have an unpleasant, sometimes burning, quality, and it may be felt in an anesthetic area. Such pain may be caused by tumor infiltration of the pelvic soft tissues or occasionally by radiation damage or chemotherapy.

When pain is neuropathic in origin, an opioid and a peripherally acting drug should be supplemented by low doses of other drugs, such as tricyclic antidepressants, anticonvulsants, or corticosteroids. Other drugs, such as *clonazepam,* or *Tegretol* also may be of value. In general, the management of neuropathic pain is difficult. The drugs used have significant side effects, and specialist assistance may well be necessary. Regional blockade with local anesthetic techniques may be worthy of consideration. Epidural *morphine* with *marcaine* is useful in carefully selected patients.

Summary

Most pain experienced by patients with gynecologic cancer can be relieved by simple means that involve oral, rectal, or subcutaneous routes of administration, without the need for infusions, or epidural techniques. There are occasional patients who will benefit from these latter techniques, however, and their availability should be assured.

Gastrointestinal Symptoms

Anorexia is a common and significant symptom with a multitude of causes and serious nutritional consequences. The latter are often not appreciated. The best initial approach includes careful preparation of small meals, elimination of reversible gastric stasis or constipation, emotional support, and direct nutritional supplements. Progestins do increase appetite without undue side effects, but the expense is considerable.

Mouth symptoms can be most distressing, and mouth care is crucial in very ill patients. Discomfort arising from oral candidiasis responds to antifungal agents such as *nystatin* mouthwashes (every 2–3 hours), *amphotericin* lozenges, or *ketoconazole* tablets. Pain from mucositis may be relieved by *sucralfate* suspension and by *acetaminophen* with *morphine* (orally or subcutaneously).

Nausea, vomiting, colic, and constipation are common in advanced gynecologic cancer. Each symptom requires precise diagnosis in order that rational therapy may be applied (14).

Nausea, with or without vomiting, is mediated finally by the vomiting center situated in the reticular formation of the medulla oblongata, an area rich in histamine receptors. The vomiting center is influenced by several connections, each of which can be the causal pathway for nausea (Fig. 20.1). These include:

1. the cerebral cortex (e.g., anxiety-conditioned responses)

2. the vestibular center, which is rich in histamine receptors (H_1) (e.g., some forms of *morphine* induce nausea, occasionally cerebral metastases)

Figure 20.1   Nausea and vomiting: Receptors, pathways, and drug therapies. (H_1 = histamine type 1 receptors; D_2 = dopamine type 2 receptors; 5-HT_3 = serotonin type 3 receptors; MCh = muscarinic-cholinergic receptors.)

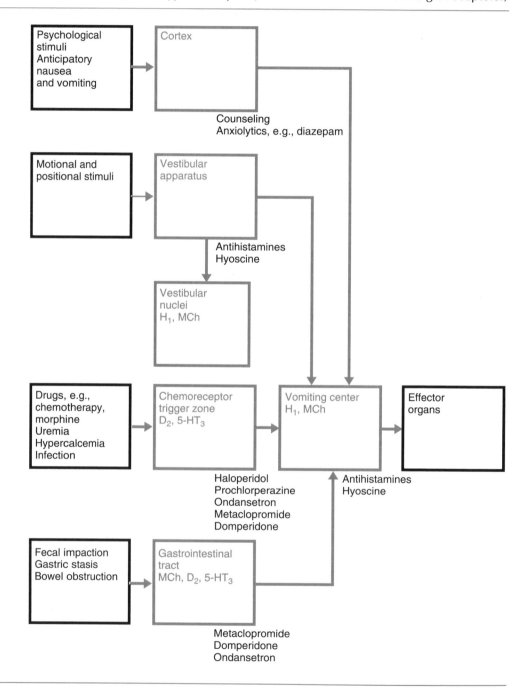

Table 20.2 Commonly Used Antinauseant Drugs

Drug	Dose	Comment
Metoclopramide	10–20 mg q 4 hours (oral or sub-cutaneous)	Avoid if patient has bowel colic
Haloperidol	1–3 mg bid or tid (oral)	Lower doses required than when used as a sedative
Prochlorperazine	5–25 mg bid or tid (oral or rectal)	May be useful if vomiting mechanism is unknown
Meclozine	10–75 mg per day in divided doses (oral)	Antihistamine with doses that produce minimal sedation
Cyclizine	10–75 mg per day in divided doses (oral, rectal, or subcutaneous)	Useful if patient has bowel obstruction
Hyoscine	0.1–0.4 mg q 6–8 hours (subcutaneous)	CNS side effects can occur, particularly drowsiness and confusion
Ondansetron	0.15 mg/kg q 4 for 3 doses IV 4–8 mg tid (oral)	Main use is for chemotherapy-related nausea Constipation can be troublesome

See text and manufacturers' information before prescribing; watch for side effects; review frequently; cease ineffective drugs.

3. the chemosensitive trigger zone (CTZ), which is rich in dopamine receptors (D_2) (e.g., nausea induced by some drugs, including chemotherapeutic agents, hypercalcemia, uremia)

4. the gastrointestinal tract (e.g., gastric stasis, intestinal obstruction, fecal impaction, abnormalities of gut motility).

Once the likely mechanism has been determined by means of a careful history, clinical examination, and investigations if indicated, the appropriate antinauseant can be prescribed (Table 20.2).

When anxiety dominates the scene, anxiolytics may be crucial in reducing the nausea. When vestibular mechanisms are suspected or when no specific pathway can be identified, relatively nonsedating antihistamines (e.g., *cyclizine* and *meclozine*), which act directly on the vomiting center and the vestibular center, may be useful. Such drugs as *prochlorperazine* have some affinity for both muscarinic and histaminic receptors and are moderately useful though less specific.

Nausea clearly related to the CTZ requires a drug with high affinity for dopamine receptors, such as *haloperidol*. A dose of 3 mg or less at night (orally or subcutaneously) may be sufficient. Nausea related to chemotherapy has become less of a problem for many patients with the introduction of new drugs such as *ondansetron*, a 5-HT (serotonin) receptor agonist (which has central and peripheral effects), but care must be taken with respect to side effects, which can include constipation.

Nausea arising from stimuli in the gastrointestinal tract associated with slowing of the gut should respond to gastrokinetic antinauseants such as *metaclopramide* or *domperidone*, which promote gastric emptying and increase gut motility. These actions will be counterproductive in a patient with a very high gastrointestinal obstruction, and vomiting will be aggravated.

Clearly, drugs available by more than one route—especially oral, subcutaneous, and rectal routes—are advantageous. Both *metaclopramide* and *haloperidol* may be used subcutaneously as well as orally, but other useful drugs (notably *prochlorperazine*) cannot be used subcutaneously.

Many other drugs have useful antinauseant activity through various mechanisms, including *amitriptyline*, which has a central action.

In addition to the established antinauseant drugs, *dexamethasone*, which acts by an unknown mechanism, is also useful in suppressing nausea, and the drug is used in some premedication programs prior to chemotherapy. It is also useful in some patients with advanced disease, but it should be used in the lowest possible dose and as an adjunct to other therapy. Small doses (e.g., 2 mg *dexamethasone*) may reduce nausea associated with tumors involving the alimentary tract, especially hepatic metastases or motility disturbances. If benefit is not obvious within 1 week, it should be discontinued (15). Caution must be exercised if the patient has a history of active peptic ulceration, tuberculosis, or diabetes mellitus.

Constipation, a common symptom, may be due to changing diet, inactivity, opioid use without laxatives, or varying degrees of tumor-induced intestinal obstruction. Fecal impaction is a common cause of major symptoms, including nausea, diarrhea, pain, and even confusion, especially in the elderly; the diagnosis should not be missed if avoidable misery is to be prevented. Opioid-induced fecal impaction is usually avoidable but, if present, requires vigorous local treatment such as rectal softeners, stimulant suppositories, or careful enemas. Laxatives, including large-bowel stimulants (e.g. *Senokot*), stool softeners (e.g., *coloxyl*), and occasionally small-bowel flushers (e.g., *lactulose*) are also essential. Constipation due to mechanical obstruction requires either surgical intervention or acceptance of the problem as an end-stage manifestation.

Medical Management of Intestinal Obstruction

Obstruction may occur at any level of the gastrointestinal tract in patients with gynecologic cancer and frequently involves several different sites of the bowel. It is a common late-stage problem, particularly in patients with ovarian cancer.

In general, the first episode of obstruction in a patient not yet exposed to reasonable chemotherapy justifies very active measures, including nasogastric suction, maintenance of fluid and electrolyte balance by intravenous therapy, and surgery if these measures fail. In patients who have exhausted reasonable chemotherapeutic options, the approach may be more conservative.

One option for conservative management is a trial of corticosteroids (e.g., *dexamethasone*, 4 mg orally or parenterally daily for 3–5 days). The obstruction may be relieved, presumably by decreasing inflammatory edema, and the maneuver may be repeated in the future. There is need for caution in the use of corticosteroids in patients with a history of diabetes mellitus, peptic ulceration, recent infection, impending bowel perforation, significant psychiatric disorder, or tuberculosis.

In a patient with end-stage obstruction, when the above measures have failed to relieve the problem, the totally symptomatic approach developed at St.

Christopher's Hospice may be helpful (16). In brief, this approach avoids the use of both a nasogastric tube and intravenous fluids. It relies on careful mouth care, with a little food and drink as desired. The patient remains mildly dehydrated, but this is beneficial and decreases the amount of vomiting. Centrally acting antinauseants are used, if necessary, in combination with low doses of analgesics. Gastrokinetic antinauseants (e.g., metoclopramide or domperidone) are contraindicated in patients with a high obstruction.

Hyoscine hydrobromide may serve multiple purposes in patients with bowel obstruction, because it acts not only on the vomiting center but also on the intestines, relaxing it and increasing the intestinal reservoir. This enables the patient with complete obstruction to avoid multiple small vomits, while having infrequent large emeses. *Hyoscine butyl bromide* is similar but lacks the central effects.

A subcutaneous butterfly needle with or without a battery-driven syringe driver can be used to deliver appropriate doses of antinauseants, such as *haloperidol*, 2–6 mg/day, as well as *hyoscine hydrobromide* or *hyoscine butyl bromide*, 0.1–0.2 mg every 6 hours. With careful calibration of dose, the patient need not be drowsy. A *hyoscine* transdermal patch may also be useful. It should be changed every 2–3 days, and the patient should be observed for central nervous system effects. *Morphine* may be given in the same syringe if necessary, but pain other than colic is rarely a problem. If colic is not controlled with a little *morphine*, additional *hyoscine* may be useful. Rectal *prochlorperazine*, 25–75 mg/day, may be tried instead of *haloperidol*. *Cyclizine* (oral, parenteral, rectal) is often very helpful, but is not available everywhere.

This treatment should abolish the nausea, but occasional vomiting, two or three times a day, will still occur. Most patients prefer bouts of even severe vomiting with the ability to drink tea or coffee to a continuous nasogastric tube. If the obstruction is very high, intermittent insertion of a nasogastric tube for a few minutes to relieve pressure may be undertaken in the last days of life, or a percutaneous gastrostomy could be considered. Under all these circumstances, electrolytes should neither be monitored nor corrected. Electrolyte imbalance becomes inevitable and should be allowed to take its course. The role of *somatostatin* in the management of end-stage intestinal obstruction is not yet clear, but the drug should be considered if, despite all the above maneuvers, there is poor control of vomiting.

This approach, although it requires considerable medical and nursing experience, has significantly improved the last phase of life for a large number of women dying with intestinal obstruction. It represents a major advance in palliative therapeutics.

Diarrhea and Tenesmus   Diarrhea in a patient with advanced gynecologic cancer is probably best considered as a sign of fecal impaction until proven otherwise. True irritative diarrhea can occur by involvement of the bowel wall. *Loperamide* is useful in the management of such patients, but corticosteroids occasionally may be used for short periods with few side effects and considerable benefit. When diarrhea is associated with a rectovaginal fistula and surgical diversion is not possible, the emphasis is on nursing procedures calculated to keep the vagina clean and comfortable and to support the patient in her quite extreme distress. The use of *somatostatin* is occasionally worthy of consideration. Antibiotics, especially *metronidazole*, locally as well as systemically, may be valuable in reducing some of the distressing odor when necrosis has occurred.

Tenesmus can occasionally be problematic but usually responds to rectal anticholinergic derivatives, (e.g., *hyoscine butyl bromide* suppositories) and also to corticosteroids and opioids.

Ascites

Abdominal distention due to intractable ascites can be a major cause of distress. Recurrent paracentesis has a limited but definite place, while shunting procedures have severe limitations. Diuretics, especially *spironolactone*, 50–150 mg per day, may prove helpful initially. Occasionally corticosteroids in very low doses may reduce fluid production and are worthy of trial. The actual discomfort is readily controlled with a combination of a peripherally acting drug such as *acetaminophen* and a low dose of an opioid. Cytotoxics (systemic or intraperitoneal) may be worthy of consideration, but in practice their potential is limited in a late-stage patient and care must be taken not to waste the patient's time and energy and increase her distress.

Respiratory Symptoms

Dyspnea is common, and the dominant cause can usually be clarified by a clinical history, physical examination, and a chest radiograph. It should be possible to differentiate between a pleural effusion, bronchial obstruction, diffuse lung involvement, reduced excursion due to massive ascites, bronchial asthma, chronic obstructive airway disease, cardiac failure, and respiratory infection.

When the dyspnea is due to diffuse lung involvement, the careful use of *morphine*, with or without a small dose of corticosteroids, may improve the situation dramatically (17). Oral *morphine* should be commenced at doses of 2–5 mg every 4 hours and increased until no further benefit is gained. In practice, this usually means doses of around 10–20 mg every 4 hours, with or without corticosteroids in low dosage. *Morphine* may improve dyspnea not only through central mechanisms but possibly also through peripheral effects. If a patient is already receiving *morphine* calibrated correctly for pain relief but becomes dyspneic because of tumor progression, *morphine* may be increased by a further 30–50% to give relief.

If medical management of dyspnea is optimal, oxygen is rarely necessary or truly advantageous, even with widespread pulmonary metastases. Anxiolytics, however, may be valuable in modest doses. *Benzodiazepines* (for example, 2 mg *diazepam* orally or 0.5 mg *lorazepam* sublingually) may have significant benefit for the anxious patient.

Urinary Tract Symptoms

Urinary tract symptoms are common in women with far-advanced gynecologic cancer. Hydronephrosis, with subsequent infection, pain, and obstructive nephropathy, may justify mechanical measures such as nephrostomy or stent insertion if the prognosis on other grounds is for at least several good-quality months of life. Although some patients clearly benefit, complications are frequent and the personal and financial costs can be considerable. Fine judgment is required in the individual case.

In the short term, patency of ureters, with a significant reduction in serum creatinine level and improved quality of life, may be achieved by short courses of modest doses of corticosteroids (e.g., oral *dexamethasone*, 4 mg daily for 3–5 days). Bladder symptoms may yield to the use of *NSAIDS* to reduce detrusor irritability or drugs with an anticholinergic action, such as tricyclic antidepressants, *flavoxate*, or *propantheline*, to reduce bladder contractility. Catheterization may be unavoidable in some circumstances.

Edema

Leg swelling due to venous or lymphatic obstruction can be distressing and may respond either to small doses of diuretics or to careful massage toward the trunk, beginning at the top of the leg. Very occasionally, the application of various pump devices or an intermittent compression apparatus may be helpful. Systematic bandaging of the legs when the edema is minimal should significantly improve the patient's comfort. Compression bandages or support hosiery should not be applied to grossly edematous legs, as venous circulation may be further compromised.

Low doses of corticosteroids may also improve the situation and probably should be tried for a few days if leg swelling is a dominant symptom unrelieved by more simple measures.

Weakness

Weakness can be a dominant symptom when there is a large tumor mass, but there are many reversible causes of weakness. These include nutritional deficiencies, hypotension, hypokalemia, hypoglycemia or hyperglycemia, hypoadrenalism, hypercalcemia, renal failure, infection, and anemia.

At least some of these may be either easily excluded or readily treated in appropriate circumstances. Nutritional deficiencies may aggravate the debility associated with advanced cancer, and some of these problems may be readily reversible. Anemia usually is not an indication for transfusion, as benefit may be short lived and not proportionate to the expenditure of resources. If the hemoglobin is very low and weakness is a dominant symptom, transfusion may be justified.

Hypercalcemia

Hypercalcemia (raised ionized plasma calcium level) is a recognized complication of malignancy, which is often, but not always, associated with bony metastases.

Hypercalcemia is a potent cause of symptoms, ranging from lethargy, weakness, and constipation to severe nausea, vomiting, and confusion. Pain, especially bone pain, may be aggravated by hypercalcemia. In general, such distressing symptoms should be reversed if possible. Specialist assistance may be wise both to clarify the diagnosis (for each of the symptoms above can have complex causes) and to supervise the treatment.

Treatment of hypercalcemia depends on both its severity and its urgency. Mild cases may respond to high oral intake of fluids. Oral phosphate (0.5–3 g per day as sodium cellulose phosphate powder) is occasionally used if the plasma phosphate level is not elevated but may cause gastrointestinal symptoms.

In severe cases, treatment may not be justified in a patient who is clearly dying, but in most instances treatment is justified at least once after due consideration of the ethical principles involved.

Urgent treatment involves:

1. Rehydration with intravenous saline solution (2–3 liters) plus a loop diuretic (such as *furosemide*), followed by

2. *Pamidronate*, 30–60 mg by intravenous infusion in 250 ml of *crystalloid* over 4–8 hours.

Improvement of symptoms with these measures can be expected within 2–3 days, with continuation of the effect for 2–3 weeks when repetition of *Pamidronate* infusion can be undertaken. The rate of relapse of hypercalcemia is partially dependent on the availability of effective therapy for the underlying tumor, as well as on the biologic characteristics and tempo of the neoplastic process.

Care of the Dying Patient

Once it is clear that the patient is dying, the goal is dignity and peace, best served by precise control of major symptoms. This usually involves continuing with indicated drugs in correct dosage, by either the subcutaneous or the rectal route. Sometimes one is justified in offering direct sedation when, in spite of adequate pain control, distress is extreme and opportunities for verbal communication no longer exist. *Phenothiazines* such as *chlorpromazine* may cause distressing dissociation, and anxiolytics of the *benzodiazepine* group are preferable. In such circumstances, sublingual *lorazepam*, 0.5–2.5 mg every 4–6 hours, may be valuable. Alternatively, parenteral *midazolam* (e.g., 2–5 mg subcutaneously or intramuscularly) may assist in achieving appropriate sedation, while a subcutaneous infusion of 30–50 mg every 24 hours may be helpful if the situation is protracted. Large doses of opioids are not appropriate for sedation of the dying.

Complex equipment should be avoided if possible, and it is consoling to both patient and family to avoid tubes of all sorts wherever possible so as to facilitate maximum physical contact with loved ones.

The process of dying is fraught with uncertainties. Space, time, privacy, and peacefulness are the essence of good care, and these are facilitated by the presentation of a clear therapeutic plan. In the face of imminent death, respect for individual religious and cultural customs is mandatory.

It is essential that medical and nursing staff accept and understand the value and personal significance of the final phase of life, even the last days. If the clinician and other professional staff regard dying as a battle failure, the patient may understandably feel like a battlefield (and some do)! If dying is regarded as "a master test of our journeyman years," as articulated by Bloch (18), then there is an implied need for space, time, and privacy to undertake such a test. If dying is regarded as a rite of passage, or a mysterious (even sacred) personal drama in which the doctor, the patient, and the rest are all participants, then there is an implied need for respect for this unique personal transition.

Ethical issues abound in relation to gynecologic oncology, as in all areas of clinical practice. Such issues include the rights of the patient, the responsibilities of the clinical staff and of society, and the requirements to ensure at least good symptomatic relief and basic care in accord with human dignity throughout the course of the illness.

Perhaps more subtle are the issues related to the obligation incumbent on the medical system to recognize as its goal the relief of human suffering. Cassell (19) has discussed the issues and offered an operational definition of suffering, which is the sense of disintegration of the self. This situation can be worsened by some aspects of medical care. As soon as incurability is recognized, palliative treatment is initiated. At this time, special attention must be paid to support the processes of personal development and the maintenance of realistic hope.

No person should die in despair. The physician should assist the patient to center hope, not on what in the end will fail (e.g., chemotherapy, radiotherapy, surgery), but on what will not fail—such as the physician's commitment to care, the control of pain and other symptoms, and the intrinsic value of the patient as a unique individual. No patient should die with hope focused on the next course of chemotherapy or on another surgical intervention. Unrealistic expectations may increase, not relieve, suffering (20).

It is the physician's responsibility and privilege to provide care, support and concern, no matter what ensues. The patient must be helped to cope with all of the stresses she encounters. She must be reassured that good decisions will be made considering all of her needs. She must be comforted that she will not suffer pain or other major symptoms. She should be encouraged in every effort she exerts to combat her cancer. If she prefers to die "raging against the dying of the light" (Dylan Thomas) rather than in peaceful acquiescence, that, too, must be respected. Good palliative care is concerned with the enrichment of life, even when facing the human task common to all, dying.

References

1. **World Health Organization:** Cancer Pain Relief and Palliative Care. Geneva, 1991.

2. **Feinstein AR (ed):** *Clinical Judgment.* Baltimore, Williams & Wilkins, 1967, pp 191–197.

3. **Twycross RG, Lack SA:** Therapeutics in terminal cancer. *Pain Relief,* Second edition. London, Churchill Livingstone, 1990.

4. **Doyle D, Hanks GW, MacDonald N (eds):** *Oxford Textbook of Palliative Medicine.* Oxford, Oxford University Press, 1993.

5. **Billings JA:** *Outpatient Management of Advanced Cancer.* Philadelphia, JB Lippincott, 1985.

6. **Walsh TD:** *Symptom Control.* Oxford, Blackwell, 1989.

7. **Hanks GW, Justins DM:** Cancer pain management. *Lancet* 339:1031, 1992.

8. **Foley KM:** Controversies in cancer pain: medical perspectives. *Cancer* 63:2257, 1989.

9. **Matthiessen HV:** Pain treatment in gynaecological cancer. *Postgrad Med J* 67 (Suppl 2):26, 1991.

10. **Conolly ME:** Recent advances in the control of pain. In Bates TD (ed): *Contemporary Palliation of Difficult Symptoms.* In *Baillière's Clinical Oncology,* vol 1. London, Baillière Tindall, 1987, pp 417–441.

11. **Ad Hoc Committee on Cancer Pain of the American Society of Clinical Oncology:** ASCO Cancer. Pain assessment and treatment curriculum guidelines. *J Clin Oncol* 10:1976, 1992.

12. **Glare PA, Walsh TD:** Clinical pharmacokinetics of morphine. *Ther Drug Monit* 13:1, 1991.

13. **Portenoy RK, Dwight EM, Rogers A, et al:** IV infusion of opioids for cancer pain: clinical review and guidelines for use. *Cancer Treat Rep* 70:575, 1986.

14. **Twycross RG, Lack SA:** *Control of Alimentary Symptoms in Far Advanced Cancer.* Edinburgh, Churchill Livingstone, 1986.

15. **Twycross RG:** Corticosteroids in advanced cancer. *Br Med J* 305:969, 1992.

16. **Baines M, Oliver DJ, Carter RL:** Medical management of intestinal obstruction in patients with advanced malignant disease: a clinical and pathological study. *Lancet* 2:990, 1985.

17. **Cowcher KC, Hanks GW:** Long term management of respiratory symptoms in advanced cancer. *J Pain Symptom Management* 5:320, 1990.

18. **Bloch E:** *Man on His Own*. Ashton EB (trans). New York, Herder & Herder, 1970, p 47.

19. **Cassell EJ:** The nature of suffering and the goals of medicine. *N Engl J Med* 306:639, 1982.

20. **Granei MD:** Ovarian cancer: unrealistic expectations. *N Engl J Med* 327:197, 1992.

Index

Note: Page numbers in *italics* refer to illustrations; page numbers followed by t refer to tables.